Nursing Assisting
A Foundation in Caregiving

Diana L. Dugan, RN

FIFTH EDITION

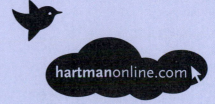

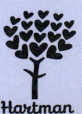

Credits

Managing Editor
Susan Alvare Hedman

Designer
Kirsten Browne

Cover Illustrator
Iveta Vaicule

Production
Elena Reznikova

Photography
Matt Pence, Pat Berrett, Art Clifton, and Dick Ruddy

Proofreaders
Kristin Calderon, Michelle Collett, Sapna Desai,
and Joanna Owusu

Editorial Assistant
Angela Storey

Sales/Marketing
Deborah Rinker-Wildey
Kendra Robertson
Erika Walker
Carol Castillo

Customer Service
Fran Desmond
Thomas Noble
Col Foley
Brian Fejer
Hank Bullis

Information Technology
Eliza Martin

Warehouse Coordinator
Chris Midyette

Copyright Information

© 2020 by Diana L. Dugan
Hartman Publishing, Inc.
1313 Iron Ave SW
Albuquerque, New Mexico 87102
(505) 291-1274
web: hartmanonline.com
email: orders@hartmanonline.com
Twitter: @HartmanPub

ISBN 978-1-60425-121-0
ISBN 978-1-60425-124-1 (Hardcover)

PRINTED IN CANADA

Notice to Readers

Though the guidelines and procedures contained in this text are based on consultations with healthcare professionals, they should not be considered absolute recommendations. The instructor and readers should follow employer, local, state, and federal guidelines concerning healthcare practices. These guidelines change, and it is the reader's responsibility to be aware of these changes and of the policies and procedures of her or his healthcare facility.

The publisher, author, editors, and reviewers cannot accept any responsibility for errors or omissions or for any consequences from application of the information in this book and make no warranty, express or implied, with respect to the contents of the book. The publisher does not warrant or guarantee any of the products described herein or perform any analysis in connection with any of the product information contained herein.

Special Thanks

A heartfelt thank you to our insightful and wonderful reviewers, listed in alphabetical order:

Melanie Ball-Pearson, MSN, RN
Royal Oak, MD

Katherine Howard, MS, RN-BC, CNE
Edison, NJ

Colby P. Hunsberger, MSN, RN
Fairmount City, PA

Charles A. Illian, BSN, RN
Orlando, FL

Gender Usage

This textbook uses gender pronouns interchangeably to denote healthcare team members and residents.

Permissions

Dedication

This book is dedicated to our newest grandchildren, our baby stars, Jack and Grace. What delightful children you are! We love and cherish our time with you, Ava, and your parents.

> Dwell on the beauty of life. Watch the stars and see yourself running with them.
> —*Marcus Aurelius Antoninus, Meditations*

To my beloved John, a heartfelt thank you for your eternal love and my endless appreciation for everything you do for our entire family every single day. Your energy and strength make our life lively and fun; onward to our next exciting adventure!

> I would not wish any companion in the world but you.
> —*William Shakespeare, The Tempest*

To our beloved children, Mark, Marissa, Carrie, and Jon, thank you for your devotion to your children and your support of our growing family. Your commitment to excellence in your work is truly an inspiration to all who know you.

To our loving extended family, thank you for your support, kindness, and good cheer. To all our dearest friends, thank you for always being there with your friendship and love.

To Mark T. Hartman, my incomparable publisher, you are truly extraordinary. Thank you for your dedication and your adherence to high standards. Wishing much happiness to you, Elliott, and Warren.

To Susan Alvare Hedman, my exceptional editor, I am profoundly thankful and grateful for your expertise and your meticulous work on behalf of our books. A sincere thank you to Mark Hedman for his remarkable support, as well as to charming Isa.

For everyone affiliated with Hartman Publishing: Kirsten Browne, Debbie Rinker-Wildey, Fran Desmond, Tom Noble, Angela Storey, Kendra Robertson, Erika Walker, Eliza Martin, Chris Midyette, Col Foley, Carol Castillo, Brian Fejer, and Henry Bullis, a huge thank you to every one of you. To our wise reviewers, thank you for your attentive help with this edition.

To the instructors, thank you for your dedication to quality care. To the students, best wishes for a bright future in the world of health care.

> All that mankind has done, thought, gained, or been; it is lying as in magic preservation in the pages of books.
> —*Thomas Carlyle, Heroes and Hero-Worship*

My warmest regards to all,

Diana

Diana L. Dugan

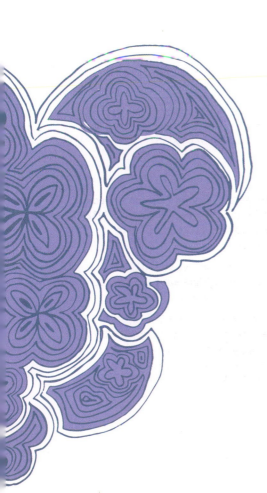

Contents

5 Diversity and Human Needs and Development

6 Infection Prevention and Control

7 Safety and Body Mechanics

Procedures

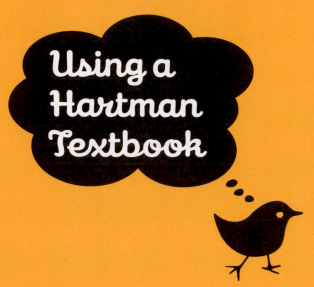

Using a Hartman Textbook

Understanding how this book is organized and what its special features are will help you make the most of this resource!

look!

Carefully chosen quotes begin each chapter and may be used for discussion. Additional information highlights how health care has changed over the years by detailing interesting events in medicine from the past.

We have assigned each chapter its own colored tab. Located on the side of every page, each colored tab contains the chapter number and title.

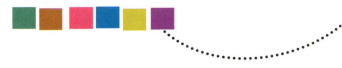

1. Explain HIPAA and related terms

Everything in this book, the student workbook, and the instructor's teaching material is organized around learning objectives. A learning objective is a very specific piece of knowledge or a very specific skill. After reading the text, if you can do what the learning objective says, you know you have mastered the material.

bloodborne pathogens

Bold key terms are located at the beginning of each chapter and then again throughout the text. These terms are defined in the text and in the glossary at the back of this book.

Making an occupied bed

All care procedures are highlighted by the same black bar for easy recognition.

Guidelines: Accurate Documentation

Guidelines and Observing and Reporting lists are colored green for easy reference.

Residents' Rights

Be patient when feeding residents
...dangerous...

Residents' Rights boxes teach important information about how to support and promote legal rights and person-centered care. Tip and Trivia boxes provide interesting and educational tidbits that you can use inside and outside of work.

Chapter Review

Chapter-ending questions test your knowledge of the information found in the chapter. We have included the textbook's learning objective numbers to make it easier for you to reread a section if you need to refresh your memory. When you see this notation after a question—(LO 3)—it refers to the particular learning objective number in the chapter on which you are working. If you have trouble answering a question, you can return to the text and reread the material.

See the Appendix at the end of the book for additional information.

Beginning and ending steps in care procedures

For most care procedures, these steps should be performed. Understanding why they are important will help you remember to perform each step every time care is provided.

Beginning Steps

Identify yourself by name. Identify the resident. Greet the resident by name.	A resident's room is his home. Residents have a right to privacy. Before any procedure, knock and wait for permission to enter the resident's room. Upon entering his room, identify yourself and state your title. Residents have the right to know who is providing their care. Identify and greet the resident. This shows courtesy and respect. It also establishes correct identification. This prevents care from being performed on the wrong person.
Wash your hands.	Handwashing provides for infection prevention. Nothing fights infection in facilities like performing consistent, proper hand hygiene. Handwashing may need to be done more than once during a procedure. Practice Standard Precautions with every resident.
Explain procedure to the resident. Speak clearly, slowly, and directly. Maintain face-to-face contact whenever possible.	Residents have a legal right to know exactly what care you will provide. It promotes understanding, cooperation, and independence. Residents are able to do more for themselves if they know what needs to happen.
Provide for the resident's privacy with a curtain, screen, or door.	Doing this maintains residents' rights to privacy and dignity. Providing for privacy in a facility is not simply a courtesy; it is a legal right.
Adjust the bed to a safe level, usually waist high. Lock the bed wheels.	Locking the bed wheels is an important safety measure. It ensures that the bed will not move as you are performing care. Raising the bed helps you to remember to use proper body mechanics. This helps prevent injury to you and to residents.

Ending Steps

Make the resident comfortable.	Make sure sheets are wrinkle-free and lie flat under the resident's body. This helps prevent pressure injuries. Replace bedding and pillows. Check that the resident's body is in proper alignment. This promotes comfort and health after you leave the room.
Return the bed to its lowest position. Remove privacy measures.	Lowering the bed provides for residents' safety. Remove extra privacy measures added during the procedure. This includes anything you may have draped over and around residents, as well as privacy screens.
Leave call light within the resident's reach.	A call light allows residents to communicate with staff as necessary. It must always be left within the resident's reach. You must respond to call lights promptly.
Wash your hands.	Handwashing is the most important thing you can do to prevent the spread of infection.
Be courteous and respectful at all times.	Say "thank you" before you leave. It is the polite and proper thing to do. Ask residents if they need anything else. Let them know that you are leaving. This promotes respect.
Report any changes in the resident to the nurse. Document procedure using facility guidelines.	You will often be the person who spends the most time with a resident, so you are in the best position to note any changes in a resident's condition. Every time you provide care, observe the resident's physical and mental capabilities, as well as the condition of the resident's body. For example, a change in a resident's ability to dress himself may signal a greater problem. After you have finished giving care, document the care using facility guidelines. Do not record care before it is given. If you do not document the care you gave, legally it did not happen.

In addition to the beginning and ending steps listed above, remember to follow infection prevention guidelines. Even if a procedure in this book does not tell you to wear gloves or other PPE, there may be times when it is appropriate.

For example, the procedure for giving a back rub does not include gloves. Gloves are usually not required for a back rub. However, if the resident has open sores on his back, gloves are necessary.

1 The Nursing Assistant in Long-Term Care

Nurses' Aides: Helping Hands During World War II

One of the earliest times nurses' aides were used in America was during World War II. Various hospitals, along with the American Red Cross, trained nurses' aides in 1941 to help deal with a shortage of nurses due to the war. Employers in the United States expected nurses' aides to volunteer during this time. The country set a goal of training 100,000 nurses' aides to assist nurses with patient care. These aides worked each day without being paid. Today it seems inconceivable that nursing assistants would work without compensation.

"A professor can never better distinguish himself in his work than by encouraging a clever pupil, for the true discoverers are among them, as comets amongst the stars."

Carl Linnaeus, 1707–1778

"If one advances confidently in the direction of his dreams, and endeavors to live the life which he has imagined, he will meet with a success unexpected in common hours."

Henry David Thoreau, 1817–1862

1. Define important words in this chapter

accountable: answerable for one's actions.

activities of daily living (ADLs): daily personal care tasks, such as bathing; caring for skin, fingernails, and hair; eating; drinking; caring for the mouth and teeth; dressing; walking; transferring; eliminating; and communicating.

acute care: 24-hour skilled care given in hospitals and ambulatory surgical centers for short-term, immediate illnesses or injuries.

adult day services: care for people who need some assistance or supervision during certain hours, but who do not live in the facility where care is given.

allergies: a condition in which the body's immune response is triggered after exposure to a substance called an *allergen*; reactions such as sneezing, difficulty breathing, and skin issues may result.

animal-assisted therapy (AAT): the practice of bringing pets into a facility or home to provide stimulation and companionship.

assisted living: residences for people who do not need 24-hour skilled care, but who do require some help with daily care.

assistive devices: special equipment that helps a person who is ill or disabled perform activities of daily living.

care team: group of people with different kinds of education and experience who provide resident care.

chain of command: the order of authority within a facility.

charge nurse: a nurse responsible for a team of healthcare workers.

chronic: long-term or long-lasting.

cite: in a long-term care facility, to find a problem through a survey.

conscientious: guided by a sense of right and wrong; principled.

continuity of care: an ongoing coordination of a resident's care over time, during which the care team regularly exchanges information and works toward shared goals.

courteous: polite, kind, and considerate.

delegation: transferring responsibility to a person for a specific task.

dementia: the serious loss of mental abilities, such as thinking, remembering, reasoning, and communicating.

diagnosis: the identification of disease or condition by its signs and symptoms and through test results.

empathetic: being able to identify with and understand the feelings of others.

first impression: a way of classifying or categorizing someone or something at the first meeting.

functional nursing: method of nursing care that involves assigning specific tasks to each team member.

holistic care: care that involves the whole person; this includes his or her physical, social, emotional, and spiritual needs.

home health care: health care that is provided in a person's home.

hospice care: holistic, compassionate care for people who have approximately six months or less to live; care is available until the person dies.

intergenerational care: caring for children and the elderly in the same setting.

Joint Commission: an independent, not-for-profit organization that evaluates and accredits different types of healthcare facilities.

length of stay: the number of days a person stays in a healthcare facility.

liability: a legal term that means a person can be held responsible for harming someone else.

licensed practical nurse (LPN) or **licensed vocational nurse (LVN):** a licensed nurse who provides skilled nursing care and gives treatments and medications.

long-term care: 24-hour skilled care provided in long-term care facilities for people with ongoing conditions.

Medicaid: a medical assistance program for people who have low incomes, as well as for people with disabilities.

Medicare: a federal health insurance program for people who are 65 or older, have certain disabilities or permanent kidney failure, or are ill and cannot work.

nursing assistant (NA): person who performs assigned nursing tasks and gives personal care.

outpatient care: care given to people who have had treatments, procedures, or surgeries and need short-term skilled care.

person-centered care: a type of care that places the emphasis on the person needing care and his or her individuality and capabilities.

policy: a course of action to be followed every time a certain situation occurs.

primary nursing: a method of nursing care in which the registered nurse provides much of the daily care to residents.

procedure: a method or way of doing something.

professionalism: the use of proper standards of behavior at work and in work-related settings.

registered nurse (RN): a licensed nurse who assesses residents, creates care plans, monitors progress, provides skilled nursing care, administers treatments and medications, and supervises the care given by nursing assistants and other members of the care team.

rehabilitation: a program of care given by specialists, such as physical therapists, to restore or improve function after an illness or injury.

resident: a person living in a long-term care facility.

sandwich generation: people responsible for the care of both their children and aging relatives.

skilled care: medically necessary care given by a skilled nurse or therapist.

subacute care: care given in hospitals or in long-term care facilities for people who need less care than for an acute (sudden onset, short-term) illness or injury but more than for a chronic (long-term) illness.

team leader: a nurse in charge of a group of residents for one shift of duty.

team nursing: method of nursing care in which a nurse acts as a leader of a group of people giving care.

trustworthy: deserving the trust of others.

2. Describe healthcare settings

Making the career choice to care for others is very rewarding. No other work is more appreciated or valued, and it makes an important difference in the lives of many people.

Nursing assistants have many job opportunities. Where someone chooses to work depends on the person, her schedule, and the type of care she prefers to give. (More information on finding a job is located in Chapter 28.)

Each healthcare setting is unique; however, some similar tasks will be performed in every setting. This textbook will focus on **long-term care** for elderly residents.

Long-term care facilities provide 24-hour skilled care for people who are no longer eligible for hospital care but are unable to be cared for at home. **Skilled care** is medically necessary care given by a skilled nurse or therapist. This care is available 24 hours a day. It is ordered by a doctor and involves a treatment plan.

Long-term care is provided for people with ongoing, chronic medical conditions and is usually given for an extended period of time. **Chronic** means long-term or long-lasting. Chronic conditions last a long period of time, even a lifetime. Examples of chronic conditions include physical disabilities, heart disease, and recovery from stroke. Other common terms for long-term care facilities are *nursing homes, skilled nursing facilities, rehabilitation centers,* or *extended care facilities.*

A long-term care facility is where a person resides or lives. This is why the people who live in these facilities are called **residents**. The facility is a resident's home, and the resident will remain there until she returns home, moves to another place, or dies (Fig. 1-1).

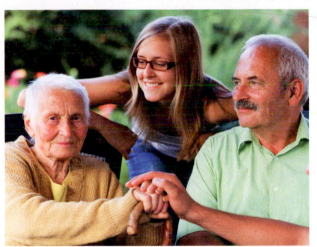

Fig. 1-1. *The care facility is the resident's home. Family and friends, as well as others, may visit the resident at the facility, just as if she were living in her own house.*

In **assisted living** facilities (sometimes referred to as *assisted living residences* [*ALRs*]), residents are generally more independent. Staff are available to provide whatever daily care residents need, such as help with bathing and dressing. Sometimes staff assist with medications. Residents in these facilities do not usually need skilled care. Many assisted living centers have different areas available if a person requires additional care. The advantage is that the resident can remain at the facility as his needs change.

Home health care is care that takes place in a person's home (Fig. 1-2). In some ways, working as a home health aide is similar to working as a nursing assistant. Almost all care in this textbook also applies to home health aides. Most of the personal care and basic nursing procedures are the same. Home health aides may also clean the home, shop for groceries, do laundry, and cook. They will work more independently, although a supervisor monitors their work, and they may have more contact with the family. The advantage of home health care is that clients do not have to leave home. They may have lived in their homes for many years, and staying at home is more comfortable for most people.

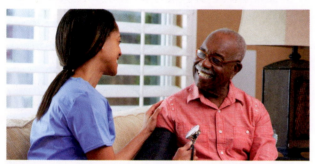

Fig. 1-2. *Home care is performed in a person's home.*

Adult day services refers to care given to people who need assistance during certain hours. The people needing this type of care do not live in the facility where care is provided. Generally, adult day services are for people who need some help but who are not seriously ill or disabled. In the past, aging family members were cared for mostly at home. Today, the **sandwich generation**—the generation caring for children and aging parents at the same time—is often unable to spend enough time at home. If no one can care for an elderly relative at home or if a person needs a break from caregiving, adult day services is an option.

Some centers have merged care for elderly adults and children in the same setting to offer **intergenerational care** (Fig. 1-3). One benefit of this kind of care is that it provides "grandparents" or "grandchildren" for those who have none or who live too far away from their own families.

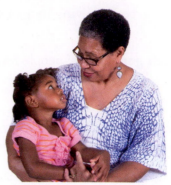

Fig. 1-3. *Intergenerational care provides an opportunity for the elderly and the young to spend time together.*

Acute care is 24-hour skilled care given in hospitals and ambulatory surgical centers. It is for people who require immediate care for illnesses or injuries. People are also admitted for short stays for surgery. The length of time the person remains depends on the illness.

Subacute care is given in hospitals or in long-term care facilities for people who need less care than for an acute illness, but a higher level of care than for a chronic illness. The cost is usually less than hospital care, but more than long-term care. Subacute care will be covered in depth in Chapter 26.

Outpatient care is given to people who have had treatments, procedures, or surgeries and need short-term skilled care. Patients do not require an overnight stay in a hospital or other care facility. They are sent home with instructions for further care. Families or friends may play a part in their recovery.

Rehabilitation is care given by specialists, including physical, occupational, and speech therapists, to help restore or improve function after an illness or injury. There is more information about these specialists in Learning Objective 9 of this chapter. Information about rehabilitation is located in Chapter 25.

Hospice care is given in facilities or homes for people who have approximately six months or less to live. Hospice workers give compassionate physical and emotional care and comfort until the person dies, while also supporting families during this process. There is more information about hospice care in Chapter 27.

Tip

Animal-Assisted Therapy (AAT)

Animal-assisted therapy (AAT), or pet therapy, is the use of different kinds of animals to brighten the days of people who are ill (Fig. 1-4). Pet Partners (petpartners.org), founded by a physician and a veterinarian under the name Delta Society in 1977, is a national organization dedicated to the therapeutic bond between animals and humans. The group welcomes inquiries from owners interested in volunteering good-natured dogs. American Humane (americanhumane.org) and the American Red Cross (redcross.org) are other organizations that may provide animal-assisted therapy. Many people love having regular contact with animals, and it may help with their treatment and recovery.

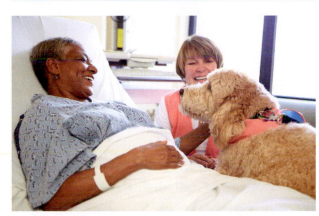

Fig. 1-4. Bringing dogs into healthcare facilities may cheer up people who are ill, as well as provide other health benefits.

3. Explain Medicare and Medicaid

The Centers for Medicare & Medicaid Services (CMS, cms.gov) is a federal agency within the United States Department of Health and Human Services. CMS runs two national healthcare programs: Medicare and Medicaid. They both help pay for health care and health insurance for millions of Americans. CMS has many other responsibilities as well.

Medicare (medicare.gov) is a federal health insurance program for people who are 65 years of age or older. Medicare also covers people of any age with permanent kidney failure or certain disabilities. Medicare has four parts. Part A helps pay for care in a hospital or skilled nursing facility or for care from a home health agency or hospice. Part B helps pay for doctor services and other medical services and equipment. Part C allows private health insurance companies to provide Medicare benefits. Part D helps pay for medications prescribed for treatment. Medicare will only pay for care it determines to be medically necessary.

Medicaid (medicaid.gov) is a medical assistance program for people who have a low income, as well as for people with disabilities. It is funded by both the federal government and each state. Eligibility is determined by income and special circumstances. People must qualify for this program.

Medicare and Medicaid pay long-term care facilities a fixed amount for services. This amount is based on the resident's needs upon admission and throughout his stay at the facility.

4. Describe the residents in long-term care facilities

There are some general statements that can be made about residents in long-term care facilities. According to a survey conducted in 2015–2016 by the National Center for Health Statistics (cdc.gov/nchs), 83.5 percent of nursing home residents in the United States are over age 65. Approximately 68 percent of residents are female. More than 75 percent are white and non-Hispanic (Fig. 1-5). About one-third of residents come from a private residence; over 50 percent come from a hospital or other facility.

The **length of stay** is the number of days a person stays in a healthcare facility. The length of stay of over two-thirds of residents in long-term care is six months or longer. These residents need enough help with their activities of daily living to require 24-hour care. Often, they did

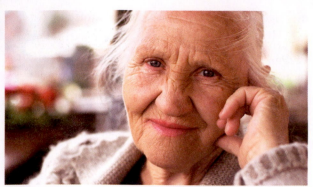

Fig. 1-5. White, non-Hispanic women make up a high percentage of residents in long-term care facilities.

not have caregivers available to give sufficient care for them to live in the community. The groups with the longest average stay are people who are developmentally disabled. They are often younger than 65. More information about developmental disabilities may be found in Chapter 5.

The other third of residents stay for fewer than six months. This group generally falls into two categories. The first category is made up of residents admitted for terminal care. Due to their diseases or conditions, they will probably die in the facility. The second category is made up of residents admitted for rehabilitation or due to temporary illness. They will usually recover and return to the community. Care of these residents may be very different than care provided for permanent residents. There is more information about rehabilitation in Chapter 25.

Dementia and other mental disorders are major causes of admissions to care facilities. **Dementia** is the serious loss of mental abilities, such as thinking, remembering, reasoning, and communicating. Various studies place the number of residents with dementia in long-term care facilities as high as 48 percent. More information about dementia may be found in Chapter 22. Many residents are admitted with other disorders as well. However, the disorders themselves are often not the main reason for admission. It is most often the lack of ability to care for oneself and the lack of a support system that lead

people into a facility. Having a support system is vital in allowing an elderly person to live outside a facility.

Some residents have very little outside support from family or friends. This is one reason it is essential to care for the whole person and her individual needs instead of only the illness or disease. Residents have many needs besides bathing, eating, drinking, and elimination. These needs will go unmet if staff do not work to meet them.

While it is helpful to understand the entire population, it is more important for nursing assistants to understand each individual for whom they will care. Residents' care should be based on their specific needs, illnesses, and preferences.

5. Describe the nursing assistant's role

A **nursing assistant (NA)** performs assigned nursing tasks. Most of the tasks deal with helping care for residents. Examples of nursing tasks include measuring residents' temperature and blood pressure. An NA also assists residents with **activities of daily living (ADLs)**, which are daily personal care tasks, such as bathing; caring for skin, fingernails, and hair; caring for the mouth and teeth; dressing; walking; transferring; eliminating; and communicating. Common NA tasks include the following:

- Serving meal trays and helping residents eat and drink (Fig. 1-6)

- Helping residents dress and undress

- Bathing residents

- Shampooing hair

- Shaving residents

- Making residents' beds

- Tidying residents' living areas

- Measuring vital signs (temperature, pulse, respiration, and blood pressure)

- Helping residents with elimination needs
- Assisting with mouth care
- Giving back rubs
- Observing and reporting changes in residents' conditions
- Reporting residents' complaints to the nurse
- Helping residents move safely around the facility
- Caring for supplies and equipment

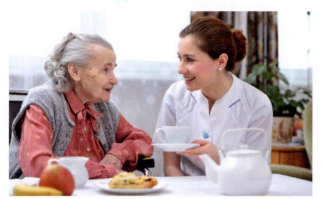

Fig. 1-6. *Helping residents eat and drink is an important part of an NA's job.*

Nursing assistants are not allowed to insert or remove tubes, give tube feedings, or change sterile dressings. Nursing assistants are not allowed to give medication; nurses are responsible for giving medication. Some states allow NAs to give medication after receiving additional, specialized training and meeting the requirements of the individual facility.

Nursing assistants can have many different titles. *Nurse aide, certified nurse aide, patient care technician,* and *certified nursing assistant* are some examples. This textbook will use the term *nursing assistant* or *NA*.

Trivia

Early Nursing Schools

Early nursing schools in the 1800s and early 1900s had very strict rules for their students. The classes were made up of women, and they normally lived together in the same building. Rigid curfews; rules restricting smoking, drinking, and profanity; separation of the sexes; and specific dress codes were strictly enforced. Generally women were not allowed to date or marry, and those who broke the rules were punished. Nursing students were expected to work long hours and, in addition to caring for patients, had to wash and wax floors and do chores that today are duties of other employees.

6. Discuss professionalism and list examples of professional behavior

Understanding how to be professional is the first step to success in the healthcare field. Professional behavior is vital in the workplace. **Professionalism** has to do with behaving properly when working. Dressing appropriately, speaking well, and being dependable and responsible are all part of professionalism. A healthcare facility is a place where professional behavior is expected.

Guidelines: Professional Behavior

G Be neatly dressed and groomed. Keep your uniform and shoes clean.

G Do not discuss personal problems or personal situations with residents. At work, conversation focuses on the resident, not the caregiver.

G Do not use your personal phone in residents' rooms or in any resident care area.

G Be on time when you are scheduled to work. Call in a timely manner if you are sick or cannot report for duty as scheduled.

G Avoid unnecessary absences. When you are absent, your coworkers have more work to complete, and without adequate staff, residents' care may suffer.

G Never leave your job early without permission. Report to the nurse in charge when leaving your unit for any reason.

G Do not report to work under the influence of illegal drugs and/or alcohol.

G Keep a positive attitude.

G Speak politely to all people in the facility. Treat all visitors with courtesy and respect.

G Address residents, family members, and visitors in the way they wish to be addressed. Never call someone "honey," "dear," or "sweetie."

G Do not use profanity or inappropriate language.

G Keep all resident information confidential. More information about confidentiality may be found in Chapter 2.

G Do not gossip or speak badly about residents, coworkers, or bosses.

G Follow all facility policies and procedures.

G Report concerns or problems to your supervisor.

G Meet and maintain all educational requirements.

G Ask questions when you do not understand something.

G Be honest. Document and report carefully and truthfully (Fig. 1-7).

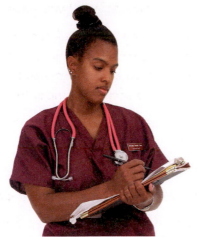

Fig. 1-7. Documenting observations is one of an NA's most important duties.

G Accept constructive feedback gracefully and learn from it. Constructive feedback is meant

to help you improve your performance. An example is, "You need to document care more accurately."

G Do not accept tips or gifts from residents, their families, or other visitors.

G Be loyal to your facility. Be a positive role model.

Behaving professionally will be an ongoing focus of this textbook. Students should pay attention to this information. Professionalism can help a person advance in his job and earn the respect of others. Not behaving professionally can result in poor performance evaluations, negative relationships with residents and other staff members, and the loss of a job.

7. List qualities that nursing assistants must have

The best nursing assistants demonstrate that they are

Patient and understanding: Working with people who are ill or disabled requires patience and understanding. People who are patient remain calm. They are able to cope with difficulties without complaining.

Honest and trustworthy: An honest person tells the truth and can be trusted. Coworkers will depend on honesty in planning care. Employers count on truthful observations and documentation. Residents count on NAs to keep their confidential information private.

Conscientious: People who are conscientious are guided by a sense of right and wrong. They always try to do their best. They are alert, observant, accurate, and responsible.

Enthusiastic: People who are enthusiastic have a positive attitude. They are encouraging. They show interest in others, including their situations and problems (Fig. 1-8). Enthusiastic people have a positive influence on others.

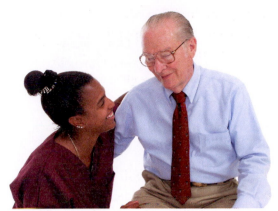

Fig. 1-8. NAs are expected to be enthusiastic, cheerful, and positive.

Courteous and **respectful**: NAs must be kind, polite, and considerate. They should respect others' beliefs, even if these beliefs are different from their own. They should value other people's individuality.

Empathetic: Empathetic people identify with the feelings of others. They care about other people's problems. They think about what it would be like to be ill and dependent on others for help.

Dependable and responsible: NAs must be at work on time and avoid too many absences. They should always follow policies and procedures. NAs must be able to be counted on to do their tasks properly.

Humble: People who are humble are willing to admit when they have made a mistake. They can accept their limitations and are open to growth. They hold themselves **accountable**. This means that they can admit when they make a mistake and apologize. They can ask others for help when they need it.

Tolerant: NAs must not judge others. They should keep their opinions to themselves and see people as individuals.

Unprejudiced: NAs work with people from many backgrounds. They must give each person quality care regardless of age, gender, sexual orientation, gender identity, religion, race, ethnicity, or condition.

8. Discuss proper grooming guidelines

Making positive **first impressions** can help a person obtain what she wants, such as getting a job. NAs must pay attention to the way they present themselves to residents, residents' family members and friends, and other staff members. Proper grooming and hygiene practices are essential to making a positive first impression.

Guidelines: Grooming and Hygiene Practices

G   Keep your uniform clean, neat, and pressed. Make sure your uniform fits you properly.

G   Bathe or shower every day. Wear deodorant or antiperspirant.

G   Brush your teeth at least twice a day.

G   Do not wear or use scented items such as perfume, cologne, aftershave, scented body washes, scented body creams and lotions, hair spray, and scented fabric softeners.

G   Keep your hair neatly tied back and away from your face.

G   Keep beards trimmed and clean.

G   Apply makeup lightly or use none at all.

G   Keep nails short, filed, and clean. Long nails may tear fragile skin, as well as harbor bacteria. Follow facility policy regarding nail polish.

G   Do not wear artificial nails (acrylic, gel, sculptured, or wraps). Artificial nails harbor bacteria, no matter how well you wash your hands.

G   Keep shoes and laces clean. Shoes should be in good condition. They should be comfortable. They should not look worn and old. Change or wash shoelaces when they become soiled.

G   Wear as little jewelry as possible. Sharp edges on jewelry can scratch or tear fragile skin. Remove rings (one smooth, plain band may be acceptable), bracelets, and necklaces while working. They collect bacteria and can cause infection. Rings and bracelets may also cause problems with wearing gloves. Confused residents may pull on necklaces and break them. Wear small earrings/studs (nothing below the earlobe) that cannot be pulled on by confused residents. Remove visible nose, lip, tongue, or other body rings/studs while working.

You will need to wear a simple, waterproof watch and an identification badge (Fig. 1-9). A watch will be used to measure a resident's pulse and respirations and record events. An identification badge (worn above the waist) identifies you to residents, visitors, and other staff members.

G   Keep tattoos covered by clothing when possible.

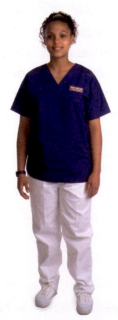

Fig. 1-9. *Wearing a clean uniform, a watch, and an identification badge are examples of professional behavior.*

> **Tip**
>
> **Perfumes, Colognes, and Other Scents**
>
> Some people do not like scents. Others may have **allergies** or illnesses that are worsened by scents. In addition, people who are ill or in pain may be bothered by smells. NAs should avoid wearing perfume, cologne, and any other scented items while at work. Putting residents' comfort first is each NA's responsibility.

9. Define the role of each member of the care team

The **care team** consists of many members who have had different training and experience in order to provide care for each resident (Fig. 1-10). The resident is the most important part—the center—of the care team. Members of the care team include the following:

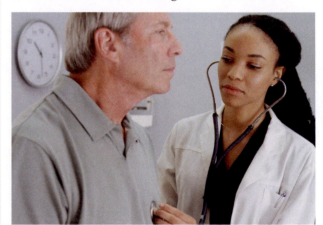

Fig. 1-10. *The care team is made up of many different types of professionals.*

Resident and Resident's Family: The care team revolves around the resident. Residents make choices about their care. They help plan their care. The resident's family and friends may also help with these decisions. In addition, family and friends may share important information about the resident with the care team. This information may include the resident's health and medical background, as well as his personal preferences, rituals, and routines. However, residents can exclude their families from the care team if they choose and are considered competent to do so.

Nurse: A nurse is a licensed health professional who assesses residents, creates the care plan, monitors progress, and gives treatments and medication. Different types of nurses include the following:

Registered Nurse (RN): A registered nurse has graduated from a state-licensed nursing program (two to four years of education). RNs have diplomas or college degrees and have passed a national licensing examination.

Licensed Practical or Licensed Vocational Nurse (LPN/LVN): A licensed practical or vocational nurse has graduated from a state-licensed nursing program (one to two years of education) and has passed a national licensing examination.

Advanced Practice Nurse (APRN): An advanced practice nurse is a registered nurse who has completed training at the postgraduate level (master's or doctoral) as a nurse practitioner (NP), nurse anesthetist (CRNA), nurse-midwife (CNM), or clinical nurse specialist (CNS). APRNs can make diagnoses and prescribe treatment. There are also other types of advanced practice nurses, such as a gerontological nurse practitioner (GNP).

Physician or Doctor (MD [medical doctor] or DO [doctor of osteopathy]): A doctor is a licensed health professional who diagnoses disease or disability and prescribes treatment. A **diagnosis** is the identification of disease or condition by its signs and symptoms and through test results. A doctor has graduated from a four-year medical school after first receiving a bachelor's degree. Many doctors also complete specialized training programs after medical school.

Physician Assistant (PA): A physician assistant is a licensed health professional who works under the supervision of a doctor. A PA performs a variety of medical duties such as diagnosing disease or illness and prescribing treatment and medications. PAs have master's degrees and have to pass national licensing examinations before they can practice.

Physical Therapist (PT or DPT): A physical therapist is a licensed health professional who develops a treatment plan to improve blood circulation, promote healing, ease pain, prevent disability, and help a resident regain or maintain mobility. A PT administers therapy in the form of heat, cold, massage, ultrasound, electrical stimulation, and exercise to muscles, bones, and joints (Fig. 1-11). A physical therapist has graduated from a graduate or doctoral degree program (doctor of physical therapy, or DPT) after receiving an undergraduate degree. PTs have to pass national licensing examinations before they can practice.

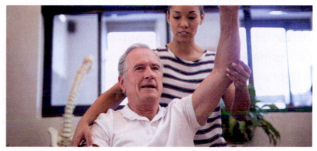

Fig. 1-11. *A physical therapist helps exercise muscles, bones, and joints to improve strength or restore abilities.*

Occupational Therapist (OT or OTD): An occupational therapist is a licensed health professional who works with people who need help adapting to disabilities and performing their activities of daily living (ADLs). An OT evaluates a person's ability to do these activities and develops a treatment plan. The OT may order **assistive devices** to help. An example of an assistive device is a special fork that helps a person feed himself (Fig. 1-12). Occupational therapists have a master's or doctoral degrees and must pass national licensing examinations before they can practice.

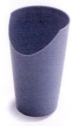 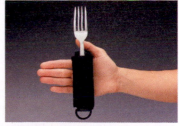

Fig. 1-12. *An occupational therapist will help residents learn to use assistive devices, such as this special cup and fork.* (PHOTO COURTESY OF NORTH COAST MEDICAL, INC., WWW.NCMEDICAL.COM, 800-821-9319)

Speech-Language Pathologist (SLP): A speech-language pathologist or speech therapist identifies communication disorders and develops a care plan to aid in improvement or recovery. An SLP teaches exercises to help the resident improve or overcome speech problems. An SLP also evaluates a person's ability to swallow food and drink. Speech-language pathologists have earned a master's degree in speech-language pathology and are licensed or certified to practice.

Registered Dietitian Nutritionist (RDN): A registered dietitian nutritionist assesses a person's nutritional status and develops a care program. A registered dietitian nutritionist creates diets for residents with special needs. These special diets can improve health and help manage illness. RDNs may supervise the preparation of food and educate people about healthy nutrition. Registered dietitian nutritionists have completed a bachelor's degree and may have completed postgraduate work. Most states require that RDNs be licensed or certified.

Respiratory Therapist (RT): A respiratory therapist is a licensed healthcare professional who provides care for people who have respiratory diseases or illnesses. Respiratory therapists have generally earned at least an associate's or a bachelor's degree and must be licensed to practice.

Medical Social Worker (MSW): A medical social worker is a licensed healthcare professional who determines residents' social needs and helps with support services, such as counseling or financial assistance. A medical social worker may help residents obtain personal items or clothing or find compatible roommates. She may help book appointments and transportation. Medical social workers have usually earned a master's degree in social work and must be licensed to work.

Activities Director: The activities director plans activities for residents to help them socialize and stay physically and mentally active. Games,

musical performances, and arts and crafts are some types of activities that the activities director plans or leads. An activities director has usually earned a bachelor's degree; however, she may have an associate's degree or qualifying work experience. An activities director may be called a *recreational therapist* or *recreation worker*, depending upon education and experience.

Nursing Assistant (NA): The nursing assistant or nurse aide performs assigned nursing or related tasks, such as measuring a resident's temperature. An NA also gives personal care, such as bathing residents, brushing their teeth, and assisting with elimination. NAs are some of the most important team members because they have the most direct contact with residents. If a resident's health changes from day to day, NAs will often be the first ones to notice this change. NAs must report any changes in a resident's condition to the nurse promptly. The federal government requires that NAs have a minimum of 75 hours of training, and many states require more than 75 hours. After completing an approved nursing assistant training program, NAs must pass a competency evaluation to be able to work in a state. More information about training requirements is located in Chapters 2 and 28.

10. Discuss the facility chain of command

The **chain of command** describes the line of authority in the facility. For example, the nurse will usually be the NA's immediate supervisor. If an NA has a problem with someone in another department, the NA will report this to the proper person. This is usually an immediate supervisor or the **charge nurse**, who is a nurse responsible for a team of healthcare workers. The NA would not go directly to the person in the other department to tell her the problem. That would not be following the chain of command (Fig. 1-13).

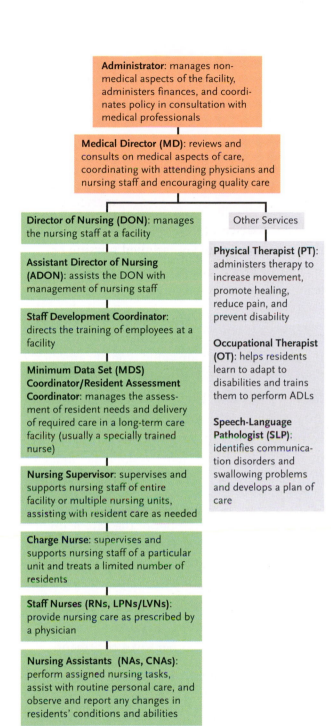

Administrator: manages non-medical aspects of the facility, administers finances, and coordinates policy in consultation with medical professionals

Medical Director (MD): reviews and consults on medical aspects of care, coordinating with attending physicians and nursing staff and encouraging quality care

Director of Nursing (DON): manages the nursing staff at a facility

Assistant Director of Nursing (ADON): assists the DON with management of nursing staff

Staff Development Coordinator: directs the training of employees at a facility

Minimum Data Set (MDS) Coordinator/Resident Assessment Coordinator: manages the assessment of resident needs and delivery of required care in a long-term care facility (usually a specially trained nurse)

Nursing Supervisor: supervises and supports nursing staff of entire facility or multiple nursing units, assisting with resident care as needed

Charge Nurse: supervises and supports nursing staff of a particular unit and treats a limited number of residents

Staff Nurses (RNs, LPNs/LVNs): provide nursing care as prescribed by a physician

Nursing Assistants (NAs, CNAs): perform assigned nursing tasks, assist with routine personal care, and observe and report any changes in residents' conditions and abilities

Other Services

Physical Therapist (PT): administers therapy to increase movement, promote healing, reduce pain, and prevent disability

Occupational Therapist (OT): helps residents learn to adapt to disabilities and trains them to perform ADLs

Speech-Language Pathologist (SLP): identifies communication disorders and swallowing problems and develops a plan of care

Fig. 1-13. The chain of command describes the line of authority in a facility and helps ensure that the resident receives proper care.

The chain of command also helps to protect staff from **liability**. Liability is a legal term that means a person can be held responsible for harming someone else. For example, imagine that a resident is injured while an NA is providing care. If the care was assigned and was done according to policy and procedure, the NA may

not be liable, or responsible, for harming the resident. However, if an NA performs a task that is not assigned to her or is not within her scope of practice and harms a resident, she could be held responsible (Chapter 2). That is why it is important for team members to follow instructions and for the facility to have a chain of command. Doing this helps promote proper care and lessen the risk of liability.

11. Explain *The Five Rights of Delegation*

When planning care, nurses decide which tasks to delegate to others, including NAs. **Delegation** means transferring responsibility to a person for a specific task. NAs do not delegate tasks; they have tasks delegated to them. Licensed nurses are accountable for care, including all delegated tasks. The National Council of State Boards of Nursing has identified *The Five Rights of Delegation*. This can be used as a mental checklist to help nurses in the decision-making process.

The Five Rights of Delegation are the *Right Task*, *Right Circumstance*, *Right Person*, *Right Direction/Communication*, and *Right Supervision/Evaluation*. Before delegating tasks, nurses consider these questions:

- Is there a match between the resident's needs and the NA's skills, abilities, and experience?

- What is the level of resident stability?

- Is the NA the right person to do the job?

- Can the nurse give appropriate direction and communication?

- Is the nurse available to give the supervision, support, and help that the NA needs?

There are questions NAs may want to consider before accepting a task:

- Do I have all the information I need to do this job? Are there questions I should ask?

- Do I believe that I can do this task? Do I have the necessary skills?

- Do I have the needed supplies, equipment, and other support?

- Do I know who my supervisor is, and how to reach her?

- Have I told my supervisor of any special needs for help and support?

- Do we both understand who is doing what?

A nursing assistant should never be afraid to ask for help. She should always ask if she needs more information or is unsure about something. If an NA feels that she does not have the skills for a task, she should talk to the nurse.

12. Describe methods of nursing care and discuss person-centered care

The nursing profession takes a holistic view of resident care. The word *holistic* comes from a Greek word meaning *whole*. **Holistic care** means considering a whole system, such as a whole person, and not dividing the system up into parts. Holistic care is caring for the whole person. This includes her physical needs, as well as other needs, such as social, emotional, intellectual, and spiritual (Fig. 1-14). Meeting these needs helps improve residents' quality of life. More information about these needs may be found in Chapter 5.

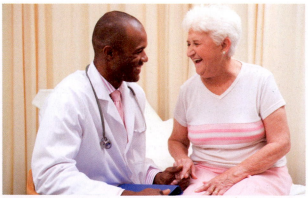

Fig. 1-14. *Caring for residents holistically means considering their emotional needs as well as their physical needs.*

Over the years, the nursing profession has changed a great deal. Many types of nursing care have been used at care facilities. Each facility utilizes the type that provides the best care for their residents:

Team Nursing: In this method of nursing care, a registered nurse functions as the **team leader**. Assignments are made, care is given, and the team members report to the team leader throughout the day. The resident's care is managed efficiently and cooperatively by using this team approach to care.

Primary Nursing: A registered nurse provides much of the daily care to residents in this method of nursing care. This type of care allows for a closer relationship between the nurse and the residents. Consistency and continuity of care are positive results. **Continuity of care** is an ongoing coordination of a resident's care. The nursing team regularly exchanges information about the resident, while working toward shared goals.

Functional Nursing: Using this method of nursing care, each member of the care team is given one or more specific tasks to complete for a large number of residents. For example, one team member is assigned to measure vital signs for all residents in the unit. Another completes all of the daily weights. One nurse administers medications, while another gives treatments. This type of care is not as organized as other methods. Staff may not have enough time to accurately observe each resident, and changes in a resident's condition may be overlooked.

Regardless of the type of nursing care utilized, many long-term care facilities promote **person-centered care** (also known as *person-directed care*). Person-centered care emphasizes the individuality of the person who needs care, and recognizes and develops his capabilities. Person-centered care revolves around the resident and promotes his individual preferences, choices, dignity, and interests. Each person's background, culture, language, beliefs, and traditions are respected. Improving each resident's quality of life and enhancing control over his care are important goals. Giving person-centered care will be an ongoing focus throughout this textbook.

Trauma Informed Care (TIC)

Trauma informed care is a way of approaching patient care that recognizes and considers trauma. Many people have experienced some form of trauma, such as having been abused or assaulted, having been the victim of a crime, or experiencing other forms of violence. Having a life-threatening illness or negative experiences in the medical setting can cause trauma. Imprisonment and military combat are additional situations that cause trauma. The goal of TIC is to be aware of the prevalence of trauma and to provide support by giving person-centered care. Each person's experiences and preferences should be taken into account. Staff must try to avoid triggers that cause discomfort and re-traumatization.

National Center for Complementary and Integrative Health (NCCIH)

The National Center for Complementary and Integrative Health (nccih.nih.gov) is a federal agency that conducts and supports scientific research about the safety and effectiveness of using complementary and integrative therapies to improve health and health care. Complementary medicine refers to treatments that are used in addition to conventional medical treatments. Alternative medicine involves practices and treatments that are used in place of conventional methods. Examples of these treatments include acupuncture, herbal therapy, massage, and meditation. Integrative health care merges conventional and complementary treatments, while emphasizing person-centered care and maintaining continuity of care between providers.

13. Explain policy and procedure manuals

All facilities have manuals outlining policies and procedures. A **policy** is a course of action to be taken every time a certain situation occurs. The policy manual has information about every facility policy. For example, one basic policy is that the chain of command must always be followed.

A **procedure** is a specific method, or way, of doing something. The procedure manual has information on the exact way to complete every procedure. For example, there will be a procedure for giving a resident a bed bath.

Everyone needs a reminder about how to perform a task from time to time. The procedure manual serves as a guide if a staff member wants to review the steps in a procedure. NAs should always look at this manual if they are unsure and ask for help if they have questions. This promotes safety. Not asking questions when unsure how to perform a procedure can be dangerous.

The policy and procedure manuals are usually kept together. Employees will be told where to find them.

14. Describe the long-term care survey process

Inspections are performed to help ensure that long-term care facilities are following state and federal regulations. Inspections are done periodically by the state agency that licenses facilities. These inspections are called *surveys*. They may be done more often if a facility has been cited for problems. To **cite** means to find a problem through a survey. Inspections may be done less often if the facility has a good record. Inspection teams include a variety of trained healthcare professionals.

Surveyors study how well the staff cares for residents. They focus on how residents' nutritional, physical, social, emotional, and spiritual needs are being met. They interview residents and families and observe the staff's interactions with residents and the care given. They review resident charts and observe meals. Surveys are one reason the documentation done by NAs is so important.

Surveyors identify violations of specific federal regulations using numbered codes called *F-Tags*.

When surveyors are in a facility, staff should try not to be nervous. They should give the same quality care they give every day and answer any questions to the best of their abilities. If an employee does not know the answer to the surveyor's question, she should be honest and never guess. She should tell the surveyor that she does not know the answer but will find out as quickly as possible. Then she should follow up with the surveyor after she has the answer.

The **Joint Commission** is an independent, not-for-profit organization that evaluates and accredits healthcare facilities. Its standards focus on improving the quality and safety of care given to patients, residents, and clients. For an organization to receive accreditation from the Joint Commission, it must undergo a comprehensive survey process at least every three years. This process includes checking performance in specific areas, such as treatment, infection prevention, and patient rights.

The Joint Commission's surveys are not associated with state inspections. Healthcare facilities are not required to participate in the Joint Commission's survey process; they may do so on a voluntary basis. Types of healthcare facilities that are accredited by the Joint Commission include hospitals, long-term care facilities, rehabilitation centers, laboratories, and other organizations.

Chapter Review

1. Whom does Medicare insurance cover (LO 3)?

2. Who makes up the majority of residents in long-term care facilities—men or women (LO 4)?

3. What are three tasks that NAs do not usually perform (LO 5)?

4. What is one way that an NA can demonstrate professionalism (LO 6)?

5. List each of the ten qualities in Learning Objective 7. For each quality, write one example of a way that an NA can demonstrate that quality (LO 7).

6. Who is the most important member of the care team (LO 9)?

7. List *The Five Rights of Delegation* (LO 11).

8. Define *person-centered care* (LO 12).

9. When surveyors visit a facility, what do they study and observe (LO 14)?

10. When a surveyor asks an NA a question she does not know the answer to, how should she respond (LO 14)?

Multiple Choice

11. Which of the following statements is true of long-term care (LO 2)?
    (A) Long-term care is only given during certain hours of the day.
    (B) Long-term care assists people with ongoing, chronic medical conditions.
    (C) Long-term care is given in an adult day services setting.
    (D) Long-term care is for people who need care for a short time after surgery.

12. One common NA task is (LO 5)
    (A) Prescribing medication
    (B) Creating residents' care plans
    (C) Managing other NAs' work
    (D) Bathing residents

13. Which of the following is true of proper grooming for an NA (LO 8)?
    (A) Gel nails should be freshly applied.
    (B) A simple waterproof watch should be worn.
    (C) Earrings can dangle just past the earlobe.
    (D) Perfume should be applied behind the ears or on both wrists.

14. If an NA is following the chain of command, to whom would she normally report a problem (LO 10)?
    (A) Nurse
    (B) Administrator
    (C) Resident
    (D) Medical social worker

15. If an NA has forgotten the correct order in which to perform a procedure, which of the following would be the best way for her to proceed (LO 13)?
    (A) The NA should review the procedure manual before beginning.
    (B) The NA should ask the resident to see if he remembers the correct order.
    (C) The NA should perform the procedure to the best of her memory, knowing that she will probably do it correctly.
    (D) The NA should consult with the administrator to find out the correct order.

2
Ethical and Legal Issues

The First Code of Ethics

An English physician named Thomas Percival wrote *Medical Ethics* in 1803. Here is a sample from that first code of ethics: "A physician ought not to abandon a patient because the case is deemed incurable, for his attendance may continue to be highly useful to the patient, and comforting to the relatives around him ." In 1847, Percival's *Medical Ethics* was used to help develop the American Medical Association's first code of ethics. The American Medical Association's *Principles of Medical Ethics* is still the code of ethics that physicians use today.

"It's a funny thing about life, if you refuse to accept anything but the best, you very often get it."

W. Somerset Maugham, 1874–1965

"Wherever there is a human being, I see God-given rights inherent in that being, whatever may be the sex or complexion."

William Lloyd Garrison, 1805–1879

1. Define important words in this chapter

abuse: purposeful or willful mistreatment that causes physical, mental, emotional, or financial pain or injury to a person.

advance directives: legal documents that allow people to decide what kind of medical care they wish to have in the event they are unable to make those decisions themselves.

assault: a threat to harm a person, resulting in the person feeling fearful that he will be harmed.

battery: the intentional touching of a person without her consent.

civil law: private law; law between individuals.

criminal law: public law; law related to committing a crime against the community.

defamation: any untrue statement (written or oral) that injures a person's reputation and/or damages the person's ability to make a living.

DNR: an abbreviation for do-not-resuscitate; an order that tells medical professionals not to perform CPR in the event of cardiac or respiratory arrest.

domestic violence: physical, sexual, or emotional abuse by spouses, intimate partners, or family members.

durable power of attorney for health care: a legal document that appoints someone to make the medical decisions for a person in the event he becomes unable to do so.

electronic health record (EHR): the electronic form of a resident's personal and health data that is used to manage and coordinate a resident's health care.

ethics: the knowledge of right and wrong; standards of conduct.

etiquette: the code of proper behavior and courtesy in a certain setting.

eviction: involuntary discharge from a facility.

exploitation: the act of taking advantage of a person for personal gain through threats or manipulation.

false imprisonment: unlawful restraint that affects a person's freedom of movement; includes both the threat of being physically restrained and actually being physically restrained.

financial abuse: improper or illegal use of a person's money, possessions, property, or other assets.

HIPAA: an abbreviation for Health Insurance Portability and Accountability Act; a federal law that sets standards for protecting the privacy of patients' health information.

intimate partner violence (IPV): physical, sexual, or emotional harm caused by a partner or spouse.

invasion of privacy: the violation of the right to be left alone and the right to control personal information.

involuntary seclusion: the separation of a person from others against the person's will.

laws: rules set by the government to help protect the public.

libel: defamation in written form.

living will: a document that states the medical care a person wants, or does not want, in case she becomes unable to make those decisions.

malpractice: professional misconduct that results in damage or injury to a person.

mandated reporters: people who are required to report suspected or observed abuse or neglect due to their regular contact with vulnerable populations, such as the elderly in long-term care facilities.

misappropriation: the deliberate misplacement, exploitation, or improper use of a resident's belongings or money without the resident's consent.

mistreatment: the inappropriate treatment or exploitation of a resident.

NATCEP: an abbreviation for Nurse Aide Training and Competency Evaluation Program; part of the Omnibus Budget Reconciliation Act (OBRA) that sets minimum requirements for training and testing nursing assistants.

neglect: failure to provide necessary care or services, resulting in physical, mental, or emotional harm to a person.

negligence: actions, or the failure to act or provide proper care for a person, resulting in unintended injury.

OBRA: an abbreviation for Omnibus Budget Reconciliation Act; law passed by the federal government that includes minimum standards for nursing assistant training, staffing requirements, resident assessment instructions, and information on rights for residents.

ombudsman: a legal advocate for residents in long-term care facilities.

physical abuse: any treatment, intentional or not, that causes harm or injury to a person's body.

protected health information (PHI): information that can be used to identify a person and relates to his past, present, or future physical or mental condition, including any health care the patient has had, or payment for that health care.

psychological abuse: emotional harm caused by threatening, frightening, isolating, intimidating, humiliating, or insulting a person.

Resident Council: a group of residents who meet regularly to discuss issues related to the long-term care facility.

Residents' Rights: rights identified in the Omnibus Budget Reconciliation Act (OBRA) that relate to how residents must be treated while living in a long-term care facility; they provide an ethical code of conduct for healthcare workers.

scope of practice: the tasks that healthcare providers are legally permitted to perform according to state or federal law.

sexual abuse: nonconsensual sexual contact of any type.

sexual harassment: any unwelcome sexual advance or behavior that creates an intimidating, hostile, or offensive working environment.

slander: defamation in oral form.

substance abuse: the repeated use of legal or illegal drugs, cigarettes, or alcohol in a way that causes harm to oneself or others.

verbal abuse: the use of language that threatens, embarrasses, or insults a person.

workplace violence: verbal, physical, or sexual abuse of staff by other staff members, residents, or visitors.

2. Define *law, ethics,* and *etiquette*

There are many legal and ethical terms that relate to resident care. **Ethics** are the knowledge of what is right and wrong; they help guide conduct. Ethics help people make decisions at home, in the workplace, or in the community. In health care, ethics guide the people giving care. For example, keeping a resident's information confidential is ethical behavior. It is also the law.

Laws are rules set by the government to help protect the public. In health care, laws protect those receiving care (Fig. 2-1). For example, there is a law against stealing a resident's belongings.

Laws can be civil or criminal. **Criminal laws** are enacted to protect society from people or organizations that try to harm them. This type of law protects the public. It is also called *public law*. **Civil law** refers to disputes between individuals. Problems with landlords, conflicts with neighbors, and divorce issues are examples of areas covered by civil law. Civil law is sometimes referred to as *private law*.

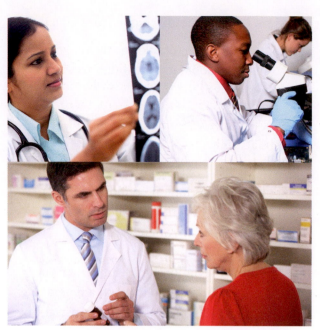

Fig. 2-1. *All healthcare providers must behave ethically and follow the law.*

Criminal law includes these types of offenses (crimes):

- A felony is a serious crime. Murder and bribery are examples of felonies. Punishment may include a long prison term, such as life without parole or even a death sentence.

- A misdemeanor is any crime that is not a felony. It is a less serious offense than a felony. Disturbing the peace is an example of a misdemeanor. Punishment may include community service time, a fine, and/or a short prison term.

Etiquette is the code of proper behavior and courtesy in a certain setting. For example, proper telephone etiquette includes identifying oneself when answering the phone at a facility. Asking "How may I help you?" is also part of proper telephone etiquette.

3. Discuss examples of ethical and professional behavior

A nursing assistant's ethics play an important part in her success as a care team member. Professional and ethical behavior is vital to the safety and well-being of the residents.

Guidelines: Legal and Ethical Behavior

G   Keep all resident information confidential (private). This is one of the Residents' Rights covered later in this chapter. All team members must keep resident information confidential. Only discuss residents with specific members of the care team.

G   Keep staff information confidential. Do not share private information about your coworkers at home or anywhere else.

G   Be honest at all times. Communicate honestly and clearly with members of the care team. Be honest when documenting resident care. Be truthful when reporting the hours you have worked. Do not take items that do not belong to you.

G   Be trustworthy. Trusting others is important in facilities. Residents must be able to trust staff members. Employers must be able to trust their employees. Employees need to trust their supervisors. One way employees can show that they are trustworthy is to be at work on time each day. When an employee often fails to show up for work, the boss cannot trust or count on that employee. Employers also trust that employees will come to them if they have a problem. This is part of following the chain of command.

G   Do not accept tips or gifts from residents or their family members or friends (Fig. 2-2).

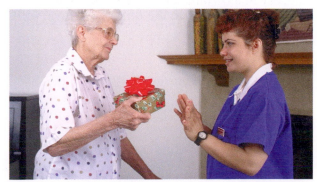

Fig. 2-2. Nursing assistants should not accept money or gifts, because it is unprofessional and can lead to conflict.

G   Report abuse or suspected abuse of residents. Learning Objective 7 of this chapter has more information about abuse.

G   Do not report to work under the influence of alcohol, illegal drugs, or chemical substances.

G   Follow all facility policies, rules, and procedures. Document care you give accurately and promptly.

G   Do your assigned tasks. If you make a mistake, report it promptly to the nurse. This can help minimize damage and prevent any further problems.

G   Be positive and professional. Residents deserve caregivers who try to make their days as pleasant as possible. A person who is positive and encouraging is someone people like to be around.

G   Be tactful. Tact is the ability to understand what is proper and appropriate when dealing with others. It is the ability to speak and act without offending others.

G   Treat all residents with respect, and be empathetic. Showing respect means allowing others to believe or act as they wish. Empathy means being able to share in and understand the feelings and troubles of others. A caring person is empathetic with a person who is ill. A caring person also respects an ill person's actions or beliefs about the illness, despite her own feelings.

G   Be patient. Nursing assistants have to deal with residents' troubles and pain without getting frustrated. Activities of daily living (ADLs), such as eating, dressing, and elimination, may take older people much longer and use up much of their energy, leaving them tired (Fig. 2-3). Residents should be allowed to do tasks at their own pace. The more patient you are, the better care you will provide.

Tip

Gifts and Tips

Accepting gifts or tips is not allowed in the health-care field. It is unprofessional and can lead to conflict. Nursing assistants and other staff members receive payment from the facility for the work they do. If a resident, family member, or visitor offers to tip an NA or tries to give an NA a gift, she should politely refuse. She can explain that it would not be ethical for her to accept it and that it is against the facility's policies.

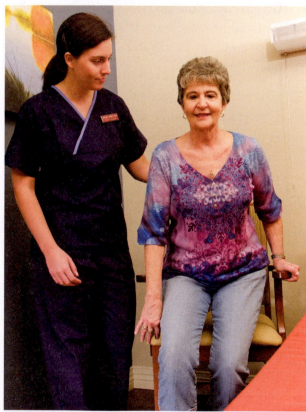

Fig. 2-3. Older adults may need extra time when performing their activities of daily living. NAs must be patient and allow them to do tasks at their own pace.

4. Describe a nursing assistant code of ethics

Many facilities have adopted a formal code of ethics that helps their employees deal with issues of what is right and what is wrong. Codes of ethics differ but all revolve around the idea that a resident, patient, or client is a valuable person who deserves ethical care. A sample code of ethics for nursing assistants follows:

1. I will strive to provide and maintain the highest quality of care for all residents. I will fully recognize and follow all Residents' Rights.

2. I will communicate well, serve on committees, and read all material as provided and required by my employer. I will attend educational in-services and join organizations relevant to nursing assistant care.

3. I will show a positive attitude toward all residents, their family members, staff, and other visitors.

4. I will always provide privacy for all residents. I will maintain confidentiality of resident, staff, and visitor information.

5. I will be trustworthy and honest in all dealings with residents, staff, and visitors.

6. I will strive to preserve resident safety. I will report mistakes I make, along with anything that I deem dangerous, to the right person(s).

7. I will have empathy for all residents, staff members, and visitors, giving support and encouragement when needed.

8. I will respect all people, without regard to age, gender, sexual orientation, gender identity, religion, race, ethnicity, economic situation, or diagnosis.

9. I will never abuse residents in any way. I will always report any suspected abuse to the proper person immediately.

10. I will strive to have the utmost patience with all people at my facility.

Tip

Nursing assistants are not nurses

Nursing assistants must *never* identify themselves as nurses. Nurses have had more education and training than NAs, and they have different responsibilities. An NA calling himself a nurse could result in injury to the NA or others, a lawsuit, and/or the NA being fired from his job. The term *nurse* should not be used lightly; NAs must always identify themselves as nursing assistants.

5. Explain OBRA

OBRA (The Omnibus Budget Reconciliation Act) is a federal law that was passed in 1987 and has been updated several times since then. OBRA was created in response to reports of poor care and abuse in long-term care facilities. Congress decided to set minimum standards of care, which included standardizing training of nursing assistants.

OBRA requires that **NATCEP** (Nurse Aide Training and Competency Evaluation Program) sets minimum requirements for nursing assistants. Nursing assistants must complete at least 75 hours of training that cover topics like basic nursing skills, personal care skills, restorative skills, mental health and social service needs, Residents' Rights, safety and emergency care, and cognitive impairment. However, many states require more training than the minimum set by the federal government. Programs may require 80 to 150 hours of training in theory and clinical skills.

Nursing assistants must also pass a competency evaluation (testing program) before they can be employed. The exam consists of both written and demonstrated nursing skills. Nursing assistants must attend regular in-service education classes (a minimum of 12 hours per year) to keep their skills updated.

OBRA requires that states keep a current list of nursing assistants in a state registry. In addition, OBRA identifies standards that instructors must meet in order to train nursing assistants. OBRA sets guidelines for minimum staff requirements and specifies services that long-term care facilities must provide.

The resident assessment requirements are another important part of OBRA. OBRA requires that complete assessments be done on every resident. The assessment forms are the same for every facility. The Minimum Data Set (MDS) is a resident assessment system that was developed in 1990 and is revised periodically. The MDS is a detailed form with guidelines for assessing residents. More information about the MDS is located in Chapter 3.

OBRA also identifies important rights for residents in long-term care facilities. Learning Objective 6 contains more information about these rights.

OBRA regulations are important to nursing assistants because they

- Give recognition through certification and registration

- Help define the nursing assistant's **scope of practice**, which specifies the tasks that nursing assistants are legally permitted to perform according to state or federal law

- Provide directions for uniformity of care

- Promote educational standards

Tip

Reciprocity

When a person has completed an approved nursing assistant course, he may be eligible for nursing assistant certification. When moving to another state, the person's certification may transfer to that state. This is called *reciprocity*. Before moving to another state, an NA should contact the proper agency to help determine if he qualifies for reciprocity. It might be necessary to gather important paperwork from the NA's original state before he leaves. Obtaining a new certificate in a new state is the NA's responsibility and will be necessary before the NA begins work there.

6. Explain Residents' Rights

Residents' Rights specify how residents must be treated while living in a facility. They provide an ethical code of conduct for healthcare workers. Facility staff give residents a list of these rights and review each right with them. In 2016, the Centers for Medicare and Medicaid Services (CMS) finalized a rule to improve the care and safety of residents in long-term care facilities. It was the first comprehensive update since 1991. It includes strengthening the rights of residents who live in long-term care facilities. NAs must be familiar with these legal rights. Residents' Rights include the following:

Quality of life: Residents have the right to the best care available. Dignity, choice, and independence are important parts of quality of life. The facility must give equal access to quality care regardless of a resident's condition, diagnosis, or payment source.

Services and activities to maintain a high level of wellness: Residents must receive the correct care. Healthcare professionals at facilities are required to develop a care plan for residents, and their care must keep them as healthy as possible. A baseline care plan for residents, which includes instructions for providing person-centered care, must be developed within 48 hours of admission. Residents' health should not decline as a direct result of the facility's care.

The right to be fully informed about rights and services: Residents must be told what services are offered and what the fee is for each service. They must be informed of charges both orally and in writing. Residents must be given a written copy of their legal rights, along with the facility's rules and regulations. Legal rights must be explained in a language that each resident can understand. Residents must be given contact information for state agencies related to monitoring the quality of care, such as the ombudsman program (more information may be found later in the chapter). When requested, survey results must be shared with residents. Residents have the right to be notified about any change of room or roommate. They have the right to communicate with someone who speaks their language. They have the right to assistance for any sensory impairment, such as hearing loss.

The resident representative is a person chosen by the resident who acts on behalf of the resident. A resident representative may help make decisions, access the resident's information and receive notifications about the resident, or manage the resident's finances. A person who is legally considered a guardian or has a power of attorney may be a resident representative.

The right to participate in their own care: Residents have the right to participate in planning their treatment, care, and discharge (Fig. 2-4). Residents have the right to see and sign their care plans after all significant changes. Residents have the right to be informed of risks and benefits of care and treatment, including treatment options and alternatives, and to choose the options they prefer. They have the right to request, refuse, and/or discontinue treatment and care. They can refuse restraints and refuse to participate in experimental research.

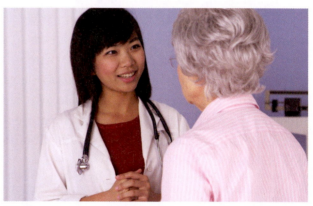

Fig. 2-4. *Residents have the right to be informed about their care and to make decisions about the kind of care they want.*

Residents have the right to be told of changes in their condition. They have the right to review their medical record. They have the right to choose and change their care providers at any time.

The right to make independent choices: Residents can make choices about their doctors, care, and treatments. They can make personal decisions, such as what to wear and how to spend their time. They can join in community activities, both inside and outside the care facility. They can vote in federal, state, and local elections. If a resident requires assistance with voting, a designated person might be needed to help the resident vote. They have the right to a reasonable accommodation of their needs and preferences. They have a right to participate in resident or family groups, such as a Resident Council.

A **Resident Council** is a group of residents who meet regularly to discuss issues related to the long-term care facility. This council gives residents a voice in facility operations. Topics of discussion may include facility policies and decisions regarding activities, concerns, and problems. The Resident Council offers residents a chance to provide suggestions on improving the quality of care. Council executives are elected by residents. Family members are invited to attend meetings with or on behalf of residents. Staff may participate in this process when invited by council members.

The right to privacy and confidentiality: Residents have the right to speak privately with anyone, the right to privacy during care, and the right to confidentiality regarding every aspect of their lives (Fig. 2-5). Their medical, personal, and financial information cannot be shared with anyone but the care team. Learning Objective 11 of this chapter contains more information about confidentiality.

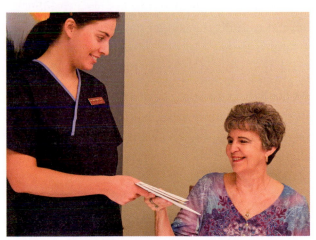

Fig. 2-5. Residents have the right to privacy, which includes being able to send and receive mail that is unopened.

The right to dignity, respect, and freedom: Residents must be respected and treated with dignity by caregivers. Residents must not be abused, mistreated, or neglected in any way.

The right to security of possessions: Residents' personal possessions must be safe at all times. Residents have the right to have secure personal property that is protected from loss or theft. Their possessions cannot be taken or used by anyone without a resident's permission. Residents have the right to file a complaint with the state agency for misappropriation of property. **Misappropriation** is the deliberate misplacement, exploitation, or improper use of a resident's belongings or money without the resident's consent. **Exploitation** is the act of taking advantage of a person for personal gain through threats or manipulation.

Residents have the right to manage their own finances or choose someone else to do it for them. They have the right to not be charged for any care that is covered by Medicaid or Medicare.

Rights during transfers and discharges: Residents have the right to be informed of and to consent to any location changes. Residents have the right to stay in a facility unless a transfer or discharge is needed. Residents can be moved or evicted from the facility due to safety reasons (their safety or others' safety), if their health has improved, or if payment for care has not been received for a determined period of time. **Eviction** is the involuntary discharge of a resident.

The facility must develop an effective discharge plan that involves each resident's goals and preferences. This plan must be regularly reviewed and updated as appropriate. Even if the resident is planning to stay at the facility long-term, a discharge plan must be created, keeping the resident's preferences in mind.

The right to complain: Residents have the right to make complaints and voice grievances without fear for their safety or care. Facilities must work quickly to address their concerns.

The right to visits: Residents have the right to visits from doctors, family members (including spouses and domestic partners), friends, ombudsmen, clergy members, legal representatives, or any other person (Fig. 2-6). Visits cannot be restricted, limited, or denied on the basis of race, color, national origin, religion, sex, gender identity, sexual orientation, or disability. In certain cases where a visitor may pose a clinical or safety risk to residents or staff, a visit may be denied, and the resident must be immediately informed.

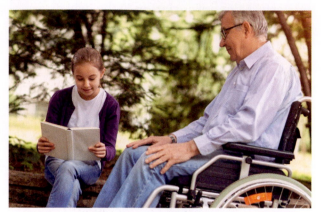

Fig. 2-6. Residents have the right to receive visitors at any reasonable hour.

Rights with regard to social services: The facility must provide residents with access to social services, including counseling, assistance in solving problems with others (mediation), and help contacting legal and financial professionals.

Blue boxes are located throughout this textbook that explain how to promote Residents' Rights and how to reinforce person-centered care.

7. Explain types of abuse and neglect

Preventing abuse and neglect of vulnerable adults is a very important part of Residents' Rights. Vulnerable adults are people over the age of 18 who are at a higher risk of harm or abuse, which includes the elderly in care facilities. **Abuse** is purposeful **mistreatment** that causes physical, mental, emotional, or financial pain or injury to someone. There are many different types of abuse, including the following:

Physical abuse is any treatment, intentional or not, that causes harm to a person's body. This includes slapping, hitting, kicking, cutting,

burning, pushing, shoving, and rough handling. Pushing a resident to move faster is one example of physical abuse. Physically restraining a resident is also considered abuse.

Psychological abuse is emotional harm caused by threatening, frightening, isolating, intimidating, humiliating, or insulting a person. Threatening to harm a resident if he tells another caregiver about a problem is one example of psychological abuse. Sharing something potentially embarrassing about a resident with another resident is another example of psychological abuse.

Verbal abuse is the use of spoken or written words, pictures, or gestures that threaten, embarrass, or insult a person.

Sexual abuse is nonconsensual sexual contact of any type. Any kind of nonconsensual sexual activity is considered sexual abuse. For example, showing sexually explicit magazines to a resident is sexual abuse. Rubbing against a resident inappropriately during personal care is also sexual abuse.

Financial abuse is the improper or illegal use of a person's money, possessions, property, or other assets. For example, offering to give a resident special care if the resident pays the nursing assistant is financial abuse. Stealing money from a resident is also considered financial abuse.

Assault is a threat to harm a person, resulting in the person feeling fearful that she will be harmed. Telling a resident that she will be slapped if she does not stop yelling is an example of assault.

Battery is the intentional touching of a person without her consent. An example is a nursing assistant hitting or pushing a resident, which is also considered physical abuse. Performing a procedure on a resident who has refused the procedure is also considered battery.

Domestic violence is abuse by spouses, intimate partners, or family members. It can be physical, sexual, or emotional. The victim can be a woman or man of any age or a child. **Intimate partner violence (IPV)** is physical, sexual, or emotional harm caused by a partner or spouse. It also includes isolating a partner or restricting the partner's access to help and information.

Workplace violence is abuse of staff by other staff members, residents, or visitors. It can be verbal, physical, or sexual. This includes improper touching and discussion about sexual subjects. A resident's family member threatening a staff member with violence is workplace violence.

False imprisonment is unlawful restraint that affects a person's freedom of movement. Both the threat of being physically restrained and actually being physically restrained are types of false imprisonment. Not allowing a resident to leave the building is also considered false imprisonment. Residents who have dementia, however, may be confined for their own safety.

Involuntary seclusion is the separation of a person from others against the person's will. An example is a nursing assistant forcing a resident to stay in her room with the door closed.

Sexual harassment is any unwelcome sexual advance or behavior that creates an intimidating, hostile, or offensive working environment. Requests for sexual favors, unwanted touching, and other acts of a sexual nature are examples of sexual harassment. Another example is a supervisor telling a team member that she will get the work schedule she wants if she has sex with him.

Substance abuse is the repeated use of legal or illegal drugs, cigarettes, or alcohol in a way that causes harms to oneself or others. Substances can be legal, or even prescribed, and still be abused. For example, alcohol and cigarettes are legal for adults but are often abused. Over-the-counter medications can be addictive and harmful (Fig. 2-7). Even paint or glue may be abused. Information on signs of substance abuse is located in Chapter 22.

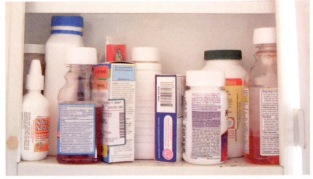

Fig. 2-7. Both prescription and non-prescription drugs can be abused.

Defamation is any untrue statement—written or oral—that injures a person's reputation and/or damages the person's ability to make a living. **Libel** is defamation in written form. **Slander** is defamation in oral form.

Neglect is the failure to provide necessary care or services, resulting in physical, mental, or emotional harm to a person. Examples include leaving a bedridden resident alone for lengthy periods, ignoring a resident's call light, or willfully denying the resident food, medication, dentures, or eyeglasses.

Negligence means actions, or the failure to act or give proper care to a person, resulting in unintended injury. An example of negligence is a nursing assistant forgetting to lock the bed wheels before transferring a resident. If the resident falls and is injured, it can be classified as negligence. **Malpractice** occurs when a negligent or improper act due to professional misconduct results in damage or injury to a person.

If an NA sees or suspects that a resident is being abused in any way, she is legally required to report it immediately to her supervisor. An NA should document any complaints of abuse reported to her and anything she witnesses. If action is not taken, she should keep reporting up the chain of command until action is taken. If no appropriate action is taken at the facility, she can call the state abuse hotline or contact the proper state agency. Abuse can be reported anonymously. These agencies are required to promptly investigate reports of abuse.

8. Recognize signs and symptoms of abuse and neglect

All care team members must observe for and report signs and symptoms of abuse and neglect.

Observing and Reporting: Abuse and Neglect

The following signs could indicate abuse:

O/R Broken bones

O/R Bruising, contusions, and welts

O/R Similar injuries that occur repeatedly, such as injuries shaped like a belt buckle

O/R Burns of unusual shape and in unusual locations, or cigarette burns

O/R Bite marks or scratches

O/R Unexplained weight loss

O/R Dehydration

O/R Dry, cracked, torn, or bleeding skin

O/R Missing hair

O/R Broken or missing teeth

O/R Blood in underwear

O/R Bruising, bleeding, or discharge from the genital area

O/R Depression or withdrawal (Fig. 2-8)

O/R Mood swings

O/R Fear and anxiety, especially when a particular caregiver is present

O/R Fear of being left alone

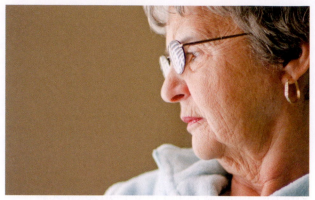

Fig. 2-8. *Withdrawing from others is an important change to report.*

The following signs could indicate neglect:

O/R Pressure injuries

O/R Weight loss or poor appetite

O/R Dehydration

O/R Frequent complaints of hunger or thirst

O/R Strong smell of urine

O/R Unclean body

O/R Dirty, matted, or unstyled hair

O/R Ragged or dirty fingernails

O/R Soiled clothes or bed linens or incontinence briefs not being changed

O/R Ripped or torn clothing

O/R Damaged or poorly-fitting hearing aids, eyeglasses, or dentures

O/R Unanswered call lights

Other signs of abuse include the following:

O/R Missing doctors' appointments

O/R Changing doctors frequently

O/R Wearing makeup or sunglasses to hide injuries

O/R Family concern that abuse is occurring

O/R Resident not taking his medication

O/R Private conversations not allowed, or the caregiver/family member is present during all conversations

Remember that nursing assistants are legally required to report abuse or suspected abuse. NAs are considered mandated reporters. **Mandated reporters** are people who are required to report suspected or observed abuse or neglect because they have regular contact with vulnerable populations, such as the elderly in long-term care facilities.

If abuse is suspected or observed, the NA should give the nurse as much information as possible. If residents want to make a complaint of abuse, NAs must assist them in every way. This includes telling them of the process and their rights. Nursing assistants must never retaliate against (punish) residents complaining of abuse. If an NA sees someone being cruel or abusive to a resident who made a complaint, she must report it. All care team members are responsible for residents' safety and should take this responsibility seriously.

9. Describe the steps taken if a nursing assistant is suspected of abuse

When a report of abuse against a nursing assistant is made, the NA is usually suspended immediately, pending investigation. The Nurse Aide Training and Competency Evaluation Program (NATCEP) is notified, as well as the facility administrator. Adult Protective Services (APS) may be notified. APS organizations help protect adults who, because of a physical or mental impairment, need help from other people for their care. A full, confidential investigation is completed. The facility will protect the resident and the person who reported the abuse from retaliation. If the investigation does not prove the claim of abuse, the NA returns to work. If the investigation shows that there might be truth to the claim, specific actions are taken.

The NATCEP outlines steps that must be followed. These steps include notification, investigation, a hearing, decision of the hearing, actions, and the appeals process. If the findings show that abuse did occur, the nursing assistant is placed on the abuse registry, in addition to facing other possible legal penalties, such as revocation of certification. The abuse registry is shared with other states. Employers check this registry before hiring nursing assistants.

10. Discuss the ombudsman's role

The word *ombudsman* originally came from a Scandinavian word. In parts of Scandinavia, an ombudsman is a government official who investigates citizens' complaints. In long-term care facilities in the United States, an **ombudsman** is the legal advocate for residents. The Older Americans Act (OAA) is a federal law that requires all states to have an ombudsman program. The ombudsman visits the facility and listens to residents. He decides what course of action to take if there is a problem. An ombudsman can help settle disputes and resolve conflicts. He provides an ongoing presence in long-term care facilities to monitor care and conditions (Fig. 2-9).

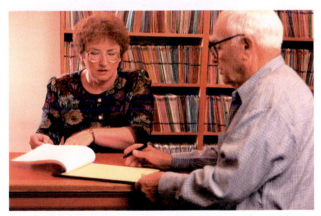

Fig. 2-9. *An ombudsman is a legal advocate for residents who visits the facility and listens to residents. He may work with other agencies to resolve complaints.*

An ombudsman typically performs these duties:

- Advocates for Residents' Rights and quality care

- Educates consumers and care providers

- Investigates and resolves complaints; works with investigators from the police, APS, and health departments

- Appears in court and/or at legal hearings
- Gives information to the public

In some states, a group of specially selected people may also investigate reports of abuse that occur in healthcare facilities. There are also state agencies that can assist people with other concerns about a facility, such as the State Department of Health and the State Department of Health and Human Services.

More information about the ombudsman program may be found by contacting The National Long-Term Care Ombudsman Resource Center (ltcombudsman.org) or a local legal aid society.

Residents' Rights

Elder Justice Act

The Elder Justice Act was passed as part of the Affordable Care Act in March of 2010. It is the first federal law designed specifically to combat elder abuse. Under the Elder Justice Act, the federal Department of Health and Human Services has established an Elder Justice Coordinating Council and an Advisory Board on Elder Abuse, Neglect, and Exploitation. These groups are intended to coordinate educational resources, support, and grant funding to aid efforts to stop elder abuse.

11. Explain HIPAA and related terms

One of the most important parts of a nursing assistant's job is to keep resident information confidential. Staff members will learn residents' health information from the residents themselves, their families, and from their medical records. They may also learn personal information about a resident's finances or relationships. This information cannot be shared with anyone except other care team members who are directly involved with the resident's care.

Congress passed **HIPAA** (Health Insurance Portability and Accountability Act, hhs.gov/hipaa) in 1996. It has been further defined and revised since then. This law sets standards for protecting the privacy of patients' health information. It identifies certain **protected health information (PHI)** that must remain confidential. It was also passed to facilitate the transfer of PHI for payment and research needs.

Protected health information is information that can be used to identify a person and relates to the patient's past, present, or future physical or mental condition; any health care that the person has had; or payment for that health care. PHI includes the patient's name, address, telephone number, medical record, social security number, email address, and other information. This information must remain secure at all times, both inside and outside of the facility. All healthcare organizations must take special steps to protect health information. Only people who must have information to give care or to process records can have access to this information (Fig. 2-10).

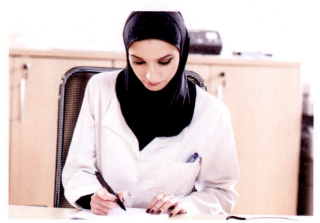

Fig. 2-10. HIPAA requires that special measures be taken to keep medical records confidential. Only people who give care or process records should have access to this information.

The Health Information Technology for Economic and Clinical Health (HITECH) Act became law at the end of 2009. It was enacted as a part of the American Recovery and Reinvestment Act of 2009. HITECH was created to expand the protection and security of consumers' **electronic health records (EHR)**. HITECH increases civil and criminal penalties for unauthorized sharing or access of PHI and expands the ability to enforce these penalties. HITECH also offers incentives to organizations to adopt the use of EHR.

HIPAA applies to all healthcare providers, including doctors, nurses, nursing assistants, and any other members of the care team. Nursing assistants must never share any protected information with anyone who is not directly involved in a resident's care unless the resident gives official consent or unless the law requires it. For example, if a friend asks an NA about a resident's condition, the correct response is "I cannot share that information. It is confidential." Only people who have a legal reason to know about the resident, such as members of the care team involved in the resident's care, can share health information.

Guidelines: Protecting Privacy

G Do not give health information on the phone unless you know you are speaking with an approved staff member.

G Do not give any personal information to any visitors, no matter who they are.

G Never share a medical record with anyone other than a staff member directly involved in the resident's care.

G Do not discuss residents in any public area, such as the dining room/cafeteria, a restaurant, store, or waiting room (Fig. 2-11). Use private areas at the facility to give reports.

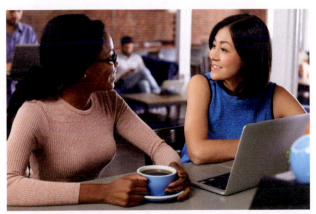

Fig. 2-11. *Do not discuss any information about residents in public places.*

G Do not bring your family or friends to the facility to meet residents.

G Make sure fax numbers are correct before faxing healthcare information. Use a cover sheet with a confidentiality statement.

G Return paper charts to their proper place after use. Hand charts directly to team members if transferring a resident to another unit or for a test.

G Dispose of personal notes regarding resident care (for example, notes taken during care reports) prior to leaving work for the day. They may need to be shredded or put in a special area. Follow facility policy.

G When finished with any computer work, log out and exit the web browser. Do not share your personal passwords with others.

G Do not give confidential information in emails. You do not know who has access to your messages.

G Do not share resident information, photos, or videos on any social networking site, such as Facebook, Instagram, or Twitter.

G Do not take photos of residents and share them, including via phones, email, social networking sites, or other websites.

G Give any documents you find with a resident's information to the nurse.

There are serious penalties for healthcare workers who violate HIPAA regulations. Team members may have to pay a fine and can be sentenced to prison. Maintaining confidentiality is a legal and ethical obligation. All healthcare workers must follow HIPAA regulations.

In addition to maintaining confidentiality, facilities are legally required to assure *full visual privacy* for residents. This means that each resident must be able to completely withdraw from public view while they are in their beds. This can be accomplished with a movable privacy screen or curtain or with a private room.

Invasion of privacy is a legal term. It means violating a person's right to be left alone or exposing information about that person without his consent. This includes releasing private facts, such as a medical record or even a photograph, without the person's consent. For example, invasion of privacy could be charged if a caregiver released medical information about a resident to the media. Discussing a resident's care or personal affairs with anyone other than care team members can be considered an invasion of privacy, which violates the law.

12. Discuss the Patient Self-Determination Act (PSDA) and advance directives

The Patient Self-Determination Act (PSDA) is a federal law passed in 1990 as an amendment to OBRA. The PSDA requires all healthcare agencies receiving Medicare and Medicaid funds to give adults, during admission or enrollment, information about their rights relating to advance directives. **Advance directives** are legal documents that allow people to decide what kind of medical care they wish to have in the event they are unable to make those decisions themselves. An advance directive can also designate someone else to make medical decisions for a person if that person is ill or disabled. Rules about how to execute these documents vary from state to state. Living wills and durable powers of attorney for health care are examples of advance directives.

A **living will** outlines the medical care a person wants, or does not want, in case he becomes unable to make those decisions. For example, a person may specify that certain measures are to be taken or withheld if he is in a coma. It is called a *living will* because it takes effect while the person is still alive. It may also be called a *directive to physicians*, *health care declaration*, or *medical directive*.

A **durable power of attorney for health care** (sometimes called a *health care proxy*) is a signed, dated, and witnessed legal document that appoints someone to make the medical decisions for a person in the event he becomes unable to do so. This can include instructions about medical treatment the person wants to avoid. Because the term *power of attorney* indicates legal issues, people may think this means that someone can take control of a person's money, property, etc. This document, however, deals only with medical issues.

A **DNR** (do-not-resuscitate) order is another way to honor wishes about health care. A DNR order instructs medical professionals not to perform cardiopulmonary resuscitation (CPR) in the event of cardiac or respiratory arrest. CPR refers to medical procedures used when the heart and lungs have stopped working. There is more information about CPR in Chapter 8. Generally these orders are used by people who are in the final stages of a terminal illness or who have a very serious condition.

These different types of advance directives may be used together, or a person may elect to use only one type or none at all. Having an advance directive is not legally required. However, it is a good way to make sure a person's wishes regarding medical care are known. An advance directive can be changed or canceled at any time, either in writing, or orally, or both.

According to the Patient Self-Determination Act, rights relating to advance directives that must be given upon admission include the following:

- The right to participate in and direct healthcare decisions

- The right to accept or refuse treatment

- The right to prepare an advance directive

- Information on the facility's policies that govern these rights

The PSDA requires that facilities give new residents the facility's policies on handling advance directives. Each facility must ask residents what advance directives they have and obtain copies of these documents. In addition, facilities must offer education to the staff about advance directives. The act prohibits discriminating against a patient who does not have an advance directive.

Tip

Wills and Living Wills
A living will is different from a will. A living will is a type of advance directive that states the medical care a person wants, or does not want, in case she becomes unable to make those decisions. A will is a legal document that details how a person wants her possessions to be distributed after her death. If a resident tells a nursing assistant that she wants to prepare a will, the NA should notify the nurse. Many facilities have a rule that staff should not witness a will, even if a resident asks the person to do so.

Chapter Review

1. What are ethics (LO 2)?

2. Give one example of a law that must be followed (LO 2).

3. Describe five elements of a typical nursing assistant code of ethics (LO 4).

4. According to the Omnibus Budget Reconciliation Act's (OBRA) requirements, how many hours of training must nursing assistants complete at a minimum (LO 5)?

5. Give one example of negligence (LO 7).

6. What is a nursing assistant's responsibility if she sees or suspects abuse (LO 8)?

7. What generally happens to a nursing assistant after a report of abuse has been made about him (LO 9)?

8. Describe some of the typical duties of an ombudsman (LO 10).

9. With whom may a nursing assistant share a resident's health information (LO 11)?

10. What does HIPAA protect (LO 11)?

11. To which members of the care team does HIPAA apply (LO 11)?

12. What are advance directives (LO 12)?

13. List four rights related to advance directives that the PSDA requires be given to new residents upon admission (LO 12).

Multiple Choice

14. Which of the following is one reason that a nursing assistant should not accept money or gifts from residents (LO 3)?
(A) The NA will start to depend on the extra income and will not be able to live within her budget without it.
(B) Receiving money or gifts is unprofessional and can lead to conflict.
(C) Receiving money or gifts is unfair because not all residents can afford to tip staff or give gifts.
(D) The NA will be unable to ask for an advance on her salary if she receives additional income from residents.

15. What is the name of the resident assessment system required by OBRA (LO 5)?
(A) Resident Information Protocols (RIP)
(B) Reporting and Recording Intake (RRI)
(C) Minimum Data Set (MDS)
(D) Evaluation Implementation Form (EIF)

16. Residents have a legal right not to be abused or mistreated. To which one of the Residents' Rights does this relate (LO 6)?
(A) Right to visits
(B) Right to dignity, respect, and freedom
(C) Right with regard to social services
(D) Right to security of possessions

17. Residents have a legal right to be told of changes in their medical condition. To which one of the Residents' Rights does this relate (LO 6)?
(A) Right to participate in their own care
(B) Right to privacy and confidentiality
(C) Right to complain
(D) Rights during transfers and discharges

18. A nursing assistant takes money from a resident's purse, planning to pay it back later. Which type of abuse is this considered (LO 7)?
    (A) Psychological abuse
    (B) Physical abuse
    (C) Substance abuse
    (D) Financial abuse

19. Emotional abuse of a resident by his wife is considered (LO 7)
    (A) Domestic violence
    (B) Physical abuse
    (C) Substance abuse
    (D) Sexual abuse

3 Communication Skills

1. Define important words in this chapter

active listening: a way of communicating that involves giving a person one's full attention while he is speaking and encouraging him to give information and clarify ideas.

adverse event: an unexpected event that causes serious injury or death; also called *sentinel event*.

barrier: a block or an obstacle.

body language: all of the conscious or unconscious messages a person's body sends as she communicates; facial expressions, gestures, and posture are examples.

care conference: a meeting to share and gather information about a resident in order to develop a care plan.

care plan: a plan for each resident created by a registered nurse that outlines the tasks that team members must perform to help the resident reach her goals of care.

charting: the act of noting care and observations; documenting.

code: in health care, an emergent medical situation in which specially trained responders provide the necessary care.

code status: formal documentation of the type and scope of care that should be provided to a particular resident in the event of a cardiac arrest, other catastrophic organ failure, or terminal illness.

critical thinking: the process of reasoning and analyzing in order to solve problems; for the nursing assistant, critical thinking means making careful observations and promptly reporting all potential problems.

culture: a set of learned beliefs, values, traditions, and behaviors shared by a social or ethnic group.

edema: swelling in body tissues caused by excess fluid.

incident: an accident, problem, or unexpected event during the course of care.

incident report: a report documenting an incident and the response to the incident; also called an *occurrence, accident, accident/incident,* or *event report.*

medical chart: legal record of all medical care a patient, resident, or client receives.

Minimum Data Set (MDS): a detailed form with guidelines for assessing residents in long-term care facilities; also details what to do if resident problems are identified.

nonverbal communication: communication without using words, such as through gestures and facial expressions.

nursing process: an organized method used by nurses to determine residents' needs, plan the appropriate care to meet those needs, and evaluate how well the plan of care is working; the five steps are assessment, diagnosis, planning, implementation, and evaluation.

objective information: factual information collected using the senses of sight, hearing, smell, and touch; also called *signs.*

orientation: a person's awareness of person, place, and time.

prefix: a word part that comes before the root to help form a new term.

prioritize: to place things in order of importance.

root: the main part of a word that contains its basic meaning or definition.

rounds: scheduled visits to each resident's room to assess the resident's condition and needs and to discuss the care plan with participating staff.

sentinel event: an unexpected event that causes serious injury or death; also called *adverse event.*

subjective information: information collected from residents, their family members, and their friends; information may not be true, but is what the person reported; also called *symptoms.*

suffix: a word part added to the end of a root or a prefix to create a new word.

verbal communication: communication involving the use of spoken or written words or sounds; also called *oral communication.*

vital signs: measurements—temperature, pulse, respirations, and blood pressure—that monitor the functioning of the vital organs of the body.

2. Explain types of communication

Communication is the process of exchanging information with others. It is a process of sending and receiving messages. People communicate with signs and symbols, such as words, drawings, and pictures; they also communicate through their behavior.

The simplest form of communication is a three-step process that takes place between two people. In the first step, the sender (the person who communicates first) sends a message. In the second step, the receiver receives the message. Receiver and sender switch roles as they communicate. The third step involves providing feedback. The receiver repeats the message or responds to it to let the sender know the message was received and understood. All three steps must occur before the communication process is complete. During a conversation, this process is repeated continuously (Fig. 3-1).

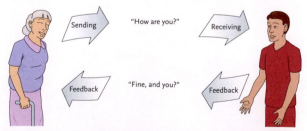

Fig. 3-1. The communication process consists of sending a message, receiving the message, and providing feedback.

Verbal communication (also called *oral communication*) involves using words. Speaking and writing are two ways of communicating verbally. Oral reports are an example of verbal communication. Verbal communication also includes the way in which words are spoken or written, including symbols such as emojis. How the voice sounds when a person speaks says as much as the words he uses. For example, if a nursing assistant sounds irritated when saying, "Let me know if you need anything else," the resident may feel that the nursing assistant does not want to be bothered. The resident may not want to communicate a need because he fears it will annoy or anger the nursing assistant. The words a person uses send a message as well.

Nursing assistants should always use a pleasant tone of voice with residents and consider their choice of words before speaking. When writing information, NAs should be clear and direct. They should make sure they are using the right words so that they will be understood.

Nonverbal communication is communication that happens without the use of words. **Body language** is a form of nonverbal communication. Body language has to do with all of the conscious or unconscious messages a person's body sends as she communicates. It includes posture, body movements, facial expressions, and gestures (Fig. 3-2). Body language can add positive or negative messages during communication.

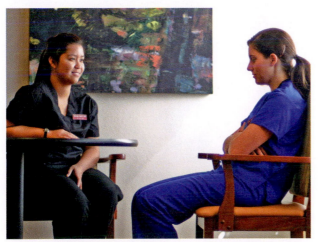

Fig. 3-2. Body language sends messages just as words do. Which of these people seems more interested in their conversation—the person on the right who is looking down with her arms crossed or the person on the left who is sitting up straight and smiling?

For example, if an NA smiles and tells a resident, "I'll be glad to help you find your glasses, Mrs. Martinez," it communicates that she is willing to help. However, if she rolls her eyes while responding, it sends a message that she is annoyed by the request.

Touch is another important part of nonverbal communication. Some people are more comfortable with being touched than others. Some find it comforting, while others are bothered by it. Nursing assistants have to touch residents during care. However, if a resident is not comfortable being touched, the NA should limit touch as much as possible. An NA should always ask permission before touching a resident. Learning Objective 4 contains more information about touch.

Examples of positive nonverbal communication include the following:

- Smiling in a friendly way

- Leaning forward to listen

- Nodding while a person is speaking

Examples of negative nonverbal communication include the following:

- Rolling eyes

- Crossing arms

- Tapping feet

- Pointing at someone while speaking

If a resident seems offended by an NA's behavior, the NA can apologize and ask how she can make the situation better. Even if the NA's body language was unintentionally negative, making positive changes will improve the way she relates to other people.

Guidelines: Proper Communication

G Use appropriate words. Make sure residents are able to understand what you say. Use proper words and terms with care team members.

G   Be aware of your body language.

G   Use a friendly, professional tone of voice. Communicate care and concern.

G   Wait for responses. Let pauses happen. Do not interrupt or try to finish the person's sentences.

G   Practice active listening. **Active listening** involves giving residents your full attention while they are speaking. Maintain eye contact. Use phrases that encourage them to keep speaking and to clarify their communication. Examples are "Yes," "Hmm," "I see," and "I understand." "Go on" is another example. Repeat the resident's message to show you have been listening closely. Active listening also includes nonverbal communication, such as nodding and smiling. Show residents you are really interested in what they have to say.

G   Use facts when communicating. A fact is something that is definitely true. An opinion is something someone believes to be true, but is not definitely true or cannot be proven. For example, "Ms. Simpson weighs 155 pounds" is a fact. "Ms. Simpson looks thinner" is an opinion. It might be true but cannot be backed up with evidence. If you give an opinion to the care team, make it clear that what you are saying is an opinion, not a fact. Both facts and opinions are valuable to the care team. However, using facts will help you communicate more effectively.

3. Explain barriers to communication

Some residents will have trouble understanding or using verbal (spoken or written) communication. This is due to a **barrier** that blocks or disrupts communication (Fig. 3-3). For example, a resident who has a hearing impairment may not understand when an NA is explaining a care procedure. These are some communication barriers and ways for nursing assistants to avoid them:

Resident does not hear NA, does not hear correctly, or does not understand. The NA should stand directly facing the resident. He should speak slowly and clearly. He should not shout, whisper, or mumble. The NA should speak in a low voice, using a pleasant tone. If the resident wears a hearing aid, the NA should check to ensure that it is on and is working properly.

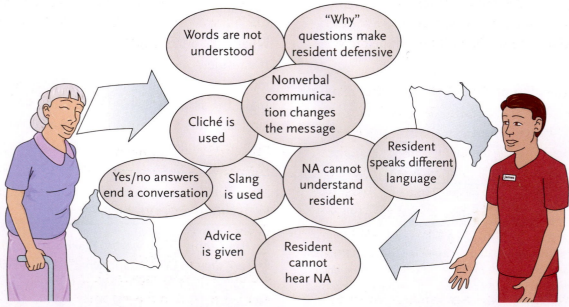

Fig. 3-3. Barriers to communication.

Resident is difficult to understand. The NA should be patient and take time to listen. He can ask the resident to repeat or explain the message, and then state the message in the NA's own words to make sure he has understood. *Reflecting* means an NA restates the words the resident uses to help ensure that they continue the conversation. *Rephrasing* means the NA paraphrases those words in order to show that he understands the resident.

NA, resident, or others use words that are not understood. An NA should not use medical terminology with residents or their families. He should speak in simple, everyday words and ask what a word means if he is not sure.

NA uses slang or profanity. The NA should avoid using slang words and expressions. These words are unprofessional and may not be understood. He should not use profanity, even if the resident does.

NA uses clichés. Clichés are phrases that are used repeatedly and do not really mean anything. For example, "Everything will be fine" is a cliché. Instead of using a cliché, the NA should listen to what a resident is really saying and respond with a meaningful message. For example, if a resident is afraid of having a bath, the NA can say, "I understand that it seems scary to you. What can I do to make you feel more at ease?" instead of saying, "Oh, it'll be over before you know it."

NA responds with "Why?" The NA should avoid asking "Why?" when a resident makes a statement. "Why" questions make people feel defensive. For example, a resident may say she does not want to go for a walk today. If the NA asks "Why not?" he may receive an angry response. Instead, he can ask "Are you too tired to take a walk? Is there something else you want to do?" The resident may then be willing to discuss the issue.

NA gives advice. The NA should not offer his opinion or give advice. Giving medical advice is not within an NA's scope of practice. It could be dangerous. Professionals with more education, such as doctors, give medical advice.

NA asks questions that only require yes/no answers. The NA should ask open-ended questions that need more than a "yes" or "no" answer. Yes and no answers end conversation. For example, if an NA wants to know what a resident likes to eat, she should not ask "Do you like vegetables?" Instead, she should ask "Which vegetables do you like best?"

Resident speaks a different language. If a resident's native language is not the same as the NA's, the NA should speak slowly and clearly. He should keep his messages short and simple. He should be alert for words the resident understands and also be alert for signs that the resident is only pretending to understand. He may need to use pictures or gestures to communicate. The NA can ask other staff members who speak the resident's language for help. The NA should be patient and calm.

NA or resident uses nonverbal communication. Nonverbal communication can change a message. The NA should be aware of his body language and gestures. He can look for nonverbal messages from residents and clarify them. For example, "Mr. Feldman, you say you're feeling fine but you seem to be in pain. Is that true? What can I do to help?"

4. List ways that cultures impact communication

The world is full of many different cultures. A **culture** is a set of learned beliefs, values, and behaviors shared by a social or ethnic group. People from different cultures communicate in diverse ways.

The use of eye contact varies from culture to culture. A person may feel it is important to look another person in the eye when speaking. She may view it as a sign of honesty or respect.

Communication Skills

Another person may think looking someone in the eye is rude or threatening. Part of providing person-centered care is learning about and respecting each resident's preferences.

As discussed earlier, touch is another important form of communication. Touch practices differ from one culture to another (Fig. 3-4). Preferences regarding touch may also just be a part of a person's personality. NAs must touch residents during daily care. However, if a resident is uncomfortable with touch, the NA should limit it when it is not necessary.

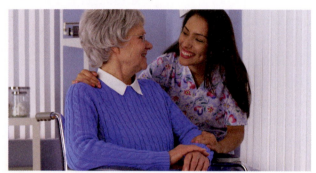

Fig. 3-4. How a person perceives touch may depend on her background.

Examples of acceptable or appropriate touch by an NA include the following:

- When providing personal care, such as bathing, dressing, feeding, and shaving

- Hugging a resident if the resident permits it or asks for it

- Holding a resident's hand when asked

Examples of unacceptable or inappropriate touch by an NA include the following:

- Sitting on a resident's lap or asking a resident to sit on the NA's lap

- Kissing a resident

- Hugging a resident who pulls away

- Rubbing against a resident or staff member or touching a person without consent

Language barriers can pose a problem when communicating. A resident's native language may be different than her nursing assistant's. One way to deal with this is to use a certified translator or interpreter. A translator is a person who speaks the resident's language and can translate words from another language to explain the message. A translator will make sure that residents can fully understand the information given to them. Picture cards and flash cards can also assist with communication.

NAs can also try to learn a few words or phrases in a resident's native language. A translator, or possibly a resident's family and friends, can help with that. A resident may be comforted by hearing a few words in her native language. When talking to another staff member in front of a resident, the NA should speak in a language that the resident understands.

5. Identify the people a nursing assistant communicates with in a facility

Nursing assistants communicate daily with many people in a facility. Some of these people are listed below.

Doctors, Nurses, Supervisors, Managers, and Other Staff Members

Nursing assistants communicate verbally and nonverbally with the care team. Charting information (manually or electronically) and using the telephone and call systems are other ways NAs communicate. NAs may also be involved in care planning. More information on each of these methods of communication is listed later in the chapter. It is important for NAs to be familiar with them, as they promote better communication with the care team.

Other Departments

Nursing assistants will communicate directly or via the phone with people in various departments, such as the dietary or housekeeping department. Maintaining a good relationship with other departments in a care facility helps promote organized care. Being positive when dealing with other departments, as well as keeping communication open and respectful, is important. Problems with other departments should be reported to the nurse.

Residents

Nursing assistants communicate with residents every day. The most important communication with residents occurs each time an NA greets them. At that time, the NA introduces herself and identifies the resident. She explains the care she will be providing and encourages the resident's participation. Facilities may use signs outside the door or photos to identify residents. Identifying residents before performing care is a vital part of promoting safety in the workplace. Explaining care before the NA gives it is an important part of person-centered care, as well as Residents' Rights.

Families and Visitors

The care team should strive to have a positive, open relationship with residents' families and friends (Fig. 3-5). One way to do this is to always respond immediately when a resident calls for help. This lets family and friends know that their loved ones are receiving proper care. Responding immediately to requests also helps prevent injury. Families are a rich source of information regarding residents' likes, dislikes, and histories. NAs can ask them about residents' preferences and experiences to help provide better care.

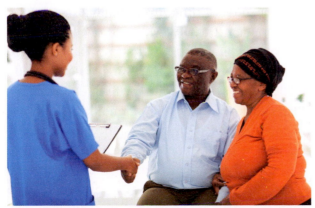

Fig. 3-5. Taking time to talk to residents' family members about residents' preferences, routines, and histories promotes better, person-centered care.

The Community

Staff may receive calls or visits from doctors' offices or clinics. An NA should refer any questions to her supervisor. She should keep all resident and staff information confidential unless she has been instructed otherwise.

6. Understand basic medical terminology and abbreviations

In order to communicate well with care team members, nursing assistants need to learn medical terminology. NAs will use medical terms for specific conditions. For example, **edema** is swelling in body tissues caused by excess fluid.

Medical terms are often made up of roots, prefixes, and suffixes. A **root** is the main part of the word that contains its basic meaning or definition. For example, the root *scope* means an instrument to look inside. The prefix *oto* means ear. An *otoscope* is an instrument used to examine the ear.

A **prefix** comes before the root to help form a new term. For example, the prefix *brady* means slow. The root *cardia* means heart. *Bradycardia* means slow heart rate or pulse.

A **suffix** is found at the end of a word and helps form a new word. By itself, a suffix does not form a full word. However, when a prefix or a root is added, the suffix turns it into a working medical term. For example, the suffix *meter* means measuring instrument. The prefix *thermo* means heat. A *thermometer* is an instrument that measures body temperature. One of the most common suffixes is *logy*, which means the study of something. It often refers to a medical specialty. For example, *cardiology* is the study of the heart.

When speaking with residents and their families, NAs should use simple, nonmedical terms. When speaking with the care team, using medical terms helps NAs give more complete information.

Abbreviations are another way to communicate more efficiently. For example, the abbreviation *prn* means *when necessary*. *Stat* means *immediately*. *BP* or *B/P* means *blood pressure*. Nursing assistants should learn the standard medical abbreviations their facility uses. They can use them to report information briefly and accurately. NAs may need to know these abbreviations to read assignments, care plans, or medical charts. If an abbreviation is unclear, an NA should always ask for clarification from a supervisor. A brief list of abbreviations follows. There is a more comprehensive list at the end of this textbook, but it is not a complete list. NAs should check with their facility about other abbreviations they must know.

Common Abbreviations

ADLs	activities of daily living
amb	ambulatory
BID, b.i.d.	two times a day
BM	bowel movement
BP, B/P	blood pressure
c̄	with
c/o	complains of
DNR	do not resuscitate
DX, dx	diagnosis
f/u, F/U	follow up
h, hr	hour
H₂O	water
I&O	intake and output
isol	isolation
IV	intravenous (within vein)
meds	medications
min	minute
mL	milliliter
NPO	nothing by mouth
p.c.	after meals
PPE	personal protective equipment

prn, PRN	as necessary
q̄	every
q.2h., q.3h., etc.	every 2 hours, every 3 hours, and so on
q.h., qh	every hour
ROM	range of motion
s̄	without
stat	immediately
T, temp	temperature
TID, t.i.d.	three times a day
TPR	temperature, pulse, and respiration
v.s., VS	vital signs
w/c, W/C	wheelchair

Residents' Rights

Using Medical Terminology

NAs should not use medical terminology when speaking to residents or their families or friends. Using medical terminology can prevent someone from understanding important information. Residents may act as if they understand even if they do not, which prevents the message from being communicated. When talking with residents, NAs should speak in simple, everyday language. They should speak in a language that residents understand.

7. Explain how to convert regular time to military time

NAs may need to document using the 24-hour clock, or military time (Fig. 3-6). Regular time uses numbers 1 through 12 to show each of the 24 hours in a day. In military time, the hours are numbered from 00 to 23. Midnight is expressed as 0000 (or 2400), 1:00 a.m. is 0100, 1:00 p.m. is 1300, and so on. Both regular and military time list minutes and seconds the same way. The minutes and seconds do not change when converting from regular to military time. The abbreviations a.m. and p.m. are used in regular time to indicate whether it is before noon or after noon. However, these are not used in military time, since specific numbers show each hour of the day.

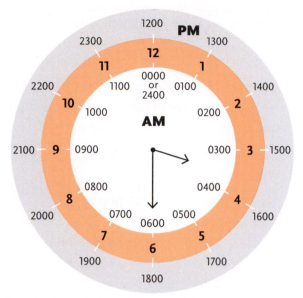

Fig. 3-6. Illustration showing the divisions in the 24-hour clock.

To change the hours between 1:00 p.m. to 11:59 p.m. to military time, add 12 to the regular time. For example, to change 4:00 p.m. to military time, add 4 + 12. The time is expressed as 1600 (sixteen hundred) hours. To change 1:42 p.m. to military time, add 1 + 12. The minutes do not change. The time is expressed as 1342 (thirteen forty-two) hours.

Midnight is the only time that differs. Midnight can be written as 0000, or it can be written as 2400. This follows the rule of adding 12 to the regular time. NAs should follow their facility's policy on how to express midnight.

To change from military time to regular time, subtract 12. The minutes do not change. For example, to change 1600 hours to standard time, subtract 12 from 16. The answer is 4:00 p.m. To change 2210 hours to standard time, subtract 12 from 22. The answer is 10:10 p.m.

Examples of the way the numbers are written follow:

Regular to Military
3:00 p.m. = 1500 (fifteen hundred hours)

Military to Regular
1115 = 11:15 a.m.

8. Describe a standard resident chart

The **medical chart**, or clinical or medical record, is the legal record of a resident's care. The chart is a legal document. What is included in the chart is considered to be what actually happened. This chart is saved as long as the law dictates that it be kept. It is saved in case other care providers need to refer to it. A provider may need medical history or information about an advance directive. Lawyers or judges may also request to see a chart if there is a legal need. The information found in the medical chart includes the following:

- Admission forms

- Resident's history and results of physical examinations

- Care plans

- Doctors' orders

- Doctors' progress notes

- Nursing assessments

- Nurses' notes

- Notes from physical therapists, occupational therapists, and other specialists

- Flow sheets (check-off sheets for documenting care; may also be called an *ADL sheet*)

- Graphic record

- Intake and output record

- Consent forms

- Lab and test results

- Surgery reports

- Advance directives

The NA's responsibility with regard to the resident's chart is to gather information and report it to the nurse. Noting observations about residents and their care is called **charting**. This information may be recorded in written format or by computer. More information about documentation is located in the next learning objective.

Some facilities allow nursing assistants to chart in a medical record. Others limit NAs' charting to certain forms. NAs should follow their facility's policies and remember that all of the information listed in a medical record is confidential.

Residents' Rights

Confidentiality

The observations NAs gather about residents are private information. They cannot be shared with anyone except specific members of the care team. Keeping resident information confidential is part of honoring dignity and being respectful. An NA can think about how she might feel if some of her private information, such as a health diagnosis or the state of her finances, was shared with others. And confidentiality is not only about promoting respect and dignity: keeping residents' information confidential is the law. All healthcare workers must obey it. More information on HIPAA is located in Chapter 2.

9. Explain guidelines for documentation

Nursing assistants chart, or document, all resident care that they provide. They also document their observations. It is very important to document accurately (Fig. 3-7). Documentation provides an up-to-date record of each resident's status and care. The medical chart is a legal document, and documentation is a legal record of all resident care. Documentation is also important for planning residents' care.

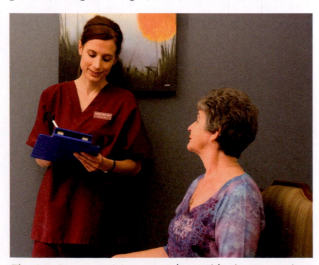

Fig. 3-7. Documenting accurately provides important information about residents to the care team.

Guidelines: Accurate Documentation

G Keep all information in the chart confidential.

G Document immediately after care is given. Record your notes carefully. Never record any care before it has been completed.

G Use black ink when documenting by hand. Write neatly.

G Sign each note you make in the chart. Sign your name and title, following facility policy. Use the correct date and time. Documentation done on a computer automatically enters the correct date and time.

G Use only facts, not opinions, when documenting. Document exactly what the person has said, or what you see, hear, smell, or touch. The words "seems," "appears to be," or "looks like" are not used in charting. For example, "The resident doesn't like the food here" is an opinion. "The resident refused her dinner tray, saying the food is too spicy" is a fact.

G If you make a mistake, draw one line through it. Write the correct information. Put your initials and the date and any other needed information, following facility policy (Fig. 3-8). Do not erase what you have written. Do not use correction fluid. Documentation done on a computer is time-stamped; it can only be changed by entering another notation.

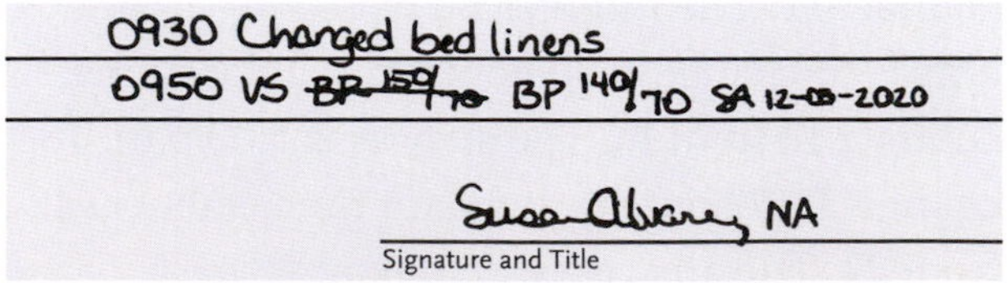

> 0930 Changed bed linens
> 0950 VS ~~BP 159/70~~ BP 140/70 SA 12-03-2020
>
> Susan Abrey, NA
> Signature and Title

Fig. 3-8. One example of how to correct a mistake.

G Use only your facility's accepted abbreviations and terms. A short list of abbreviations is located earlier in this chapter, and a longer list is located at the end of this book.

G Use comparisons to describe size instead of words like "large," "medium," or "small." For example, "There is a spot of blood on her bandage the size of a dime."

All facilities will have policies and procedures for documenting and NAs should follow them. Some facilities will require documentation on a "check-off" sheet. This is also called an *ADL* (activities of daily living) or *flow sheet* (Fig. 3-9). More about ADLs is located in Chapter 12.

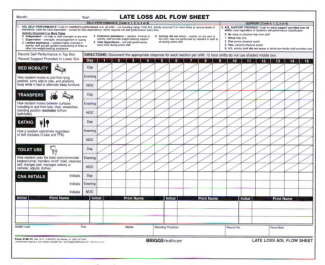

Fig. 3-9. *Some facilities use ADL flow sheets for documenting care.* (REPRINTED WITH PERMISSION OF BRIGGS HEALTHCARE®, 800.247.2343, BRIGGSHEALTHCARE.COM)

Tip

Abbreviations

Many abbreviations are derived from Latin. Here are a few examples:

et al. (Latin *et alia*): means *and other things*. Only *al* has a period at the end.

i.e. (Latin *id est*): means *that is*. Both letters have a period.

e.g. (Latin *exempli gratia*): means *for example*. Both letters have a period.

---

10. Describe the use of computers in documentation

Some care facilities require that computers be used to document information. Computers can easily store information that can be retrieved when it is needed. This is usually faster and more legible than writing by hand.

Some facilities have a computer in every resident's room. Staff input information each time they enter and leave the room. In other facilities, a computer or tablet is moved from room to room. Computer documentation replaces time-consuming paper charting, although some paperwork may still need to be done.

Facilities will train staff on computer use. Even when facilities require electronic/computer documentation, training often includes how to document by hand in case there is a system failure. Legal guidelines apply to both electronic and paper charts. Here are some general rules for electronic/computer documentation:

Guidelines: Electronic/Computer Documentation

G Do not share personal passwords or login IDs with anyone. Do not have a coworker enter information for you, even if it is more convenient.

G Be careful about who can see private or protected health information (PHI) or electronic health records (EHR) on the computer screen while you are working; HIPAA privacy guidelines apply to electronic documentation.

G Make sure you are logged into the correct resident's chart before beginning to document. Log out and/or exit the resident's chart when finished with documentation.

G If the computer software has an autofill feature (automatically completes certain fields that have been entered before), be sure that entries are accurate. Check your entries again before exiting the resident's chart.

G Change passwords when prompted.

G Do not print documents unless directed to do so, and shred documents as instructed.

G Do not send confidential information via email.

- **G** Exit the web browser when finished with charting or using the computer.
- **G** Do not access your personal accounts or browse the internet from work computers.

11. Explain the Minimum Data Set (MDS)

The **Minimum Data Set (MDS)** manual is an assessment tool developed by the federal government. It gives long-term care facilities a structured, standardized approach to care. The original edition was produced in 1990. The manual is revised periodically.

The MDS is a detailed form with guidelines for assessing residents. It also lists what to do if resident problems are identified. The manual provides examples and definitions to help nurses complete the assessments accurately (Fig. 3-10).

Resident ______ Identifier ______ Date ______

Section D Mood

D0100. Should Resident Mood Interview be Conducted? – Attempt to conduct interview with all residents

Enter Code
0. **No** (resident is rarely/never understood) → Skip to and complete D0500-D0600, Staff Assessment of Resident Mood (PHQ-9-OV)
1. **Yes** → Continue to D0200, Resident Mood Interview (PHQ-9©)

D0200. Resident Mood Interview (PHQ-9©) CAA

Say to resident: *"Over the last 2 weeks, have you been bothered by any of the following problems?"*

If symptom is present, enter 1 (yes) in column 1, Symptom Presence.
If yes in column 1, then ask the resident: *"About **how often** have you been bothered by this?"*
Read and show the resident a card with the symptom frequency choices. Indicate response in column 2, Symptom Frequency.

1. Symptom Presence
   0. **No** (enter 0 in column 2)
   1. **Yes** (enter 0-3 in column 2)
   9. **No response** (leave column 2 blank)
2. Symptom Frequency
   0. **Never or 1 day**
   1. **2-6 days** (several days)
   2. **7-11 days** (half or more of the days) 30.01
   3. **12-14 days** (nearly every day) 30.01

	1. Symptom Presence	2. Symptom Frequency
	↓ Enter Scores in Boxes ↓	
A. *Little interest or pleasure in doing things* 30.01	7 10	8
B. *Feeling down, depressed, or hopeless* 30.01		8
C. *Trouble falling or staying asleep, or sleeping too much*		8
D. *Feeling tired or having little energy*		8
E. *Poor appetite or overeating*		8
F. *Feeling bad about yourself – or that you are a failure or have let yourself or your family down*		8
G. *Trouble concentrating on things, such as reading the newspaper or watching television*		8
H. *Moving or speaking so slowly that other people could have noticed. Or the opposite – being so fidgety or restless that you have been moving around a lot more than usual*		8
I. *Thoughts that you would be better off dead, or of hurting yourself in some way*	8	8

D0300. Total Severity Score CAA

Enter Score
Add scores for all frequency responses in Column 2, Symptom Frequency. Total score must be between 00 and 27.
Enter 99 if unable to complete interview (i.e., Symptom Frequency is blank for 3 or more items). 00-27 = 8 3 10-27 = 30.01

D0350. Safety Notification – Complete only if D0200I1 = 1 indicating possibility of resident self harm

Enter Code
Was responsible staff or provider informed that there is a potential for resident self harm?
0. **No**
1. **Yes**

Copyright© Pfizer Inc. All rights reserved. Reproduced with permission.

7 Psychosocial Well-Being
8 Mood State
8 3 Mood State, 3 or More Items Trigger
10 Activities
30.01 Residents who have depressive symptoms

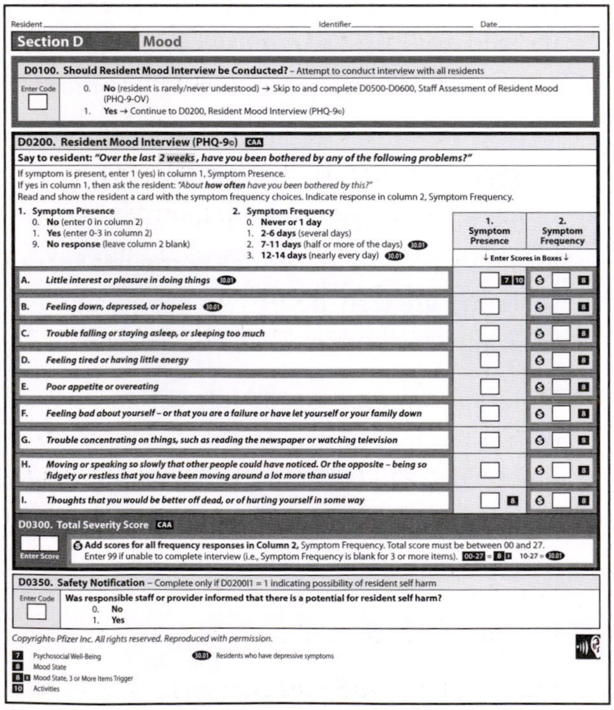

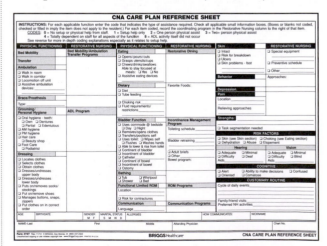

Fig. 3-10. *A sample MDS form.* (REPRINTED WITH PERMISSION OF BRIGGS HEALTHCARE®, 800.247.2343, BRIGGSHEALTHCARE.COM)

Nurses must complete the MDS for each resident within 14 days of admission and again each year. In addition, the MDS for each resident must be reviewed every three months. A new MDS is done when there is any significant change in a resident's condition.

The MDS helps the care team identify health problems. NAs should always report changes they notice to the nurse. Changes may be a sign of a problem or illness. The reporting an NA does may trigger a needed assessment.

12. Describe how to observe and report accurately

Nursing assistants spend more time with residents than other members of the care team. They may observe changes in residents that other team members have not noticed. Reporting these observations accurately is very important and is vital to the resident's care.

The resident's care is managed with a **care plan**, which is developed by a registered nurse, using data collected from the resident, his family, and care team members. Person-centered care places emphasizes the importance of the resident's input. The plan outlines the steps and tasks that the care team must perform to help the resident achieve his goals (Fig. 3-11). The care plan must be followed very carefully.

CNA CARE PLAN REFERENCE SHEET

INSTRUCTIONS: For each applicable function enter the code that indicates the type of assistance required. Check all applicable small information boxes. (Boxes or blanks not coded, checked or filled in imply the item does not apply to the resident.) For each item coded, record the coordinating program in the Restorative Nursing column to the right of that item.
CODES: **0** = No setup or physical help from staff. **1** = Setup help only **2** = One person physical assist **3** = Two+ person physical assist **4** = Totally dependent on staff for all aspects of the function **8** = ADL activity itself did not occur
See reverse for more in depth coding explanations especially as it relates to setup help.

PHYSICAL FUNCTIONING | RESTORATIVE NURSING
- Bed Mobility | Bed Mobility/Ambulation Transfer Programs
- Transfer
- Ambulation: ❑ Walk in room ❑ Walk in corridor ❑ Locomotion off unit ❑ Assistive ambulation devices: ______
- Brace/Prosthesis — Type: ______
- Grooming/Personal Hygiene | ADL Program: ❑ Oral hygiene - teeth: ❑ Own ❑ Dentures ❑ Partial ❑ Edentulous ❑ AM hygiene ❑ PM hygiene ❑ Hair care ❑ Beauty shop ❑ Foot Care ❑ Podiatrist
- Dressing: ❑ Locates clothes ❑ Selects clothes ❑ Obtain clothes ❑ Dresses/undresses upper body ❑ Dresses/undresses lower body ❑ Puts on/removes socks/stockings ❑ Put on/remove shoes ❑ Manages buttons, snaps, zippers ❑ Put clothes on in correct order

PHYSICAL FUNCTIONING | RESTORATIVE NURSING
- Eating: ❑ Opens/pours/cuts ❑ Grasps utensils/cups ❑ Chews/drinks/swallows — Able to stay focused at meals: ❑ Yes ❑ No ❑ Assistive eating devices | Restorative Dining
- Dietary: ❑ Diet ______ ❑ Tube feeding ______ ❑ Choking risk ______ ❑ Fluid requirements/restrictions ______ | Favorite Foods:
- Bladder Function: ❑ Uses commode @ bedside ❑ Day ❑ Night ❑ Removes/opens clothes ❑ Transfers/positions self ❑ Uses toilet: ❑ Wipes self ❑ Flushes ❑ Washes hands ❑ Able to lower & rise from toilet ❑ Continent of bladder ❑ Incontinent of bladder ❑ Catheter ______ ❑ Continent of bowel ❑ Incontinent of bowel ❑ Ostomy | Incontinence Management Program: Toileting schedule ______ Bladder retraining ______ ❑ Adult briefs ❑ Other ______ Bowel program:
- Bathing: ❑ Tub ❑ Whirlpool ❑ Shower ❑ Bed
- Functional Limited ROM: Location ______ ❑ Risk for contractures | ROM Programs
- Communication: Language ______ | Communication Programs

Skin: ❑ Intact ❑ Risk for breakdown ❑ Ulcers ❑ Skin problems - foot | RESTORATIVE NURSING: ❑ Special equipment ❑ Preventive schedule ❑ Other ______
Behavior | Approaches:
Depression
Pain: Location ______ Relieving approaches
Strengths: ______ ❑ Task segmentation needed

RISK FACTORS: ❑ Skin (see Skin section) ❑ Choking (see Eating section) ❑ Dehydration ❑ Abuse ❑ Elopement
Hearing: ❑ Adequate ❑ Minimal ❑ Difficulty ❑ Deaf Aids ______
Vision: ❑ Adequate ❑ Minimal ❑ Difficulty ❑ Blind Aids ______
COGNITIVE: ❑ Alert ❑ Ability to make decisions ❑ Confused ❑ Oriented ❑ Comatose
CUSTOMARY ROUTINE: Cycle of daily events ______ Family/friend visits ______ Preferred NH activities ______

AGE | BIRTHDATE | GENDER M F | MARITAL STATUS S M W D | ALLERGIES | HOW COMMUNICATES: | NICKNAME
NAME–Last | First | Middle | Attending Physician | Chart No.

BRIGGS Healthcare — CNA CARE PLAN REFERENCE SHEET

Fig. 3-11. *A sample resident care plan.* (REPRINTED WITH PERMISSION OF BRIGGS HEALTHCARE®, 800.247.2343, BRIGGSHEALTHCARE.COM)

In order to plan care, nurses collect information from staff. Nursing assistants report signs and symptoms that they observe. This information will be either objective or subjective.

Objective information is information based on what a person sees, hears, touches, or smells. It is collected using four of the five senses: sight, hearing, smell, and touch. It is also called *signs*. **Subjective information** is information collected from something that residents or their families reported, and it may or may not be true. It is also called *symptoms*. Subjective information is something a person cannot or did not observe. This is information the subject is relaying, so it is an opinion. Objective information may confirm subjective information.

An example of objective information is "Mr. Hartman is rubbing his temples and holding his head." A subjective report of the same situation might be, "Mr. Hartman says he has a headache." Both objective and subjective reports are valuable.

In order to report accurately, NAs must observe residents accurately. They should use medical terminology when making and recording observations. To observe accurately, they need to use as many senses as possible to gather information (Fig. 3-12). Some examples follow:

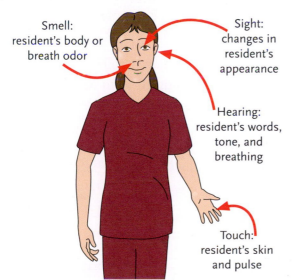

Smell: resident's body or breath odor

Sight: changes in resident's appearance

Hearing: resident's words, tone, and breathing

Touch: resident's skin and pulse

Fig. 3-12. Reporting what you observe means using four of your senses.

Sight: The NA should look for changes in the resident's appearance, such as redness, swelling, rashes, discharge, changes in the eyes or ears, and changes in mobility.

Hearing: The NA should listen to what the resident says. Is the resident making sense? Is his breathing normal? Does he cough, groan, or cry? Does he appear to be angry or sad?

Smell: Are there any odors coming from the resident's body? Odors can indicate infection, a need for bathing, incontinence, or poor mouth care.

Touch: Does the resident's skin feel hot or cool, moist or dry?

Observing and Reporting: The Resident

O/R Note any change in orientation. **Orientation** is a person's awareness of person, place, and time. Does the resident know who he is, who you are, where he is, and what year it is?

O/R Check to see if the resident's vital signs are normal or abnormal. **Vital signs** are the measurements—temperature, pulse, respirations, and blood pressure—that monitor the functioning of the vital organs of the body. (Vital signs will be covered in depth in Chapter 13.)

O/R Report any change in ability. Has there been a change in the resident's ability to move any part of her body? Can the resident perform all of the activities today that she could yesterday? Are the resident's senses of sight, hearing, smell, touch, and taste the same today?

O/R Report other important changes, such as changes in weight or overall appetite, changes in ability to urinate or have a bowel movement, and changes in mood.

Accurate documentation and prompt reporting are important to residents' well-being. Determining what to report immediately to the nurse and what can wait until later involves critical thinking. Nursing assistants do not try to solve problems or make decisions about a resident's health. This is the nurse's or doctor's role. However, while working, NAs must determine whether any information they collect regarding residents could mean a problem is developing or has already occurred. For nursing assistants, **critical thinking** means making careful observations, evaluating resident information, and immediately reporting all potential problems. Reporting these types of changes in a resident's condition may lead to the quick diagnosis and treatment of a potentially serious problem.

Signs and symptoms that should be reported will be discussed throughout this book. In addition, anything that endangers residents should be reported immediately, including the following:

- Falls
- Wheezing
- Difficulty breathing
- Chest pain or pressure
- Pain in calf or leg
- Blurred vision
- Slurred speech
- Vomiting
- Sudden limp or change in ability to walk
- Numbness or loss of feeling in one side of the body or in arms or legs
- Abdominal pain
- Change in vital signs
- Sudden or severe headache
- Change in mental status, such as confusion or disorientation

Sometimes a nurse will ask a nursing assistant to report every change in a resident, no matter what the change is. If this is the case, the NA will report each change as it happens.

13. Explain the nursing process

To communicate with other care team members, nurses use the **nursing process**. This is an organized method used by registered nurses to determine residents' needs, plan the appropriate care to meet those needs, and evaluate how well the plan of care is working. The process has five steps:

- **Assessment**: getting information from many sources, including medical history and physical assessment, and reviewing this information; the purpose is to identify actual or potential problems

- **Diagnosis**: identifying health problems after looking at all the resident's needs; completed to create a care plan

- **Planning**: setting goals and creating a care plan in accordance with the resident's and/or the family's preferences to meet the resident's needs

- **Implementation**: putting the care plan into action; giving care

- **Evaluation**: examining carefully to see if goals were met or progress was achieved; if progress is slow or if the problem worsened, the care plan must be changed

The nursing process allows for constant adjustment as new information is collected. Clear communication among all team members and the resident is vital to ensure the success of the process. The nursing assistant's accurate observations and reports are an important part of planning and evaluating care.

14. Discuss the nursing assistant's role in care planning and at care conferences

Nursing assistants have an important role in care planning. Care plans are prepared from the observations of staff caring for the resident. At care planning meetings, NAs should not be afraid to share their observations; they can speak to the nurse before the meeting to determine what is important to share.

Care plans may be written at a special care conference. The **care conference** is a meeting to share and gather information. This is done in order to develop care plans for residents. Care team members attend to share information used to create or add to the care plan. Residents and their families and friends may also attend the care conference. Members of the community, such as ombudsmen, sometimes share helpful information too. Care plans are kept at the nurse's station or near the resident's room.

HIPAA privacy guidelines apply to care plans. Team members should not share a resident's information with anyone not directly involved with the resident's care.

15. Describe incident reporting and recording

An **incident** is an accident, problem, or unexpected event during the course of care. It is something that is not part of the normal routine. A mistake in care, such as feeding the resident from the wrong meal tray, is an incident. A resident fall or injury is another type of incident. Accusations made by residents against staff, as well as employee injuries, are other types of incidents.

State and federal guidelines require that incidents be recorded in an incident report (Fig. 3-13). An **incident report** (also called an *occurrence, accident, accident/incident,* or *event report*) is a report that documents the incident and the response to it. This report is a factual, objective account of what happened. The information in an incident report is confidential and is intended for internal use to help prevent future incidents. When documenting incidents, NAs should complete the report as soon as possible and give it to

the charge nurse. This is important so that they do not forget any details.

An NA must always complete an incident report if she is injured in any way, no matter how slightly, while on the job. This protects the NA and identifies that the injury occurred at work. Nurses may add information to an incident report. The nurse will complete these reports for any accident or injury to residents or visitors. The NA may be asked to add information regarding residents or visitors. When completing an incident report, the NA should do the following:

- Include exactly what she saw

- State the time and the mental and physical condition of the person

- Describe the person's reaction to the incident

- State the facts; the NA should not give her opinion

- Not include "Incident report filed" in the resident's medical record

- Not make any photocopies of the incident report

Tip

Incident Reports

A nursing assistant should not let anyone try to talk her out of completing an incident report. It is important to have these reports on file. Reporting and documenting incidents are done to protect everyone involved. The NA should complete the report the same day the incident occurs, as soon as possible.

Tip

Sentinel Event

A **sentinel event**, or **adverse event**, is an unexpected event that causes serious injury or death. A *sentinel* is a guard who stands watch, and the phrase *sentinel event* is used to emphasize the need for immediate investigation and response. An example of this type of event is a medication error that results in a resident's death. A sentinel event is required to be reported to the proper agency.

INCIDENT/ACCIDENT REPORT

PERSON INVOLVED	(Last name)	(First name)	(Middle initial)	○ Adult ○ Child	○ Male ○ Female	Age_____

Date of incident/accident	Time of incident/accident ○ AM ○ PM	Exact location of incident/accident ○ Resident's room (No._____)	○ Dining Area ○ Hallway ○ Bathroom ○ Other Specify_____

○ RESIDENT
Record diagnosis if contributed to incident/accident:

Resident's condition before incident/accident ○ Normal ○ Confused ○ Disoriented
☐ Sedated (Medication_____ Dose_____ Time of most recent dose_____ ○ AM ○ PM Other (Specify)_____

Were bed rails ordered? ○ No ○ Yes	Were bed rails present? ○ No ○ Yes	If Yes, were bed rails ○ Up ○ Down	Was height of bed adjustable? ○ No ○ Yes	If Yes, was bed ○ Up ○ Down

Was a restraint in use at time of incident/accident? ○ No ○ Yes
☐ Physical restraint Type_____ ☐ Chemical restraint Specify_____

○ EMPLOYEE	Department	Job title	Length of time in this position

○ VISITOR ○ OTHER _____	Home address	Home phone: Cell phone:
	Occupation	Reason for presence at this facility

☐ Equipment involved Describe:_____
☐ Property involved Describe:_____

Was person authorized to be at location of incident/accident? No ○ Yes ○

Describe exactly what happened, why it happened and what the cause was, if known. If injured, record part of body injured. If property or equipment damaged, describe damage.

Indicate location of injury on diagrams below:

Temp._____ Pulse_____ Resp._____
B/P_____

TYPE OF INJURY
1. None apparent ☐
2. Abrasion ☐
3. Skin tear ☐
4. Laceration ☐
5. Hematoma ☐
6. Swelling ☐
7. Burn ☐
8. Sprain ☐
9. Fracture ☐
10. Other (specify below) ☐

_____

LEVEL OF CONSCIOUSNESS

Name of Physician notified	Time of notification ○ AM ○ PM	Time Physician responded ○ AM ○ PM
Name and relationship of family member/resident representative notified	Time of notification ○ AM ○ PM	Time responded ○ AM ○ PM

Was person involved seen by a physician? No ○ Yes ○ Physician's name	If No, why not?	Where	Date	Time ○ AM ○ PM
Was first aid needed? No ○ Yes ○ If needed, type of care provided	By whom?	Where	Date	Time ○ AM ○ PM
Was person involved taken to a hospital? No ○ Yes ○ If Yes, hospital name	By whom?	Manner of transport	Date	Time ○ AM ○ PM

Name, title (if applicable), address & phone number of witness(es)	Additional comments and/or steps taken to prevent recurrence

SIGNATURE/TITLE/DATE	**SIGNATURE/TITLE/DATE**
Person Preparing Report	Medical Director
Director of Nursing/Health Services	Administrator/Manager

Form 3322/2R Rev. 2/18 © 1991 BRIGGS, Des Moines, IA (800) 247-2343
Unauthorized copying or use violates copyright law. www.BriggsHealthcare.com

BRIGGS Healthcare®

INCIDENT/ACCIDENT REPORT

Fig. 3-13. *A sample incident report.* (REPRINTED WITH PERMISSION OF BRIGGS HEALTHCARE®, 800.247.2343, BRIGGSHEALTHCARE.COM)

16. Explain proper telephone etiquette

When nursing assistants use the telephone during their shifts, whether making or answering a call, they are representing their facility to the community. It is important that they follow rules for proper telephone etiquette.

Guidelines: Telephone Communication

G When greeting a caller, cheerfully say "Good morning," "Good afternoon," or "Good evening."

G Identify your facility: "Evergreen Facility."

G Identify yourself and your position: "Deserae Jenkins, Nursing Assistant."

G Listen closely to the caller's request. Write down messages. Ask for the correct spelling of names. In emergencies, take appropriate action immediately.

G Get a telephone number if needed.

G Say "Thank you" and "Goodbye."

G Do not give out any information about staff or residents over the phone. For example, if someone calls and asks if a specific person works at the facility, respond with "Please hold and I will get my supervisor to help you." Employers may have this policy to protect employees who may be victims of domestic violence or stalking. Creditors may also call looking for people who owe them money. People may call to ask about a resident's condition. Remember that all resident information is confidential. This type of call should also be referred to a supervisor.

G Place a caller on hold if you need to get someone to take the call. Ask the caller if she can hold first. You may have to transfer a call. Ask for help and training on transferring calls if you need it.

G Follow your facility's policy on personal phone calls and cell phone use.

17. Describe the resident call system

Residents signal staff that they need them by using the facility call system. Other terms for this system are *call light* or *signal light*. This system allows residents to call for help when needed by relaying a notification to a central work station or directly to a staff member (Fig. 3-14). Nursing assistants must think of this system as a resident's lifeline. A lifeline is something that connects a person to help when it is needed; it can literally save someone's life. NAs should always respond to call lights promptly, even for residents who are not assigned to them. NAs should not ignore call lights. Ignoring a call light can be considered abusive or neglectful behavior. The call light should always be left within the resident's reach before the NA leaves the resident's room.

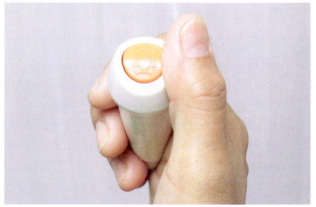

Fig. 3-14. Call lights allow residents to signal staff when needed. Other types of call systems are available for residents who are not able to push buttons. Nursing assistants must always respond to call lights promptly.

18. Describe the nursing assistant's role in change-of-shift reports and rounds

There are two types of shift reports: a start-of-shift report and an end-of-shift report. Nursing assistants usually are asked to attend start-of-shift reports. This is when the care team gathers to discuss and plan a resident's care for a shift. Nurses are present for both types of reports. Shift length varies by facility; a shift may be 8, 10, or 12 hours long.

Guidelines: Shift Reports

For start-of-shift reports

G   Arrive on time.

G   Each staff member is given his assignment for the shift. This assignment lists each resident and the staff member who will be responsible for that resident during that shift. Every resident, however, is considered every NA's responsibility. This means you must respond to any resident who needs your help. Listen for important information about all of the residents in your area.

G   The staff listens to a nurse from the prior shift who reports on the care of each resident. Examples of information passed to the next shift are falls that occurred, appetite problems, difficulties with urination, complaints of pain, or changes in the ability to move. Listen carefully to this information.

G   The nurses give special instructions to the other staff members who will be providing resident care. Ask any questions you have. Special information shared during a report may include new admissions and transfers or discharges from the facility.

For end-of-shift reports

G   Report resident information to the nurses before the end-of-shift report. Examples are changes in pulse or temperature and skin changes that could signal the start of a pressure injury. Nurses will share this information with the staff for the next shift.

Some facilities use a method of reporting called **rounds**. Staff members make scheduled visits to each resident's room to assess the resident's condition and needs and to discuss the care plan. A nursing assistant may be involved in rounds at his facility. If so, he should listen closely and take notes. He can also share information about residents to staff, but should keep his voice low when doing so.

The Handoff Transfer Process

A handoff is the transfer of a resident and all of the care responsibilities for that resident to another caregiver or team of caregivers. A handoff also involves the acceptance of that resident by the receiving caregiver or team. The goal is an effective transfer of the resident's care and the thorough transmission of resident information. The handoff process involves senders and receivers. Senders are caregivers transferring care of the resident, and receivers are caregivers accepting the care of the resident. The Joint Commission works to improve handoff communication in order to provide safer, higher quality care. Periodic updates are released with new recommendations to improve the handoff communication process.

19. List the information found on an assignment sheet

An assignment sheet lists residents and all of the tasks that must be done for them. Certain tasks are done daily. These daily tasks are called *activities of daily living* (*ADLs*). Range of motion (ROM) exercises may be listed on the sheet. These are exercises done to bring joints through a full range of movement. A resident's **code status** tells the staff the type and scope of care that should be provided in the event of a cardiac arrest, other catastrophic organ failure, or terminal illness. In health care, a **code** is an emergent medical situation in which specially trained responders provide the necessary care. An assignment sheet contains the following information:

•   The resident's name and room number

•   The medical diagnosis

•   Code status

•   Activity level/transfer status

•   Range of motion (ROM) exercises

•   Bathing information

•   Diet orders

•   Fluid orders

•   Bowel and bladder information

- How often to measure vital signs

- Treatments to be performed

- Special tests and other procedures to be performed

> **Tip**
>
> **NAs Must Show Up**
>
> Assignments are based on the number of residents and the number of staff members available on that shift. It is important for NAs to work every day they are scheduled. Missing a day can compromise both residents' and staff members' safety.
>
> If an NA is sick, she should call her supervisor to discuss taking a day off, as she could transmit her illness to others. Illnesses can be more serious for elderly people.
>
> If an NA must be absent, she should call her facility as early as possible to let the charge nurse know. This may make it easier for the supervisor to find someone else to work that shift.

20. Discuss how to organize work and manage time

Following the start-of-shift report, nursing assistants begin their day of caring for residents. Staff members have duties to complete at certain times of the day. In order to complete assignments properly each day, NAs must learn to organize their work. Here is an example of how a work day might be organized:

After receiving her assignment, the NA can make rounds on all of her residents. She can check to see if any residents require immediate help or care. If residents have their call lights within reach and do not need immediate help, anything important related to their care needs should be listed on the assignment sheet. Any needed reminders can be listed on a notepad. For example, the NA can list special tests a resident needs. She can ask the nurse if there are any special orders that need to be added to the resident's plan of care. When the NA feels she has all of the necessary information, she can decide which resident she will care for first.

Here are some other basic tips for organization and time management:

Plan ahead. It is important to list everything that needs to be done, including special tasks. NAs must take the time to check to see if they have all the supplies needed for a procedure. Often just making the list and rechecking it will help a caregiver feel more prepared.

Prioritize. An NA should identify the most important things to get done and do those first.

Make a schedule. Many people find it useful to write out the hours of the day and fill in what needs to be done and when. This allows for a more realistic schedule.

Combine activities. NAs can talk with residents while providing care, which combines two important tasks. It is important to work more efficiently whenever possible.

Get help. It is a simple reality that it is not possible for a nursing assistant to do everything. Sometimes an NA will need help to ensure a resident's safety, and she should not be afraid to ask for help. If an assignment cannot be completed, the NA should notify the nurse.

Each facility will have its own schedule of events and care. Duties at the beginning of a shift include setting up residents for mealtime, bathing residents, and measuring residents' vital signs. During a shift, duties may include measuring vital signs, helping with elimination and other personal care tasks, and responding to resident requests. End-of-shift tasks may include measuring vital signs and giving reports on residents.

These are only a few of the duties an NA may have on a given day. Many things can happen to affect the work day. Adapting quickly to changing situations will help things run more smoothly. A new resident, a staff member going home, or a resident transferring to a hospital are some things that can change the plans for the day.

Tip

Organizing Work

It is important for nursing assistants to prioritize and organize their work every day. Many methods can help with this, including listing items in a small notebook. Careful organization helps ensure tasks are completed efficiently.

Chapter Review

1. What is the difference between verbal and nonverbal communication (LO 2)?

2. Why should a nursing assistant avoid asking yes or no questions (LO 3)?

3. A resident tells a nursing assistant that he is scared of a medical test that is going to be performed. How could the NA respond without using a cliché such as "Oh, everything will be fine" (LO 3)?

4. What can help an NA overcome a language barrier with a resident (LO 4)?

5. What should an NA do each time he greets a resident (LO 5)?

6. Convert 8:33 p.m. to military time (LO 7).

7. Convert 11:10 a.m. to military time (LO 7).

8. With whom can a nursing assistant's observations about residents be shared (LO 8)?

9. When should care be documented (LO 9)?

10. Do HIPAA guidelines apply to computer use (LO 10)?

11. How does a nursing assistant's reporting impact a resident's Minimum Data Set (MDS) assessment (LO 11)?

12. List the four senses that are used in accurate observing and reporting (LO 12).

13. What is an incident (LO 15)?

14. When should an incident report be completed (LO 15)?

15. Give an example of a proper greeting when answering the phone (LO 16).

16. Describe the NA's role in rounds at a facility (LO 18).

17. Give an example of how to combine activities to manage time better (LO 20).

Short Answer

For each of the following five statements, decide whether it is an objective sign or subjective symptom observation. Write S for subjective or O for objective (LO 12).

18. Resident says she has a sore throat. ___

19. Resident has dark red urine. ___

20. Resident states, "I have a hard time catching my breath." ___

21. Resident is running a fever. ___

22. Resident has blisters on her feet. ___

Multiple Choice

23. Which of the following is the correct abbreviation for *nothing by mouth* (LO 6)?
    (A) NBM
    (B) NPO
    (C) ZVM
    (D) NFF

24. What does the abbreviation *PRN* stand for (LO 6)?
    (A) Every hour
    (B) When needed
    (C) Two times per day
    (D) Immediately

25. How does a nursing assistant contribute to care planning (LO 14)?
    (A) By giving her suggestions regarding medication changes
    (B) By diagnosing the resident's current condition
    (C) By sharing her observations of residents
    (D) By demonstrating the types of treatment she gives to the resident for the resident's family

26. Where should the call light be left when a nursing assistant leaves a resident's room (LO 17)?
    (A) By the door leading to the hallway
    (B) Next to the toilet in the bathroom
    (C) On the resident's windowsill
    (D) Within the resident's reach

27. Which of the following is typically found on an assignment sheet (LO 19)?
    (A) Resident's last known address
    (B) Resident's television preferences
    (C) Names of the resident's closest living relatives
    (D) Resident's diet order

4
Communication Challenges

The Navajo Code Talkers

During World War II, the Japanese were able to break almost any American military code. So in 1942, a young Navajo man approached top-ranking US military officials with the idea of using the Navajo language as a code. He believed the code would help communicate military messages securely. Many Native Americans, including some teenagers, became Marines and went to work as "Code Talkers." They used a form of the Navajo language to send top-secret messages during the war. In 1943, there were about 200 Navajo Code Talkers, and ultimately, around 400 Code Talkers were sent to the Pacific to serve in World War II. The code was never broken. The Navajo Code Talk remained classified information until 1968. The Navajo Code Talkers played a vital role in the victory of the United States in World War II, and some have since been awarded Congressional Medals. August 14 has been designated as "National Navajo Code Talker Day." Memorials have been built to honor the Navajo Code Talkers.

"A wise old owl sat on an oak,
The more he saw the less he spoke;
The less he spoke the more he heard;
Why aren't we like that wise old bird?"

Edward Hersey Richards, 1874–1957

"The important thing is to not stop questioning."

Albert Einstein, 1879–1955

1. Define important words in this chapter

airway: the natural passageway for air to enter into the lungs.

anxiety: unease or worry, often about a situation or condition.

artificial airway: any tube inserted into the respiratory tract for the purpose of maintaining an airway and facilitating ventilation.

coma: state of unconsciousness in which a person is unable to respond to any change in the environment, including pain.

combative: violent or hostile.

confusion: the inability to think clearly and logically.

defense mechanisms: unconscious behaviors used to release tension and/or help a person cope with stress.

disorientation: confusion about person, place, or time; may be permanent or temporary.

dyspnea: difficulty breathing.

impairment: a partial or complete loss of function or ability.

major depressive disorder: an illness that causes social withdrawal, lack of energy, and loss of interest in activities, as well as other symptoms.

masturbation: to touch or rub sexual organs in order to give oneself or another person sexual pleasure.

tracheostomy: a surgically-created opening through the neck into the trachea.

ventilation: in medicine, the exchange of air between the lungs and the environment.

2. Identify communication guidelines for visual impairment

An **impairment** is a partial or complete loss of function or ability. Some residents for whom nursing assistants care have a visual impairment. Several diseases can cause visual impairment or blindness. Glaucoma and diabetes are two examples. More information about these diseases may be found in Chapters 22 and 23. A visual impairment is also something that can exist at birth. People of all ages can be visually impaired, and one or both eyes can be affected.

Guidelines: Visual Impairment

G   Knock on the door, announce yourself, and greet the resident as soon as you enter the room. Do not touch the resident before you have identified yourself. Explain why you are there and what you plan to do.

G   Face the resident the entire time you are speaking with him. Keep talking to him while giving care.

G   Make sure there is proper lighting in the room.

G   Do not shout.

G   Use the face of an imaginary clock as a guide to explain the position of objects. If you are taking the resident to a new area, orient him to the room. For example, "There is a table with four chairs around it at 3 o'clock. There is a sofa at 7 o'clock." Describe the things you see around you. Try not to use words such as "see," "look," and "watch."

G   If the resident wears eyeglasses, make sure they are on. Check to see that the eyeglasses are clean, fit properly, and are in good condition (Fig. 4-1). If they are damaged or do not fit well, report it to the nurse.

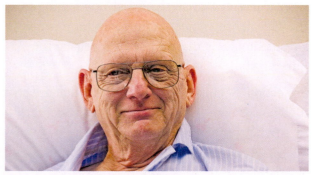

Fig. 4-1. Eyeglasses must fit properly, be clean, and be in good condition.

G   Vision loss can cause falls. Do not move personal items or furniture. Put everything back where you found it.

G   Read menus to the resident if needed.

G   Encourage the resident to use his other senses, such as smell, touch, and hearing.

G   Let the resident know when you are leaving the room or area.

G   If a resident has a guide dog, do not play with, distract, or feed the dog.

G   There are many helpful items for people with visual impairments. Audiobooks, large-print books, digital books, and large clocks are examples. Offer them when available.

G   Be empathetic. Try to imagine what it feels like to not be able to see or see well.

3. Identify communication guidelines for hearing impairment

There are different types of hearing loss. A person may have been born with an impairment or may have lost his hearing gradually. He may have a partial loss in one ear or may be completely unable to hear anything. Some hearing loss is temporary, such as that caused by sinus congestion or wax buildup.

Most hearing loss occurs gradually. The person will notice changes over time. The following list shows some symptoms of hearing loss that should be reported to the nurse.

Observing and Reporting: Hearing Loss

O/R   Trouble hearing high-pitched noises

O/R   Trouble hearing soft consonants, such as "s" and "t"

O/R   Trouble hearing what is said in a setting that has background noise

O/R   Not understanding the meaning of words

O/R   Being unable to hear people when they are not in the same room

O/R Favoring one ear over the other one

O/R Avoiding movies or special events due to difficulty hearing the dialogue

O/R Complaining of ringing in the ears

O/R Complaining of pain in one or both ears

Guidelines: Hearing Impairment

G Get the resident's attention before speaking. Do not approach her from behind, as she may not hear you come in. Walk in front of her or touch her lightly on the arm to let her know you are near.

G Stand or sit so that the resident can see your face. Make sure there is proper lighting in the room. The light should be on your face, not on the resident's face (Fig. 4-2).

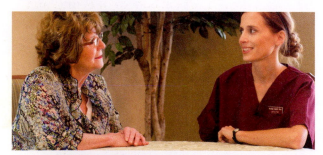

Fig. 4-2. When communicating with a resident who has a hearing impairment, the nursing assistant should speak face-to-face in good light.

G Look directly at the resident while speaking. A resident who has a hearing impairment may read lips.

G If the resident uses a hearing aid, make sure the resident is wearing it and it is turned on (Fig. 4-3). More information on hearing aids is in Chapter 22.

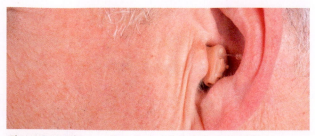

Fig. 4-3. Make sure hearing aids are worn and are turned on.

G Turn off televisions or radios.

G Speak clearly and do not shout. If the person favors one ear, speak to that side.

G Lower the pitch of your voice.

G Do not chew gum, eat, or cover your mouth with your hand while speaking.

G Do not exaggerate pronunciation of words or mouth the words in an exaggerated way.

G Use simple words and short sentences.

G Use pen and paper or picture cards when needed.

4. Explain defense mechanisms as methods of coping with stress

Communicating with residents who are under stress requires empathy and sensitivity. Words must be carefully chosen. Residents who are stressed may use defense mechanisms. **Defense mechanisms** are unconscious behaviors used to release tension and/or help a person cope with stress. They help to block uncomfortable or unpleasant feelings that may cause anxiety.

Defense mechanisms prevent a person from facing the real reason a situation has occurred. Overuse of these mechanisms keeps a person from understanding his emotional issues and actions. They include the following:

Denial: Blocking reality; rejecting the thought or feeling—for example, a resident refuses to believe his diagnosis of cancer.

Displacement: Transferring a strong feeling to a less threatening object or person—for example, a resident who is mad at her aunt yells at the nursing staff.

Projection: Seeing feelings in others that are actually one's own—for example, a staff member says that a resident does not like her.

Rationalization: Making excuses to justify something—for example, an elderly man fails a driving test and says the test was "unfair."

Repression: Blocking painful events or feelings from the mind—for example, not remembering a traumatic experience.

Regression: Going back to behavior from the past for comfort—for example, a resident who is stressed starts to rock back and forth.

5. List communication guidelines for anxiety

Anxiety is unease or worry, often about a situation or condition. It can be a response to an environmental stimulus or an internal stimulus. However, a person may not always know why she feels anxious. Anxiety is a vague emotional state. The feelings may be caused by uncertainty or concern about something or a future event. Feeling anxious is not the same as feeling afraid. When a person is fearful, she is dealing with a specific and immediate danger.

Anxiety causes physical symptoms such as nausea, shaking, sweating, chest pain, and rapid heartbeat. When communicating with a person who is anxious, it is important to try to reduce anxiety and stress.

Guidelines: Anxiety

G Knock on the door, announce yourself, and greet the resident as soon as you enter the room. Do not touch the resident before you have identified yourself. Use touch only if it does not upset him.

G Speak softly. Reduce the noise level.

G Speak slowly and calmly.

G Listen to the resident. Be patient. Ask gentle questions to try to identify the cause of the anxiety.

G Be empathetic. Be calm and reassuring.

G Avoid demanding behavior.

More information on anxiety disorders may be found in Chapter 22.

6. Discuss communication guidelines for depression

Major depressive disorder, also called *clinical depression*, is a type of mental health disorder that causes withdrawal, lack of energy, and loss of interest in activities, as well as other symptoms. It can be managed or even cured. There are different types and degrees of depression, and more information is located in Chapter 22.

Residents who have recently moved into a facility may be depressed. They have experienced significant changes and losses, such as the loss of a spouse or friend. They may also be dealing with the loss of health, independence, mobility, and the ability to care for themselves.

Residents may have moved out of their familiar homes and into a facility full of strangers. Their family and friends may not be able to visit. Residents will probably have to share a room with a new person, possibly for the first time in their lives. One of these factors can be enough to make a person depressed. However, residents may have to deal with all of these problems at the same time. It is not surprising that some become depressed.

Major depressive disorder is not something people can overcome by choosing to be well. It is a disorder like any other disorder. The nursing assistant's role is to be supportive and compassionate. The NA should try to make each day as pleasant an experience as possible for residents.

Guidelines: Major Depressive Disorder

G Be pleasant, respectful, and supportive.

G Use touch if it helps comfort the resident.

G Sit down and listen carefully. Lean forward and maintain eye contact. This body language helps show you are interested (Fig. 4-4).

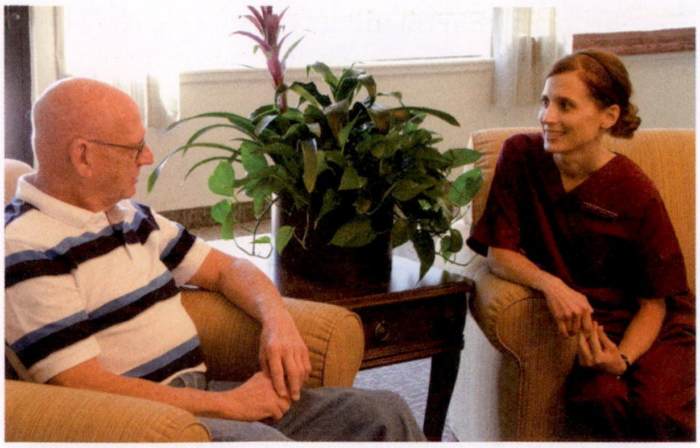

Fig. 4-4. Nursing assistants should maintain eye contact, sit at a normal distance, and practice active listening when communicating with residents who are depressed.

- G Think before you speak. Try to empathize with the resident's feelings and situation.
- G Use a normal tone of voice when speaking. Use simple, clear statements. Do not talk to adults as if they were children.
- G Talk about feelings if the resident wishes.
- G Encourage social interaction.

NAs should report any signs of possible depression to the nurse immediately. A list of signs of depression to report is located in Chapter 22.

7. Identify communication guidelines for anger

Anger is a natural human emotion. Residents, their families and friends, and staff members may express anger. Anger has many causes. Residents may feel angry due to illness, fear, pain, grief, loneliness, or a loss of independence. Even minor things, such as a change in the dinner menu, can trigger anger. Anger may also just be a part of someone's personality.

Some people express anger by yelling, throwing things, being sarcastic, pacing, and threatening others. Narrowed eyes and clenched or raised fists are other signs of anger. Anger can also be expressed by withdrawing, being silent, or sulking. Anger can be difficult to handle. Nursing assistants should always report angry behavior to the nurse immediately.

If a resident becomes angry frequently or if his anger is difficult to manage, a care conference may be scheduled. Care plans can be developed to reduce the behavior. An NA's input at a care conference is valuable. She can offer ideas to help identify the cause of the anger and give suggestions for reducing the behavior.

Guidelines: Angry Behavior

- G Be pleasant and supportive. Let the resident know you are available to help.
- G Try to find out what caused the resident's anger. Using silence may help him explain. Listen closely as he speaks. Note the exact words the resident uses.
- G Observe the resident's body language.
- G Empathize with the resident. Try to understand what he is feeling.
- G Do not argue with an angry resident. Choose your words carefully. Stay calm. Speak in a normal tone of voice.
- G Treat the resident with dignity and respect.
- G Answer call lights promptly.
- G If the resident's anger increases, get the nurse immediately. Stay at a safe distance if the resident becomes violent.
- G Try to involve the resident in activities, such as taking a walk or listening to music, after she has calmed down.

Tip

Assertive vs. Aggressive Behavior

Assertiveness is a desired trait, both in and out of the workplace. Being assertive means being confident when dealing with other people. Expressing thoughts and feelings in a direct, honest, and respectful way shows assertive behavior. For example, an NA who asks for help with a resident when needed is being assertive.

Aggressiveness is different from assertiveness. Aggressiveness means expressing thoughts and feelings in a way that humiliates or overpowers another person. Aggressive behavior does not show respect for the needs or feelings of others.

Being assertive at work is important for providing the best care for residents. An NA should share her feelings, thoughts, and observations in a respectful way. However, she should not behave aggressively in the workplace. Aggressive behavior can result in both physical and emotional harm.

8. Identify communication guidelines for combative behavior

When anger increases, a person may become combative. **Combative** means violent or hostile. Such behavior includes raising one's voice, yelling, hitting, shoving, kicking, throwing things, biting, spitting, insulting others, and resisting care.

Combative behavior may be the result of a disease affecting the brain, such as dementia. It may be due to worsening anger or frustration. Medication, pain, illness, or changes in health are other causes of this behavior. Combativeness may be linked to behaviors seen or practiced in a person's childhood. In general, combative behavior is not a reaction to the caregiver and should not be taken personally.

Even though the behavior is most likely not personal, a resident who is combative may be a threat to staff members, other residents, and visitors. To promote safety, the nursing assistant can observe for early signs of possible combativeness, such as pacing, tensing the body, a flushed face, and an angry look. If a nursing assistant sees that a resident is becoming combative, he should report it to the nurse immediately. Combative behavior may require special techniques to manage it.

Guidelines: Combative Behavior

G Call for the nurse immediately or get someone to call the nurse. Use the call light if you need to contact someone. Try not to leave the resident alone.

G Keep yourself and other people at a safe distance from the resident. If a resident tries to hit you or does hit you, never hit back (Fig. 4-5).

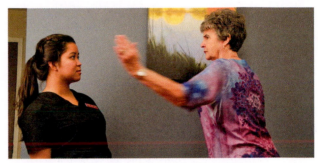

Fig. 4-5. *When dealing with combative residents, nursing assistants should step out of the way, but never hit back.*

G Stay calm. Try not to appear threatening to the resident.

G Be reassuring. Consider what might have triggered the behavior.

G Stay neutral. Do not respond to insults and do not argue with the resident.

G Follow the direction of the nurses.

G Report facts you observed.

G When the resident has calmed down, stay with her if she wishes to talk.

Residents' Rights

Combative Behavior

Elderly people are sometimes abused by their caregivers. This abuse is often the result of a stressful situation, such as the person being combative. No matter how angry, hurt, or afraid nursing assistants are, they can never hit residents. NAs should remain calm and professional and report this behavior to the nurse.

9. Identify communication guidelines for inappropriate sexual behavior

Older adults, like all humans, are sexual beings. Residents have the right to make choices about sex and how they express their sexuality. In all age groups, there is a variety of sexual behavior. This is also true of residents.

However, sometimes residents will show inappropriate sexual behavior. This behavior includes sexual advances and comments to staff or other residents. The behavior does not seem normal and makes the person to whom the advances are directed feel uncomfortable. Inappropriate behavior also includes things like residents removing clothing in public places, such as the dining room or hallway.

This behavior can be caused by illness, dementia, confusion, or medication. Changes in the brain may make a person unable to tell the difference between proper and improper behavior.

Guidelines: Inappropriate Sexual Behavior

G　If you encounter an embarrassing situation, do not overreact. Be professional. Remain calm and try to distract the person. If this does not work, gently direct the resident to a private area. Tell the nurse.

G　Do not judge the behavior and do not gossip about it with other staff members or residents.

G　A resident who is confused may sometimes exhibit inappropriate behavior that is caused by a rash; clothes that are too tight, too hot, or too scratchy; or the need to go to the bathroom. Watch for these problems.

G　Always report all inappropriate behavior to the nurse.

It is important to remember that residents may engage in normal, appropriate sexual behavior. All human beings need love and affection. Residents are sexual beings and can express their sexual needs. They have the right to engage in mutually-agreed-upon sexual relationships. Residents also have the right to masturbate. **Masturbation** means to touch or rub sexual organs in order to give oneself or another person sexual pleasure. Masturbation is a normal expression of sexual needs in all people, including the elderly. If an NA witnesses a sexual situation between

consenting adults, she should provide privacy and leave the area. Chapter 5 contains more information about sexual needs.

10. Identify communication guidelines for disorientation and confusion

Disorientation is confusion about person, place, or time. This condition may be permanent, due to an injury or disorder in the brain. It can also be temporary, due to dehydration, constipation, hypoxia (lack of oxygen to the brain), or medication. Orientation was first discussed as a way to observe residents accurately in Chapter 3. When a resident is oriented, it means he can identify who he is and who his caregiver is (person); the city, state, and facility he is in (place); and the correct time (time of day, year, or season, e.g., spring). A resident who is disoriented may not be able to express one or more of these things.

Confusion is the inability to think clearly and logically. A confused person has trouble focusing his attention and may feel disoriented. A confused resident may not remember to finish his meal or may not be able to locate his room. Confusion interferes with the ability to make decisions and may change a person's personality. When a resident is confused, he may not be able to identify his name, the date, other people, or where he is. Confusion can be a temporary or permanent state.

Confusion is often due to a physical problem, such as a stroke. More information about strokes, also called *cerebrovascular accidents (CVAs)*, is found in Chapter 22. Confusion can also be caused by any of the following:

- Urinary tract infection (UTI)
- Low blood sugar
- Head trauma or head injury
- Dehydration
- Nutritional problems
- Fever
- Sudden drop in body temperature

- Lack of oxygen
- Medication
- Infection
- Brain tumor
- Illness
- Loss of sleep
- Seizures
- Not using a hearing aid when it is necessary

Guidelines: Disorientation or Confusion

G Do not leave the resident alone.

G Stay calm. Provide a quiet environment.

G Speak in a lower tone of voice. Speak clearly and slowly.

G Introduce yourself each time you see the resident. Remind the resident of her location, her name, and the date. A calendar can help (Fig. 4-6).

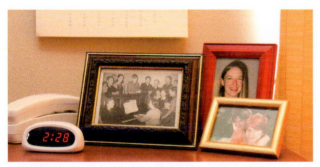

Fig. 4-6. Personal photos and a calendar can help remind a resident who she is and what the date is.

G Explain what you are going to do, using short, simple sentences. Break tasks into steps.

G Be patient with the resident. Do not rush her.

G Listen closely and observe how the resident is communicating. Pay attention to his body language. Do not focus on his words alone.

G Tell the resident about plans for the day. Keeping a routine may help.

G Encourage the use of eyeglasses and hearing aids. Make sure they are clean and are not damaged.

G Tell the resident when you are leaving the area. Repeat if needed.

G Report observations to the nurse.

11. Identify communication guidelines for a resident who is comatose

Nursing assistants may be assigned to care for residents who are comatose. A **coma** is a state of unconsciousness. A person in a coma cannot respond to any change in the environment, including pain. It usually occurs due to an illness, such as meningitis; a condition, such as a drug overdose; or an injury, such as a motor vehicle accident. A resident who is comatose deserves the same respect as an alert resident.

Guidelines: Resident Who is Comatose

G Introduce yourself when entering the resident's room.

G Explain each procedure you will be performing. List the steps you will take.

G Do not hold personal discussions while caring for the resident.

G Let the resident know when you are going to leave the room.

Related Terms

A coma is a state of unconsciousness in which a person is unable to be aroused, even by powerful stimulation. The person does not respond to pain, does not open his eyes, and does not speak.

A person in a coma can transition to a *persistent vegetative state* (PVS), which means the person may have some level of consciousness. He may open his eyes and have some facial movements, but these are mostly involuntary reactions and not a response to external stimuli.

A *minimally conscious state* (MCS) is different from a coma or vegetative state. The person exhibits some cognitive behavior and shows sporadic signs of consciousness, such as crying or laughing appropriately.

Communication Challenges

Unconscious Residents

Even when people are unconscious, they may be able to hear what is going on around them. Unconscious people have been known to regain consciousness and relate many of the things they heard while they were unconscious. NAs should limit their discussions to appropriate subjects. They should speak respectfully and explain what they are doing, as they would with any resident.

12. Identify communication guidelines for functional barriers

Functional problems can interfere with the ability to speak. Causes of these problems include difficulty breathing **(dyspnea)**, physical problems with the mouth or lips, or an artificial airway. Physical problems of the lips, mouth, and tongue include the following:

- Lip, mouth, or tongue sores

- Missing teeth, mouth pain, or recent dental work

- Poorly-fitting dentures (artificial teeth)

- Birth defects like cleft palate (an opening or split in the roof of the mouth)

- Paralysis of one side of the mouth due to stroke

An **airway** is the passageway for air to move into and out of the lungs. An **artificial airway** is any tube inserted into the respiratory tract for the purpose of maintaining an airway and facilitating ventilation. **Ventilation** is the exchange of air between the lungs and the environment. An artificial airway is needed when the airway is obstructed due to illness, injury, secretions, or inhaling fluid into the lungs. An artificial airway may be necessary when a person has surgery or is unconscious.

A **tracheostomy** is a common type of artificial airway seen in long-term care. An opening is made in the neck, either surgically or percutaneously (through the skin, usually in an emergency), into the trachea (windpipe), so that air can reach the person's lungs. This procedure can be temporary or permanent. A tracheostomy may be used while a person is recovering from an acute illness. Some types of head and neck cancers require a tracheostomy. It may also be necessary when a person needs a ventilator. While a tracheostomy is in place, the person may be unable to speak. More information about artificial airways is located in Chapter 26.

Guidelines: Functional Barriers

G   Give the resident plenty of time to speak. Allow pauses between words and sentences. Be patient.

G   Ask the resident to write down anything you do not understand.

G   Allow for rest periods if the resident becomes tired.

G   Do not remove a resident's oxygen for any reason. Only nurses remove oxygen.

G   Report mouth sores, poorly fitting dentures, or complaints of mouth pain to the nurse.

G   Use other methods of communication if the resident cannot speak. Try writing notes, drawing pictures, and using communication boards (Fig. 4-7). Watch for hand and eye signals. For example, use one blink for "yes" and two blinks for "no."

G   Be reassuring and calm. Be empathetic. It can be frightening and uncomfortable to have an artificial airway. Some residents may choke or gag. Imagine how it might feel to have a tube in your nose, mouth, or throat.

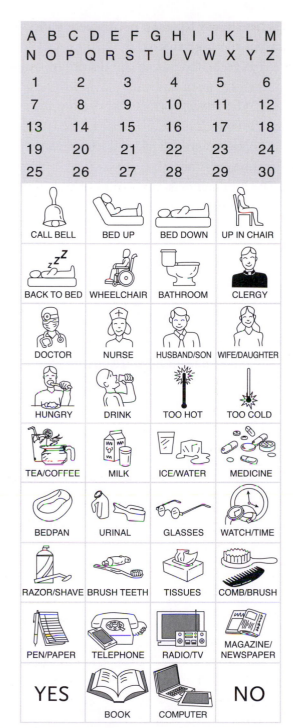

Fig. 4-7. A sample communication board.

Chapter Review

1. What should the nursing assistant do first when dealing with a resident who has a visual impairment (LO 2)?

2. How can a nursing assistant explain the position of objects to a resident who is visually impaired (LO 2)?

3. When speaking with a hearing-impaired resident, whose face should the light be on—the nursing assistant's or the resident's (LO 3)?

4. Why should a nursing assistant explain procedures and introduce herself to a resident who is unconscious (LO 11)?

5. What are other possible methods of communication if a person cannot speak (LO 12)?

6. What is an artificial airway (LO 12)?

Multiple Choice

7. A resident starts sleeping with a doll she had when she was a little girl. This is an example of which defense mechanism (LO 4)?
   (A) Repression
   (B) Regression
   (C) Displacement
   (D) Rationalization

8. A resident refuses to believe her diagnosis of a terminal illness. This is an example of which defense mechanism (LO 4)?
   (A) Denial
   (B) Projection
   (C) Displacement
   (D) Repression

9. Which of the following is true of anxiety (LO 5)?
   (A) Feeling anxious is the same as feeling afraid.
   (B) Anxiety produces only mental and emotional symptoms; it does not cause physical symptoms.
   (C) A person may not always know why she feels anxious.
   (D) Speaking loudly and quickly is helpful for a person who is anxious.

10. Major depressive disorder is also known as (LO 6)
    (A) Clinical depression
    (B) Anxiety disorder
    (C) Mood therapy
    (D) Minor regression

11. Which of the following statements best describes anger (LO 7)?
    (A) Anger is only experienced by people who have a mental health disorder.
    (B) Nursing assistants do not need to report angry behavior by residents.
    (C) Anger is the first sign of an anxiety disorder.
    (D) Anger is a natural emotion with many causes.

12. If a resident becomes combative, the best response by the nursing assistant would be to (LO 8)
    (A) Let the resident know what he did was wrong
    (B) Stay at a safe distance from the resident
    (C) Startle the resident into stopping the behavior
    (D) Threaten the resident by withholding something he likes

13. If a resident exhibits inappropriate sexual behavior, what would be the best response by the nursing assistant (LO 9)?
    (A) The NA should let the resident know that he is embarrassing himself.
    (B) The NA should tell other NAs what the resident is doing so that they can avoid him.
    (C) The NA should tell the resident that he is being inappropriate.
    (D) The NA should try to distract the resident.

14. What should a person be able to identify when she is oriented (LO 10)?
    (A) Favorite foods, city she resides in, mother's maiden name
    (B) Who she is, correct year, facility she lives in
    (C) Medication she takes, doctor's name, correct time
    (D) Her diagnosis, the names of her family members, and the date

15. Which of the following is a common cause of confusion (LO 10)?
    (A) Anxiety
    (B) Anger
    (C) Urinary tract infection
    (D) Diabetes

16. The medical term for difficulty breathing is (LO 12)
    (A) Dyspnea
    (B) Ventilation
    (C) Combative
    (D) Mechanism

5
Diversity and Human Needs and Development

The Black Death: The Plague That Didn't Discriminate

The bubonic plague, also known as the *Black Death*, first reared its ugly head in the 14th century. The name *Black Death* came from the black areas on the skin commonly seen on plague patients. It is thought to have developed in the Far East. This plague moved across Asia and into North Africa, slipping into Europe by way of Italy. At that time, Italian merchants traveled to Asia searching for beautiful wares to sell. When they set sail for home, they carried the disease with them to Italy without realizing it. The plague spread from Italy across Europe to England. An estimated 60 million people died of the plague from 1340 to 1350. The plague killed people from many cultures and ethnic groups. Disease can strike anyone from any age group. It truly does not discriminate.

"The great law of culture is: Let each become all that he was created capable of being."

Thomas Carlyle, 1795–1881

"Religion is a great force—the only real motive force in the world: but what you fellows don't understand is that you must get at a man through his own religion and not through yours."

George Bernard Shaw, 1856–1950

1. Define important words in this chapter

ageism: stereotyping of, prejudice toward, and/or discrimination against the elderly.

agnostic: a person who believes that he does not know or cannot know if God exists.

atheist: a person who believes that there is no God.

Buddhism: a religion that follows the teachings of Buddha.

Christianity: a religion that follows the teachings of Jesus Christ.

cultural competence: an ongoing process of learning about other cultures and applying that knowledge to provide better health care.

cultural diversity: the variety of people living and working together in the world.

developmental disability: a chronic condition that restricts physical and/or mental abilities.

health: state of physical, mental, and social well-being.

Hinduism: a religion that believes in the unity of everything and that all are a part of God.

Islam: a religion that follows the prophet Muhammad and the Five Pillars of Islam.

Judaism: a religion that follows the teachings of God as given to Moses in laws and commandments.

mores: the accepted traditional customs of a particular social group.

need: something necessary or required.

psychosocial needs: needs that involve social interaction, emotions, intellect, and spirituality.

puberty: the period during which a person develops secondary sex characteristics.

religion: a set of beliefs concerning the cause and nature of the universe that often includes a moral code and usually involves specific rituals and practices.

spirituality: of or relating to concerns of the spirit, the sacred, or the soul.

stereotype: a biased generalization about a group that is usually based on opinions and distorted ideas.

transcultural nursing: the study of various cultures with the goal of providing care specific to each culture.

wellness: successfully balancing things that happen in everyday life; includes five different types: physical, social, emotional, intellectual, and spiritual.

2. Explain health and wellness

The World Health Organization (who.int) has defined **health** as "a complete state of physical, mental, and social well-being, and not merely the absence of disease or infirmity." This view of health looks at the whole person. It also takes the emphasis off disease and redirects it to healthy attitudes and lifestyles. In recent years, many cultures have increased focus on healthy living.

Wellness has to do with successfully balancing things that happen in everyday lives. There are five types of wellness: physical, social, emotional, intellectual, and spiritual. Physical wellness includes things like being able to complete everyday tasks. Social wellness has to do with relating to other people. Emotional wellness involves managing stress and expressing feelings. Intellectual wellness deals with growing and learning throughout the life span. Spiritual wellness includes religious beliefs, ethics, values, and mores. **Mores** are the accepted traditional customs of a particular social group.

3. Explain the importance of holistic health care

Holistic health care was first introduced in Chapter 1. Care team members should view resident care in a holistic way. Holistic health care involves considering the whole person, which includes his physical and psychosocial needs (Fig. 5-1). **Psychosocial needs** include social contact, emotions, thought, and spirituality. Caring for a person holistically is part of providing person-centered care. Person-centered care revolves around the resident and promotes her individual preferences, choices, dignity, and interests. A simple example of holistic health care is taking time to talk with residents while helping them bathe. The nursing assistant is meeting a physical need with the bath and meeting the psychosocial need for interaction with others at the same time.

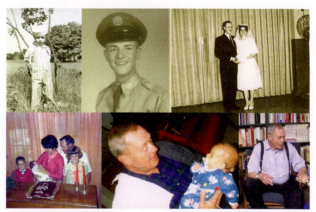

Fig. 5-1. *Residents are people, not just lists of illnesses and disabilities. They have many needs, like other people. Many have had rich lives with wonderful experiences. Nursing assistants should take the time to know and care for each resident as a whole person.*

Health care is developed around the idea that harmony or balance in one's life promotes health. If the balance is disturbed, illness can result. Holistic health care supports harmony, which can improve a resident's chances of living a better life.

4. Identify basic human needs and discuss Maslow's Hierarchy of Needs

All human beings have the same basic physical needs. A **need** is something necessary for a person to survive and grow. Physical needs include the following:

- Food and water

- Protection and shelter

- Activity

- Sleep and rest

- Comfort, especially freedom from pain

Human beings also have psychosocial needs. Although they are not as easy to define as physical needs, psychosocial needs include the following:

- Love and affection

- Acceptance by others

- Self-reliance and independence in daily living

- Contact with others

- Success and self-esteem

Abraham Maslow, a psychologist and researcher of human behavior, developed a model to show how physical and psychosocial needs are arranged in order of importance. He believed that physical needs must be met before psychosocial needs can be met. His theory is called *Maslow's Hierarchy of Needs* (Fig. 5-2).

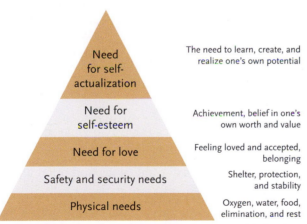

Fig. 5-2. *Maslow's Hierarchy of Needs is a model developed by Abraham Maslow to show how physical and psychosocial needs are arranged in order of importance.*

The needs at the bottom of the pyramid are physical needs. They are the ones that must be met to survive. For example, a person can live only a few days without water. NAs can help residents meet these needs by encouraging them

to eat and drink. NAs can provide a quiet place for residents to rest. They can also help residents with elimination needs whenever needed.

The second level is safety and security needs. These include shelter, protection, and stability. For example, moving a person from her home into a facility can cause anxiety. Because it is not yet a stable environment, new residents may find it hard to adapt. It may take time for them to feel comfortable in their new homes. NAs can help residents by being compassionate and empathetic. They can listen to residents when residents want to talk. NAs can reassure residents that they are receiving quality care.

The third level is love, acceptance, and belonging. When residents move into a facility, they may be separated from their loved ones. Living in a new place with strangers can be very lonely. This is especially true if loved ones do not visit as often as before. Residents need to feel as if they belong in their new home. NAs can help by welcoming them and making them feel listened to and cared for. NAs can encourage residents to interact with other residents and staff.

The fourth level is the need for self-esteem. Residents may feel less of a sense of self-worth as they become dependent on others. They will need help with tasks they have performed independently all their lives. NAs can help by encouraging residents to be as independent as possible. The more residents can care for themselves, the better they will feel about themselves. NAs should praise successes, no matter how small. This maintains dignity and self-esteem.

According to Maslow's theory, self-actualization is the highest need a person can achieve. A person must reach her highest potential to become self-actualized. People rarely reach this level in every single part of their lives. Residents will each be at different stages in this process. Some residents will be content with the level they have reached in life. Other residents will still be striving to do more. For example, a resident might help other residents read mail or write letters, or volunteer to oversee special activities.

5. Identify ways to accommodate cultural differences

As described in Chapter 3, *culture* refers to a set of learned beliefs, values, and behaviors. The world is full of many different groups of people. Each group has a unique way of looking at the world. NAs will have the opportunity to take care of people from many cultures. Having an understanding of cultures will help NAs give better care to residents. Each person's culture greatly influences her in many ways.

Cultural diversity has to do with the wide variety of people throughout the world. Each culture may have different customs, traditions, religions, behaviors, and lifestyles. Culture and background often have an impact on how a person behaves when she is ill. **Transcultural nursing** is the study of various cultures with the goal of providing care specific to each culture. **Cultural competence** is a method of learning about each individual's views and behaviors and applying that knowledge to health care. It is an ongoing process of understanding other cultures to help provide better care. This is part of person-centered care. The use of cultural competence can help make nursing care more equitable. It can reduce misunderstandings and improve resident care.

NAs should be sensitive to differences and respect and value each person as an individual. It is important for NAs to respond to new ideas with acceptance, not prejudice.

There are more cultures than can be listed here. There are thousands of different groups in the United States alone (Fig. 5-3). Some examples are Japanese Americans, American Indians (Native Americans), and Latinos. The US also has people from many different regions. Each region has its own culture and traditions. For example, the rural US is different from the urban US. The culture of the Northeast is not the same as the culture of the South.

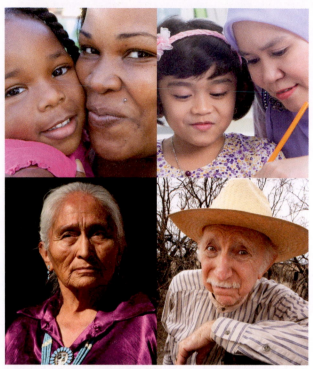

Fig. 5-3. *There are many different cultures in the US.*

Culture can affect ideas about touch or eye contact, as well as the language people use. A person's culture also influences his food choices. For example, some Korean people eat *kimchi*, which is a spicy fermented vegetable dish. Some Mexican people eat *queso fresco*, which is a type of cheese. There is more information about food choices in Chapter 14.

Culture also influences the way people seek health care or discuss health issues. Some people are very comfortable with and open about discussing their health. Others feel hesitant about doing this and are embarrassed by it. NAs must be sensitive to differences in how residents feel about discussing their health.

NAs should become familiar with each resident's culture. Residents may be happy to talk about their backgrounds and educate others about their beliefs and customs. NAs can ask residents and their families and friends about special traditions. When NAs are sensitive to cultural differences, residents benefit.

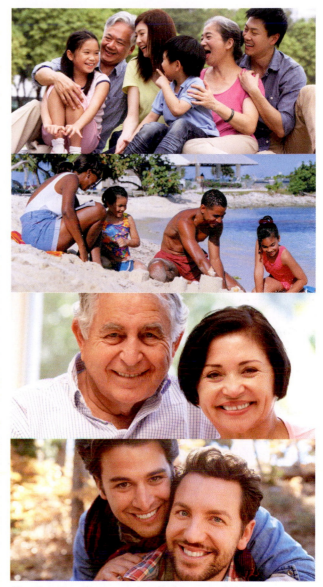

NAs must never make fun of or disrespect any culture, behavior, or belief. When people accept and do not judge others' beliefs or choices, they can learn new ideas and create lasting relationships.

Residents' Rights

Rights Regarding Language

Residents have the right to communicate with someone who speaks their language. They must understand all documents before signing them. They also must understand all care before it is performed. In some languages a change in pronunciation will change the meaning of what is said. An NA should inform the nurse if he feels a translator is needed to make sure his meaning is clear.

6. Discuss the role of the family in health care

Families play an important part in most people's lives. The concept of family is always changing. Often a family is defined more by the support people give each other rather than by the particular people involved. There are many different kinds of families (Fig. 5-4):

- Nuclear families (two parents and one or more children)

- Single-parent families (one parent and one or more children)

- Married or committed couples of the same sex or opposite sex, with or without children

- Extended families (parents, children, grandparents, aunts, uncles, cousins, other relatives, and even friends)

- Blended families (divorced or widowed parents who have remarried and have children from previous relationships and/or the current marriage)

NAs must respect all kinds of families. NAs should not judge families, even if they are different from their own ideas of family. No family is a right or wrong kind of family.

Fig. 5-4. Families come in all shapes and sizes.

Families have an important role in residents' health care. They may provide some of their loved one's care. Friends may also help with care. They both help in many other ways:

- Helping residents make care decisions

- Relating routines and preferences to care team members

- Connecting residents to what is going on outside of the facility

- Reading mail and helping to prepare cards, letters, and gifts

- Helping to prepare menus

- Taking residents on walks

- Going with residents to activities or outside functions

- Bathing or helping with other personal care

- Washing residents' clothes at home

- Shopping for special items, gifts, or cards

When families visit, NAs should do all they can to help residents prepare. NAs can help by getting residents dressed, applying makeup, or anything else residents require. The NA can help find a private place for the visit if needed. She should pay attention to the resident's and family's needs during the visit and report questions from the family promptly to the nurse.

7. Explain how to meet emotional needs of residents and their families

NAs may be of great help to residents and their families and friends. Because NAs are the primary caregivers, they play an important role in the comfort and well-being of residents.

NAs may be the people residents or their family members turn to when they are scared, angry, or stressed. They may go to NAs during an emotional crisis. For example, if a resident's friend dies, he may seek out an NA for comfort or to talk. If a resident dies, his family may do the same.

When a resident wants to discuss problems or needs with an NA, the NA should listen closely to what the resident says without interrupting. The NA can offer support and encouragement. She should not respond with clichés, such as "You will be fine." The resident may not be fine. It is more comforting to respond with a meaningful message, such as "How can I help?" If it is within her scope of practice, the NA can answer questions that are asked. However, if questions have to do with medical issues or advice, they should be reported to the nurse.

Residents sometimes feel that NAs are a part of their family. However, it is important for NAs to maintain professional boundaries. Understanding the limits of professional relationships with residents means behaving in an ethical and responsible way. Residents who are ill and lonely may feel that they need more from staff than what is appropriate. Staff who are overworked, have poor relationships at home, or are prone to substance abuse may be at risk for inappropriate relationships with residents. It is important for NAs to be aware of these factors. If an NA is unsure about how to maintain a proper emotional distance from a resident, a supervisor can help.

NAs should be available for residents' family members or friends, too. Families often seek out NAs because they see them more than other staff members. NAs can provide comfort and compassion. Sitting quietly and listening may be the best help an NA can give (Fig. 5-5).

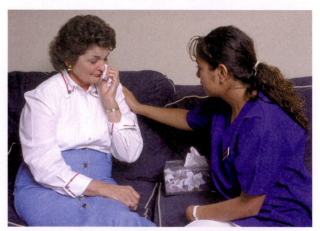

Fig. 5-5. *Sometimes listening to a resident's family member is the best way to provide emotional support.*

A family member may ask questions about a resident's care, such as when the resident is bathed or when meals are offered. The NA can answer these types of questions. However, when a family member wants to know about a resident's diagnosis, treatments, and therapies, he should be referred to the nurse. The nurse should also be notified if an NA has concerns about a resident's safety around one or more family members.

8. Explain ways to help residents with their spiritual needs

Residents may have many different spiritual needs and beliefs. These beliefs can help them cope with illness and problems they face. Residents may feel strongly about their spiritual beliefs. Spirituality is a sensitive area, and NAs should always treat residents' needs and practices with respect.

Residents' beliefs will vary. Some may consider themselves deeply religious, while others may think of themselves as spiritual but not religious. Other residents may not consider themselves religious or spiritual at all. Residents may believe in God or may not believe in God. The important thing for NAs to remember is to respect all residents' beliefs, whatever they are. NAs must never make judgments about residents' spiritual beliefs or try to push their own beliefs on residents.

Understanding a little bit about common **religions** and religious groups may be useful. Some people belong to a religious group but do not believe or practice everything that religion teaches. There are many different faiths, and within each of these, there are many different beliefs. An NA's job is to accommodate religious practices and requests when possible. Common religions, listed alphabetically, follow:

Buddhism: Buddhism evolved from Siddhartha Gautama, who reached enlightenment and took the title of Buddha. Buddhists believe that morality, meditation, and wisdom are the path to enlightenment. They believe in reincarnation and that people must travel through birth, life, and death. After these travels, a person can reach Nirvana. Nirvana is the state of peace, happiness, and freedom from worry and pain. It is the highest spiritual plane a person can reach. There are many Buddhist texts. The Tipitaka, also called the Pali Canon, is the standard scripture collection. The Dalai Lama is considered to be the highest spiritual leader.

Christianity: Christians generally believe in a single God made up of the Trinity—the Father, Son (Jesus Christ), and Holy Spirit. Christians believe that they receive forgiveness for their sins through a relationship with God. They believe that Jesus Christ was the son of God and that he rose from the dead after being crucified. Christians believe in eternal life. There are many subgroups or denominations, such as Baptist, Episcopalian, Evangelical, Lutheran, Methodist, Presbyterian, and Roman Catholic. Many Christians participate in rituals they consider holy, like baptism or communion. The Bible is the sacred text. Religious leaders may be called *priests*, *preachers*, *pastors*, or *ministers*.

Hinduism: Hindus believe in the unity of everything, called *Brahman*. According to Hindu beliefs, there are four purposes of life: acting morally and ethically (Dharma), pursuing prosperity (Artha), enjoying life (Kama), and accomplishing enlightenment (Moksha). People move through birth, life, death, and rebirth. How a person moves toward enlightenment is determined by karma. Karma is the result of actions in past lives, and actions in this life can determine one's destiny in future lives. Good thoughts and deeds can cause one to be reborn at a higher level, while bad thoughts and deeds can cause a person to be born at a lower level. The Vedas are the primary texts of Hinduism. Holy men are called *sadhus*.

Islam: Muslims are followers of the prophet Muhammad [Mohammed]. Muslims worship God; the Arabic term for God is *Allah*. The Five Pillars of Islam include reciting the profession of faith, ritual prayer five times daily at certain times of the day, fasting during the month called *Ramadan*, charitable donations to the poor and needy, and pilgrimage to Mecca. Mecca is the Muslim holy city. Muslims worship at mosques and follow specific religious practices related to food and drink. For example, Muslims do not eat pork or drink alcohol. The sacred text of Islam is the Qur'an [Koran]. The Qur'an is believed to be the literal word of God as revealed to Muhammad. Titles of Islamic religious leaders include *ayatollah, caliph, imam, mufti,* and *mullah.*

Judaism: Judaism is the religion of the Jewish people. It is divided into Reform, Conservative, and Orthodox movements. Jewish people believe that God gave them laws and commandments through Moses in the form of the Torah (the sacred text). Jewish services are held on Friday evenings and sometimes on Saturdays in synagogues or temples. The Sabbath day, called *Shabbat,* is a special day of rest and contemplation. Jewish people may not do certain things, such as work or drive, on the Sabbath, which lasts from Friday sundown to Saturday sundown. Religious leaders are called *rabbis.*

Spirituality concerns a person's beliefs about the spirit, the sacred, or the soul. Some people consider themselves to be spiritual but not religious. Others believe that their spiritual self is the same as their religious self. Spirituality centers around thoughts of a spiritual aspect of life and nature beyond worldly things. It may be associated with inner peace and well-being. It may refer to a person's beliefs about the overall meaning or purpose of life.

Many American Indian (Native American) tribes follow their own spiritual traditions. Their beliefs include the idea that everything—people, animals, oceans, trees, and other things—has a spirit. The importance of community and a reverence for the environment are emphasized, and there are many varied practices and rituals.

As mentioned earlier, some people have varying beliefs in religion, spirituality, and God. Some people may not believe in God or a higher power and identify themselves as **agnostic**. Agnostics believe that they do not know or cannot know if God exists. They do not deny that God might exist, but they feel there is no true knowledge of God's existence.

Atheists are people who believe that there is no God. This is different from what agnostics believe. Atheists actively deny the existence of any deity (higher power). For many atheists, this belief is as strongly held as any religious belief.

Guidelines: Respecting Spiritual Needs

G   Honor dietary restrictions. Dietary restrictions are rules about what and when followers can eat. For example, some Muslims do not eat shellfish. Many Catholics choose not to eat meat on Fridays during Lent. Jewish people may eat only kosher foods and may not eat pork. Many Buddhists are vegetarians. Do not judge any dietary restrictions. Report fasting requests to the nurse.

G   Report requests to see clergy to the nurse promptly. Give privacy for clergy visits.

G   Respect all religious items (Fig. 5-6). Handle religious items carefully. When asked, help residents apply religious articles of clothing.

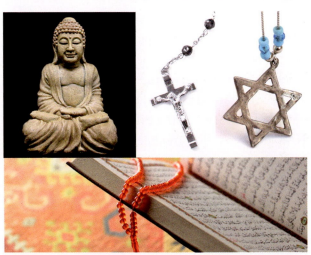

Fig. 5-6. These are just a few examples of different religious items residents may have. Respect their religious items and handle them carefully.

G   Allow time and privacy for prayer. If you are asked to do so, read religious materials aloud.

G   Make sure residents who want to attend religious services are ready on time and are helped to the proper site.

G   Report to the nurse or social worker if a resident needs help finding spiritual resources.

G   Do not do any of the following:

- Try to change someone's religion or tell a resident that his belief or religion is wrong

- Express judgments or say anything negative about a religious group

- Insist that a resident join in a religious activity

- Interfere with a religious practice

- Discuss your personal beliefs or opinions, either directly or indirectly

G   Spiritual needs are different for each person. Respect residents' religions or beliefs. Respect for residents' beliefs regarding religion and spirituality is an essential way in which NAs provide person-centered care. Listen when residents want to discuss their beliefs.

9. Identify ways to accommodate sexual needs

Humans are sexual beings, and they continue to have sexual needs throughout their lives (Fig. 5-7). Sexual needs encompass more than just having sex; having one's sexuality respected and acknowledged is an important need for all ages. Sex and sexuality have been defined in this way: sex is something a person does, while sexuality is something a person is.

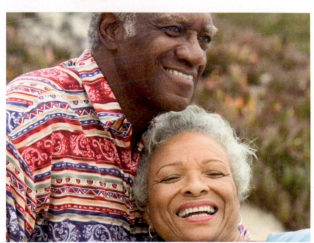

Fig. 5-7. *Human beings continue to have sexual needs and desires throughout their lives.*

Sexual orientation is a person's physical, emotional, and/or romantic attraction to another person. Sexual orientation plays a big part in human sexuality. *Gender identity* is a deeply felt sense of one's gender. A person may have the gender identity of a man or a woman, or may not fit into either of those two categories. Terms related to sexual orientation and gender identity, listed alphabetically, include the following:

- Asexual: A person who does not experience sexual attraction to any gender.

- Bisexual, Bi: A person whose physical, emotional, and/or romantic attraction may be for people of the same gender or different gender.

- Celibate: A person who abstains from sexual activity.

- Coming out: A continual process of revealing one's sexual orientation or gender identity to others.

- Cross-dresser: Typically refers to a heterosexual man who sometimes wears clothing and other items associated with women; cross-dressing is not associated with men who permanently wish to change their sex.

- Gay: A person whose physical, emotional, and/or romantic attraction is for people of the same sex.

- Heterosexual: A person whose physical, emotional, and/or romantic attraction is for people of the opposite sex; also known as *straight*.

- Lesbian: A woman whose physical, emotional, and/or romantic attraction is for other women.

- LGBT: Acronym for lesbian, gay, bisexual, and transgender.

- LGBTQ: Acronym for lesbian, gay, bisexual, transgender, and queer.

- Transgender: A person whose gender identity conflicts with his or her birth sex (sex assigned at birth due to anatomy); transgender identity is not dependent on someone having undergone medical measures like hormones or surgery.

- Transition: The process of changing genders, which can include legal procedures, such as changing one's name and/or sex on documents, and medical measures, such as hormone therapy and surgery; it can also include telling others and using new pronouns.

Residents' Rights

LGBTQ Residents

The Administration for Community Living (acl.gov) cites research suggesting that older lesbian, gay, bisexual, transgender, and queer (LGBTQ) adults often face discrimination due to their sexual orientation as well as their age (Fig. 5-8). NAs must treat every resident with respect, no matter what their personal or religious feelings regarding sexuality may be. Part of respecting each resident's sexual orientation and gender identity is not making the assumption that all residents are heterosexual. NAs must use terms and pronouns that residents prefer (using "she," for example, to refer to a resident who is physically male but identifies as female). More information may be found at the National Resource Center on LGBT Aging's website (lgbtagingcenter.org) or at GLAAD's website (glaad.org).

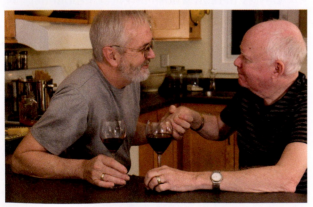

Fig. 5-8. *The number of lesbian, gay, bisexual, transgender, and queer older adults continues to increase. It is important for NAs to treat all residents with respect.*

common myth is that elderly people no longer sexual needs or desires. That is not true. urges do not end due to age or admis-care facility. Many things can affect

residents' sexual needs. Illness and disability can affect sexual desires, needs, and abilities. Sexual desire may not be lessened by a disability, although the ability to meet sexual needs may be limited. Many people who use wheelchairs can have sexual and intimate relationships, although adjustments may have to be made. NAs should not assume they know what impact a physical disability has had on sexuality.

Sexual needs may also be affected by residents' living environments. A lack of privacy and no available partner are often reasons for a lack of sexual expression in care facilities. NAs should always be sensitive to privacy needs.

Guidelines: Respecting Sexual Needs

G   Always knock and wait for permission to enter before going into residents' rooms. Honor *Do Not Disturb* signs if your facility uses them.

G   If you encounter any sexual situation between consenting adult residents, provide privacy and leave the room. Do not discuss what you saw with other staff members. Residents are allowed to meet their sexual needs however they choose, such as through masturbation and sexual relationships.

G   Do not judge residents' sexual choices, sexual orientation, or gender identity. Do not judge the sexual orientation or gender identity of residents' family members or friends.

G   When possible, ask transgender residents which pronouns they would like you to use and use them. Be patient if a resident takes time to decide which pronouns are best for him or her. The resident may decide a set of pronouns works for a time and then prefer a different set later.

G   Always use a transgender person's chosen name.

G   If you ever see sexual abuse occurring, remove the resident from the situation immediately. Take the resident to a safe place, and report to the nurse right away.

G Do not treat any expression of sexuality by the elderly as disgusting or cute. That attitude is inappropriate and deprives residents of their right to dignity and respect.

G If a sexual situation is disturbing or inappropriate, ask a nurse for help. Tips on dealing with inappropriate sexual behavior are in Chapter 4. More information on the sexual needs of the elderly is in Chapter 17.

10. Describe the stages of human growth and development

Human growth and development is an ongoing and complex process. Growth refers to the physical changes that can be measured. Development means the emotional, social, and physical changes that occur. Each person's growth and development will differ. One child may walk at nine months old, while another will not walk until over a year old.

Many things affect growth and development. These include the parents' involvement, the child's surroundings, nutrition, exercise, medical care, and overall lifestyle.

There are different types of development. Cognitive development focuses on how children think and learn. Language development focuses on gaining language skills. Moral development deals with forming a sense of right and wrong. Motor development is gaining an ability to do things like grasp items, use scissors, and draw. Physical development deals with the changes that happen to the body during growth. Sexual development has to do with the reproductive changes that occur when people reach puberty. Social development is the process of learning to relate to other people.

The age ranges given here provide a general idea of developmental stages, not an exact description.

Infancy (Birth to 12 months)

Babies grow quickly during the first year. Infants tend to triple birth weight in the first year of life. Physical development in infancy moves from the head down (Fig. 5-9). For example, infants gain control over the muscles of the neck before the muscles in their shoulders. Infants learn to grasp, lift their heads, and crawl. They are able to pick up objects, usually between four and eight months of age. Infants are totally dependent on others for care. Touch is important as a communication tool. Touch helps babies grow and thrive.

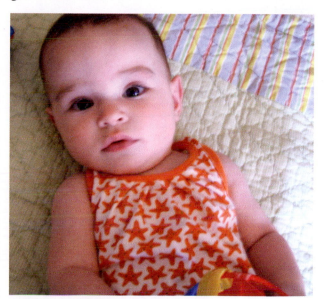

Fig. 5-9. An infant's physical development moves from the head down.

Toddler (Ages 1 to 3)

Toddlers grow fast between the ages of one and three. Most toddlers can move about quickly, run, and jump. During the toddler years, speech improves. Toddlers gain coordination of their limbs and learn to control their bladders and bowels (Fig. 5-10). It is important to protect toddlers as they explore their world, for they often take risks. They do not understand what can harm them. Parents begin to teach them language, the difference between right and wrong, and acceptable behavior.

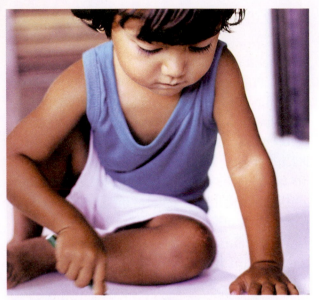

Fig. 5-10. *Toddlers gain coordination of their limbs.*

Preschool (Ages 3 to 5)

Preschool-age children become more independent and have social relationships. They play better with other children, and they can play in groups (Fig. 5-11). Their language abilities improve. Preschoolers learn to care for themselves. They become more physically coordinated, and their sense of imagination develops. Playing dress-up in parents' clothing is common.

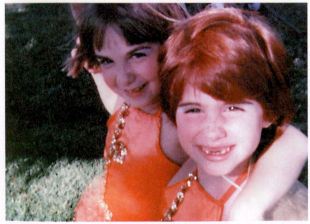

Fig. 5-11. *Children in preschool years develop social relationships.*

School Age (Ages 5 to 10)

School-age children's development centers on cognitive and social development. Entering school is a big adjustment for children and their families. Children learn to get along with each other. They begin to develop a conscience, morals, and self-esteem. During this time, boys develop more muscle, but girls may be taller than boys.

Preadolescence (Ages 10 to 12)

During the ages between 10 and 12, children begin to view life more realistically. They use reason to analyze situations and may begin questioning authority. They become more independent. Social relationships become very important. Growth spurts and hormonal changes occur, and preadolescents become more self-conscious. Girls may reach puberty in the later years of this stage. During **puberty**, a person develops secondary sex characteristics. In females, secondary sex characteristics include growth of body hair and development of breasts and hips. In males, they include growth of body hair, growth of the testes and the penis, broadening of the shoulders, and a lower voice.

Adolescence (Ages 12 to 18)

During adolescence, people of both genders become sexually mature. Boys tend to reach puberty during this stage. If girls did not reach puberty during the prior stage, it will start here. Adolescents may have a hard time adapting to changes caused by puberty (Fig. 5-12).

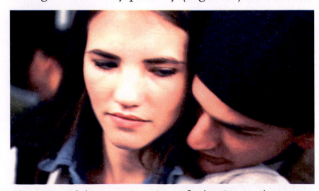

Fig. 5-12. *Adolescence is a time of adapting to change.*

This group becomes more independent. They must make important decisions, mostly by themselves, each day. Moral values that the child has learned play a part in these decisions. Adolescents can sometimes become stubborn and difficult for their parents to handle. They may have mood swings. They are concerned with acceptance from others.

Young Adulthood (Ages 18 to 40)

Physical growth has usually been completed by this time, although boys can continue to grow up to the age of 25. Psychological and social development continues. During young adulthood, people make decisions about whether to continue their education or join the work force. They may meet a life partner. Many couples marry (Fig. 5-13). Some people have children during this time.

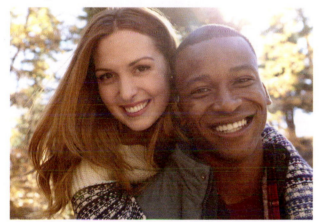

Fig. 5-13. *Young adulthood often involves finding long-term mates and may involve having children.*

Middle Adulthood (Ages 40 to 65)

In general, during middle adulthood people become more comfortable and stable than in previous stages. Their children may have left home to go to college or to live on their own. However, as some people are waiting longer to have children, they may be having children or rearing them at the beginning of this stage. This can be a very happy time for people (Fig. 5-14). They may find there is more time and money to spend on themselves. Couples may take trips and spend more time together. A person may decide to begin a second career.

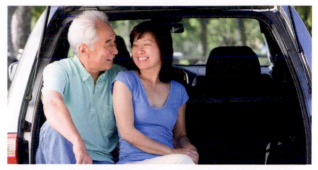

Fig. 5-14. *Middle adulthood can offer more free time to take trips and pursue hobbies.*

Some people may find themselves in a midlife crisis during this stage. This is a period of unrest due to a desire for change and fulfillment of unmet goals. It has to do with the reality of getting older. A midlife crisis can occur in both men and women. People may change the way they dress, act, or behave during this time.

Late Adulthood (65 years and older)

People in late adulthood may see many changes. They may retire from jobs. Medical care may be needed for problems that develop during this time. People may have to cope with a loved one's illness or death. Staying connected to others is vital to remaining healthy and mentally alert (Fig. 5-15). Hobbies and volunteering can help people stay connected. People in this stage should continue to be active and involved. Figure 5-16 outlines the developmental tasks that are required throughout all stages of life.

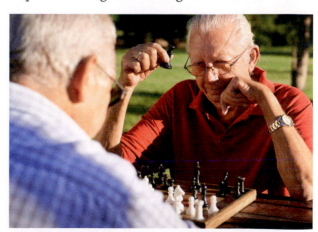

Fig. 5-15. *In late adulthood, it is important to stay connected with others to help remain healthy and active.*

Human Growth and Development

Infant (Birth to 12 months)	Toddler (Ages 1 to 3)	Preschool (Ages 3 to 5)	School Age (Ages 5 to 10)	Preadolescence (Ages 10 to 12)
• Rapid physical growth • Physical development moves from the head down • Learns to lift head and grasp • Begins to crawl and climb • Picks up objects • Smiles, cries, coos, babbles, and laughs	• Learns to walk, run, and jump • Speech improves • Gains coordination of limbs • Learns to control bladder and bowels	• Becomes more independent • Has social relationships • Language ability improves • Learns to care for self • Becomes more physically coordinated	• Learns to get along with other children • Begins to develop a conscience, morals, and self-esteem	• Views life more realistically • Uses reason to analyze situations • Social relationships very important • Growth spurts occur • Girls may reach puberty in the later years of this stage

Adolescence (Ages 12 to 18)	Young Adulthood (Ages 18 to 40)	Middle Adulthood (Ages 40 to 65)	Late Adulthood (65 years and older)
• Boys reach puberty • Girls reach puberty if they have not before • May have a difficult time adapting to changes caused by puberty • Becomes more independent • Makes important decisions • Can become stubborn • Has mood swings • Concerned with acceptance from others	• Growth is usually complete • Makes decisions about education or careers • Selects a mate • May marry • May have children	• More comfortable and stable • Some changes of aging appear • Children may have left home • Some people have children at beginning of this stage • May travel more	• Retires from jobs • Changes of aging more apparent • May require medical care for problems • Mobility can become limited • Copes with illness and/or death of loved ones and friends

Fig. 5-16. The stages of human growth and development.

11. Discuss stereotypes of the elderly

It is common for people to have false beliefs about the elderly. A **stereotype** is a biased generalization about a group. These generalizations are usually based on opinions and distorted ideas and often come from television shows or movies. These unfair ideas create prejudices against the elderly. Stereotyping of, prejudice toward, and/or discrimination against the elderly is called **ageism**. Common stereotypes of the elderly include the following:

• They cannot remember things.

• They are totally dependent on others.

• They do not have an active sex life.

• They do not like to leave home.

• They are grumpy or grouchy.

• They cannot manage their money.

• They are less intelligent than younger people.

• They have no friends.

• They have no interests.

These ideas are not true of most elderly people. Research has shown that most older people are active and have many interests (Fig. 5-17). They exercise, continue to learn, work, manage their finances, and have intimate relationships. They are relatively independent.

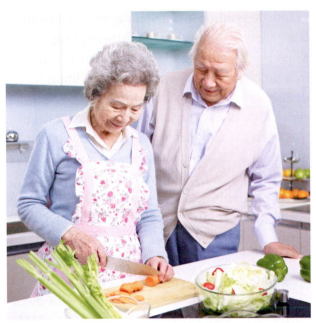

Fig. 5-17. Most older people lead active lives.

Aging is a normal process. There are many emotional and physical changes that occur as people age. These normal changes of aging do not mean that a person will always become ill or dependent. NAs must be able to know what is true about the aging process and what is not true. Distinguishing normal changes of aging from signs of illness will allow NAs to better help residents.

12. Discuss developmental disabilities

Developmental disabilities are disabilities that are present at birth or emerge during childhood, up to age 22. A **developmental disability** is a chronic condition; it will exist throughout a person's life. Developmental disabilities restrict physical and/or mental ability. These disabilities prevent a child from developing at a normal rate. These disabilities include intellectual disabilities, cerebral palsy, spina bifida, autism spectrum disorder, and fragile X syndrome.

Developmental disabilities cause problems with language, mobility, learning, and the ability to perform self-care. For example, a person may struggle with eating, bathing, walking, or speaking. A brief description of some developmental disabilities follows:

Intellectual Disability: The most common developmental disability is an intellectual disability (formerly called *mental retardation*). An intellectual disability is neither a disease nor a mental health disorder. People with an intellectual disability develop at a below-average rate. They have below-average mental functioning. They experience difficulty with social skills (interpersonal communication, making friends, and empathizing with others). They have problems with conceptual skills (reading, writing, reasoning, and memory). The ability to develop practical skills, such as performing activities of daily living (bathing, eating, moving, and positioning) is affected.

People with an intellectual disability need some support in their day-to-day lives. Working and living independently may be an option, depending upon the severity of the disability.

There are four different degrees of this disability: mild, moderate, severe, and profound. The level of care required for individuals with an intellectual disability can range from relatively independent living with mild intellectual disability to a need for skilled, 24-hour care for a person who has profound intellectual disability.

Some residents and their families will use the term *intellectually disabled*, while others may use *challenged* or *developmentally delayed*. NAs should respect each resident's wishes about how to refer to this disability.

Cerebral Palsy (CP): Cerebral palsy is a developmental disability that affects movement and balance. It can also cause intellectual disabilities. A person with cerebral palsy suffered brain damage while in the uterus or during birth. This damage can be caused by birth trauma, infection, or a head injury. The part of the brain that was damaged controls muscle tone. People with CP may lack control of their head and have trouble using their arms and hands. They can have poor balance or posture. They may be stiff or limp. CP can cause problems with speech and may affect intelligence.

CP generally does not worsen as the person gets older. Cerebral palsy includes four types: ataxic, athetoid, spastic, and mixed. Most people with CP have spastic cerebral palsy. This means they might move awkwardly and have stiff muscles.

Signs and symptoms of CP can be different for each person. Some people have very mild symptoms. Others are much more severe. Some people with CP also have other disorders, such as hearing or visual impairment or a seizure disorder.

Spina Bifida: Spina bifida is a neural tube defect that occurs when the spinal cord and spine do not develop properly. Damage can occur to the spinal cord and nerves, causing a range of problems, such as problems with ambulation, bowel and bladder function, and orthopedic issues. Complications of spina bifida may also cause learning disabilities. The risk of spina bifida can be significantly decreased if women take daily folic acid during pregnancy.

Autism Spectrum Disorder (ASD): Autism spectrum disorder is a developmental disability that affects social and communication skills. People with ASD exhibit repetitive behavior (for example, putting things in a certain order). Intensely focused interests (for example, learning everything about trains) are also common. Changes in routine or surroundings may cause people with ASD to become extremely upset.

There is no known exact cause of ASD, although studies suggest that genetics and environment play a part. Males are more likely to have ASD. Making a diagnosis involves a comprehensive process. Many people with ASD have some degree of intellectual disability. They may also have sensory, sleep, and nutritional problems and seizures, among other issues.

Treatment includes physical, speech, and occupational therapy, along with social skills training. Dietary and allergy evaluation and careful nutritional management can also benefit people with ASD.

Fragile X Syndrome (FXS): Fragile X syndrome is a genetic disorder causing inherited intellectual disability. Fragile X syndrome is caused by a problem with a gene needed for brain development. Some people with FXS show no signs. Others may experience significant cognitive, social, emotional, speech, and language problems. FXS affects both males and females; females, however, can have milder symptoms. Other problems are associated with fragile X syndrome, including intellectual disability and autism spectrum disorder. Diagnosis is made through a blood test. There is no cure for this syndrome. Certain types of therapy, such as physical, speech, or behavioral, along with medication, may help. Early intervention may provide a higher degree of success and a better quality of life.

Guidelines: Developmental Disabilities

G   Treat adult residents as adults, regardless of their intellectual abilities.

G   Praise and encourage often, especially positive behavior.

G   Help teach the resident to perform ADLs by dividing a task into small steps.

G   Repeat words to ensure understanding.

G   Talk to residents even if they cannot speak. Use alternate methods of communication as directed.

G   Promote independence while ensuring safety. Assist with safe activities and motor functions that are difficult.

G   Prevent falls in residents who have balance problems.

G   Encourage residents to follow special diets and know any food allergies residents may have.

G   Encourage social interaction.

G   Always be patient.

Chapter Review

1. What do the terms *health* and *wellness* mean (LO 2)?

2. Describe what holistic health care involves (LO 3).

3. What are psychosocial needs (LO 3)?

4. What is cultural diversity (LO 5)?

5. What is cultural competence (LO 5)?

6. If an NA encounters a sexual situation between two consenting residents, what should she do (LO 9)?

7. What should an NA do if she sees a resident being sexually abused (LO 9)?

8. What is a stereotype (LO 11)?

9. Why should stereotyping be avoided (LO 11)?

10. Why is it important for NAs to treat residents who are developmentally disabled as adults, regardless of their behavior (LO 12)?

Multiple Choice

11. Which of the following is an example of a physical need (LO 4)?
(A) Acceptance
(B) Sleep
(C) Success
(D) Affection

12. Which of the following is an example of a psychosocial need (LO 4)?
(A) Water
(B) Rest
(C) Independence
(D) Food

13. According to Maslow, which of the following needs must be met first (LO 4)?
(A) Physical needs
(B) Safety needs
(C) Psychosocial needs
(D) Need for self-esteem

14. Which of the following terms describes a family made up of one parent and one child (LO 6)?
(A) Blended family
(B) Extended family
(C) Nuclear family
(D) Single-parent family

15. Which of the following is the best example of an extended family (LO 6)?
(A) Mother, grandmother, and aunt living together
(B) Father and son living together
(C) Mother, father, and daughter living together
(D) Divorced mother and daughter living together

16. Which of the following would be the best response by the NA if a resident wants to discuss health concerns he has (LO 7)?
(A) "Everything works out for the best."
(B) "I understand you're scared. Can you tell me more?"
(C) "I read about a new medication that could help you."
(D) "It's better for you to talk to your daughter rather than me."

17. Which of the following sentences is true of spiritual beliefs (LO 8)?
(A) All residents have the same spiritual needs.
(B) NAs should let residents know when they do not agree with residents' beliefs.
(C) NAs should give privacy for prayer if residents request it.
(D) NAs should insist that residents attend church services when residents seem lonely.

18. During which stage of human development might girls reach puberty (LO 10)?
(A) Young adulthood
(B) School-age
(C) Preadolescence
(D) Preschool

6
Infection Prevention and Control

It Was Handwashing, Plain and Simple!

Ignaz Semmelweis (1818-1865) was a Hungarian doctor who practiced and taught medicine in Vienna, Austria during the mid-1800s. He noted that the death rate from childbed fever, or puerperal fever (a bacterial infection of the female reproductive organs after giving birth), was higher on a certain maternity ward than on a similar ward at the same facility. The only difference he could find was that doctors and medical students came to the ward where the death rate was higher right after dissecting corpses in the autopsy rooms. The second ward, where the midwives worked, had a much lower death rate. The midwives did not go into the autopsy rooms.

Semmelweis asked the doctors and the medical students to first wash their hands and then soak them in a special solution before and after examining the maternity patients. After this process was initiated, the death rate from childbed fever dropped dramatically. Semmelweis eventually wrote a book on his groundbreaking discovery.

"Cleanliness is a great virtue."
Charles B. Fairbanks, 1827–1859

"The biggest problem in the world could have been solved when it was small."
Witter Bynner, 1881–1968,
The Way of Life According to Laotzu

1. Define important words in this chapter

antimicrobial: an agent that destroys, resists, or prevents the development of pathogens.

autoclave: an appliance used to sterilize medical instruments or other objects by using steam under pressure.

bloodborne pathogens: microorganisms found in human blood that can cause infection and disease.

Bloodborne Pathogen Standard: federal law requiring that healthcare facilities protect employees from bloodborne health hazards.

body fluids: tears, saliva, sputum (mucus coughed up), urine, feces, semen, vaginal secretions, pus or other wound drainage, and vomit.

carbapenem-resistant *Enterobacteriaceae* (CRE): bacteria (*Enterobacteriaceae*) that have developed resistance to carbapenems, which is a category of antibiotics.

carrier: person who carries a pathogen, usually without signs or symptoms of disease, but who can still spread the disease.

catheter: tube inserted through the skin or into a body opening that is used to administer or drain fluid.

C. difficile or C. diff: an abbreviation for *Clostridioides difficile* (formerly *Clostridium difficile*); a bacterium that is spread by spores in feces that are difficult to kill; it causes symptoms such as diarrhea and nausea and can lead to serious inflammation of the colon (colitis).

Centers for Disease Control and Prevention (CDC): federal government agency responsible for improving the overall health and safety of the people in the United States.

clean: in health care, a condition in which an object is not contaminated with pathogens.

communicable disease: an infectious disease transmissible by direct contact or by indirect contact.

contagious disease: a type of communicable disease that spreads quickly from person to person.

contaminated: soiled, unclean; having disease-causing organisms or infectious material on it.

cross-infection: the physical movement or transfer of harmful bacteria from one person, object, or place to another, or from one part of the body to another.

dehydration: an excessive loss of water from the body; a condition that occurs when fluid loss is greater than fluid intake.

direct contact: way to transmit pathogens through touching the infected person or his secretions.

dirty: in health care, a condition in which an object has been contaminated with pathogens.

disinfection: process that destroys most, but not all, pathogens and other types of microorganisms.

doff: to remove.

don: to put on.

drainage: flow of fluids from a wound or cavity.

exposure control plan: plan that outlines specific work practices to prevent exposure to infectious material and identifies step-by-step procedures to follow when exposures do occur.

exposure incident: specific eye, mouth, other mucous membrane, nonintact skin, or parenteral contact with blood or other potentially infectious materials that results from the performance of an employee's duties.

fomite: an object that is contaminated with a pathogen and can spread the pathogen to another person.

hand hygiene: washing hands with either plain or antiseptic soap and water and using alcohol-based hand rubs.

hand rub: an alcohol-containing preparation designed for application to the hands for reducing the number of microorganisms on the hands.

healthcare-associated infection (HAI): an infection acquired within a healthcare setting during the delivery of medical care.

hepatitis: inflammation of the liver caused by certain viruses and other factors, such as alcohol abuse, some medications, and trauma.

immunity: resistance to infection by a specific pathogen.

incubation period: the period of time between exposure to a pathogen and the time it causes visible signs and symptoms of disease or illness.

indirect contact: way to transmit pathogens by touching something contaminated by the infected person.

infection: the state resulting from pathogens invading the body and multiplying.

infection prevention: set of methods used to prevent and control the spread of disease.

infectious disease: any disease caused by growth of a pathogen.

isolate: to keep something separate, or by itself.

localized infection: an infection that is limited to a specific location in the body and has local symptoms.

malnutrition: a serious condition in which a person is not getting proper nutrition.

medical asepsis: measures used to reduce, remove, and control the spread of pathogens.

microbe: a living thing or organism that is so small that it is only visible under a microscope; also called *microorganism*.

microorganism (MO): a living thing or organism that is so small that it is only visible under a microscope; also called *microbe*.

MRSA: an abbreviation for *methicillin-resistant Staphylococcus*; bacteria (*Staphylococcus aureus*) that have developed resistance to the antibiotic methicillin.

mucous membranes: the membranes that line body cavities that open to the outside of the body, such as the linings of the mouth, nose, eyes, rectum, or genitals.

multidrug-resistant organisms (MDROs): microorganisms, mostly bacteria, that are resistant to one or more antimicrobial agents that are commonly used for treatment.

noncommunicable disease: a disease not capable of being spread from one person to another.

nonintact skin: skin that is broken by abrasions, cuts, rashes, acne, pimples, lesions, surgical incisions, or boils.

normal flora: microorganisms that normally live in and on the body and do not cause harm in a healthy person, as long as the flora remain in that particular location.

Occupational Safety and Health Administration (OSHA): a federal government agency that makes and enforces rules to protect workers from hazards on the job.

pathogens: microorganisms that are capable of causing infection and disease.

perineal care: care of the genitals and anal area.

personal protective equipment (PPE): equipment that helps protect employees from serious workplace injuries or illnesses resulting from contact with workplace hazards.

reinfection: being infected again with the same pathogen.

resistance: the body's ability to prevent infection and disease.

sanitation: ways individuals and communities maintain clean, hygienic conditions that help prevent disease, such as the disposal of sewage and solid waste.

Standard Precautions: a method of infection prevention in which all blood, body fluids, nonintact skin, and mucous membranes are treated as if they were infected with an infectious disease.

sterilization: cleaning measure that destroys all microorganisms, including pathogens.

surgical asepsis: the state of being completely free of microorganisms; also called *sterile technique.*

systemic infection: an infection that is in the bloodstream and is spread throughout the body, causing general symptoms.

transmission: the way and means by which disease is spread.

vaccine: a product that is administered to produce immunity to a specific disease.

VRE: an abbreviation for *vancomycin-resistant Enterococcus*; bacteria (*enterococci*) that have developed resistance to the antibiotic vancomycin.

2. Define *infection prevention* and discuss types of infections

Individuals and communities strive to maintain clean conditions in order to help prevent the spread of disease. This is known as **sanitation**. In care facilities, **infection prevention** is the set of methods used to prevent and control the spread of disease. Facilities must have an infection preventionist on staff. This licensed health professional is responsible for the infection control program in the facility. Infection prevention and control is the responsibility of all care team members. Nursing assistants must know and follow their facility's policies relating to infection prevention; these policies help protect staff members, residents, visitors, and others from disease.

A **microorganism (MO)** is a living thing or organism that is so small that it is only visible under a microscope. It is also called a **microbe**. Microorganisms are always present in the environment (Fig. 6-1). **Infections** are caused by **pathogens**, which are harmful microorganisms. For infections to develop, pathogens must invade and grow within the human body.

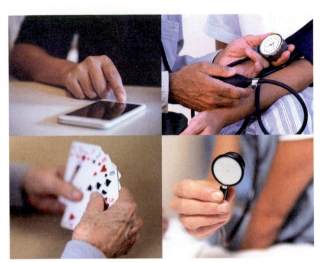

Fig. 6-1. Microorganisms are always present in the environment. They are on almost everything a person touches.

There are two main types of infections, localized and systemic. A **localized infection** is limited to a specific location in the body. It has local symptoms, which are near the site of infection. For example, if the eye becomes infected, the area around it might be red, swollen, painful, and warm. A **systemic infection** occurs when pathogens enter the bloodstream and move throughout the body. It causes general symptoms, such as fever, chills, or mental confusion. Sepsis is a condition caused by a systemic infection. There is more information about sepsis later in this chapter and in Chapter 26.

A special type of infection that can be localized or systemic is a **healthcare-associated infection (HAI)**. A healthcare-associated infection is an infection acquired within a healthcare setting during the delivery of medical care. Healthcare settings include long-term care facilities, hospitals, ambulatory care settings, and home care. HAIs can be mild or life-threatening.

Observing and Reporting: Infection

Signs and symptoms of infection must be reported to the nurse promptly. Not reporting immediately can put residents at risk for more serious infections. If you forget to report a resident's

symptoms before leaving the facility, by the time you return, the infection might have traveled into the bloodstream and become systemic. Always report the following signs and symptoms right away.

Signs and symptoms of a localized infection include the following:

O/R Redness

O/R Swelling

O/R Pain

O/R Heat

O/R **Drainage** (fluid from a wound or cavity)

Signs and symptoms of a systemic infection include the following:

O/R Fever

O/R Chills

O/R Headache

O/R Change in other vital signs

O/R Nausea, vomiting, and diarrhea

O/R Mental confusion

An **infectious disease** is a disease caused by a pathogen. The pathogen will cause an infection if conditions are right. Pathogens grow best in warm, dark, and moist places where food is present and in hosts who have low resistance. **Resistance** is the body's ability to prevent infection and disease. There are two types of infectious diseases: communicable and noncommunicable.

A **communicable disease** is an infectious disease that is transmitted by direct contact with the infected person or his secretions, or indirectly, by touching objects contaminated by the infected person. An example of a communicable disease is influenza. A **contagious disease** is a type of communicable disease that spreads quickly from person to person. Measles is an example of a contagious disease. A **noncommunicable disease** is a disease not capable of being spread from one person to another. For example, a person who has emphysema, a disease of the lungs, is not contagious to others.

By using proper infection prevention methods, NAs can help prevent residents, visitors, and staff members from acquiring an infection from another person, object, place, or from one part of the body to another. This is called **cross-infection**, or cross-contamination. Infection prevention methods will also help protect a person from being infected again with the same pathogen, called **reinfection**.

3. Discuss terms related to infection prevention

Infection prevention is about breaking the chain of infection, which is discussed in the next learning objective. **Transmission** of disease can be blocked by using proper infection prevention practices, such as handwashing, which are a part of **medical asepsis**. Medical asepsis is used in all healthcare facilities. Before asepsis is explained in more detail, some terms must be understood.

In health care, an object can be called **clean** if it is not **contaminated** with pathogens. An object that is **dirty** has been contaminated with pathogens.

Cleaning measures like disinfection and sterilization decrease the spread of pathogens that could cause disease. **Disinfection** means that most, but not all, pathogens are destroyed. **Sterilization** means all microorganisms are destroyed, including those that form spores. Spore-forming microorganisms are a special group of organisms that produce a protective covering that is difficult to penetrate. An **autoclave** is a type of special equipment used to sterilize objects and kill pathogens that form spores. This machine creates hot steam under pressure for a period of time to kill all microorganisms. There are other types of devices used to kill

microorganisms. These sterilizing devices use toxic gases, dry heat, strong chemical solutions, or radiation.

The goal of medical asepsis is to prevent the spread of pathogens by keeping a facility as clean as possible. This does not mean that the facility is free from all microorganisms. The only way to make an area or object completely free of microorganisms is to use **surgical asepsis**, also known as *sterile technique*. Surgical asepsis makes an object or area sterile. This means it is completely free of all microorganisms. There may be times when NAs will assist a nurse with a procedure that requires sterile technique. Special training may be required to help with this type of procedure. Chapter 18 has more information on the sterile field, sterile gloves, and sterile dressings. These are all used in surgical asepsis.

Facilities have separate rooms or areas for clean and dirty items, such as equipment, linen, and supplies. They are normally called the *clean* and the *dirty* or *contaminated* utility rooms. NAs should wash their hands before entering clean rooms. This helps keep the equipment in this room clean.

The contaminated or dirty utility room is separate from the clean utility room. It is used to store equipment that is not needed by the resident. Supplies in this room, such as trash bags, are not considered clean. A sink is usually in this room. NAs should wash their hands before leaving dirty rooms so that pathogens are not transferred to other areas in the facility. After washing hands, NAs should not touch anything in the dirty utility room, including the door handle. If this occurs, hands must be washed again.

NAs will be told where these rooms are located and what types of equipment and supplies are found in each room. More information about handling linen and equipment is located in Learning Objective 9 of this chapter.

4. Describe the chain of infection

The chain of infection describes how disease is transmitted from one human being to another (Fig. 6-2). There are six links in the chain of infection:

- Link 1: Causative agent
- Link 2: Reservoir
- Link 3: Portal of exit
- Link 4: Mode of transmission
- Link 5: Portal of entry
- Link 6: Susceptible host

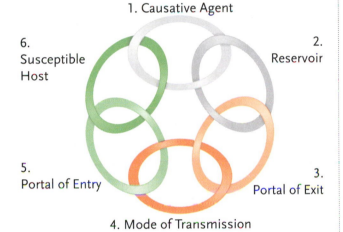

Fig. 6-2. The chain of infection.

If one of the links in the chain of infection is broken, transmission of infection can be prevented.

Chain Link 1: The causative agent is a pathogenic microorganism that causes disease. Microorganisms are small living bodies that cannot be seen without a microscope. They are everywhere—on skin, in food, in the air, and in water. Causative agents include bacteria, viruses, fungi, and parasites.

Normal flora are the microorganisms that normally live in and on the body without causing harm to a healthy person, as long as the flora remain in that particular location. When they enter a different part of the body, they may cause an infection.

There is a waiting period between the time the body is exposed to the pathogen and the time it causes visible signs and symptoms of disease or illness. This period is called an **incubation period**. Examples of incubation periods include the following

- Chickenpox: 10–21 days
- Influenza (flu): 1–4 days
- Measles: 7–21 days

Chain Link 2: A reservoir is where the pathogen lives and multiplies. A reservoir can be a human, an animal, a plant, soil, or a substance. Warm, dark, and moist places are the ideal environments for microorganisms to live, grow, and multiply. Some microorganisms need oxygen to survive while others do not. The blood and the lungs are examples of reservoirs.

The human reservoir may be a person with an active disease or a person carrying the disease (a **carrier**). A human carrier carries the disease, but usually does not show any signs or symptoms at the time he spreads the disease. This carrier may or may not get the disease later.

Chain Link 3: There can be different exit routes, or portals of exit, from a reservoir. The portal of exit is any opening on an infected person that allows pathogens to leave (Fig. 6-3). These include the nose, mouth, eyes, or a cut in the skin.

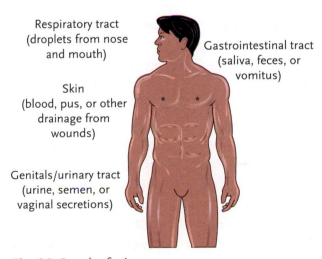

Fig. 6-3. Portals of exit.

Chain Link 4: The mode of transmission describes how the pathogen travels. The transmission of an infectious disease occurs in different ways. The main routes of transmission are contact, droplet, and airborne transmission. The primary route of disease transmission within the healthcare setting is via the hands of healthcare workers.

Contact transmission occurs through contact with the person's blood or body fluids that are contaminated by the pathogen. **Body fluids** include tears, saliva, sputum (mucus coughed up), urine, feces, semen, vaginal secretions, pus or other wound drainage, and vomit. **Direct contact** happens by touching the infected person or her secretions. **Indirect contact** results from touching an object contaminated by the infected person. These objects are also called *fomites*. A **fomite** is an object that has been contaminated with a pathogen. Fomites may be things like infected food, water, food utensils, bedpans, needles, dressings, or bed linens.

Droplet transmission occurs when the pathogen travels short distances after being expelled. Droplets normally do not travel more than six feet. Droplets can be created when the infected person coughs, sneezes, or talks. Laughing, suctioning, singing, and spitting may also transmit droplets. A susceptible host (Link 6) inhales contaminated droplets and may get an infection.

In airborne transmission, the pathogen is transmitted through the air after being expelled. The pathogen is carried a distance on air currents. A pathogen can also be carried by dust. A susceptible host (Link 6) inhales contaminated moisture or dust, which may cause an infection.

Chain Link 5: Pathogens enter the human host through different portals of entry. The portal of entry is any body opening on an uninfected person that allows pathogens to enter (Fig. 6-4). These include the nose, mouth, eyes, and other mucous membranes, cuts in the skin, and cracked skin. **Mucous membranes** are the

membranes that line body cavities that open to the outside of the body. These include the linings of the mouth, nose, eyes, rectum, and genitals.

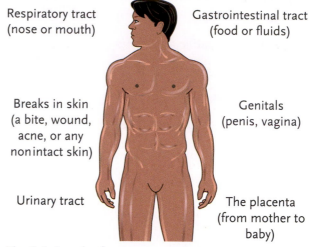

Respiratory tract (nose or mouth)

Gastrointestinal tract (food or fluids)

Breaks in skin (a bite, wound, acne, or any nonintact skin)

Genitals (penis, vagina)

Urinary tract

The placenta (from mother to baby)

Fig. 6-4. Portals of entry.

When a pathogen invades the body, it can cause an infection. Many areas of the body are protected from invading pathogens. A sort of body "armor" works with the immune system to help protect the body from harmful bacteria. The box below describes how the body keeps itself healthy.

The Human Body's Defenses

Nasal passages: Mucous membranes have cilia, tiny hairs in the nose that trap microorganisms.

Epidermis: As long as skin stays intact and undamaged, microorganisms cannot get inside.

Lungs: Cilia move microbes, mucus, and debris up and out of the airways.

Mouth: Saliva has a protein called *lactoferrin* that blocks the growth of pathogens.

Eyes: The eyes have tears that protect them by cleaning out microorganisms.

GI (gastrointestinal) tract: The GI tract has "good" microorganisms, called *normal flora*, that prevent the growth of "bad" microorganisms, or pathogens. In addition, the strong acid environment of the gastrointestinal tract prevents many microorganisms from surviving.

Vagina: The vagina has a low pH of about 3.5 to 4.5, which blocks the growth of pathogens.

Urethra: Urine rinses out pathogens from the urinary tract.

Blood cells: White blood cells defend the body from microorganisms and play a role in the secretion of antibodies.

Chain Link 6: A susceptible host is an uninfected person who could become ill. A person becomes a susceptible host when her resistance to disease decreases. Some reasons for lowered resistance include age, existing illnesses, fatigue, poor nutrition, lack of adequate fluid intake, certain medications, and stress. The elderly have weaker immune systems and lower resistance to pathogens. When a pathogen invades the body, it will start reproducing itself, causing tissue invasion and tissue damage.

Vaccines are products that are administered to produce **immunity** to a specific disease without causing illness or disease. The immunity may not last forever.

Trivia

Edward Jenner's Amazing Discovery

In 18th-century England, smallpox was a very common, horribly disfiguring disease. A doctor at that time, Edward Jenner (1749–1823), noticed that people who were exposed to cowpox, such as the milkmaids who milked cows, would develop a small sore and then never get smallpox. He then developed a vaccine from the cowpox sores to give immunity to smallpox. After he injected the matter from the sore into a boy, James Phipps, he tested the vaccine by trying to give James the disease more than once. Each time, Jenner found that little James was immune to the disease.

5. Explain why the elderly are at a higher risk for infection

Residents are at a greater risk of acquiring infections while living in a facility. As people age, multiple changes occur to increase susceptibility to infection (Fig. 6-5). Elderly people are hospitalized more often, which increases their chances

for acquiring a healthcare-associated infection (HAI). In addition, the elderly may have more serious infections with longer recovery times.

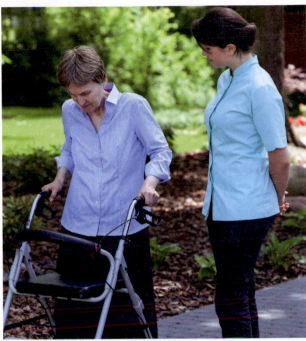

Fig. 6-5. *The elderly are at higher risk for infection due to weaker immune systems, limited mobility, thinner skin, slow wound healing, and many other reasons.*

As people age, their skin becomes less elastic. The skin's oil glands become less productive, leading to dryness and thinning of the skin layers. This can cause skin to tear easily and delays the healing process. Skin changes and limited mobility increase the risk of pressure injuries and skin infections.

Bones become more brittle and can break more easily. Broken bones increase the risk of infection. Decreased circulation and slow wound healing also contribute to infections in the elderly.

Elderly people may require catheters for urinary elimination. **Catheters** and other types of tubing, such as feeding tubes, can greatly increase the risk of infections.

Older adults are at risk for dehydration and **malnutrition**. A person who is malnourished is not getting the proper nutrition. **Dehydration** occurs when there is an excessive loss of water from the body. Both dehydration and malnutrition are serious problems. They may be caused by a lack of thirst and appetite, certain illnesses, weakness, or medications. When cells do not get proper nutrients and fluids, the chance of infection greatly increases.

One method of reducing infection is to keep residents as healthy as possible by promoting healthy habits and using proper infection prevention methods. This is required of all staff members. There is more information about how to keep residents infection-free in Chapter 24.

6. Describe Centers for Disease Control and Prevention (CDC) and explain Standard Precautions

Centers for Disease Control and Prevention (**CDC**, cdc.gov) is a federal government agency that issues guidelines to protect and improve health. It promotes public health and safety through education and tries to prevent and control disease. In 1996, the CDC created a new infection prevention system to reduce the risk of contracting infectious diseases in healthcare settings. In 2007, some additions and changes were made to this system.

There are two levels of precautions within the infection prevention system recommended by the CDC: Standard Precautions and Transmission-Based Precautions.

Following **Standard Precautions** means treating blood, body fluids, nonintact skin, and mucous membranes as if they were infected. Body fluids include tears, saliva, sputum (mucus coughed up), urine, feces, semen, vaginal secretions, pus or other wound drainage, and vomit. They do not include sweat.

Standard Precautions must be used with every resident. An NA cannot tell by looking at residents or even by reading their medical charts if they have a communicable disease such as tuberculosis or hepatitis.

Guidelines: Standard Precautions

G **Wash your hands** before putting on gloves. Wash your hands immediately after removing gloves. Do not touch clean objects with your used gloves.

G **Wear gloves** if you may come into contact with any of the following: blood, body fluids, secretions or excretions, broken or open skin, human tissue, or mucous membranes (linings of the eyes, nose, mouth, vagina, penis, or rectum).

G **Remove gloves** immediately when finished with a procedure and wash your hands.

G **Immediately wash all skin surfaces that have been contaminated** with blood and body fluids.

G **Wear a disposable gown** that is resistant to body fluids if you may come into contact with blood, body fluids, or secretions or excretions, or when splashing or spraying blood or body fluids is likely.

G **Wear a mask, protective goggles, and/or face shield** if you may come into contact with blood, body fluids, or secretions or excretions, or when splashing or spraying blood or body fluids is likely.

G **Wear gloves and use caution when handling razor blades, needles, and other sharps.** Avoid nicks or cuts when shaving residents. Place sharps carefully in a biohazard container for sharps. Biohazard containers used for sharps are puncture-resistant, leakproof containers. They are clearly labeled and warn of the danger of the contents inside (Figs. 6-6 and 6-7). There are also biohazard bags that are used for biomedical waste that is not sharp, such as soiled dressings, contaminated tubing, and other items. The Occupational Safety and Health Administration (OSHA) recommends that biomedical/biohazard waste be disposed of at the *point of origin*, or where the waste occurs.

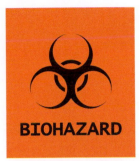

Fig. 6-6. *This label indicates that the material is potentially infectious.*

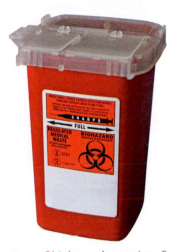

Fig. 6-7. *One type of biohazard container for sharps.*

G **Never attempt to recap needles or sharps after use**. You might stick yourself. Dispose of them in a biohazard container for sharps.

G **Bag all disposable contaminated supplies**. Dispose of them according to your facility's policy. Special containers are used for disposal. Place nondisposable contaminated supplies, such as linens and reusable equipment, in the proper container.

G **Clean all surfaces that may be contaminated with infectious waste**. Follow facility policy. Examples of these areas are overbed tables, beds, wheelchairs, and shower chairs.

G **Remember that Standard Precautions must be practiced on every single person in your care.** Standard Precautions help reduce the risk of acquiring or transmitting disease.

In addition to Standard Precautions, here are general guidelines for preventing infection in a facility:

Guidelines: Additional Ways to Prevent Infection

G Clean a cut or break in your skin immediately with a facility-approved disinfecting product.

G Turn your head away from others and cover your mouth and nose with a tissue when coughing or sneezing. Immediately dispose of tissues in the nearest no-touch waste container. If you do not have a tissue, cough or sneeze into your upper sleeve or elbow, not your hands. After coughing or sneezing, wash your hands immediately or use an alcohol-based hand rub.

G Never share a resident's personal items with another resident. Keep all personal items separate and labeled with the resident's name and room number.

G Never transfer personal items or any kind of equipment from one room to another. An exception is something like your stethoscope. You must disinfect the part of your stethoscope that touches a resident after each use.

G Hold all equipment, personal care items, and soiled laundry and linens away from your uniform while carrying them.

G Do not use equipment that has been dropped on the floor. Dispose of it properly and obtain new/clean items.

G Clean all equipment used by residents after use. Follow the facility's guidelines for disinfection.

G Clean all common areas (areas used by more than one resident) after use.

G Remove food or soiled eating utensils in residents' rooms after food trays have been picked up.

G Change water cups often. Write the date on the cup each time it is changed, along with the resident's name and room number.

G Clean residents' toothbrushes and shaving equipment often, following facility policy.

Place in the proper container that is clearly labeled following use.

G   Never place contaminated items like bedpans or any other dirty items on the overbed table. There is more information about unit equipment in Chapter 10.

G   When cleaning anything, move from the cleanest to the dirtiest area.

Respiratory Hygiene/Cough Etiquette

As part of Standard Precautions, the CDC developed guidelines for all persons entering facilities who show any signs of respiratory illnesses. The guidelines are listed below:

• Covering the nose and mouth with a tissue when coughing or sneezing, or coughing or sneezing into the upper sleeve or elbow, not the hands

• Promptly disposing of tissues in the nearest no-touch waste container

• Cleaning hands after coughing or sneezing by washing them with soap and water or using an alcohol-based hand rub or antiseptic handwash

• Wearing special masks and turning one's head away from others when coughing

• Encouraging coughing persons to sit at least three feet from others in common waiting areas

7. Define *hand hygiene* and identify when to wash hands

NAs use their hands constantly while they work. Microorganisms are on everything they touch. The single most common way for healthcare-associated infections (HAIs) to be spread is via the hands of healthcare workers. Handwashing is the most important thing NAs can do to prevent the spread of disease (Fig. 6-8).

The CDC has defined **hand hygiene** as washing hands with either plain or antiseptic soap and water or using alcohol-based hand rubs. Alcohol-based hand rubs (often referred to as a **hand rub** or *hand sanitizer*) include gels, rinses, and foams that do not require the use of water.

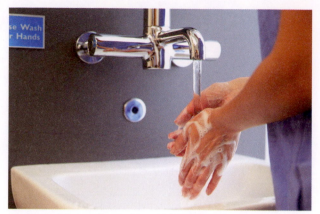

Fig. 6-8. *All people working in health care must wash their hands often. Handwashing is the most effective measure in preventing the spread of disease.*

Alcohol-based hand rubs have proven effective in reducing bacteria on the skin. However, they are not a substitute for frequent, proper handwashing. When hands are visibly soiled, they should be washed using plain or antimicrobial soap and water. An **antimicrobial** agent destroys, resists, or prevents the development of pathogens. Hand rubs can be used in addition to handwashing any time hands are not visibly soiled. When using a hand rub, the hands must be rubbed together until the product has completely dried. Hand lotion can help prevent dry, cracked skin.

NAs should keep their nails short, smooth, and clean. Artificial nails (acrylic, gel, or wraps) should not be worn, because they harbor bacteria and increase the risk of contamination even if hands are washed often. NAs should not wear rings and bracelets while working, because they may increase the risk of contamination. These items should be left at home.

NAs should wash their hands at these times:

• When first arriving at work

• Whenever hands are visibly soiled

• Before, between, and after all contact with residents

• Before putting on gloves and after removing gloves

• Before and after touching meal trays and/or handling food

- Before and after feeding residents
- Before entering a clean supply room
- Before getting clean linen
- Before leaving a dirty supply room
- Before and after eating
- After contact with blood or any body fluids, mucous membranes, nonintact skin, or wound dressings
- After changing incontinence pads
- After handling contaminated items
- After contact with any object, including medical equipment, in the resident's room
- After touching garbage
- After cleaning spills or picking up anything from the floor
- Before and after using the toilet
- After blowing the nose, wiping the nose, or coughing or sneezing
- After smoking
- After touching areas on the body, such as the nose, mouth, eyes, face, ears, or hair
- After touching jewelry
- After handling animals/pets and after contact with pet care items
- Before leaving the facility and after arriving home from work, before touching anything or anyone

Washing hands (hand hygiene) ▶

Equipment: soap, paper towels

1. Turn on the water at the sink. Keep your clothes dry because moisture breeds bacteria. Do not let your clothing touch the outside portion of the sink or counter.

2. Wet your hands and wrists thoroughly (Fig. 6-9).

3. Apply soap to your hands.

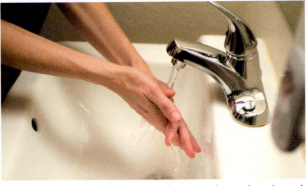

Fig. 6-9. *Keeping arms angled downward, wet hands and wrists thoroughly.*

4. Keep your hands lower than your elbows and your fingertips down. Rub hands together and fingers between each other to create a lather. Lather all surfaces of wrists, fingers, and hands, using friction for at least 20 seconds (Fig. 6-10).

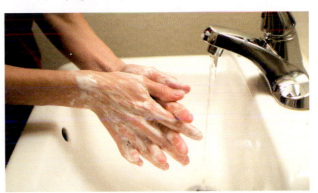

Fig. 6-10. *Using friction for at least 20 seconds, lather all surfaces of fingers and hands.*

5. Clean your nails by rubbing them in the palm of your other hand.

6. Keep your hands lower than your elbows and your fingertips down. Being careful not to touch the sink, rinse thoroughly under running water. Rinse all surfaces of your wrists and hands. Run water down from your wrists to your fingertips. Do not run water over unwashed arms down to clean hands.

7. Use a clean, dry paper towel to dry all surfaces of your fingers, hands, and wrists, starting at the fingertips. Do not wipe the towel on unwashed forearms and then wipe your

clean hands. Discard the paper towel in the waste container without touching the container. If your hands touch the sink or wastebasket, start over.

8. Use a clean, dry paper towel to turn off the faucet (Fig. 6-11). Discard the towel in the waste container. Do not contaminate your hands by touching the surface of the sink or faucet. Avoid touching door handles when leaving bathrooms. Use a paper towel to open the door.

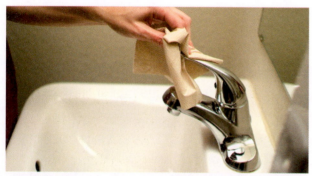

Fig. 6-11. Use a clean, dry paper towel to turn off the faucet so that you do not contaminate your hands.

Residents' Rights

Handwashing

NAs must always wash their hands before and after giving resident care. Microorganisms are on everything a person touches. Washing hands frequently helps prevent the spread of disease.

8. Discuss the use of personal protective equipment (PPE) in facilities

Personal protective equipment (PPE) is equipment that helps protect employees from serious workplace injuries or illnesses resulting from contact with workplace hazards. In long-term care facilities, PPE helps protect NAs from contact with potentially infectious material.

Personal protective equipment includes gloves, gowns, masks, goggles, and face shields. Gloves protect the hands and are the type of PPE used most often by all caregivers. Gowns protect the skin and/or clothing. Masks protect the mouth and nose. Goggles protect the eyes, and face shields protect the entire face—the eyes, nose, and mouth.

Employers are responsible for providing NAs with the appropriate PPE to wear. OSHA requires that PPE be easy to access and readily available in a variety of sizes. The type of PPE worn depends on what kind of exposure may be encountered. For example, a chance of coming into contact with spraying or splashing blood or body fluids requires a gown, gloves, and a mask and goggles or face shield. PPE selection also depends on the type of Transmission-Based Precautions that are ordered for a resident. More information about these precautions may be found in Learning Objective 11.

NAs have a responsibility to know how to put on **(don)**, use, and remove **(doff)** PPE correctly. NAs must always perform hand hygiene before and after removing and disposing of PPE.

Gloves

There are two types of gloves: nonsterile and sterile. Nonsterile gloves are used for basic care in a facility. They come in different sizes and may be made of nitrile or vinyl. Gloves should fit the hands comfortably and should not be too loose or too tight.

Gloves should always be worn for the following tasks:

- Any time the caregiver may come into contact with blood or any body fluid, open wounds, or mucous membranes

- When performing or helping with mouth care or care of any mucous membrane

- When performing or helping with **perineal care** (care of the genitals and anal area)

- When performing care on **nonintact skin**—skin that is broken by abrasions, cuts, rashes, acne, pimples, lesions, surgical incisions, or boils

- When the caregiver has any open sores or cuts on his hands

- When shaving a resident

- When disposing of soiled bed linens, gowns, dressings, and pads

- When having direct contact with residents who require Contact Precautions (a type of Transmission-Based Precaution; information is in Learning Objective 11)

- When touching surfaces or equipment that either are visibly contaminated or may be contaminated

Disposable gloves can only be worn once; they cannot be washed or reused. Gloves should be changed immediately if they become wet, worn, soiled, or torn. Gloves should also be changed before contact with mucous membranes or broken skin. After removing gloves, the NA should wash his hands before donning new gloves.

Nonintact areas should be covered with bandages or gauze before putting on gloves; this is known as wearing or applying a double barrier. When wearing gloves, the NA should always work from the cleanest to the dirtiest area. This means that clean surfaces or areas should be touched before contaminated ones. The NA should not adjust PPE or touch his face while wearing gloves.

Putting on (donning) gloves ▶

1. Wash your hands.

2. If you are right-handed, slide one glove on your left hand (reverse if left-handed).

3. Using your gloved hand, slide the other hand into the second glove.

4. Interlace your fingers to smooth out folds and create a comfortable fit.

5. Check for tears, holes, cracks, or discolored spots. Replace the glove if needed.

6. Adjust the gloves until they are pulled up over your wrists and fit correctly. If wearing a gown, pull the cuffs of the gloves over the sleeves of the gown (Fig. 6-12).

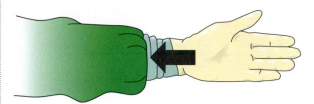

Fig. 6-12. *Adjust gloves until they are pulled up over the sleeves of the gown.*

Gloves should be removed immediately after use and before caring for another resident. The NA should wash his hands. He should be careful not to contaminate his skin or clothing when removing gloves. Gloves are worn to protect the skin from becoming contaminated. After giving care, gloves are contaminated. If an NA opens a door with a gloved hand, the doorknob becomes contaminated. Later, anyone who opens the door with an ungloved hand will be touching a contaminated surface. Before touching surfaces or leaving residents' rooms, the NA must remove gloves and wash his hands. Afterward, new gloves can be donned if needed.

Removing (doffing) gloves ▶

1. Touch only the outside of one glove. With one gloved hand, grasp the other glove at the palm and pull the glove off (Fig. 6-13).

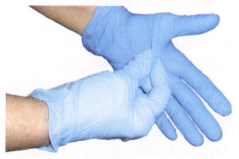

Fig. 6-13. *Grasp the glove at the palm and pull it off.*

2. With the fingertips of your gloved hand, hold the glove you just removed. With your un-gloved hand, slip two fingers underneath the cuff of the remaining glove at the wrist. Do not touch any part of the outside of the glove (Fig. 6-14).

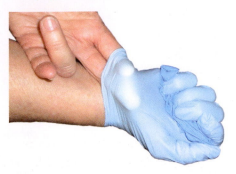

Fig. 6-14. Reach inside the glove at the wrist, without touching any part of the outside of the glove.

3. Pull down, turning this glove inside out and over the first glove as you remove it.

4. You should now be holding one glove from its clean inner side. The other glove should be inside it.

5. Drop both gloves into the proper container without contaminating yourself.

6. Wash your hands.

Gowns

Gowns protect the skin and the clothing from contamination. An NA should wear a gown in these circumstances:

- If he may come into contact with blood, body fluids, secretions or excretions, or tissue, or if splashing or spraying blood or body fluids is likely

- If his clothing will have direct contact with a resident or any contaminated equipment or surfaces that may have come into contact with the resident

- When handling any equipment that is visibly soiled or may have had contact with blood or body fluids

Gowns should fully cover the torso. They should fit comfortably over the body and have long sleeves that fit snugly at the wrists. If a gown does not fit properly, the NA should report it to the supervisor. Two gowns may need to be worn if one gown is too small to safely and completely cover the torso. If this is the case, the underlying gown is donned with the opening to the front, and the top gown is donned with the opening to the back.

Gowns are made of a fluid-resistant material. If a gown becomes wet or soiled during care, it should be discarded and a new gown should be donned. A gown can only be worn once. It should be discarded after care, before leaving the resident's room.

Putting on (donning) and removing (doffing) gown ▶

1. Wash your hands.

2. Open the gown. Hold it out in front of you and allow it to open/unfold. Do not shake the gown or touch it to the floor (Fig. 6-15). Facing the back opening of the gown, place an arm through each sleeve.

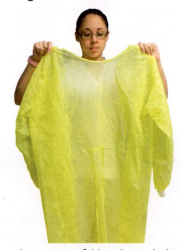

Fig. 6-15. Let the gown unfold without shaking it.

3. Fasten the neck opening.

4. Reach behind you. Pull the gown until it completely covers your clothing. Secure the gown at your waist (Fig. 6-16).

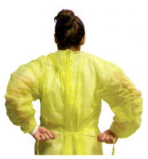

Fig. 6-16. *Reaching behind you, secure the gown at the waist.*

5. Use a gown only once and then remove and discard it. If gown becomes wet or soiled during care, remove it and put on a new gown.

6. Put on your gloves after putting on the gown. The cuffs of the gloves should overlap the cuffs of the gown (Fig. 6-17).

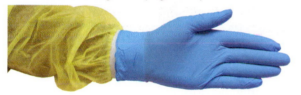

Fig. 6-17. *The cuffs of the gloves should overlap the cuffs of the gown.*

7. When removing a gown, first remove and discard gloves properly. Then unfasten the gown at the neck and waist. Remove the gown without touching the outside of the gown. Roll the dirty side in, while holding the gown away from your body. Discard the gown properly and wash your hands. Avoid touching any surface in the room with your uniform or your skin before exiting the room.

Masks and Goggles

Masks can prevent inhalation of microorganisms through the nose or mouth. They protect the nose, mouth, and mucous membranes from contamination during resident care. Masks should be worn when caring for residents who cough or sneeze or have respiratory illnesses. They should also be worn when it is likely that contact with blood or body fluids may occur.

Masks should fully cover the nose and mouth and fit snugly to prevent fluid penetration. Masks can only be worn once before they need to be discarded. If a mask becomes wet or soiled, it must be changed immediately. NAs must always remove masks after a procedure and must change masks before providing care to a different resident. Masks should not be worn in the hall; they should be discarded after care, before leaving the resident's room.

Goggles are worn with a mask and are used whenever it is likely that blood or body fluids may be splashed or sprayed into the eye area or into the eyes. Eyeglasses alone do not provide proper eye protection. Goggles should fit snugly over and around the eyes or eyeglasses.

Putting on (donning) mask and goggles ▶

1. Wash your hands.

2. Pick up the mask by the top strings or the elastic strap. Do not touch the mask where it touches your face.

3. Pull the elastic strap over your head, or if the mask has strings, tie the top strings first, then the bottom strings. Do not wear a mask hanging from only the bottom ties or straps. Masks must always be dry or they must be replaced.

4. Pinch the metal strip at the top of the mask (if part of the mask) tightly around your nose so that it feels snug (Fig. 6-18). Fit the mask snugly around your face and below the chin.

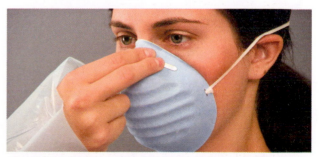

Fig. 6-18. *Adjust the metal strip until the mask fits snugly around your nose.*

5. Place the goggles over your eyes or eye-glasses. Use the headband or earpieces to secure them to your head. Make sure they fit snugly.

6. Put on your gloves after putting on the mask and goggles.

___

Gloves should be removed before removing a mask or goggles. The NA should not touch her clothing or her skin with the mask or goggles when removing them. The pieces used to secure the mask or goggles to the head are considered clean and can be touched with ungloved hands. The mask and goggles themselves are considered contaminated.

Some respiratory diseases, such as tuberculosis (TB), require special PPE to be worn. Special masks must be worn because a standard mask does not protect the caregiver from TB. These masks, called *respirators*, have a filter that protects the face and lungs. An N95 respirator is one type of special mask. The caregiver must be fitted for this mask. At least annually and any time a new model or type of mask is worn, a fit test must be done to minimize the leaking of any air from around the respirator. NAs will receive training on how to perform this check. Respirators are the only type of PPE not removed before leaving the resident's room. They must be removed after leaving the room and closing the door. More information about TB is located in Chapter 20.

Face Shields

Face shields may be worn when blood or body fluids may be splashed or sprayed into the eyes or eye area. Face shields may be worn with a mask. The face shield should cover the forehead, go below the chin, and wrap around the side of the face. The headband can secure it to the head.

Gloves should be removed before removing a face shield. The NA should not touch his clothing or his skin with the face shield when removing it. The pieces used to secure the shield are considered clean and can be touched with ungloved hands. The face shield itself is considered contaminated. Face shields should not be worn outside a resident's room.

The NA's employer will provide PPE as needed. It is the NA's responsibility to know where it is kept and how to use it. A specific order must be followed when donning and doffing PPE. The order depends on what PPE is worn and whether special precautions have been ordered.

Donning and doffing a full set of PPE

Donning (Fig. 6-19):

1. Wash your hands.

2. Put on gown.

3. Put on mask or respirator.

4. Put on goggles or face shield.

5. Put on gloves.

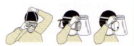

SEQUENCE FOR PUTTING ON PERSONAL PROTECTIVE EQUIPMENT (PPE)

The type of PPE used will vary based on the level of precautions required, such as standard and contact, droplet or airborne infection isolation precautions. The procedure for putting on and removing PPE should be tailored to the specific type of PPE.

1. GOWN
- Fully cover torso from neck to knees, arms to end of wrists, and wrap around the back
- Fasten in back of neck and waist

2. MASK OR RESPIRATOR
- Secure ties or elastic bands at middle of head and neck
- Fit flexible band to nose bridge
- Fit snug to face and below chin
- Fit-check respirator

3. GOGGLES OR FACE SHIELD
- Place over face and eyes and adjust to fit

4. GLOVES
- Extend to cover wrist of isolation gown

USE SAFE WORK PRACTICES TO PROTECT YOURSELF AND LIMIT THE SPREAD OF CONTAMINATION
- Keep hands away from face
- Limit surfaces touched
- Change gloves when torn or heavily contaminated
- Perform hand hygiene

Fig. 6-19. *Sequence for putting on personal protective equipment.* (IMAGE REPRINTED FROM THE CDC'S WEBSITE, WWW.CDC.GOV/HAI/PDFS/PPE/PPE-SEQUENCE.PDF)

All PPE must be removed before exiting the resident's room except a respirator, if worn. A respirator is removed after leaving the room and closing the door.

Doffing (Fig. 6-20):

1. Remove and discard gloves.

2. Remove goggles or face shield.

3. Remove and discard gown.

4. Remove and discard mask.

5. Wash your hands. Performing hand hygiene is always the final step after removing and discarding PPE. Hand hygiene should also be performed between steps if hands become contaminated at any time.

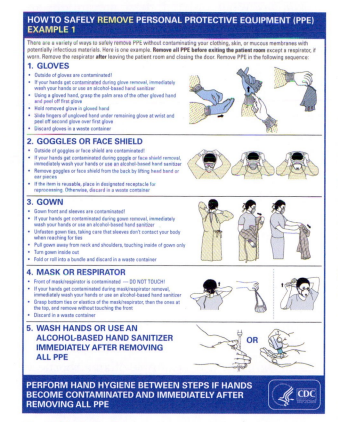

Fig. 6-20. *Order for removing personal protective equipment.* (IMAGE REPRINTED FROM THE CDC'S WEBSITE, WWW.CDC.GOV/HAI/PDFS/ PPE/PPE-SEQUENCE.PDF)

9. List guidelines for handling linen and equipment

Facilities follow guidelines set by the CDC for storing and disposing of linen and equipment. Facilities have separate areas for clean and dirty items. Soiled linen and equipment will be placed in separate containers to be cleaned or discarded. Within the dirty utility room there will be disposal containers for

- Linen

- Trash

- Equipment

- Infectious waste

Guidelines: Handling Linen and Equipment

G Wear gloves when handling, transporting, and processing soiled linens.

G When removing linen, handle it carefully. Check linen to make sure no items are left inside, especially sharps, as you remove it from the bed. Fold or roll linen so that the dirtiest area is inside and away from you.

G Hold and carry dirty linen away from your uniform.

G Do not shake dirty linen or clothes.

G Place or dispose of linen, trash, used equipment, and infectious waste in the proper containers. All sharps must be safely placed in puncture-resistant biohazard containers for sharps.

G Do not touch the inside of any disposal container.

G Do not use reusable equipment again until it has been properly cleaned and reprocessed. Dispose of all single-use, or disposable, equipment properly.

G Wear gloves when cleaning and disinfecting surfaces. Clean and disinfect beds, bedrails and all bedside equipment. Clean all frequently touched surfaces, such as doorknobs.

10. Explain how to handle spills

In a healthcare facility, spills are a threat to safety. Spilled blood, body fluids, and other fluids increase the risk of infection and, in addition, spills put residents and staff at risk for falls. NAs must clean spills using the proper equipment and follow the proper procedures.

Guidelines: Cleaning Spills

G Don gloves immediately. You may need to use special heavy-duty gloves, depending on the spill.

G First, absorb the spill with whatever product is used by the facility. It may be an absorbing powder.

G Scoop up the absorbed spill and dispose of it in a designated container.

G Apply the proper disinfectant to the spill area. Allow it to stand wet for the proper length of time, following directions on the label.

G Be careful if any glass or other sharp objects are in the spill. Get help when picking up and disposing of sharps and other objects. Never pick up broken glass, even with gloved hands. If you do accidentally cut yourself, follow exposure incident guidelines (see Learning Objective 13).

G For large spills, call for the nurse, and she will follow your facility's policy for large spill clean-up. Dispose of gloves and cleaning supplies according to facility policy.

G If you spill a substance on your body, immediately wash that area using the proper cleaning agent. Follow exposure incident guidelines.

G Wash your hands after cleaning spills.

Some facilities have special areas that contain equipment to handle spills. Colored cones are placed to identify the area where the spill occurred. Pads that come in different sizes are placed over the spill. Then the proper department is notified to clean the area.

11. Discuss Transmission-Based Precautions

The CDC set forth a second level of precautions beyond Standard Precautions. These guidelines are used for persons who are infected or may be infected with certain infectious diseases. These precautions are known as *Transmission-Based Precautions*. When ordered, these precautions are used in addition to Standard Precautions.

There are three categories of Transmission-Based Precautions: Airborne Precautions, Droplet Precautions, and Contact Precautions. The category used depends on what type of pathogenic microorganism or disease the person has or may have and how it spreads. These precautions may also be used in combination for diseases that have multiple routes of transmission.

Airborne Precautions

Airborne Precautions prevent the spread of pathogens that travel through the air after being expelled (Fig. 6-21). The pathogens are able to remain suspended in the air for extended periods of time. They are carried by moisture, air currents, and dust. An example of an airborne disease is tuberculosis (TB). TB is a highly contagious disease that usually affects the lungs and is carried on mucous droplets suspended in the air. Droplets are released when an infected person talks, coughs, breathes, laughs, or sings. TB can be fatal if not treated. More information on TB is found in Chapter 20.

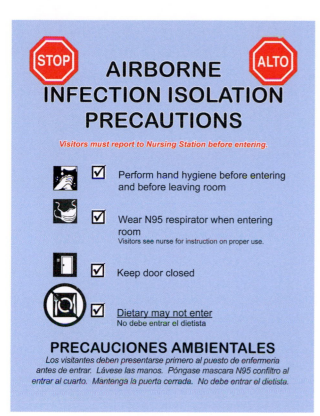

Fig. 6-21. *Airborne Precautions are used for diseases that can be transmitted through the air. The infection prevention guidelines will often be posted on a resident's door.* (IMAGE COURTESY OF STATEWIDE PROGRAM FOR INFECTION CONTROL AND EPIDEMIOLOGY (SPICE), UNC, CHAPEL HILL, SPICE.UNC.EDU)

Guidelines: Airborne Precautions

G   Follow Standard Precautions.

G   Residents will be placed in an *airborne infection isolation room (AIIR)*. These rooms have a controlled flow of air. All of the air inside the room will be exhausted directly to the outside, or all air will first be recirculated through a special HEPA filter before returning to circulation. Within this ventilation system, air flows into the room from the hallways or other adjacent areas when the door to the room is opened. This helps ensure that contaminated air does not enter other parts of the facility.

G   Keep windows in these rooms closed. Keep doors to these rooms closed except when someone must enter or exit the room. When

entering an airborne infection isolation room, do not open or close the door rapidly. This pulls contaminated room air into the hallway.

G   Wear a special mask (respirator) during resident care. All people entering the room must wear a special mask, such as an N95 respirator, prior to entering the AIIR. Respirators are specially designed to help prevent a person from inhaling droplets.

G   Residents who have TB must wear regular surgical masks if they must leave the room to help reduce the number of droplets they exhale into the air.

Droplet Precautions

Droplet Precautions are used for diseases that are spread by droplets in the air. Droplets normally do not travel farther than six feet. Talking, singing, sneezing, laughing, breathing, or coughing can spread droplets (Fig. 6-22). An example of a droplet disease is influenza (flu).

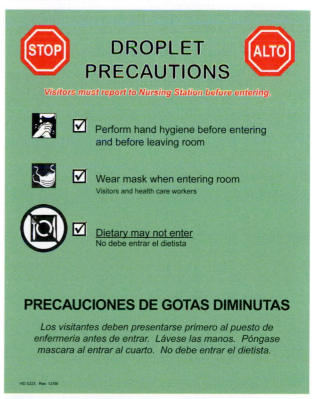

Fig. 6-22. *Droplet Precautions may be in place for some residents with illnesses such as influenza.* (IMAGE COURTESY OF STATEWIDE PROGRAM FOR INFECTION CONTROL AND EPIDEMIOLOGY (SPICE), UNC, CHAPEL HILL, SPICE.UNC.EDU)

Infection Prevention and Control

Guidelines: Droplet Precautions

G Follow Standard Precautions.

G Don a mask before entering the room. Wear the mask during resident care.

G Facilities should limit the transport of residents outside of the room to medical necessities. Residents must wear masks if they leave the room and should avoid close contact with others.

G Cover your mouth and nose with a tissue when coughing or sneezing. Ask others to do the same. Immediately dispose of tissues in a no-touch waste container. Do not place used tissues in your pocket for future use. If you do not have a tissue, cough or sneeze into your upper sleeve or elbow, not your hands. After coughing or sneezing, wash your hands immediately or use an alcohol-based hand rub.

G Visits from uninfected people may be restricted.

Contact Precautions

Contact Precautions are used when a resident may spread an infection by direct contact with another person or object. The infection can be spread when an NA touches a contaminated area on a resident's body or touches a resident's contaminated blood or body fluids (Fig. 6-23). It may also be spread by touching contaminated personal items, linen, equipment, or supplies. Conjunctivitis (pink eye) and *Clostridioides difficile* (*C. diff*) are examples of situations that require Contact Precautions. *Clostridioides difficile* is discussed later in the chapter.

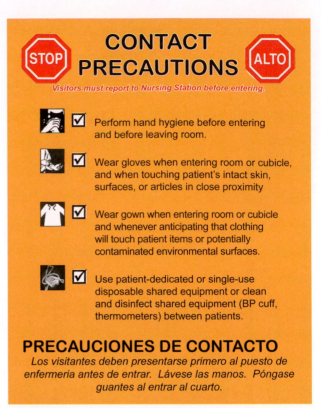

Fig. 6-23. *Contact Precautions can help prevent the spread of dangerous illnesses that can be transmitted by touch.* (IMAGE COURTESY OF STATEWIDE PROGRAM FOR INFECTION CONTROL AND EPIDEMIOLOGY (SPICE), UNC, CHAPEL HILL, SPICE.UNC.EDU)

Guidelines: Contact Precautions

G Follow Standard Precautions.

G Put on a gown before entering a resident's room. Remove and discard the gown before leaving the room. Wash your hands after removing the gown, before leaving. Do not touch any surface in the room with your uniform or your skin before exiting.

G Put on gloves before entering a resident's room. Change your gloves if they become contaminated with infectious material. Remove your gloves before leaving the room.

G While still in the room, wash your hands with an antimicrobial soap after removing your gloves. Do not touch any surface with your hands before exiting.

G Do not share residents' equipment with other residents. Any equipment that must be used by more than one resident will be disinfected before being used again.

G Do not share residents' towels, bedding, or clothing with other residents.

G Residents will most likely be placed in a private room or placed with another resident who has the same infection.

12. Describe care of the resident in an isolation unit

Residents who require Transmission-Based Precautions are referred to as being "in isolation." To **isolate** means to keep something separate, or by itself. Isolation is ordered when it is necessary to protect residents, staff, and visitors, but the method of isolation must be the least restrictive possible. A sign should be on the door indicating the type of precaution and alerting people to see the nurse before entering the room. Tuberculosis and chickenpox are examples of diseases requiring isolation.

Guidelines: Residents in Isolation

G You may assist the nurse in setting up an isolation unit. Before doing anything in the isolation area, wash your hands and don clean gloves. Follow the nurse's instructions, which may include the following:

- Adjust the bed to the proper height.

- Put away clean towels and other supplies.

- Leave clean pajamas or a gown in an easy-to-reach spot.

- Check to make sure these are in working order: the bed controls, including the call light; lights in the room; the television and radio controls; telephone; closet and dressers/cabinets; and windows and latches.

- Restock bathroom supplies as needed. Notify the proper department if trash needs to be emptied or if anything is damaged and not working properly.

G If asked to set up an isolation cart outside of the resident's room, make sure the cart is stocked with all PPE needed. This includes gloves, gowns, masks, goggles, and face shields. Gather extra plastic bags and laundry bags.

G Some facilities use an anteroom just outside of the isolation room. This anteroom may have a sink. Follow facility policy when using the anteroom. Special steps may need to be taken in that room.

G Apply proper PPE before entering the isolation room.

G Use disposable supplies that can be discarded after use whenever possible. Use dedicated (only for use by one resident) equipment when disposable is not an option. Staff may not be allowed to take their own equipment, such as stethoscopes, into the room. If so, there will be a stethoscope that stays in the isolation room at all times. Disinfect the stethoscope with alcohol wipes before and after using each time.

G Dispose of trash in proper containers.

G Dispose of waste containing blood or body fluids and sharps in biohazard containers.

G Bag used linen and equipment so that the contaminated items do not touch the outside of the bag. Tie or seal the bag. Should you accidentally touch the outside of the bag with the contaminated items, you will need to double-bag the item. To double-bag something, drop the contaminated bag into a clean second bag that a coworker is holding just outside the resident's room. The coworker will seal the bag and dispose of it properly.

G Disinfect all furniture and surfaces (e.g., doorknobs, sinks, other bathroom surfaces) regularly.

G   Assist visitors to put on gowns and masks as needed.

G   Before you leave the room, make sure the TV, telephone, and radio are all in working order.

G   Encourage the use of reading material that can be disposed of, such as magazines and newspapers. Make sure the resident has access to eyeglasses if needed.

G   Always place the call light within the resident's reach when leaving the isolation room.

G   Residents in isolation units experience significant changes. They may not be able to move about freely because they may be separated from others. Empathize with them. Think about how you would feel if you were in isolation. Spend as much time with the resident as possible, if allowed. This can help reduce loneliness and gives her a connection to the outside world. Listen to residents and encourage them to talk about their feelings and concerns. Reassure residents that it is the disease, not the person, that is being isolated. Explain why these special steps are being taken.

Information on collecting specimens from a resident in isolation will be discussed in Chapter 15.

Residents' Rights

Residents in Isolation

Residents' rights must be protected when they are in isolation. Their dignity, privacy, and confidentiality must be maintained at all times. Residents can participate in their care as much as possible. They have the right to choose what care they receive and to file complaints. They have the right to visits from family, friends, or clergy. Visitors must receive training on the safe and proper use of PPE before entering the isolation room.

13. Explain OSHA's Bloodborne Pathogen Standard

Bloodborne pathogens are microorganisms found in human blood that can cause infection

and disease in humans. They may also be found in body fluids, draining wounds, and mucous membranes. These pathogens are transmitted when infected blood enters the bloodstream, or if infected semen or vaginal secretions contact mucous membranes. Having sexual contact with someone carrying a bloodborne disease can also transmit the disease. Sexual contact includes sexual intercourse (vaginal and anal), contact of the mouth with the genitals or anus, and contact of the hands with the genital area. Sharing infected drug needles is another way to spread bloodborne diseases. Infected pregnant women may transmit bloodborne disease to their babies in the womb or at birth.

In health care, contact with infected blood or body fluids is the most common way to be infected with a bloodborne disease. Infections can be spread through contact with contaminated blood or body fluids, skin, needles or other sharp objects, or contaminated supplies or equipment.

The **Occupational Safety and Health Administration** (**OSHA**, osha.gov) is a federal government agency that is responsible for the safety of workers in the United States. OSHA makes and enforces rules to protect workers from hazards on the job. OSHA conducts workplace inspections to check on worker safety and updates safety standards. OSHA also provides training for employers and employees on workplace safety. The employer is responsible for meeting all safety standards and providing a workplace that is free of hazards. Employees are responsible for doing their jobs in a way that meets OSHA's safety standards.

OSHA sets standards for equipment use and special techniques to use when working in facilities. One of these standards is the **Bloodborne Pathogen Standard**. It requires that healthcare facilities protect employees from bloodborne health hazards.

By law, employers must follow these rules to reduce or eliminate the risk of exposure to infectious diseases. The standard also guides employers and employees through the steps to follow if exposed to infectious material. Types of waste that are considered infectious include blood, body fluids, and human tissue. Significant exposures include the following:

- Exposure by injection; a needle stick

- Mucous membrane contact

- A cut from an object containing a potentially infectious body fluid (includes human bites)

- Having nonintact skin (OSHA includes acne in this category)

Employers must also follow these guidelines:

- Employers must provide in-service training on the risks from bloodborne pathogens and updates on any new safety standards at the time of hire and annually to all employees.

- Employers must have an exposure control plan should an employee accidentally become exposed to any infectious waste. The **exposure control plan** outlines specific work practices to prevent exposure to infectious material and identifies step-by-step procedures to follow when exposures do occur. This plan must be accessible to all employees, and they must receive training on this plan.

- Employers must give all employees, visitors, and residents proper personal protective equipment (PPE) to wear when needed at no cost. Employers must make sure PPE is available in the appropriate sizes and is readily accessible.

- Employers must place biohazard containers in each resident's room and in other areas in the facility to dispose of equipment and supplies contaminated with infectious waste. These containers must be puncture-resistant, labeled or color-coded, and leakproof.

- Biohazard bags must be used for biomedical waste (Fig. 6-24). The bag must be sealed tightly before leaving the resident's room.

Bags must be safely taken to the proper area for biohazard infectious waste.

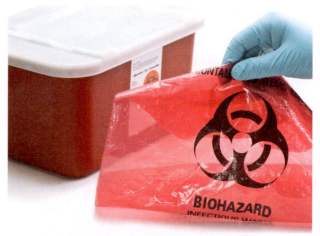

Fig. 6-24. *Biohazard bags are used for biomedical waste and must be sealed tightly before leaving a resident's room.*

- Employers must keep a log of injuries from contaminated sharps. The information recorded must protect the confidentiality of the injured employee. Employers are also required to select safer needle devices and to involve employees in choosing these devices.

- Employers are required to provide a free hepatitis B vaccine to all employees after hire.

When an employee is exposed to blood or other potentially infectious material, it is called an **exposure incident**. After an exposure incident, the person must take these specific steps:

- Immediately follow facility policy regarding a spill, splash, or cut. (More information on skin and eye splashes is in Chapter 7.)

- Report the exposure immediately to her supervisor.

- Fill out an exposure report form. Exposure reports help employees receive the necessary follow-up care after an exposure. They also help employers find ways to prevent future exposures.

- Go to the employer's health department to get any needed tests.

14. Discuss two important bloodborne diseases

Two major bloodborne diseases in the United States are acquired immunodeficiency syndrome (AIDS) and the viral hepatitis family.

HIV stands for human immunodeficiency virus, and it is the virus that can cause AIDS. Over time, HIV weakens the immune system so that the body cannot effectively fight infections. These types of infections are called *opportunistic infections*. In addition to these infections, tumors and central nervous system symptoms may appear. This stage of the disease is known as *AIDS*, which is the final stage of HIV infection. People with AIDS lose all ability to fight infection. They can die from illnesses that a healthy immune system could handle.

HIV is transmitted by blood, by infected needles, and from mother to fetus. It is also a sexually transmitted disease. More information about HIV and AIDS is located in Chapter 24.

Hepatitis is an inflammation of the liver caused by certain viruses and other factors, such as alcohol abuse, some medications, and trauma. Liver function can be permanently damaged by hepatitis. Several different viruses can cause hepatitis, including hepatitis A, B, C, D, and E. The most common types of hepatitis are hepatitis A, B, and C. Hepatitis B and C are bloodborne diseases that can cause death. Many more people have hepatitis B (HBV) than HIV. In the United States today, the risk of contracting hepatitis is greater than the risk of contracting HIV.

The virus causing hepatitis A (HAV) is spread by the fecal-oral route, which means through food or water contaminated by stool from an infected person. HAV can survive outside the body for months. Symptoms of HAV include fever, loss of appetite, vomiting, jaundice (yellow skin or eyes), dark urine, and joint pain. There is a vaccine available for hepatitis A.

Hepatitis B (HBV) is a bloodborne form of hepatitis. HBV is spread through sexual contact, by sharing infected needles, from a mother to her baby during delivery, through improperly sterilized needles used for tattoos and piercings, and through grooming supplies, such as razors, nail clippers, and toothbrushes. It is also spread by exposure at work from accidental contact with infected needles or other sharps or from splashing blood.

The hepatitis B virus can survive outside the body at least seven days and can still cause infection in others during that time. HBV may cause few symptoms or may become a severe infection. Some of the symptoms are fatigue, nausea, vomiting, diarrhea, jaundice, lack of appetite, joint pain, and abdominal pain. Hepatitis B can lead to serious problems with the liver, such as cirrhosis (liver damage) or liver cancer. In some cases, HBV can be fatal.

HBV poses a serious threat to healthcare workers. It is important for NAs to use proper PPE and to handle sharps carefully to help prevent HBV. Equally important is getting the vaccine for hepatitis B when it is offered. Employers must offer NAs a free vaccine to protect against hepatitis B. The hepatitis B vaccine is usually given as a series of three shots.

Hepatitis C (HCV) is also transmitted through blood or body fluids. Many people who have hepatitis C experience no symptoms. If symptoms do occur, they include fatigue, nausea, jaundice, dark urine, lack of appetite, and abdominal pain. Hepatitis C can be fatal if it leads to serious illness, such as liver cancer or cirrhosis. A liver transplant may be required. There is no vaccine for hepatitis C, but HCV can be cured using medications (sometimes in combination).

Less common types of hepatitis in the United States are hepatitis D (HDV) and hepatitis E (HEV). Hepatitis D is transmitted by blood. A person must have the hepatitis B virus in order to get hepatitis D, and HDV worsens HBV. Symptoms of HDV include fatigue, nausea, vomiting, jaundice, dark urine, lack of appetite, joint pain, and abdominal pain. There is no vaccine for hepatitis D.

Hepatitis E is spread by the fecal-oral route, mostly through contaminated water. Symptoms include fatigue, nausea, vomiting, jaundice, dark urine, lack of appetite, and abdominal pain. Currently there is no vaccine for hepatitis E.

15. Discuss MRSA, VRE, *C. difficile*, and CRE

Multidrug-resistant organisms (MDROs) are microorganisms, mostly bacteria, that are resistant to one or more antimicrobial agents that are commonly used for treatment. An antimicrobial agent destroys, resists, or prevents the development of pathogens. There has been an increase in MDROs in healthcare facilities, and it is a serious problem. Two common types of MDROs are MRSA and VRE.

MRSA stands for methicillin-resistant *Staphylococcus aureus*. *Staphylococcus aureus* is a common type of bacteria that can cause infection. Methicillin is a powerful antibiotic often used in healthcare facilities. MRSA is an antibiotic-resistant infection to methicillin. This type of MRSA is also known as *HA-MRSA*, which stands for *hospital-associated MRSA*.

Community-associated methicillin-resistant *Staphylococcus aureus* (CA-MRSA) is a type of MRSA infection that occurs in people who have not recently been admitted to healthcare facilities

and who have no past diagnosis of MRSA. Often CA-MRSA manifests as skin infections, such as boils or pimples. This type of infection is becoming more common.

MRSA is almost always spread by direct physical contact with infected people. This means that if a person has MRSA on her skin, especially on the hands, and touches another person, she may spread MRSA. Spread also occurs through indirect contact by touching equipment or supplies (for example, towels, wound dressings, clothes) contaminated by a person with MRSA.

Common MRSA infection sites include the skin, the respiratory tract, surgical wounds, the urinary tract, the perineum, and the rectum. Symptoms of MRSA infection include drainage, fever, chills, and redness. Residents with MRSA are placed in contact isolation, and possibly under additional precautions are needed, depending upon the site of the infection.

NAs can help prevent MRSA by practicing proper hygiene. Handwashing, using soap and warm water, is the single most important measure to control the spread of MRSA. NAs should wash their hands frequently and should assist residents to wash their hands as well. Chlorhexidine (CHG) bathing is another method that may be used to help prevent MRSA. CHG is a substance used to kill microbes and its use has been proven effective against MRSA. NAs must always follow Standard Precautions, along with Transmission-Based Precautions as ordered.

VRE stands for vancomycin-resistant *Enterococcus*. *Enterococci* are bacteria that live in the digestive and genital tracts. Although they normally do not cause problems in healthy people, they can sometimes cause infections. Vancomycin is a powerful antibiotic used to treat infections caused by *enterococci*. If the *enterococci* become resistant to vancomycin, then it is called *VRE*.

VRE is spread through direct and indirect contact. Symptoms of VRE infection include fever, fatigue, chills, and drainage. VRE infections are often difficult to treat and may require the use of several medications. Residents with VRE may be placed in contact isolation.

Preventing VRE infection is much easier than trying to treat it. Proper hand hygiene can help prevent the spread of VRE. NAs must always follow Standard Precautions, along with Transmission-Based Precautions as ordered.

Clostridioides difficile (formerly *Clostridium difficile*) infection is commonly known as **C. diff** or **C. difficile**. It is a spore-forming bacterium which can be part of the normal intestinal flora. When the normal intestinal flora is altered, *C. difficile* can flourish in the intestinal tract and can cause infection. It produces a toxin that causes a watery diarrhea. Enemas, nasogastric tube insertion, and GI tract surgery increase a person's risk of developing the disease. The elderly are at a higher risk of getting *C. difficile* infection. The overuse of antibiotics may alter the normal intestinal flora and increase the risk of developing *C. difficile* infection. *C. difficile* can also cause colitis, a more serious intestinal condition. It can cause sepsis, a condition caused by an infection, which can be fatal. More information about sepsis can be found in Chapter 26.

When released in the environment, *C. difficile* can form a spore that makes it difficult to kill. These spores can be carried on the hands of people who have direct contact with infected residents or with environmental surfaces (floors, bedpans, toilets, etc.) contaminated with *C. difficile*. Touching an object contaminated with *C. difficile* can transmit *C. difficile*. Alcohol-based hand sanitizers are not considered effective on *C. difficile*. Soap and water must be used each time hand hygiene is performed.

Symptoms of *C. difficile* infection include frequent, foul-smelling, watery stools. Other symptoms are fever, diarrhea that contains blood and mucus, nausea, lack of appetite, and abdominal cramps. Proper handwashing with soap and water, especially after using the toilet and before

eating or drinking, is vital in preventing the spread of the infection. Handling contaminated wastes properly can also help prevent the spread of the infection. Additional Transmission-Based Precautions are used with residents who have *C. difficile* infection. Cleaning surfaces and items used for care with an appropriate disinfectant, such as a bleach solution, can also help reduce transmission.

Residents who have *C. difficile* infection should have a private room if possible. They should have dedicated equipment, such as blood pressure monitors. All caregivers and visitors must be advised to take proper precautions before having any contact with a resident who has *C. difficile*. They should don gloves and gowns when entering the resident's room.

There is a quick test that can diagnose *C. difficile* infection. If an NA notes any of the symptoms, she should promptly report them to the nurse. The risks of serious illness and potential transmission to others increase if the infection is not identified and cared for promptly. Treatment of *C. difficile* infection includes certain antibiotics, as well as discontinuing the use of other antibiotics. Treatment may also include fecal microbiota transplant (FMT), which involves transplanting the stool from a healthy person to the colon of a person who has *C. difficile* infection.

Enterobacteriaceae are bacteria that are part of the normal flora of the intestines, but can also grow out of control and cause infections. Examples of *Enterobacteriaceae* include *Klebsiella* species and *Escherichia coli* (*E. coli*). Sometimes these bacteria can spread and cause serious infections. Carbapenems are powerful antibiotics used to treat certain serious infections. When *Enterobacteriaceae* infections are not controlled by carbapenems, it is referred to as **carbapenem-resistant *Enterobacteriaceae* (CRE)**.

CRE is normally spread through direct contact with an infected person, especially with the person's wounds or stool. Residents who have catheters or ventilators, or who receive intravenous therapy are at greater risk of acquiring these infections.

Because these infections are highly resistant to antibiotics, healthcare providers find CRE infections difficult to treat. However, antibiotics and other measures can be used to treat CRE infections.

CRE has been shown to have a high death rate, up to 50 percent. Proper, frequent handwashing is the most effective way to prevent CRE. For residents who have CRE infection, Contact Precautions will be ordered, and residents should be placed in private rooms if possible.

Other Infections

Influenza, also known as *the flu*, is a contagious respiratory illness. Older people are at a higher risk for experiencing complications from influenza, such as pneumonia. Influenza is generally spread by droplets, but it can also spread if a person touches a surface that has the virus on it and then touches his eyes, nose, or mouth. Symptoms include fever, chills, muscle aches, sore throat, runny nose, and headaches. Treatment includes medication, rest, and increased fluids. A flu vaccine is available and can help prevent the flu. Measures for prevention include maintaining a distance of at least six feet from an infected person, frequent handwashing, and covering the nose and mouth when sneezing. Touching the eyes, nose, and mouth should be avoided.

Norovirus is a highly contagious virus. It causes more cases of acute gastroenteritis in the United States than any other virus. A person can get norovirus from contaminated surfaces, food, or water, or from a person infected with the virus. Symptoms include diarrhea, vomiting, nausea, and stomach pain. Fever, headache, and body aches are other symptoms. Treatment focuses on preventing dehydration by drinking plenty of liquids. Performing proper handwashing is the most effective way to prevent norovirus. Soap and water should be used for washing hands. Hands should be washed often, including after using the toilet, after changing diapers, and before preparing food or eating. Proper handwashing will need to continue to be done for at least two weeks after symptoms disappear. A person should avoid touching his face, as the mouth is the portal of entry for the virus. Fruits and vegetables must be washed well before eating them. Seafood should be cooked properly before consuming it. Contaminated surfaces must be cleaned with the proper disinfectant (often this is a bleach solution).

Group A Streptococcus (*GAS*) is a bacterium that can cause many infections. Infections can range from mild (strep throat or impetigo) to serious (pneumonia or necrotizing fasciitis). GAS can be spread through direct contact with an infected person (such as with the person's mucus, infected wounds, or sores on the skin). The elderly are at a higher risk for GAS infections. Symptoms include sore throat, fever, rash, redness, swelling, and drainage or pain associated with a wound. Antibiotics are used to treat GAS. Proper handwashing can help prevent the spread of GAS. A person who has a sore throat should be tested to find out whether or not it is strep throat. Wounds should be kept clean and closely observed for signs of infection.

Chapter Review

1. Describe the difference between the terms *clean* and *dirty* (LO 3).

2. What is sterilization? What is disinfection (LO 3)?

3. List four reasons the elderly are at a higher risk for infection (LO 5).

4. On whom should Standard Precautions be practiced (LO 6)?

5. What is hand hygiene (LO 7)?

6. Why should NAs avoid using artificial nails (LO 7)?

7. When should gowns be worn (LO 8)?

8. When should a mask and goggles be worn (LO 8)?

9. In what order should personal protective equipment (PPE) be put on and removed (LO 8)?

10. How should soiled linen be carried (LO 9)?

11. When can reusable equipment be used again (LO 9)?

12. How are bloodborne diseases transmitted (LO 13)?

13. What is hepatitis (LO 14)?

14. What does HIV do to the immune system (LO 14)?

15. How is hepatitis B (HBV) spread (LO 14)?

16. What is one of the best ways to prevent the spread of MRSA and VRE (LO 15)?

17. What are two ways to help prevent the spread of *C. difficile* (LO 15)?

18. How is carbapenem-resistant *Enterobacteria-ceae* (CRE) usually spread (LO 15)?

Multiple Choice

19. Which of the following is true of microorganisms (LO 2)?
    (A) They are only present in healthcare facilities.
    (B) They are on almost everything a person touches.
    (C) They are not present in a person's home, as long as the home is cleaned regularly.
    (D) They are only found on the human body.

20. In a care facility, who has the responsibility for preventing infection (LO 2)?
    (A) All care team members
    (B) Doctors
    (C) Nursing assistants
    (D) The dietary department

21. Which type of infection is limited to a specific location in the body and has symptoms that are near the site of infection (LO 2)?
    (A) Cross-infection
    (B) Healthcare-associated infection
    (C) Systemic infection
    (D) Localized infection

22. Which link in the chain of infection refers to any body opening on an infected person that allows pathogens to leave (LO 4)?
    (A) Reservoir
    (B) Susceptible host
    (C) Mode of transmission
    (D) Portal of exit

23. Which of the following is the primary route of disease transmission within the health-care setting (LO 4)?
    (A) On the stethoscopes of care team members
    (B) On the hands of healthcare workers
    (C) On the elimination equipment used by residents
    (D) On the food trays served to residents

24. Under Standard Precautions, which of the following is not considered a body fluid (LO 6)?
    (A) Vomit
    (B) Feces
    (C) Sweat
    (D) Pus

25. What is the first step the NA should take when cleaning a spill (LO 10)?
    (A) The NA should scoop up the spill.
    (B) The NA should don gloves.
    (C) The NA should apply a disinfectant to the spill area.
    (D) The NA should place an absorbing powder on the spill.

26. Which of the following precautions is used for pathogens that are carried by moisture, by air currents, and by dust and remain floating for some time (LO 11)?
    (A) Airborne Precautions
    (B) Contact Precautions
    (C) Droplet Precautions
    (D) Standard Precautions

27. Which of the following is true of disposable supplies (LO 12)?
    (A) They should be avoided when a resident is in isolation.
    (B) They can be used once before they must be discarded.
    (C) They can be reused as long as they are disinfected between uses.
    (D) They can be reused as long as they are sterilized between use.

7 Safety and Body Mechanics

The Great Chicago Fire and Daisy the Cow

Legend has it that a cow named Daisy kicked over a lantern and started the Great Chicago Fire of October 8, 1871. That fire killed more than 300 people and left 100,000 more homeless, including patients at Deaconess Hospital of Chicago (later Passavant Memorial Hospital), who were forced to flee for their lives as the fires burned out of control.

Two weeks after the fire, Reverend Passavant arrived in Chicago to survey the damage and assist the homeless and destitute. He observed that "ruin reigns supreme." In fact, the remains of the hospital were sold for the pathetic sum of $8.50.

If the story of Daisy the Cow is true, then the fire that devastated the nation's fourth-largest city in 1871 did not have to happen. The Great Chicago Fire could have been prevented with a little care and caution.

Adapted from *To Be a Nurse*
by Susan M. Sacharski

"When you see a rattlesnake poised to strike, you do not wait until he has struck before you crush him."

Franklin Delano Roosevelt, 1882–1945

"In them and in ourselves our safety lies."

William Shakespeare, 1564–1616
King Henry VI, Part III, Act III

1. Define important words in this chapter

aspiration: the inhalation of food, fluid, or foreign material into the lungs.

atrophy: weakening or wasting away of muscles.

body mechanics: the way the parts of the body work together when a person moves.

chemical restraint: medications used to control a person's mood or behavior.

combustion: the process of burning.

contracture: the permanent and painful shortening of a muscle, tendon, or ligament that can restrict movement.

cyanosis: blue or pale skin and/or mucous membranes due to decreased oxygen in the blood.

dysphagia: difficulty swallowing.

flammable: easily ignited and capable of burning quickly.

hoarding: collecting and putting things away in a guarded way.

intravenous therapy: the delivery of medication, nutrition, or fluids through a person's vein.

PASS: acronym for use of a fire extinguisher; stands for Pull-Aim-Squeeze-Sweep.

physical restraint: any method, device, material, or equipment that restricts a person's freedom of movement.

RACE: acronym for steps taken during a fire; stands for Rescue-Activate-Contain-Extinguish.

restraint: a physical or chemical way to restrict voluntary movement or behavior.

restraint alternatives: measures used in place of a restraint or that reduce the need for a restraint.

restraint-free care: an environment in which restraints are not kept or used for any reason.

Safety Data Sheet (SDS): sheet that provides information on the safe use and hazards of chemicals, as well as emergency steps to take in the event chemicals are splashed, sprayed, or ingested.

scalds: burns caused by hot liquids.

suffocation: the stoppage of breathing from a lack of oxygen or excess of carbon dioxide in the body; may result in unconsciousness or death.

2. List common accidents in facilities and ways to prevent them

Many types of accidents can occur in a long-term care facility. Nursing assistants should always be observant to try to keep residents, staff members, visitors, and themselves safe. Being proactive is the goal. Being proactive means trying to *prevent* an accident from occurring. It is much better than being reactive. Reacting or responding to an accident means that it has already taken place. Prevention is the key to safety.

Maintaining safety is also a way to protect residents' rights. Residents have the legal right to be safe and secure. The environment must be as free of hazards as possible. Residents must have adequate supervision and assistance to prevent accidents from occurring.

Some common accidents that may occur in a facility include the following:

- Falls
- Failing to identify residents before performing procedures or serving food
- Burns and scalds
- Poisoning
- Choking
- Cuts

Fall Prevention

Falls make up the majority of accidents that occur in a facility. A fall is any sudden, uncontrollable descent from a higher to a lower level,

with or without injury resulting. Many things increase the risk of falls. Unsafe environments, loss of abilities, diseases, and medications increase a person's risk of falls. Problems with walking, muscle weakness, poor vision, hearing loss, and disorientation, which is confusion about person, place, or time, are other factors that increase the risk of falls. Preventing falls is very important.

Guidelines: Preventing Falls

G Know which residents are at risk for falls (the nurse should let you know this). Report unsteadiness to the nurse.

G Keep frequently-used items close to residents, including call lights. Respond to call lights promptly (Fig. 7-1). Make sure eyeglasses and hearing aids are on and are not damaged.

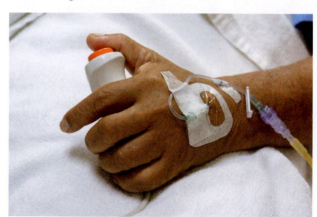

Fig. 7-1. Keep call lights within reach of residents so they can use them when needed. Respond to call lights promptly.

G Wipe up spills immediately or ask someone to get you supplies needed to wipe it up. Do not leave spill area until the spill is gone.

G Remove clutter from walkways. Keep all equipment, such as linen carts, food carts, etc., on one side of the hallway. Pick up anything that has fallen on the floor right away. If you see loose electrical cords or wires, notify the nurse. Make sure purses, bag straps, and linens are not dangling or on the floor.

G   Get help when moving a resident. Never assume you can handle it alone. When in doubt, ask for help.

G   Lock bed wheels before giving care. Lock bed wheels before moving a resident into or out of bed.

G   Lock wheels before helping residents into or out of wheelchairs (Fig. 7-2).

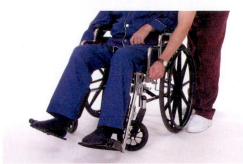

Fig. 7-2. Always lock a wheelchair and remove footrests before a resident transfers into or out of it.

G   Return beds to their lowest position when you are finished with care.

G   Residents should wear clothing that is not too long. Make sure residents are wearing nonskid, sturdy shoes with the laces tied. Report if shoes seem unsafe.

G   Report any rugs or mats that move. Use non-skid mats in the bath or shower each time residents bathe. If allowed, stay with residents while they are showering or in the tub.

G   Report loose handrails in halls or rooms immediately. Report cracks or holes in floors, tile, walls, furniture, bathrooms, ceilings, or stairwells.

G   Report damage to outdoor furniture or benches, walkways, or ramps in outdoor common areas.

G   Use brightly colored tape to mark uneven areas on stairs or the floor. Point out any uneven areas when walking with residents.

G   Keep walkers and canes close to residents. Allow residents to sit for short periods before getting up to prevent lightheadedness.

G   Do not move furniture without an order from the nurse. Tell the resident before moving furniture.

G   Offer trips to the bathroom often. Respond to residents' requests for bathroom assistance promptly.

G   Report any areas that are not well lit or any problems with lighting.

G   If a resident begins to fall, do not try to stop it or catch her. Use your body to slide her to the floor safely (Fig. 7-3). If you try to stop a fall, you may injure yourself or the resident.

G   Whenever a resident falls, it must be reported to the nurse. Always complete an incident report, even if the resident says she feels fine.

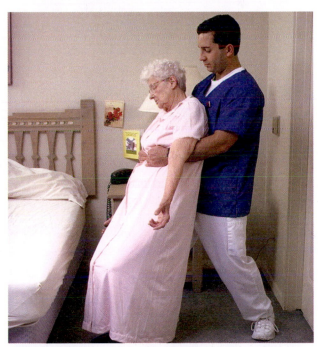

Fig. 7-3. If a resident starts to fall, do not try to stop the fall. Bring the resident's body close to you to break the fall. Bend your knees and support the resident as you gently lower her to the floor.

Tip

Safety with Wheelchairs

NAs should lock wheelchairs and remove footrests before moving residents into or out of them. Wheelchairs should be pushed slowly and carefully. This helps to ensure safety, as well as making residents feel more secure.

Resident Identification

NAs must always identify residents before providing care or serving food. Failing to identify residents can result in serious problems, illnesses, and even death.

Some facilities use photos to identify residents, while others have signs outside residents' doors (Fig. 7-4). NAs must identify each resident before providing care or serving food. The diet card should be checked against the resident's identification to make sure they match. The resident should be called by name and asked to state her name if she is able.

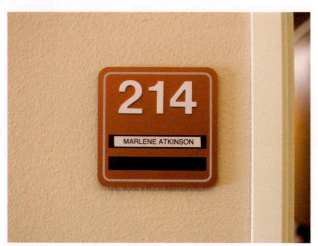

Fig. 7-4. *A resident's name may be displayed outside the room to identify who is living in that room. Before giving any care, nursing assistants must always identify residents.*

> **Tip**
>
> **Alarm Bands**
> Special bands are sometimes used for residents who are disoriented or confused. The bands have alarms on them, and the alarm will sound when a resident tries to leave the facility. If a resident wears an alarm band, the alarm should be checked regularly to make sure it is turned on and working correctly.

Burn/Scald Prevention

Burns can have many causes, such as hot electrical appliances, hot liquids or steam, or chemicals. **Scalds** are burns caused by hot liquids, such as coffee or hot water. It does not take long for a serious burn to occur. When the temperature of a liquid reaches 140°F, it can take five seconds or less to cause a serious burn.

Burns are extremely painful. They can require surgery. They can cause a resident's condition to deteriorate quickly, depending on his physical state prior to the burn. Elderly people and people who have a loss of sensation (such as from paralysis or diabetes) are at the greatest risk for burns. Preventing burns is very important.

Guidelines: Preventing Burns and Scalds

G Check water temperature with a water thermometer or on your wrist before giving a resident a bath or shower. The temperature should not be over 105°F. Do not allow a resident to get into a bath or shower without checking the water temperature first.

G Follow instructions for proper temperature of warm water applications, such as warm packs. A resident's skin is fragile. Warm or cold water applications should only be applied for 20 minutes at a time. (Chapter 18 contains more information.)

G Use low settings on hair dryers.

G Spills can cause burns. Residents may spill drinks on themselves if they are unsteady. Drinking hot liquids can also cause burns. Make sure the drink has cooled before encouraging the resident to drink.

G Serve residents drinks only after they are seated.

G Let residents know when you are about to pour or set down hot liquids.

G Pour hot drinks away from residents. Keep hot drinks and liquids away from edges of tables. Use lids on hot liquids if possible.

G If plate warmers are used to keep food warm, check the plates carefully. They may be hot. Warn residents if plates are hot.

G Make sure anything that was left in the sun, such as a wheelchair, has cooled off completely before letting a resident sit in it. Residents themselves should not be left out in the sun too long. Use sunscreen and hats when residents are going outside.

G Tell residents about smoking precautions. Although many healthcare facilities do not permit smoking, some may allow smoking in specific areas. Serious burns, and even fires, can occur if a resident falls asleep with a cigarette, pipe, or cigar burning.

Poisoning Prevention

There are many poisonous items in facilities that should not be ingested. Cleaning products, glue, soaps, perfumes, and paints are some examples. These items might be consumed by a confused resident. Medication can also be poisonous if taken in the wrong amount or by the wrong person.

Guidelines: Preventing Poisoning

G Keep fresh flowers or plants away from disoriented or confused residents. Store or lock away items like nail polish remover, soaps, perfumes, or hair products. Lock up cleaning products and paints. Do not leave cleaning products in residents' rooms. The number of the Poison Control Center should be posted by all telephones.

G Check expiration dates of foods to ensure that they are fresh.

G Check bedside table drawers for food that was hoarded and has spoiled. Residents who are confused or have dementia may hoard items; **hoarding** is collecting and putting things away in a guarded way.

G Residents can be overcome by fumes when chemical products are being used. Make sure there is proper ventilation. Always report to the nurse any situation that you believe to be unsafe.

Choking Prevention

Residents must be observed during meals for signs of choking. Residents who are weak or who have dysphagia are at a high risk for choking. **Dysphagia** means difficulty swallowing. Swallowing problems may cause a resident to choke on her food or drink. Inhaling food, fluid, or foreign material into the lungs is called **aspiration**, which can cause pneumonia or death. Residents who have swallowing problems may have special diets consisting of liquids thickened to the consistency of nectar, honey, or pudding. Thickened liquids are easier to swallow. Chapter 14 contains more information about dysphagia, thickened liquids, and aspiration.

Guidelines: Preventing Choking

G Whether in bed or a chair, residents should sit upright, at 90 degrees, while eating (Fig. 7-5).

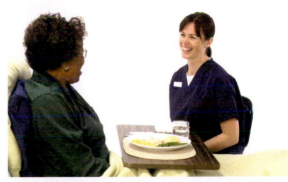

Fig. 7-5. Residents must be sitting up straight when eating, whether in a bed or a chair.

G Assist with feeding slowly. Never rush a resident during a meal.

G Alternate between food and drink.

G Cut food into small pieces.

G If you believe a resident would be helped by softer foods or thickened liquids, report this to the nurse.

G   Make sure dentures are in place and fit properly.

G   Know any swallowing precautions residents have.

Cuts and Other Injuries

Cuts, tears, and scrapes can happen quickly. These guidelines can help prevent injuries:

Guidelines: Preventing Cuts, Scrapes, and Other Injuries

G   Do not leave any sharp objects, such as razors, out. Put them away after use.

G   Prevent skin tears when dressing residents by carefully guiding clothing over the body.

G   When approaching doors, move slowly. If there is a window in the door, check the other side before opening it.

G   When moving residents in wheelchairs or stretchers, protect their arms and legs. Hands and feet can be hit or bumped into walls or doors. Fingers may be caught in a wheelchair. Make sure arms and legs are inside of the chair or stretcher (gurney).

G   Push wheelchairs forward; do not pull them behind you. When entering elevators, turn the chair around so that residents are facing forward. Watch for doors closing before arms and legs are safely inside.

In addition to all of the guidelines listed above, here are some general safety guidelines:

Guidelines: General Safety

G   Do not run in a facility. Pay attention to your environment. Look for wet areas or things that you might trip over. Wipe up spilled liquids right away. Remove clutter from walkways.

G   Do not stick your hand into a bed or anywhere else without looking first. Be on the lookout for sharp objects or needles.

G   Ask for help any time you feel you need it when lifting or assisting residents. Follow facility guidelines for lifting. Use proper equipment provided for lifting.

G   Know which residents are combative and try to learn what triggers this behavior. If a resident tries to hit you, step out of the way. Do not hit back.

G   Follow facility policy if your skin is exposed to potentially dangerous chemicals. Immediately rinse your skin with large amounts of water.

G   Follow facility policy if anything splashes in your eyes. If no eye wash station is available, immediately rinse your eye with large amounts of water at a sink. If an eye wash station is available, follow directions listed there (Fig. 7-6). If you need to use an emergency eye wash, flip the cup lid open. Open your eyelid with your thumb and index finger. Press cup against eye and squeeze bottle repeatedly. Notify the nurse as soon as possible and get checked by a doctor.

G   Report all injuries immediately.

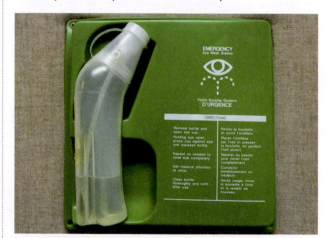

Fig. 7-6. *This is one type of eye wash station.*

3. Explain the Safety Data Sheet (SDS)

The Occupational Safety and Health Administration (OSHA, osha.gov) is responsible for the safety of employees at work. OSHA requires that all dangerous chemicals have a **Safety Data Sheet (SDS)** (formerly called *Material Safety*

Data Sheet, or *MSDS*). These sheets are required to be placed where all staff can easily access them.

The SDS contains the following important information:

- The chemical ingredients of the product

- The dangers of the product

- Pictograms (graphic symbols used to convey information about the chemical's hazards)

- The protective items to wear when using the chemical

- The correct method of using and cleaning up a chemical

- The emergency response actions to be taken when a chemical is splashed, sprayed, or ingested by a person

- The safe handling, storage, and disposal procedures for the product

Some facilities use a toll-free number to access SDS information. Employers will have an SDS for every hazardous chemical used. NAs must know where they are located and how to read them. NAs should ask for help if they do not know how to do this. Some facilities provide annual training for SDSs, and NAs should attend this class when it is offered.

4. Describe safety guidelines for sharps and biohazard containers

As explained in Chapter 6, sharps and biohazard containers are the containers that hold sharp objects and infectious waste. Here are safety guidelines to follow when using these containers:

Guidelines: Safe Use of Sharps and Biohazard Containers

G   Always don, or put on, gloves before touching a sharps container because there is a chance you could come into contact with blood or other body fluids.

G   When dropping an object into the sharps or biohazard container, keep your hands clear of the opening (Fig. 7-7). If you need to carry the container, carry it by the bottom. Make sure it is closed.

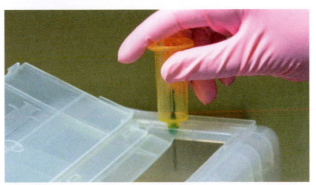

Fig. 7-7. *Wear gloves and keep your fingers above the opening of a sharps container.*

G   Request that the sharps container be replaced when it is ¾ full (or follow your facility policy).

G   Remove gloves and wash your hands after putting anything into the sharps container.

G   Use a biohazard container or bag for anything contaminated with infectious waste (blood, body fluids, or human tissue), except for anything sharp.

G   Always wear gloves when disposing of infectious waste.

G   Remove gloves and wash your hands after putting anything into the biohazard container or bag.

5. Explain the principles of body mechanics and apply them to daily activities

Back and body injuries are serious problems for nursing assistants. They are common risks of working in a facility. Preventing injury by using proper techniques is very important. Every time a nursing assistant moves, lifts, or transfers a resident, he will need to use proper body mechanics. In addition, he will need to use provided equipment properly. More information about moving and lifting equipment may be found in Chapter 11.

Body mechanics is the way the parts of the body work together when a person moves. Using proper body mechanics helps save energy and prevent injury and muscle strain. When muscles are used correctly to push and lift objects, it reduces the risk of injury.

Alignment: Alignment is based on the word *line*. When a person stands up straight, a vertical line could be drawn right through the center of his body and his center of gravity (Fig. 7-8). When the line is straight, the body is in alignment. Whether standing, sitting, or lying down, the body should be in alignment. This means that the two sides of the body are mirror images of each other, with body parts lined up naturally and properly supported. A person can maintain correct body alignment when lifting or carrying an object by keeping it close to his body. His feet and body should be pointed in the direction he is moving. He should avoid twisting at the waist.

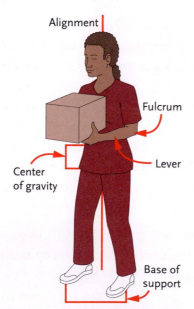

Fig. 7-8. *Proper body alignment is important when standing or sitting.*

Base of support: The base of support is the foundation that supports an object. The feet are the body's base of support. The wider the support, the more stable a person is. Standing with legs

shoulder-width apart allows for a greater base of support. This is more stable than someone standing with his feet together.

Center of gravity: The center of gravity in the body is the point where the most weight is concentrated (Fig. 7-9). This point will depend on the position of the body. When a person stands, weight is centered in the pelvis. A low center of gravity gives a more stable base of support. Bending the knees when lifting an object lowers the pelvis and, therefore, lowers a person's center of gravity. This gives the person more stability and makes him less likely to fall or strain the working muscles. When an NA moves or transfers a resident, the center of gravity includes the resident. When transferring a resident, the resident needs to be as close to the NA's body as possible.

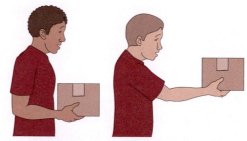

Fig. 7-9. *Holding things close to the body moves weight toward the center of gravity. In this illustration, who is more likely to strain his back muscles?*

Some activities that require nursing assistants to move or lift something include the following:

- Lifting a resident

- Picking up a resident's bag of laundry

- Carrying a new resident's luggage

- Taking heavy trash bags to the appropriate site

- Cleaning a floor

- Moving a resident's bed into another room

Each task could cause serious injury if done without using proper body mechanics. Even a simple task, such as picking up something light from the floor, could cause injury to the back.

By applying the principles of body mechanics to daily activities, injury can be avoided.

Guidelines: Using Proper Body Mechanics

G   Raise beds to a safe working level before making them. This is usually waist high.

G   Stand close to the object.

G   Stand with a wide base of support.

G   Push or slide objects rather than lifting them.

G   Use the strong, large muscles in your thighs, upper arms, and shoulders to lift an object.

G   Bend at your knees (squat) instead of bending at your waist (Fig. 7-10).

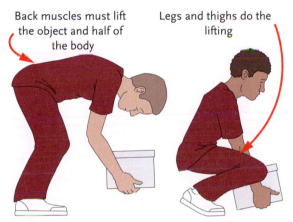

Back muscles must lift the object and half of the body

Legs and thighs do the lifting

Fig. 7-10. In this illustration, which person is lifting correctly?

G   Avoid twisting or choppy movements; keep movements smooth. Face the object or person you are moving. Pivot your feet instead of twisting at the waist.

G   Do not try to lift with just one hand. Use both arms and hands to lift, push, or carry objects.

G   Hold objects close to your body when you are lifting or carrying them.

G   Avoid bending and reaching.

G   Get help from coworkers when lifting or helping residents.

G   Talk to residents before moving them. Let them know what you will do, so that they can

help if possible. Agree on a signal, such as counting to three. Lift or move on three so that everyone moves together.

Tip

Bending Knees for Ease

When preparing to move or position a resident in bed, the NA should always bend her knees. She should be able to feel the bed with her knees before beginning the procedure. If knees are not bent, injuries to the back can occur.

6. Define two types of restraints and discuss problems associated with restraints

A **restraint** is a physical or chemical way to restrict voluntary movement or behavior. A **physical restraint** is any method, device, material, or equipment that restricts a person's freedom of movement. Common types of physical restraints are vest restraints, belt restraints, wrist/ankle restraints, and mitt restraints. **Chemical restraints** are medications used to control a person's mood or behavior.

An *enabler* is equipment or a device that promotes a resident's independence, mobility, comfort, or safety. Wheelchairs with laptop trays, geriatric chairs with tray tables attached, cushions and pillows, and certain types of assistive devices, such as special utensils, are examples of enablers. However, if a person cannot remove an enabler independently, it may be considered a restraint.

Raised bed/side rails on beds may be considered enablers or physical restraints, depending upon their intended use and the resident's condition or abilities (Fig. 7-11). Raised bed rails increase the risk of *entrapment*, which occurs when a resident becomes trapped in the bed rail or between the bed rail and the mattress, headboard, footboard, or bed frame. Bed rails require periodic maintenance. If the bed rail does not appear to be working properly, the NA should report it immediately.

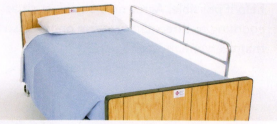

Fig. 7-11. *Raised bed rails may be considered restraints, depending upon their intended use and on the resident's condition.*

In the past, restraints were routinely used to prevent falls, to keep confused people from wandering, to keep people from hurting themselves or others, or to prevent people from pulling out tubing. Restraints were often overused by caregivers, and residents were injured. This led to new laws restricting the use of restraints.

Today, long-term care facilities are prohibited from using restraints unless they are medically necessary. If a restraint is needed, it can only be used with a doctor's order, and the least restrictive restraint possible must be chosen. It is against the law for staff to apply restraints for convenience or to discipline residents. Very specific guidelines apply to restraint use, including frequent monitoring of the resident's vital signs, skin condition, and mental status. This is important because residents have been severely injured and have died due to improper restraint use and lack of monitoring. There is more information about what must be done if a resident is restrained in Learning Objective 8.

There are many serious complications associated with restraint use, including the following:

- Bruises and cuts
- Pressure injuries
- Risk of suffocation or strangulation (**suffocation** is the stoppage of breathing from a lack of oxygen or excess of carbon dioxide in the body that may result in unconsciousness or death)
- Entrapment
- Pneumonia

- Reduced blood circulation
- Stress on the heart
- Blood clots
- Poor appetite and malnutrition
- Dehydration
- Incontinence
- Urinary tract infection
- Constipation
- Muscle **atrophy** (weakening or wasting away of the muscle) and **contractures** (permanent and painful shortening of a muscle, tendon, or ligament that can restrict movement)
- Loss of bone mass
- Nerve injuries
- Decreased mobility
- Falls
- Fractures
- Depression and/or withdrawal
- Social isolation
- Loss of self-esteem
- Sleep disorders
- Loss of dignity
- Loss of independence
- Stress and anxiety
- Increased agitation
- Confusion
- Severe injury
- Death

7. Discuss restraint alternatives

Restraint usage has significantly decreased in facilities. State and federal agencies encourage facilities to take steps to create restraint-free environments. **Restraint-free care** means that restraints are not kept or used for any reason. Creative ideas that help avoid the need for restraints are being used instead. **Restraint**

alternatives are measures used in place of a restraint or that reduce the need for a restraint.

Many scientific studies have shown that restraints are not needed. People tend to respond better to the use of creative ways to reduce tension, pulling at tubes, wandering, and boredom. If nursing assistants have ideas about ways to avoid using restraints, they should share them with the nurse. Examples of restraint alternatives include the following:

- Make sure call lights are within reach and answer call lights immediately.

- Use fall prevention and other safety techniques, such as improving lighting.

- Certain types of grab bars can assist residents with moving in bed and getting out of bed.

- Take the resident on a walk. The doctor or nurse may add exercise into the care plan.

- Let confused residents wander in designated safe areas.

- Provide activities for those who wander at night.

- Give frequent help with elimination needs. Help with cleaning immediately after an episode of incontinence. Make sure residents are clean, dry, and comfortable.

- Encourage independence with all tasks. Provide meaningful activities.

- Encourage participation in social activities. Escort the resident to social activities when needed. Increase visits and social interaction.

- Offer reading materials that the resident enjoys. Read to the resident if needed.

- Increase the number of familiar caregivers with family members and volunteers. Family members may decrease tension just by being with residents.

- Offer food or drink.

- Decrease the noise level. Offer back rubs or use relaxation techniques.

- Listen to soothing music. Music has been shown to have a calming effect on some people.

- Monitor the resident closely and report complaints of pain to the nurse immediately.

There are also several types of pads, belts, special chairs, and alarms that can be used instead of restraints. If a resident is ordered to have an alarm on his bed or chair, the NA should make sure it is there and is turned on and working properly.

> **Tip**
>
> **Music Soothes**
>
> Residents may enjoy listening to music. The music they prefer varies, and part of providing person-centered care is taking into account each resident's preferences when possible. When new residents are admitted, staff can ask questions to find out if they enjoy music and which type of music they like. Listening to music may also help with medical conditions. For example, some studies indicate it may lower blood pressure.

8. Identify what must be done if a restraint is ordered

OBRA sets specific rules for restraint use. Restraints are used only after everything else has been ruled out and only with a doctor's order. Restraints cannot be used for staff convenience or discipline.

Guidelines: Restraints

Here is a partial list of guidelines for restraint use:

G When a resident is physically restrained, he must be monitored regularly. Complications due to the use of physical restraints must be prevented. Follow the care plan and the nurse's instructions for monitoring.

G Place the call light or required signaling device within the resident's reach. Respond to call lights immediately.

G Residents in physical restraints must be checked at least every 15 minutes. At a minimum, every two hours the restraint must be released and the resident must be given appropriate care:

- Check for physical and psychological status and comfort.

- Provide help with elimination and related hygiene needs, food and/or fluids, skin care, and range of motion exercises.

- Measure vital signs.

- Check for blue-tinged, gray, or pale skin **(cyanosis)**, which could mean lack of oxygen in the blood. With darker skin, check for purple or darkening skin. In addition, notify the nurse if redness or swelling is noted in any area of the body.

G Document the following when restraints are used:

- Type of restraint and time applied

- Each time of removal

- Care given when released, including vital signs measurements

- Any circulation, skin, behavioral, or other problems

9. List safety guidelines for oxygen use

Oxygen therapy is the administration of oxygen to increase the supply of oxygen to the lungs. This increases oxygen to the body cells. Oxygen therapy is used to treat breathing problems. It is prescribed by a doctor. Nursing assistants do not turn off or adjust oxygen levels. This is the nurse's responsibility. There is more information about oxygen in Chapter 20.

Combustion means the process of burning. Oxygen is a dangerous fire hazard because it supports combustion (makes other things burn). Working around oxygen requires special safety precautions.

Guidelines: Safety with Oxygen

G Post *No Smoking* and *Oxygen in Use* signs. These should be posted on each door. **Never allow smoking anywhere around oxygen equipment.** If you find smoking materials in a room where oxygen is in use or on a resident who is using oxygen, report to the nurse immediately.

G Remove fire hazards from the room. These include electrical equipment, such as electric razors and hair dryers. Tell the nurse if residents do not want fire hazards removed.

G Remove flammable liquids from the area. **Flammable** means easily ignited and capable of burning quickly. Alcohol and nail polish remover are examples of flammable liquids. Read the label on liquids if you are unsure. If it says *flammable*, remove it from the area.

G Do not burn candles, light matches, or use lighters around oxygen. Any type of open flame that is present around oxygen is a dangerous fire hazard.

G Check the nasal area, cheeks, and behind the ears often and report signs of irritation from the tubing from the nasal cannula or face mask (Fig. 7-12).

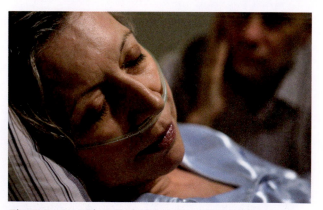

Fig. 7-12. A resident with a nasal cannula.

G Do not use any petroleum-based products, such as Vaseline or ChapStick, on the resident or on any part of the cannula or mask.

G Make sure that the resident is not lying on the oxygen tubing and that there are no kinks in it. Make sure nothing is pressing on the tubing.

G In case of a fire, you may be trained to turn off oxygen. Follow facility policy.

10. Identify safety guidelines for intravenous (IV) lines

Intravenous therapy, often called *IV therapy*, is the delivery of medication, nutrition, or fluids through a person's vein. When a doctor prescribes IV therapy, a nurse inserts an IV catheter into a vein. This gives direct access to the bloodstream. Medication, nutrition, or fluids either drip from a bag suspended on a pole or are pumped by a portable pump through a tube and into the vein (Fig. 7-13).

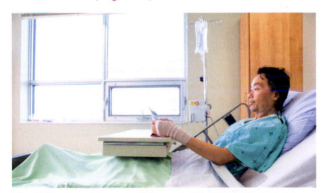

Fig. 7-13. A resident receiving medication intravenously.

Guidelines: Intravenous (IV) Therapy

G Always wear gloves if you have to touch the IV area.

G Do not do any of the following when caring for a resident with an IV line:

- Measure blood pressure on an arm with an IV line.

- Get the IV site wet.

- Pull on or catch the tubing on anything, such as clothing, during positioning.

- Leave the tubing kinked.

- Lower the IV bag below the IV site.

- Touch the clamp.

- Disconnect the IV line from the pump or turn off the alarm.

G Report to the nurse if any of the following occurs:

- The needle or catheter has fallen out or moves out of the vein. If an IV catheter comes out of the vein, it can cause an infiltration. An *infiltration* is the administration of fluids into surrounding tissue. Symptoms of infiltration include tissue swelling, cool or cold skin, red or warm skin, pain, tenderness, bleeding, and leaking of fluid from the IV site.

- The armboard or handboard (device taped to the arm or hand, used to help keep the IV catheter properly positioned inside the vein) becomes loose.

- The tubing is disconnected.

- Blood appears in the tubing.

- The IV fluid in the bag or container is gone or almost gone.

- The IV fluid is not dripping, is leaking, or the bag breaks.

- The IV pump is beeping.

- The resident complains of pain, has difficulty breathing, or has a fever. Pain and fever may indicate phlebitis, which is inflammation of a vein (Chapter 19).

- The resident pulls out or attempts to pull out the IV line.

Residents' Rights

Oxygen and IVs

Residents who use oxygen or have IVs have the continued right to freedom of movement and the right to safety with the use of these devices.

11. Discuss fire safety and explain the RACE and PASS acronyms

There are many causes of fire. For a fire to occur, three elements must be present:

1. Heat: makes the flame

2. Fuel: the object that burns

3. Oxygen: gas that will keep the fire burning

There are many potential fire hazards in facilities, including the following:

*   Smoking

*   Frayed or damaged electrical cords

*   Electrical equipment in need of repair

*   Overloaded electrical sockets

*   Oxygen use

*   Unattended candles

*   Flammable liquids or rags with oils on them

*   Stacks of newspapers or other clutter

All facilities have fire safety plans. Guidelines regarding fires and evacuations will be explained to all employees. Evacuation routes are posted in facilities. Nursing assistants should read and review them often and should attend fire and disaster in-service trainings when they are offered.

Guidelines: Reducing Fire Hazards and Responding to Fires

G   If the facility allows smoking, never leave smokers unattended. Check ashtrays for lit cigarettes or matches. Put out burning cigarettes. Make sure cigarettes or other smoking materials have not fallen anywhere. Before emptying an ashtray, make sure there are no hot ashes, matches, or cigarette butts in the ashtray.

G   Residents may use electronic cigarettes (e-cigarettes, e-cigs). E-cigarettes do not contain tobacco. Most e-cigarettes heat a nicotine-containing liquid until it becomes a vapor that can be inhaled. Matches or lighters are not needed to light this type of cigarette. They use a battery to turn the nicotine solution into a vapor. Fires involving e-cigarettes have been reported due to the battery overcharging or overheating. Follow your facility's policies with regard to these devices.

G   Report immediately if electrical equipment or cords are damaged or frayed. Check to see that cords are not too short. Do not use cords that have electrical tape around them. Report damaged equipment to the nurse promptly.

G   If you smell gas, report it immediately. Avoid using light switches, candles, matches, or cell phones until you have been informed that it is safe to do so.

G   Make sure you know the location of fire alarms in your facility. The **RACE** acronym outlines what to do in case of a fire:

Remove anyone in danger if you are not in danger.

Activate alarm or call 911.

Contain the fire by closing all doors and windows if possible.

Extinguish the fire, or fire department will extinguish. Evacuate if instructed to do so.

G   Every facility has multiple fire extinguishers (Fig. 7-14). Learn where they are located. In order to understand how to use an extinguisher, follow the **PASS** acronym:

Pull the pin.

Aim at the base of the fire when spraying.

Squeeze the handle.

Sweep back and forth at the base of the fire.

When a fire occurs, remember these guidelines:

G   Know the location of the fire evacuation plan.

G   Remain calm. Do not panic.

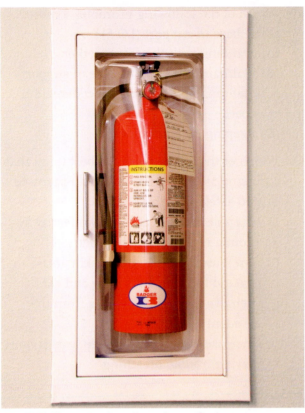

Fig. 7-14. *Know the locations of your facility's fire extinguishers and how to use them.*

G   Remove all persons in the immediate area of the fire.

G   Stay low in a room to escape a fire.

G   If a door is closed, always check for heat coming from it before opening it. If the door or doorknob feels hot, stay in the room if there is no safe exit. Plug the doorway (use wet towels or clothing) to prevent smoke from entering. Stay in the room until help arrives.

G   Use a damp covering over the face to reduce smoke inhalation.

G   If clothing is on fire, use the *stop, drop, and roll* fire safety technique to put out the fire. Stop running or stay still. Drop to the ground, lying down if possible. Roll on the ground to try to extinguish the flames.

G   Never get into an elevator during a fire unless directed to do so by the fire department.

G   In case of fire, nursing assistants may be asked to turn off all oxygen and electrical equipment in the area. Follow your facility's policies.

12. List general safety steps for working in a healthcare facility

Living or working in a healthcare facility may put a person at risk of being a victim of a crime. Many people go in and out of a facility at all hours. Delivery people, visitors, clergymembers, temporary workers, and others may enter facilities regularly. Unfortunately not everyone is honest and trustworthy. All staff members should observe and report any suspicious behavior.

Guidelines: Safety in a Facility

G   If you notice anything suspicious, report it immediately.

G   Keep valuable personal items at home.

G   Ask the nurse to lock up residents' valuable items.

G   If any visitor or staff member makes you uneasy, do not leave a resident alone with the person. Report this immediately.

G   Follow guidelines for the number of visitors allowed at one time in a resident's room.

G   Do not share your personal information with anyone. Do not share residents' or other staff members' information with anyone.

G   Report any situation or person who makes you feel unsafe or concerned to your supervisor immediately.

Chapter Review

1.   What important information does the Safety Data Sheet (SDS) provide about chemicals (LO 3)?

2. What items should be disposed of in a bio-hazard container or bag (LO 4)?

3. Should objects be held close to the body or far away from the body when lifting or carrying them (LO 5)?

4. When lifting, is it better to bend at the waist or at the knees (LO 5)?

5. Why was restraint use restricted (LO 6)?

6. What are restraint alternatives (LO 7)?

7. When can a restraint be applied (LO 8)?

8. List six signs to report to a nurse about intra-venous (IV) therapy (LO 10).

9. What three things need to be present for a fire to occur (LO 11)?

10. Identify what the acronyms *RACE* and *PASS* stand for (LO 11).

11. If a fire has started, what should the nursing assistant do before opening a closed door (LO 11)?

12. List two general safety steps to protect residents in a facility (LO 12).

Multiple Choice

13. The most common accidents that occur in a healthcare facility are (LO 2)
    (A) Burns
    (B) Falls
    (C) Cuts
    (D) Poisonings

14. The best position for a resident to be in while eating is (LO 2)
    (A) Sitting upright
    (B) Lying on his left side
    (C) Reclining with his head tilted back
    (D) On his stomach

15. Which of the following promotes a more stable base of support (LO 5)?
    (A) Standing with the feet together
    (B) Maintaining a narrow base of support
    (C) Standing with the feet shoulder-width apart
    (D) Keeping the knees locked

16. Which of the following is the best thing that a nursing assistant can do to help promote oxygen safety (LO 9)?
    (A) Keep lit matches at least two feet away from a resident using oxygen
    (B) Use Vaseline on irritated skin areas around the resident's nose and ears
    (C) Remove flammable liquids from the resident's room
    (D) Increase a resident's oxygen level if he is having trouble breathing

8
Emergency Care, First Aid, and Disasters

Emergency Transfer of Victims During the 1500s

Compare the rescue of a traveler in the 1500s to the care our emergency squads give today. "The misfortune befell me in the manner which follows: wishing to pass across the water and trying to make my hackney enter a boat, I struck [the horse] . . . with a riding crop [and] the animal gave me such a kick that she broke entirely the two bones of my left leg. . . . I was quickly carried into the boat to cross to the other side in order to have me treated. But its shaking almost made me die, because the ends of the broken bones rubbed against the flesh, and those who were carrying me could not give it fit posture. From the boat, I was carried into a house of the village with greater pain than I had endured in the boat. . . . Finally, however, they placed me on a bed to regain my breath a little. . . while my dressing was being made."

from *Ten Books of Surgery* by Ambroise Paré

"It is by presence of mind in untried emergencies that the native metal of a man is tested."

James Russell Lowell, 1819–1891

"The truly noble and resolved spirit raises itself, and becomes more conspicuous in times of disaster and ill fortune."

Plutarch, 46–120 AD

1. Define important words in this chapter

abdominal thrusts: a method of attempting to remove an object from the airway of someone who is choking.

cardiac arrest: sudden stopping/cessation of the heartbeat.

code team: group of people chosen for a particular shift to respond to resident emergencies.

conscious: having awareness of surroundings, sensations, and thoughts.

CPR: an abbreviation for *cardiopulmonary resuscitation*; medical procedures used when a person's heart and lungs have stopped working.

diabetic ketoacidosis (DKA): a life-threatening complication of diabetes that can result from undiagnosed diabetes, infection, not enough insulin, hyperglycemia (high blood sugar), eating too much, not getting enough exercise, and stress.

emesis: the act of vomiting, or ejecting stomach contents through the mouth and/or nose.

epistaxis: a nosebleed.

expressive aphasia: difficulty communicating through speech or writing.

first aid: care given to an injured person by the first people to respond to an emergency.

hemiparesis: weakness on one side of the body.

hemiplegia: paralysis of one side of the body.

hemorrhage: bleeding; blood loss.

hyperglycemia: high blood glucose (blood sugar).

hypoglycemia: low blood glucose (blood sugar); also known as *insulin reaction* or *insulin shock*.

insulin reaction: a life-threatening complication of diabetes that can result from either too much insulin or too little food; also known as *hypoglycemia* or *insulin shock*.

myocardial infarction (MI): a condition in which blood flow to the heart is blocked and muscle cells die; also called *heart attack*.

obstructed airway: a condition in which the tube through which air enters the lungs is blocked.

receptive aphasia: difficulty understanding spoken or written words.

respiratory arrest: stopping/cessation of breathing.

shock: a condition that occurs when there is decreased blood flow to organs and tissues.

syncope: temporary loss of consciousness; also called *fainting*.

2. Demonstrate how to respond to medical emergencies

Medical emergencies can happen when least expected (Fig. 8-1). Choking, diabetic emergencies, falls, poisoning, heart attacks, strokes, stab wounds, and gunshot wounds are all medical emergencies. The most serious medical emergencies involve these situations:

- The person is unconscious or unresponsive.

- The person is not breathing.

- The person has no pulse.

- The person is bleeding severely.

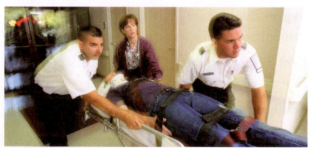

Fig. 8-1. *Medical emergencies can happen at any time. Being calm and prepared is the best way to respond to emergencies.*

In an emergency, responders should remain calm, act quickly, and communicate clearly. When an emergency occurs, the responder should take two pairs of gloves and a barrier face mask with her. She should look around to make sure the area is safe before providing care. Once gloves are on, these actions show the correct response to emergencies:

- **Assess the situation.** The responder should notice the time. She should try to find out what has happened.

- **Assess the victim.** The responder should ask the injured or ill person what has happened. If the person is unable to respond, he may be unconscious. Being **conscious** means having awareness of surroundings, sensations, and thoughts. Tapping the person and asking if he is all right helps to determine if a person is conscious. The responder should speak loudly and use the person's name if she knows it. If there is no response, she should assume the person is unconscious. This is an emergency situation. She should call for help right away or send someone else to call.

If a person is conscious and able to speak, then he is breathing and has a pulse. The responder should talk with him about what happened and check the person for any of the following:

- Severe bleeding

- Changes in consciousness

- Irregular breathing

- Unusual color or feel to the skin

- Swollen places on the body

- Medical alert tags

- Pain

If any of these exist, professional medical help may be needed. A nursing assistant should always get help. She should call the nurse before doing anything else. If the injured or ill person is conscious, he may be frightened. The responder should listen to the person and tell him what is being done to help him. A calm and confident response will help reassure him.

After the emergency, while still on duty, the NA will need to document the emergency and complete an incident report. It is important to include as many details as possible and report only facts. For example, if the NA thinks a resident suffered a heart attack, she should document only the signs and symptoms she observed and the actions she took. Understanding the kind of information the NA will have to document will help her remember the important facts during the emergency. For instance, it is especially important to remember the time at which a resident became unconscious.

> **Tip**
>
> **PPE SCC**
>
> Performing first aid is something for which many people are not prepared. This acronym is helpful when a nursing assistant must perform first aid: PPE SCC.
>
> - **PPE**: Grab and apply personal protective equipment.
> - **S**afety first! Are you safe?
> - **C**all for help or point to person and say: "You, get help now!"
> - **C**are for victims.

> **Trivia**
>
> **Flying Ambulances**
>
> Napoleon invaded Italy in 1796. During that invasion, Dominique Jean Larrey (1766–1842) developed "flying ambulances." These were horse-drawn wagons that were able to quickly remove the wounded from the front lines for treatment. During the American Civil War, around 1863, "ambulance trains" similar to the legendary wagon trains of western lore appeared.

3. Demonstrate knowledge of first aid procedures

Emergency situations can happen to anyone at any time. When a person is involved in a serious accident, such as drowning or choking, respiratory arrest can occur. **Respiratory arrest** means that breathing stops. If the person is not helped quickly, cardiac arrest may soon follow. **Cardiac arrest** is when the heart stops. When respiratory arrest occurs, rescue breathing must be initiated. When respiratory arrest and cardiac arrest occur, CPR is necessary. **CPR** refers to medical procedures used when the heart and lungs have stopped working and is used until medical help arrives.

Quick action is essential. The first few minutes of any emergency can determine the victim's ability to survive the incident. CPR must be started immediately to help prevent or minimize

brain damage. Brain damage can occur within four to six minutes after breathing stops and the heart stops beating.

In an emergency situation, NAs should never do anything that is beyond their ability or training. They should give basic first aid until the emergency medical team arrives. **First aid** is the care given to an injured person by the first people to respond to an emergency.

Employers often arrange for nursing assistants to be trained in CPR. If not, the NA can contact the American Heart Association (heart.org) or Red Cross (redcross.org) for more information. CPR is an important skill to learn.

Nursing assistants need to know their facility's policies on initiating CPR if they have been trained to do so. Some facilities do not allow nursing assistants to begin CPR without direction of the nurse. This is due, in part, to residents' advance directives. Some people have made the decision that they do not want CPR. The nurse should be notified immediately if an emergency occurs.

> **The AED**
>
> An automated external defibrillator, or AED, may be used for a cardiac arrest. The AED is a computerized device that can restore the heart rhythm by giving the heart an electrical shock. When using this device, a clear, computerized voice takes the user through each step that must be performed. Lights and text messages may also relay instructions.
>
> AEDs are available at healthcare facilities and are also located in airplanes, offices, shopping malls, and other places. AED training will be given during CPR classes. Care must be taken when using this device near oxygen. Fires can occur due to sparks.
>
> AEDs must be maintained for best performance. Regular checks should be scheduled to ensure the AED is in proper working order.

> **Residents' Rights**
>
> **CPR**
>
> During CPR, nursing assistants should provide for privacy, which helps maintain the resident's dignity.

Choking

Residents who have difficulty chewing or swallowing, have dentures that do not fit well, are confused, or have poor vision may be at risk of choking. When something is blocking the tube through which air enters the lungs, the person has an **obstructed airway**. When people are choking, they usually put their hands to their throats (Fig. 8-2). As long as the resident can speak, cough, or breathe, the NA should only encourage her to cough as forcefully as possible to get the object out. The NA should ask someone to get a nurse and should stay with the resident.

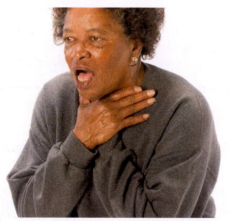

Fig. 8-2. A common sign of choking is when a person puts her hands to her throat.

If a resident can no longer speak, cough, or breathe, or turns blue, the NA should call for help immediately by using the call light or emergency cord. Time is of extreme importance. The choking victim should not be left alone. **Abdominal thrusts** are a method of attempting to remove an object from the airway of someone who is choking. These thrusts work to remove the blockage upward, out of the throat.

The NA should make sure the person needs help before starting to give abdominal thrusts. The person must show signs of a severely obstructed airway. These signs include poor air exchange, an increase in difficulty breathing, silent coughing, blue-tinged (cyanotic) skin, or an inability to speak, cough, or breathe. The NA should ask, "Are you choking? I know what to do. Can I help you?" If the resident nods her head "Yes,"

she has a severe airway obstruction and needs immediate help. The NA should begin giving abdominal thrusts if her facility allows this. This procedure should never be performed on a person who is not choking because it can cause injury.

Performing abdominal thrusts for the conscious person

1. Stand behind the person and bring your arms under her arms. Wrap your arms around the person's waist.

2. Make a fist with one hand. Place the flat, thumb side of the fist against the person's abdomen, above the navel but below the breastbone (Fig. 8-3).

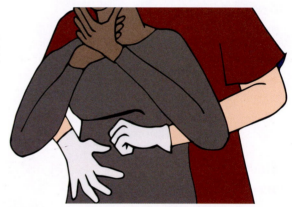

Fig. 8-3. The flat, thumb side of the fist against the person's abdomen is the correct placement for abdominal thrusts.

3. Grasp the fist with your other hand. Pull both hands toward you and up (inward and upward), quickly and forcefully.

4. Repeat until the object is pushed out or the person loses consciousness.

If the person becomes unconscious while choking, she should be helped to the floor gently. She should be lying on her back on a hard surface with her face up. The NA should begin CPR for an unconscious person if trained and allowed to do so. The NA should make sure help is on the way. The resident may have a completely blocked airway and may need medical help immediately. The NA should stay with the victim until help arrives.

Shock

Shock occurs when organs and tissues in the body do not receive an adequate blood supply. Bleeding, heart attack, severe infection, and falling blood pressure can lead to shock. Shock can become worse when the person is frightened or in severe pain.

Shock is a dangerous, life-threatening situation. Signs of shock include pale or cyanotic (bluish) skin, staring, increased pulse and respiration rates, low blood pressure, and extreme thirst. An NA should always call for help if she suspects a resident is in shock.

Responding to shock

1. Notify the nurse immediately. Victims of shock should always receive medical care as soon as possible.

2. If you need to control bleeding, put on gloves first. The next procedure will explain how to do this.

3. Have the person lie down on her back. If the person is bleeding from the mouth or vomiting, turn or logroll her on her side (Chapter 11). Elevate the legs about 8 to 12 inches unless the person has a head, neck, back, leg, spinal, or abdominal injury; breathing difficulties; or fractures (Fig. 8-4). Elevating the legs allows blood to flow back to the brain (and other vital areas). Never elevate a body part if a broken bone exists or if it causes pain.

4. Check pulse and respirations if possible (Chapter 13). Begin CPR if breathing and pulse are absent and if you are trained to do so.

5. Keep the person as calm and comfortable as possible. Loosen clothing or ties around the neck and any belts or waist strings.

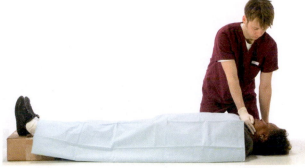

Fig. 8-4. *If the person is in shock, elevate the legs, unless the person has head, neck, back, leg, spinal, or abdominal injuries; breathing difficulties; or fractures.*

6. Maintain normal body temperature. If the weather is cold, place a blanket around the person. If the weather is hot, provide shade.

7. Do not give the person food or liquids.

Bleeding

Severe bleeding, or **hemorrhage**, can cause death quickly and must be controlled.

Controlling bleeding

1. Notify the nurse immediately.

2. Put on gloves. Always take time to do this. If the person is able, he can hold his bare hand over the wound until you can put on gloves.

3. Hold a thick sterile pad, clean cloth, or clean towel against the wound.

4. Press down hard directly on the bleeding wound until help arrives. Do not decrease pressure (Fig. 8-5). Put additional pads over the first pad if blood seeps through. Do not remove the first pads.

5. If you can, raise the wound above the level of the heart to slow the bleeding. Prop up the limb if the wound is on an arm, leg, hand, or foot, and there are no head, neck, back, spinal, or abdominal injuries; breathing difficulties; or fractures. Use towels or other absorbent material.

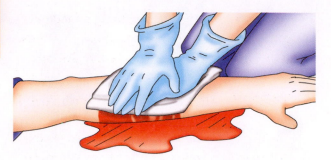

Fig. 8-5. Press down hard directly on the bleeding wound; do not decrease pressure.

6. When bleeding is under control, secure the dressing to keep it in place. Check the person for symptoms of shock (pale skin, staring, increased pulse and respiration rates, low blood pressure, and extreme thirst). Stay with the person until help arrives.

7. Remove and discard gloves and wash hands thoroughly when finished.

There are also special bandages and sponges for controlling bleeding that may be available for use.

Burns

There are three types of burns: first degree (superficial), second degree (partial thickness), and third degree (full thickness) burns. Care of a burn depends on its depth, size, and location. Chapter 18 contains more information.

Treating burns

To treat a minor burn:

1. Notify the nurse immediately. Put on gloves.

2. Use cool, clean water to decrease the skin temperature and prevent further injury. Do not use ice or ice water, as ice may cause further skin damage. Dampen a clean cloth with cool water, and place it over the burn.

3. Once the pain has eased, cover the area with a dry, clean dressing or nonadhesive sterile bandage.

4. Remove and discard gloves properly. Wash your hands.

5. Never use any kind of ointment, salve, or grease on a burn.

For more serious burns:

1. Remove the person from the source of the burn. If clothing has caught fire, have the person stop, drop, and roll, or smother the fire with a blanket or towel to put out flames. Protect yourself from the source of the burn.

2. Notify the nurse immediately. Put on gloves.

3. Check for breathing, pulse, and severe bleeding. If the person is not breathing and has no pulse, begin CPR if trained and allowed to do so. Do not put pillows under the head, as this may obstruct the airway.

4. Do not use any type of ointment, water, salve, or grease on the burn.

5. Do not try to pull away any clothing from burned areas. Cover the burn with sterile gauze or a clean sheet. Apply the gauze or sheet lightly. Do not rub the burned area.

6. Take steps to prevent shock.

7. Do not give the person food or liquids.

8. Monitor vital signs and wait for emergency medical help.

9. Remove and discard gloves properly. Wash your hands.

Fainting (Syncope)

Fainting, or **syncope**, occurs as a result of decreased blood flow to the brain, causing a temporary loss of consciousness. Fainting may be the result of an abnormal heart rhythm, decreased blood supply to the brain, hunger, **hypoglycemia** (low blood glucose), dehydration, fear, pain, fatigue, standing for a long time, poor ventilation, pregnancy, or overheating. Signs and symptoms of fainting include dizziness, nausea, perspiration, pale skin, weak pulse, shallow respirations, and blackness in the visual field.

Responding to fainting

1. Notify the nurse immediately.

2. Have the person lie down or sit down before fainting occurs.

3. If the person is in a sitting position, have him bend forward (Fig. 8-6). He can place his head between his knees if he is able. If the person is lying flat on his back, and there are no head, neck, back, spinal, or abdominal injuries; breathing difficulties; or fractures, elevate the legs about 12 inches.

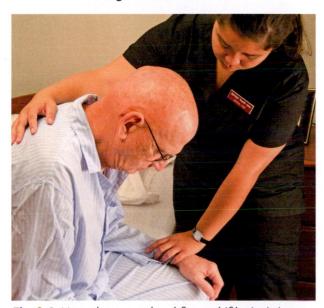

Fig. 8-6. Have the person bend forward if he is sitting.

4. Loosen any tight clothing.

5. Have the person stay in this position for at least five minutes after symptoms disappear.

6. Help the person get up slowly. Continue to observe him for symptoms of fainting. Help him to sit down if needed. Stay with him until he feels better. If you need help but cannot leave him, use the call light.

7. If a person does faint, lower him to the floor or other flat surface. Position him on his back. If he has no head, neck, back, spinal,

or abdominal injuries; breathing difficulties; or fractures, elevate his legs about 12 inches. If unsure about injuries, leave him flat on his back. Check to make sure the person is breathing. (If the person is not breathing and has no pulse, begin CPR if trained and allowed to do so.) He should recover quickly, but keep him lying down for several minutes. Report the incident to the nurse immediately. Fainting may be a sign of a more serious medical condition.

Poisoning

Facilities contain many harmful substances that should not be swallowed. Poisoning may be suspected when a resident vomits; has heavy, difficult breathing; is very drowsy; is confused; or has burns or red areas around the mouth. Some of these signs and symptoms can mimic other conditions as well. If an NA suspects poisoning, he should notify the nurse immediately. The NA may be asked to don gloves and look for a container that will help determine what the resident has taken or eaten.

Nosebleed

A nosebleed can occur suddenly when the air is dry, when injury has occurred, or when a person has taken certain medications. The medical term for a nosebleed is **epistaxis**.

Responding to a nosebleed

1. Notify the nurse immediately.

2. Elevate the head of the bed, or tell the resident to remain in a sitting position, leaning forward slightly. Offer tissues, a clean cloth, or an emesis basin to catch the blood. Do not touch blood or bloody clothes, tissues, or cloths without gloves.

3. Put on gloves. Apply firm pressure on both sides of the nose, on the soft part, up near the bridge. Squeeze the sides with your

thumb and forefinger (Fig. 8-7). Have the resident do this until you are able to put on gloves.

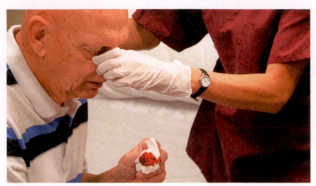

Fig. 8-7. With gloves on, squeeze the bridge of the nose with your thumb and forefinger.

4. Apply pressure until the bleeding stops.

5. Use a cool cloth or ice wrapped in a cloth over the bridge of the nose to help slow the flow of blood. Never apply ice directly to skin.

6. Keep person still and calm until help arrives.

7. Remove and discard gloves and wash your hands.

Vomiting

Vomiting, or **emesis**, is the act of ejecting stomach contents through the mouth and/or nose. It can be a sign of a serious illness or injury. Because an NA may not know when a resident is going to vomit, he may not have time to explain what he will do ahead of time. The NA should talk to the resident soothingly as he helps him clean up. He should tell the resident what he is doing to help him.

Responding to vomiting

1. Notify the nurse immediately.

2. Put on gloves.

3. If the resident is sitting up, place an emesis basin under the chin. If the resident is lying on his back, turn his head to the side to help prevent choking and aspiration, and place

the basin under the chin. If an emesis basin is not nearby, use the wash basin. Remove it when vomiting has stopped.

4. Remove soiled linens or clothes and set aside. Replace with fresh linens or clothes.

5. Note amount, color, and consistency of vomitus. Look for blood in vomitus, blood-tinged vomitus, or medication (pills) in vomitus. Find out if a specimen should be sent to the laboratory. Show the nurse the vomitus before discarding if blood or pills are noted.

6. Flush vomitus down the toilet and wash and store the basin.

7. Remove and discard gloves properly.

8. Wash your hands.

9. Put on fresh gloves.

10. Provide comfort to the resident. Wipe his face and mouth (Fig. 8-8). Position him comfortably, and offer a drink of water or a sip to swish in the mouth and spit. Provide oral care (see Chapter 12). It helps get rid of the vomit taste in the mouth.

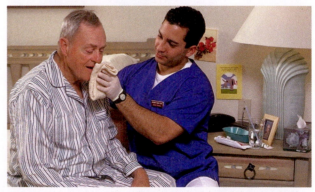

Fig. 8-8. Be calm and comforting when helping a resident who has vomited.

11. Put the soiled linen in proper containers.

12. Remove and discard gloves properly.

13. Wash your hands again.

14. Document time, amount, color, odor, and consistency of vomitus.

Myocardial Infarction or Heart Attack

When blood flow to an area of the heart is blocked, oxygen and nutrients fail to reach its cells. Waste products are not removed and the muscle cells die. This is called a **myocardial infarction (MI)**, or heart attack. The area of dead tissue may be large or small. This depends on the artery or arteries involved. A myocardial infarction is an emergency that can result in serious heart damage or death. The following are signs and symptoms of MI:

- Sudden, severe pain, pressure, squeezing, or fullness in the chest, usually on the left side or in the center, behind the breastbone

- Pain or discomfort in other areas of the body, such as one or both arms, the back, neck, jaw, or stomach

- Indigestion or heartburn

- Nausea and vomiting

- Shortness of breath

- Dizziness

- Lightheadedness

- Pale, gray, or cyanotic skin color or mucous membranes, indicating lack of oxygen

- Perspiration

- Cold and clammy skin

- Weak and irregular pulse rate

- Low blood pressure

- Anxiety and a sense of doom

- Denial of a heart problem

The pain of a heart attack is commonly described as a crushing, pressing, squeezing, stabbing, piercing pain, or, "like someone is sitting on my chest." The pain may go down the inside of the left arm. A person may also feel it in the neck and/or in the jaw. The pain usually does not go away.

As with men, women may experience chest pain or discomfort. Women, though, can have heart attacks without chest pressure. Women are more likely to have shortness of breath, nausea, vomiting, lightheadedness, fainting, dizziness, stomach pain, sweating, fatigue, and back, neck, or jaw pain. Some women's symptoms seem more flu-like, and women are more likely to deny that they are having a heart attack. An NA must take immediate action if a resident experiences any of these symptoms.

Responding to a myocardial infarction

1. Notify the nurse immediately.

2. Place the resident in a comfortable position. Encourage him to rest. Reassure him that you will not leave him alone.

3. Loosen clothing around the person's neck (Fig. 8-9).

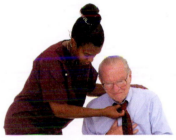

Fig. 8-9. *Loosen the clothing around the person's neck if you suspect he is having an MI.*

4. Do not give the person food or liquids.

5. Monitor the person's breathing and pulse. If the person is not breathing and has no pulse, begin CPR if trained and allowed to do so.

6. Stay with the person until help arrives.

Chapter 19 contains more information on myocardial infarctions.

Insulin Reaction and Diabetic Ketoacidosis

Insulin reaction and diabetic ketoacidosis are complications of diabetes that can be life-threatening. **Insulin reaction**, or hypoglycemia, can result from either too much insulin or too little food. It occurs when insulin is given and the person skips a meal or does not eat all the food required. Even when a regular amount of food is eaten, physical activity may cause the body to rapidly absorb the food. This causes too much insulin to be in the body. Vomiting and diarrhea may also lead to insulin reaction in people who have diabetes.

The first signs of insulin reaction include feeling weak or different, nervousness, dizziness, and perspiration. The NA should immediately report these signs to the nurse. These signal that the resident needs food in a form that can be rapidly absorbed. If the person is conscious and is able to swallow, a glass of milk, fruit juice, or water with sugar dissolved in it should be consumed right away. A glucose tablet is another quick source of sugar. Other signs and symptoms include the following:

- Headache
- Blurred vision
- Numbness of the lips and tongue
- Cold, clammy skin
- Trembling
- Hunger
- Rapid pulse
- Low blood pressure
- Confusion
- Unconsciousness

Hypoglycemia can also occur without causing any symptoms. Blood glucose levels fall, but the person does not experience any symptoms. This is known as *hypoglycemia unawareness*. The person may not realize he is experiencing hypoglycemia. In order to try to prevent this from occurring, a doctor may increase or adjust the person's blood glucose goals.

Having too little insulin in the body causes **diabetic ketoacidosis (DKA)**. It can result from undiagnosed diabetes, infection (especially a urinary tract infection), going without insulin or not taking enough insulin, **hyperglycemia**

(high blood glucose), eating too much, not getting enough exercise, or physical and emotional stress.

The signs of onset of diabetic ketoacidosis include increased hunger, thirst, or urination; abdominal pain; deep or labored breathing; and breath that smells sweet or fruity. The nurse should be notified immediately if a resident shows signs of DKA. Other signs and symptoms include the following:

- Headache
- Blurred vision
- Dry skin, dry mouth
- Flushed cheeks
- Nausea and vomiting
- Loss of appetite
- Rapid, weak pulse
- Low blood pressure
- Shortness of breath or air hunger (person gasping for air and being unable to catch his breath)
- Weakness
- Drowsiness
- Confusion
- Unconsciousness

If left untreated, DKA can lead to diabetic coma and death. Chapter 23 has more information.

Concussion

A concussion can occur after a head or body injury. Signs and symptoms of a concussion include headache, sleepiness, forgetfulness, confusion, vision changes, changes in the size of the pupil of the eye, problems with balance, weakness, numbness, slurred speech, and nausea and/or vomiting. Chapter 22 contains more information about care for people with head injuries.

Seizures

Seizures are involuntary, often violent, contractions of muscles. They can involve a small area or the entire body. Seizures are caused by an abnormality in the brain. They can occur in young children who have a high fever. Older children and adults who have a serious illness, fever, head injury, or a seizure disorder such as epilepsy may also have seizures.

The main goal of a caregiver during a seizure is to make sure the resident is safe. During a seizure, a person may shake severely and thrust arms and legs uncontrollably. He may clench his jaw, drool, and be unable to swallow. Most seizures last a short amount of time.

Responding to seizures

1. Note the time. Put on gloves. If the person is wearing eyeglasses, remove them.

2. Lower the person to the floor. Cradle and protect his head. If a pillow is nearby, place it under his head. Loosen clothing to help with breathing. Try to turn him to one side to lower the risk of choking. This may not be possible during a violent seizure.

3. Have someone call the nurse immediately or use the call light. Do not leave the person unless you must do so to get medical help.

4. Move furniture away to prevent injury.

5. Do not try to stop the seizure or restrain the person.

6. Do not force anything between the person's teeth. Do not place your hands in his mouth for any reason. You could be bitten.

7. Do not give the person food or liquids.

8. When the seizure is over, note the time. Gently turn the person onto his left side unless he has a head, neck, back, leg, spinal or abdominal injury; breathing difficulties; or fractures. Turning the person reduces the risk of choking or aspirating on vomit or saliva. If the person begins to choke, get help immediately. Check for adequate breathing and pulse. If the person is not breathing and has no pulse,

begin CPR if trained and allowed to do so. Do not begin CPR during a seizure.

9. Remove and discard gloves and wash your hands.

10. Report the length of the seizure and your observations to the nurse.

CVA or Stroke

The medical term for a stroke is cerebrovascular accident (CVA). A stroke (sometimes called *brain attack*) occurs when the blood supply to a portion of the brain is cut off. A clot, a ruptured blood vessel, or pressure from a tumor compressing a vessel may cause a stroke.

Quick response to a suspected stroke is critical. Tests and treatment need to be given within a short time of the stroke's onset (ideally within an hour). Early treatment may be able to reduce the severity of the stroke.

A transient ischemic attack, or TIA, is a warning sign of a CVA. It is the result of a temporary lack of oxygen in the brain. Symptoms may last up to 24 hours. They include difficulty speaking, weakness on one side of the body, temporary loss of vision, and numbness or tingling. These symptoms should not be ignored. They should be reported to the nurse immediately. These are also signs that a TIA or stroke is occurring:

- Facial numbness, weakness, or drooping, especially on one side

- Paralysis on one side of the body **(hemiplegia)**

- Arm or leg numbness or weakness, especially on one side **(hemiparesis)**

- Trouble walking, loss of balance

- Slurred speech or inability to speak **(expressive aphasia)**

- Inability to understand spoken or written words **(receptive aphasia)**

- Use of inappropriate words

- Severe headache
- Blurred vision or trouble seeing in one or both eyes
- Ringing in the ears
- Redness in the face
- Noisy breathing
- Slow pulse rate
- Elevated blood pressure
- Nausea or vomiting
- Loss of bowel and bladder control
- Seizures
- Dizziness
- Loss of consciousness

In addition to the symptoms listed previously, women may have these symptoms:

- Pain in the face, arms, and legs
- Hiccups
- Shortness of breath
- Palpitations
- Chest pain
- Agitation
- Hallucinations
- Disorientation

F.A.S.T.

The acronym **F.A.S.T.** can be used as a way to remember the sudden signs that a stroke is occurring.

(F)ace: Is one side of the face drooping? Is it numb? Ask the person to smile. Is the smile uneven?

(A)rms: Is one arm numb or weak? Ask the person to raise both arms. Check to see if one arm drifts downward.

(S)peech: Is the person's speech slurred? Is the person unable to speak? Can the person be understood? Ask the person to repeat a simple sentence and see if the sentence is repeated correctly.

(T)ime: Time is of the utmost importance when responding to a stroke. If the person shows any of the symptoms listed above, report to the nurse immediately.

The website for the American Stroke Association (strokeassociation.org) has more information. Chapter 22 in this textbook contains more information about strokes.

4. Explain the nursing assistant's role on a code team

Facilities often use codes to inform staff of emergencies without alarming residents and visitors. For example, *Code Red* usually means fire, and *Code Blue* usually means cardiac arrest. Nursing assistants will be taught the codes for their facilities.

When staff members are given their assignments at the beginning of shifts, some facilities also assign positions on the code team. The **code team** is the team chosen for that shift to respond in case of a resident emergency. Staff on the code team may be asked to get a special cart or other emergency equipment, such as a suction machine, CPR equipment, oxygen, or other items. Although nursing assistants will not do many of the code team procedures, they may be asked to perform chest compressions during CPR.

If a nursing assistant is on the code team for a particular shift and a code is called, the NA should respond from wherever she is in the facility. It is important for responders to remain calm and not panic when a code is announced. If the NA is caring for a resident, she should get another staff member to take over before responding to the code. Classes regarding updated procedures for responding to codes may be held periodically in healthcare facilities.

Residents' Rights

Responding to Codes

When a resident goes into respiratory or cardiac arrest, it can be difficult for staff, other residents, and visitors. When a code occurs, the staff's main concern is the victim's survival. However, it is also important to consider the impact on other people in a facility.

Staff members not involved in responding to the code can move other people away from the area until the problem has been resolved. In some facilities a *Code Watcher* team will respond to a code and deal only with the emotional concerns of residents, staff, and visitors. This team may be made up of nursing staff, social workers, trained volunteers, health unit coordinators, and administrative staff.

When a code occurs, roommates should be removed from the room or area if possible. Unconscious residents who are nearby may also be aware of everything that is happening. They should be reassured, too, during emergency situations.

5. Describe guidelines for responding to disasters

Disasters can include fire, flood, earthquake, hurricane, tornado, or severe weather. Man-made dangers, such as acts of terrorism, are also considered disasters.

Nursing assistants are expected to respond calmly and skillfully to disasters. Facilities will have an area-specific disaster plan available for employees to learn. Nursing assistants should know their facility's plan and what to do in the event of a disaster. There will be general guidelines to follow, as well as area-specific guidelines. For example, NAs working where hurricanes occur, such as Florida, need to know guidelines for hurricanes, as well as other disasters.

During an emergency, a nurse or the administrator will give directions. NAs should listen carefully and follow instructions. The following guidelines apply in any disaster situation:

- Remain calm.
- Know the locations of all exits and stairways.
- Know where the fire alarms and extinguishers are located.
- Know the appropriate action to take in any situation.

Being educated and prepared for emergencies helps decrease panic and ensure a timely and appropriate response. This helps to protect everyone. Annual in-service education and disaster drills are often held at facilities. NAs should take advantage of these sessions and pay close attention to instructions.

The Federal Emergency Management Agency (FEMA) has more information about disaster preparedness at fema.gov. The American Red Cross also has information at redcross.org.

Tip

Blackouts

If a blackout occurs, emergency generators should automatically begin working. If a generator fails, emergency battery packs may be needed for some electrical equipment, such as ventilators and IV pumps. Supplies like flashlights, portable radios, and portable clocks with extra batteries should be readily available.

Tip

Evacuation Carries

An evacuation carry is a way to remove an immobile resident safely from a dangerous situation. Nursing assistants should attend emergency care and disaster plan in-services at their facility. Evacuation carries may be practiced during disaster drills. A person's local fire department can be contacted for information and/or training.

Chapter Review

1. List the two steps to follow in an emergency after making sure the area is safe and putting on gloves (LO 2).

2. What is the difference between respiratory and cardiac arrest (LO 3)?

3. How soon can brain damage occur after the heart stops beating and breathing stops (LO 3)?

4. In what position should a person be placed if he is in shock (LO 3)?

5. If blood seeps through the first pad over a wound, should the first pad be removed before applying a second pad (LO 3)?

6. If a person feels faint and is sitting down, what should the nursing assistant do (LO 3)?

7. After putting on gloves, what should a nursing assistant do for a person who has a nosebleed (LO 3)?

8. What symptoms are women more likely to experience than men if they are having an MI (LO 3)?

9. What are the first signs that a resident is experiencing diabetic ketoacidosis (LO 3)?

10. What are three things a nursing assistant should never do when a person is having a seizure (LO 3)?

11. What is a transient ischemic attack (TIA) (LO 3)?

12. What does the term *Code Blue* usually mean (LO 4)?

13. List five examples of disasters (LO 5).

Multiple Choice

14. What document will need to be completed after an emergency occurs (LO 2)?
    (A) Incident report
    (B) Safety data set report
    (C) Cardiopulmonary resuscitation report
    (D) Activities of daily living report

15. Which of the following is appropriate to apply to a minor burn (LO 3)?
    (A) Ice
    (B) Butter
    (C) Herbal ointment
    (D) Water

16. When a resident is choking but can speak, cough, or breathe, what should the nursing assistant do (LO 3)?
    (A) The NA should begin cardiopulmonary resuscitation (CPR).
    (B) The NA should encourage the person to cough as forcefully as possible.
    (C) The NA should find an automated external defibrillator (AED) and follow its prompts.
    (D) The NA should put an oxygen mask on the resident.

17. What is the medical term for vomiting (LO 3)?
    (A) Hemiplegia
    (B) Epistaxis
    (C) Syncope
    (D) Emesis

18. What color is the skin if it is cyanotic (LO 3)?
    (A) Yellow
    (B) Red
    (C) Blue
    (D) Pink

9 Admission, Transfer, Discharge, and Physical Exams

Medieval Medicine

The old ward of St. John's Hospital, Bruges, housed patients continuously from the 12th century, when its first section was built, until the 20th. . . . A division was customary in medieval times . . . forming two wards side by side with separate entrances; or two wards built one above the other to separate the sexes. . . .The . . . hospital of the 18th century was a dangerous place, mortality there was higher than among patients nursed at home, and therefore it catered only to wretches with no alternative; but among these, many got better. The bonneted beldame at the rear of the center aisle, being shown out the door with a pat on the shoulder, is very likely being discharged "cured."

Excerpt from "A Walk Through a Ward of the Eighteenth Century" by Grace Goldin. From *Journal of the History of Medicine and Allied Sciences*, Volume XXII, Number 2, 1967. Reprinted with permission of Oxford University Press.

"Where we love is home,
Home that our feet may leave,
but not our hearts."
Oliver Wendell Holmes, 1809–1894

"The best thing we can do is to make wherever we're in look as much like home as we can."
Christopher Fry, 1907–2005

1. Define important words in this chapter

admission pack: personal care items supplied upon a resident's admission.

admit: the entrance of a person to a healthcare facility, beginning care.

baseline: initial value that can be compared to future measurements.

bedridden: confined to bed.

discharge: the release of a person from a health-care facility, ending care.

dorsal recumbent: position in which a person is flat on her back with knees flexed and slightly separated and her feet flat on the bed.

kilogram: a unit of mass equal to 1000 grams; one kilogram equals 2.2 pounds.

knee-chest: position in which a person is lying on his abdomen with knees pulled up toward the abdomen and with legs separated; arms are pulled up and flexed and the head is turned to one side.

lithotomy: position in which a person is on her back with her hips at the edge of the exam table; legs are flexed and feet are in padded stirrups.

metric: system of weights and measures based upon the meter and the kilogram.

pound: a unit of weight equal to 16 ounces.

return: the readmittance of a resident to the care facility.

transfer: moving a person from one place to another; a formal handoff of care from one health-care professional to another.

2. List factors for families choosing a facility

Choosing the right facility for a loved one can be a challenging, emotional, and difficult process. To help guide their choice, family and friends may review information from federal agencies, such as the Centers for Medicare & Medicaid

Services (medicare.gov/nursinghomecompare). They may ask for recommendations from friends. Families may review facilities' results from past state surveys or inspections. They may check to see if the facility has been accredited by the Joint Commission.

Early in the process, families usually visit each facility they are considering. In some cases, a single visit is enough to decide if a facility is right or not. For example, if a strong smell of urine is present, they may not return again to see if it was an isolated incident. These are some questions that are considered before placing a loved one in a care facility:

- Do the staff seem courteous and friendly?

- Do most of the staff speak the resident's native language? Is a translator available?

- Are there enough staff members on duty at the facility? What is the ratio of nurses and nursing assistants to residents? How is the facility staffed on evenings and weekends?

- Are foul odors present?

- What is the food like at the facility? Is attention paid to individual food preferences? Is a dietician available for meetings?

- Are residents up and dressed in the morning?

- Do staff interact positively with the residents?

- Do staff speak courteously to other staff members?

- Do residents look groomed, taken care of, and happy (Fig. 9-1)?

- How are residents' complaints resolved?

- Is the facility licensed?

- Have the state survey and other inspection results been satisfactory?

- Does the facility explain Residents' Rights?

- Does the facility provide assistance with activities of daily living (ADLs)? If so, how is it provided, and what are the associated fees?

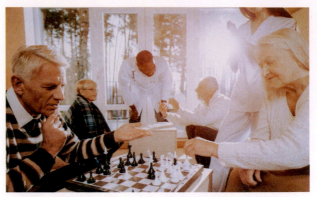

Fig. 9-1. *Before choosing a facility for a loved one, families often tour the facility. They may observe the environment, how the residents look, and what types of activities are offered.*

- Are physical, occupational, and speech therapists available?

- How often do falls, infections, and pressure injuries occur?

- Do volunteers work with residents? If so, are their interactions positive?

- How involved can the family be in creating the resident's care plan?

- Does the facility provide the level of care the resident needs? What about future needs?

- Is the environment safe, functional, and homelike?

- Does the facility have a common area? CMS has defined *common area* as any location that is not a part of a resident's room, where residents can gather with other people or do things individually. These areas can be located in living rooms, dining rooms, activity rooms, or outdoor spaces.

- Is there an activities department? What kinds of activities are offered?

- What are the steps to take if a resident wants to move out of the facility?

- What policies does the facility have on advance directives and end-of-life decisions?

These are only some factors families consider when choosing a facility for a loved one.

3. Explain the nursing assistant's role in the emotional adjustment of a new resident

Moving into a facility requires a big adjustment. New residents may have been living independently for a long time, or they may be moving from a family member's home. Either way, residents undergo a huge emotional adjustment.

Residents have had to make many life-altering changes. They had to leave their homes and get rid of some of their personal belongings (Fig. 9-2). The move may have been sudden due to health reasons. They may have had to give away beloved pets. Loved ones may have died. Due to all of these things, new residents are experiencing many losses and emotions, such as fear, anger, and uncertainty, along with a decline in health and independence.

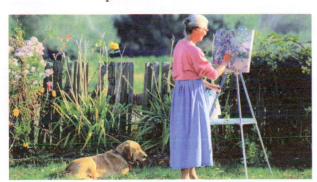

Fig. 9-2. Staff members should remember that many residents had to make major changes when moving into a care facility, such as leaving familiar places, personal items, and beloved pets.

Nursing assistants should empathize with new residents. They can think about how they might feel if they had to give up many things and move into an unfamiliar place filled with people they do not know. Understanding some of what residents are going through will help NAs provide compassionate, person-centered care. Residents will need compassion during those early days and weeks in their new home.

Nursing assistants are the team members most involved with residents on a daily basis. They play an important role in helping new residents feel comfortable in the facility.

Guidelines: Helping New Residents Adjust

G Have a positive attitude. New residents, like most people, want to be near others who are pleasant and positive. Residents want to feel comfortable around staff who provide their care. Residents should not feel as though they are a burden to staff.

G Be tactful. Think before you speak.

G Communicate clearly. Giving a simple reminder about meal times helps the resident feel more connected.

G Show respect for residents' belongings. New residents may be frightened of their new surroundings. They may feel very protective of their personal items. Treat items carefully. Show that you are trustworthy.

G Be responsible. If you make a mistake with resident care, report it to the nurse immediately. People respect and trust you more when you admit mistakes.

G Be honest. Do not make promises you cannot keep. If you tell residents you are coming by to visit, they will look for you. If you forget, apologize, and reschedule the visit as soon as possible.

G Listen to residents if they want to talk. New residents may want to express their feelings about what they are going through (Fig. 9-3). They may want to share some of their stories and backgrounds. Make time to listen.

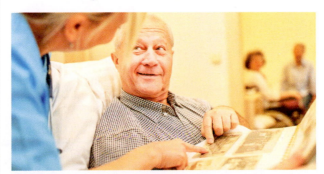

Fig. 9-3. A new resident must leave familiar places. He may have just lost someone very close to him. He may be experiencing other losses as well. Nursing assistants should be supportive and welcoming.

G   Pay attention to residents' wishes. For example, if a resident wants to be alone instead of joining others for an activity, let him do that. You can say, "Maybe next time," and leave him alone. Residents have the right to make choices about what to do and how to spend their time. If they choose to be alone, honor this decision.

G   Respect residents' privacy. The right to privacy is a legal right, and it is always important. It can be especially important when residents are first admitted. Make sure residents have as much privacy as possible.

G   Be patient and kind. A new resident might have a good day followed by a not-so-good day. Allow residents to adapt at their own pace. Everyone is different. The process of adjusting may take some time. Dealing with multiple losses initiates the grieving process (Chapter 27).

Tip

The Welcome Committee

To assist new residents with the transition into a facility, a "Welcome Committee" can be helpful. Team members from each department can be chosen to greet the new resident. Each department can make or buy a card for the resident. The special cards can be brought to the resident's new room one by one or all at once. This idea can be expanded to include other niceties, such as having flowers or a plant waiting for a resident in her new room. Small acts of showing care and warmth can help new residents feel better about the transition to a facility.

4. Describe the nursing assistant's role in the admission process

Admission is often the first time a nursing assistant meets a new resident. To **admit** a resident means that the resident has been allowed entry into a healthcare facility, beginning care. Sometimes residents are readmitted to a care facility. This is called a **return**.

For a resident who is newly admitted, staff will be told the approximate time that the resident

will arrive. When the resident arrives, the NA should try to make sure the resident has a positive impression of him and his facility. The resident should be warmly welcomed. The NA should introduce himself to the resident and any family members. The NA can answer any questions that are within his scope of practice. In order to provide person-centered care, NAs should ask new residents questions to find out their personal preferences, history, and routines. Family members are great sources of information about residents; NAs can also ask them questions.

Guidelines: Admission

G   Wash your hands, then gather any necessary equipment to bring to the resident's room. This equipment may include the following:

   • An **admission pack** or kit contains personal care items for the resident (Fig. 9-4). The pack usually has a wash basin, emesis basin, bedpan, urinal (for male residents), toothpaste, soap, tissues, and a water pitcher and cup. Other items may be in the pack, such as a toothbrush, comb, and special lotions or soaps.

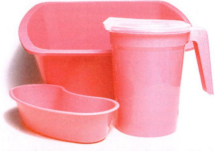

Fig. 9-4. An admission pack is usually placed in a resident's room before she is admitted. It may contain personal care items that the resident will need.

   • A stethoscope and a sphygmomanometer (used to measure blood pressure; you will learn about this in Chapter 13)

   • A thermometer

   • A facility gown or pajamas, depending upon the resident

G　Prepare the resident's room before the resident arrives. This helps her to feel expected and welcome. Know the resident's condition. Know if she is bedbound or is able to walk.

G　Make the bed according to the nurse's instructions. Open the curtains or blinds. Make sure the room is tidy.

G　When the resident arrives, introduce yourself. State your position. Call the person by her formal name until she tells you what she wants to be called.

G　Do not rush the process or the resident. She should not feel as if she is an inconvenience. Make sure that the new resident feels welcome and wanted.

G　Introduce the new resident to her roommate and other residents in the rooms on either side and across the hall. This helps the resident feel more comfortable. It may also help the family feel better.

G　Explain day-to-day life in the facility. Offer to take the resident and her family on a tour. Show them the dining room, chapel, and all other important areas, such as the activity room. If available, show them activity schedules. Review posted dining schedules and point out information about menus. During the tour, introduce residents to all staff and residents you see.

G　Show the resident how to work the bed controls.

G　Make sure the call light is close to the bed. Show the resident how to work the call light and explain its use. Ask the resident to demonstrate that she is able to work the call light.

G　Explain how to work the television and the telephone.

G　Handle all of the resident's personal items with care and respect. These are the items she has chosen to bring with her to the facility. Treat them carefully. Help the resident unpack everything. Ask her where she wants the items placed and how she would like the room set up (Fig. 9-5).

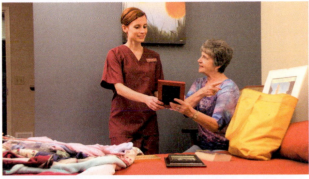

Fig. 9-5. Handle a resident's personal items carefully, and set up the room as the resident prefers.

Admitting a resident

Equipment: may include admission paperwork (checklist and inventory form), gloves, vital signs equipment

1.　Identify yourself by name. Identify the resident. Greet the resident by name.

2.　Wash your hands.

3.　Explain procedure to the resident. Speak clearly, slowly, and directly. Maintain face-to-face contact whenever possible.

4.　Provide for the resident's privacy with a curtain, screen, or door (Fig. 9-6). Ask the family to step outside until the initial admission process is complete. Show them where they may wait and let them know approximately how long they will have to wait. Tell them where they can get refreshments.

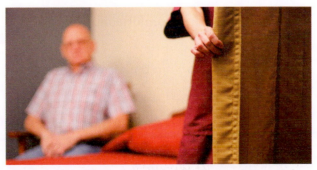

Fig. 9-6. All residents have a legal right to privacy, and providing privacy is part of doing your job professionally. Your professional, respectful behavior can help put a new resident at ease.

5. If instructed, do these things:

    Measure the resident's height, weight, and vital signs. (Height and weight procedures follow; vital signs procedures are located in Chapter 13.) Most facilities require baseline height, weight, and vital signs measurements. **Baseline** measurements are initial values that can be compared to future measurements. Document on admission form and elsewhere per facility policy.

    Obtain a urine specimen if required (see Chapter 16).

    Complete the paperwork. Take an inventory of all of the personal items. Help the resident put personal items away. Label each item if it is facility policy. If the resident has valuables, ask the nurse for instructions.

    Fill the water pitcher with fresh water if allowed. Add ice if requested.

6. When the initial portion of the admission is complete, locate the family and let them know they may return to the resident's room.

7. Show the resident the room and bathroom. Explain how to work the bed controls and the call light. Show the resident the lights, telephone, and television controls and how to work them. Give the resident information on menus, dining times, and activity schedules.

8. Introduce the resident to his roommate if there is one. Introduce other residents and staff.

9. Make the resident comfortable. Remove privacy measures.

10. Leave call light within the resident's reach.

11. Wash your hands.

12. Be courteous and respectful at all times. Let the resident know when you are leaving. Ask if he needs anything else.

13. Document procedure using facility guidelines.

Residents' height and weight will be checked when they are admitted. Nursing assistants also check weight as part of regular care (Fig. 9-7). Height is usually not checked as often as weight. Changes in a resident's weight can be a sign of illness. NAs must report any weight loss or gain, no matter how small.

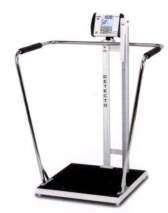

Fig. 9-7. *This is a bariatric scale that may be used for weighing residents who are overweight or obese.* (PHOTO COURTESY OF DETECTO, WWW.DETECTO.COM, 800-641-2008)

Weight will be measured using pounds or kilograms. A **pound** is a unit of weight equal to 16 ounces. Kilograms are units of **metric** measurement. A **kilogram** is a unit of mass equal to 1000 grams; one kilogram equals 2.2 pounds. Residents who are unable to get out of bed independently **(bedridden)** will need to be weighed, too.

Measuring and recording weight of an ambulatory resident ▶

Equipment: standing/upright scale, pen and paper

1. Identify yourself by name. Identify the resident. Greet the resident by name.

2. Wash your hands.

3. Explain procedure to the resident. Speak clearly, slowly, and directly. Maintain face-to-face contact whenever possible.

4. Provide for the resident's privacy with a curtain, screen, or door.

5. Make sure resident is wearing nonskid shoes that are fastened before walking to the scale.

Admission, Transfer, Discharge, and Physical Exams

6. Start with the scale balanced at zero before weighing the resident (Fig. 9-8). If you do not know how to balance the scale, ask the nurse.

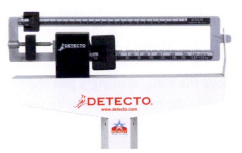

Fig. 9-8. *This scale is balanced at zero.* (PHOTO COURTESY OF DE-TECTO, WWW.DETECTO.COM, 800-641-2008)

7. Help the resident step onto the center of the scale, facing the scale. Be sure she is not holding, touching, or leaning against anything.

8. Determine the resident's weight. This is done by making the balance bar level. Move the small and large weight indicators until the bar balances. Read the two numbers shown (on the small and large weight indicators) when the bar is balanced. Add these two numbers together. This is the resident's weight.

9. Help the resident to safely step off the scale before recording weight.

10. Remove privacy measures.

11. Leave call light within the resident's reach.

12. Wash your hands.

13. Be courteous and respectful at all times.

14. Report any changes in the resident to the nurse. Record the resident's weight in pounds (lb) or kilograms (kg), depending on facility policy. Document procedure using facility guidelines.

When residents are not able to get out of wheelchairs easily, they are weighed using a wheel-

chair scale. Wheelchairs are rolled directly onto this type of scale (Fig. 9-9). For some wheelchair scales, the NA will need to subtract the weight of the wheelchair from a resident's weight. If the weight of the wheelchair is not listed on the chair, the NA should weigh the empty wheelchair first. The footrests should be attached if they will be attached when the resident is in the chair. Then he should subtract the wheelchair's weight from the total. Some scales automatically adjust for the wheelchair's weight.

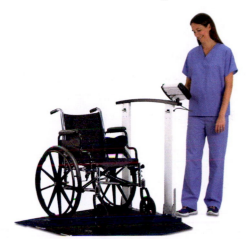

Fig. 9-9. *Wheelchairs can be rolled directly onto wheelchair scales to determine weight.* (PHOTO COURTESY OF DETECTO, WWW.DETECTO.COM, 800-641-2008)

When residents cannot get out of bed, they are weighed on special bed scales (Fig. 9-10). Before using a bed scale, the NA should know how it works and how to use it properly and safely. Below is a general procedure for weighing someone on a bed scale.

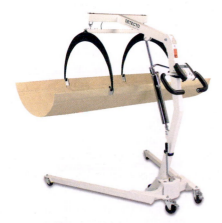

Fig. 9-10. *A type of bed scale.* (PHOTO COURTESY OF DETECTO, WWW.DETECTO.COM, 800-641-2008)

Measuring and recording weight of a bedridden resident

Equipment: scale, pen and paper

Have a coworker assist you.

1. Identify yourself by name. Identify the resident. Greet the resident by name.

2. Wash your hands.

3. Explain procedure to the resident. Speak clearly, slowly, and directly. Maintain face-to-face contact whenever possible.

4. Provide for the resident's privacy with a curtain, screen, or door.

5. Adjust the bed to a safe level, usually waist high. Lock the bed wheels.

6. Start with the scale balanced at zero before weighing the resident. If you do not know how to balance the scale, ask the nurse.

7. Examine the sling, straps, chains, and/or pad for any damage. Do not use the scale if you see damage.

8. Turn linen down so that it is off the resident.

9. Have the resident turn toward you. If the resident cannot do this, you must turn him toward you (see Chapter 11). Be sure the resident cannot roll off the bed. If a flat pad scale is used, slide the resident onto the pad using a helper. If a sling is used, remove it from the scale and place it underneath the resident without wrinkling it.

10. When using a sling, turn the resident back on his back and straighten the sling.

11. Attach the sling to the scale or, if using a flat pad scale, position resident securely on the pad.

12. Check the straps or other connectors, and raise the sling or the pad until the resident is clear of the bed. With some scales, you can keep the resident directly over the bed while weighing him. With others, you have to move the scale away from the bed. Make sure the resident is secured before moving the scale.

13. For digital scales, turn them on and note the reading. For other scales, move the weights until you get a reading. Note the weight.

14. Lower the resident back down on the bed. If using a sling, turn resident to both sides to remove the sling. If using a pad scale, carefully slide the resident back onto the bed.

15. Make the resident comfortable. Replace bed linens.

16. Return the bed to its lowest position. Remove privacy measures.

17. Leave call light within the resident's reach.

18. Wash your hands.

19. Be courteous and respectful at all times.

20. Report any changes in the resident to the nurse. Record the resident's weight in pounds (lb) or kilograms (kg), depending on facility policy. Document procedure using facility guidelines.

For measuring height, the rod measures in inches and fractions of inches. The NA should record the total number of inches. Because there are 12 inches in one foot, dividing the height in inches by 12 gives the height in feet (60 inches equal five feet).

Measuring and recording height of an ambulatory resident

Equipment: standing/upright scale, pen and paper

1. Identify yourself by name. Identify the resident. Greet the resident by name.

2. Wash your hands.

3. Explain procedure to the resident. Speak clearly, slowly, and directly. Maintain face-to-face contact whenever possible.

4. Provide for the resident's privacy with a curtain, screen, or door.

5. Make sure the resident is wearing nonskid shoes that are fastened before walking to the scale.

6. Help the resident to step onto the scale, facing away from it.

7. Ask the resident to stand straight if possible. Help as needed.

8. Pull up the measuring rod from the back of the scale. Gently lower the rod until it rests flat on the resident's head (Fig. 9-11).

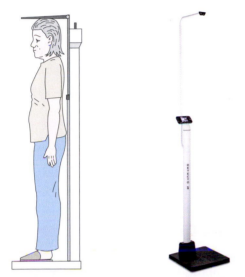

Fig. 9-11. *On the left is an illustration of how to determine height on a traditional standing scale. On the right is a photo of a scale that measures height with a sonar rod, which measures height and weight automatically and displays the measurements on the screen.* (PHOTO ON THE RIGHT COURTESY OF DETECTO, WWW.DETECTO.COM, 800-641-2008)

9. Determine the resident's height.

10. Help the resident to step off the scale. Make sure the measuring rod does not hit the resident in the head while doing so.

11. Remove privacy measures.

12. Leave call light within the resident's reach.

13. Wash your hands.

14. Be courteous and respectful at all times.

15. Report any changes in the resident to the nurse. Record the resident's height. Document procedure using facility guidelines.

Measuring and recording height of a bedridden resident

Equipment: tape measure (Fig. 9-12), pencil, pen and paper

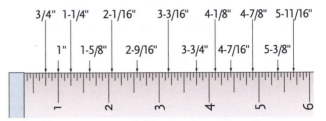

Fig. 9-12. *An illustration of a tape measure with markings.*

1. Identify yourself by name. Identify the resident. Greet the resident by name.

2. Wash your hands.

3. Explain procedure to the resident. Speak clearly, slowly, and directly. Maintain face-to-face contact whenever possible.

4. Provide for the resident's privacy with a curtain, screen, or door.

5. Adjust the bed to a safe level, usually waist high. Lock the bed wheels.

6. Turn linen down so it is off the resident.

7. Position the resident lying straight in the supine position (flat on her back). Be sure the bed sheet is smooth underneath the resident.

8. Using a pencil, make a small mark on the bottom sheet (or bath blanket that is underneath the resident) at the top of the resident's head.

9. Make another pencil mark at the resident's heel on the bottom sheet (or bath blanket that is underneath the resident).

10. Using the tape measure, measure the distance between the pencil marks. This is the resident's height.

11. Make the resident comfortable. Replace bed linen.

12. Return the bed to its lowest position. Remove privacy measures.

13. Leave call light within the resident's reach.

14. Wash your hands.

15. Be courteous and respectful at all times.

16. Report any changes in the resident to the nurse. Record the resident's height. Document procedure using facility guidelines.

Some residents cannot lie straight due to contractures. A contracture is the permanent and painful shortening of a muscle, tendon, or ligament. One way that height can be measured for residents who have contractures is by using a tape measure to follow the curves of the spine and legs. The number of inches is totaled and recorded. This is the least accurate way of measuring height.

5. Explain the nursing assistant's role during an in-house transfer of a resident

Residents may need to be transferred to another room within a facility. A **transfer** is moving a person from one place to another or a formal handoff of care from one healthcare professional to another. Transfers may be needed because of the health or safety of the resident or her roommates. For example, if someone develops a communicable disease, a transfer might be warranted. A transfer might also be needed due to weather emergencies or other types of disasters. Whatever the reason for the transfer, it may be a difficult time for the resident. Change is always hard, but this is especially true if the resident is ill or if her condition has worsened. Nursing assistants should try to make the transfer as smooth as possible for residents.

A resident should be informed of the transfer as soon as possible so that she can begin to adjust to the idea. The nurse will tell the resident about the transfer and should explain how, where, and, when, and why the transfer will occur. Any questions the resident has should be answered.

Nursing assistants are usually responsible for packing all of the resident's belongings. Packing all of the items may take some time, and the NA should pack personal items carefully so that nothing breaks, is damaged, or is lost.

The resident may be transferred in a bed, in a stretcher, or in a wheelchair. To aid with planning, the NA should find out how the resident will be transferred beforehand.

After the resident is in her new room, the NA should introduce her to everyone. If unpacking the resident's belongings, the NA should handle them carefully. Recreating the way the belongings were set up in the former room may help the resident feel more comfortable. An orientation in the new area should be promptly completed by the receiving staff. This information should be communicated in a language and via a method that the resident can understand. It is a good idea for the NA to check on the resident later in the day to make sure she is settled. After that, stopping by occasionally to say hello can help the resident feel connected and cared for.

When leaving the resident's room, the NA should report to the nurse in charge of that resident. That will signal a formal transfer or handoff of responsibility to staff at the new unit.

Residents' Rights

Transfers, Discharges, and AMA

Residents have the legal right to receive advance notice before being transferred or discharged from a facility. The written notice must contain the specifics of where and why they are being transferred or discharged. It must be in a language residents can understand. Staff must provide proper preparation for the transfer or discharge.

Residents can refuse to be transferred if the transfer is due to staff convenience. If residents are involuntarily discharged from a healthcare facility, it is called an *eviction*.

Sometimes a resident decides to leave a facility without the approval of the doctor. This is called leaving *against medical advice*, or AMA. When this occurs, a process must be followed to protect the facility and staff. The resident will be asked to sign a form that says she has been informed of and understands the risks of leaving the facility. If a resident says that she is leaving the facility, the NA must notify the charge nurse immediately.

Transferring a resident to a new room

Equipment: may include wheelchair or stretcher, cart for belongings, all of the resident's packed personal items

1. Identify yourself by name. Identify the resident. Greet the resident by name.

2. Wash your hands.

3. Explain procedure to the resident. Speak clearly, slowly, and directly. Maintain face-to-face contact whenever possible.

4. Provide for the resident's privacy with a curtain, screen, or door.

5. Collect the items to be moved onto the cart, and ask another staff member to help take them to the new location.

6. Lock the wheelchair or stretcher wheels. Help the resident into the wheelchair or onto the stretcher. Take him to the proper area.

7. Introduce new residents and staff.

8. Provide for the resident's privacy with a curtain, screen, or door.

9. Lock the wheelchair or stretcher wheels. Transfer the resident to the new bed if needed.

10. Unpack all belongings. Help the resident put personal items away.

11. Make the resident comfortable. Remove privacy measures.

12. Leave call light within the resident's reach.

13. Wash your hands.

14. Be courteous and respectful at all times.

15. Report to the charge nurse when the transfer is complete. Report any changes in the resident to the nurse. Document procedure using facility guidelines.

6. Explain the nursing assistant's role in the discharge of a resident

A **discharge** is the release of a person from a healthcare facility, ending care. It is official after the doctor orders the discharge, releasing the resident to leave the facility to go home or to another facility. The nurse will then complete instructions for the resident to follow after discharge. These instructions may include future doctor appointments, medications, ambulation instructions, and special dietary requirements. They may also contain exercises that the resident should do, as well as community resources for the resident (Fig. 9-13).

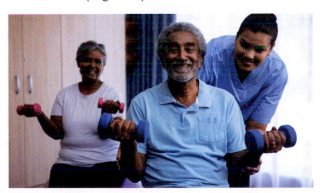

Fig. 9-13. *After a resident is discharged, he may have instructions to exercise.*

Nursing assistants help by collecting belongings and personal care items and packing them carefully. Each item should be checked against the inventory list completed during admission. The NA may need to ask a nurse to obtain valuables from a secure area.

A resident who is going home may be happy, although she may be unsure if she is ready for this important change. The nursing assistant can help by being positive and reassuring. However, if a resident has specific questions about care, the NA should inform the nurse.

Admission, Transfer, Discharge, and Physical Exams

The NA should know what the resident's condition is at the time of discharge and find out if the resident will be using a wheelchair or stretcher. The NA is responsible for the resident until she is safely in the vehicle with her belongings and the doors of the vehicle are closed.

Discharging a resident

Equipment: may include a wheelchair or stretcher; cart for belongings; the discharge paperwork, including the inventory list from admission; resident's personal care items; vital signs equipment

1. Identify yourself by name. Identify the resident. Greet the resident by name.

2. Wash your hands.

3. Explain procedure to the resident. Speak clearly, slowly, and directly. Maintain face-to-face contact whenever possible.

4. Provide for the resident's privacy with a curtain, screen, or door.

5. Measure the resident's vital signs.

6. Compare the inventory list to the items being packed. Ask the resident to sign if all items are there.

7. Carefully put the packed items onto the cart, and ask another staff member to help transport items to the pick-up area.

8. Help the resident dress in clothing of her choice. Make sure the nurse has removed all dressings and tubing that need to be removed prior to discharge.

9. Lock wheelchair or stretcher wheels. Help her safely into the wheelchair or onto the stretcher (Chapter 11) if used.

10. Help the resident say her goodbyes to other residents and the staff.

11. Take resident to the pick-up area. Lock the wheelchair or stretcher wheels. Help the resident into the vehicle. Transfer personal items into the vehicle.

12. Say goodbye to the resident. You are responsible for the resident until she is safely in the vehicle and the door is closed.

13. Wash your hands.

14. Document procedure using facility guidelines.

7. Describe the nursing assistant's role during physical exams

Some residents need a physical exam when arriving at a facility to help determine their needs and to provide important information for the care plan. Others need a physical exam periodically after they have been at the facility for a while. Doctors or nurses will perform the exam. Nursing assistants may help by bringing the resident to the proper area, gathering equipment, and providing emotional support.

Exams can make people anxious. They may fear what the examiner will do or what she will find. Exams can cause discomfort and embarrassment. Nursing assistants can provide support during this process by listening to residents or holding their hands.

Residents' Rights

Residents' Rights During Exams
Residents have the right to know why exams are being performed and who is performing the exams. Residents have the right to choose examiners and to have family members present during exams.

Nursing assistants are often responsible for gathering equipment for the nurse or doctor. Examples of equipment that may be needed include the following:

- Sphygmomanometer (for blood pressure)

- Stethoscope

- Alcohol wipes

- Flashlight

- Thermometer

- Tongue depressor

- Eye chart for vision screening

- Tuning fork (tests hearing with vibrations)

- Reflex hammer (taps body parts to test reflexes)

- Otoscope (lighted instrument that examines the outer ear and eardrum)

- Ophthalmoscope (lighted instrument that examines the eye)

- Specimen containers

- Lubricant

- Hemoccult card (tests for blood in stool)

- Vaginal speculum for females (opens the vagina so that it and the cervix can be examined)

- Gloves

- Drape

Nursing assistants may need to place residents in the correct position and drape them for the exam. Drapes cover the parts of the body that are not being examined. Some exam positions are embarrassing and uncomfortable. The nursing assistant can help by explaining why the position is needed and how long the resident can expect to stay in the position. In addition to draping the resident, the NA should close the door to the room and/or pull the privacy curtain to protect the resident's privacy. The NA should explain to the resident that she will not be exposed more than necessary during the exam. Common positions used during physical exams include the following:

- The **dorsal recumbent** position is used to examine the breasts, chest, abdomen, and perineal area. A resident in the dorsal recumbent position is flat on her back with her knees flexed and feet flat on the bed. The drape is put over the resident, covering her body. Her head remains uncovered (Fig. 9-14).

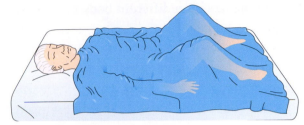

Fig. 9-14. *The dorsal recumbent position.*

- The **lithotomy** position is used to examine the vagina. The resident lies on her back and her hips are brought to the edge of the exam table. Her legs are flexed and her feet are in padded stirrups. The drape is put over the resident, covering her body. Her head remains uncovered. The drape is also brought down to cover the perineal area and tops of the thighs (Fig. 9-15).

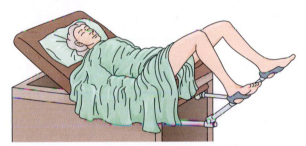

Fig. 9-15. *The lithotomy position.*

- The **knee-chest** position may be used to examine the rectum or the vagina. A resident in the knee-chest position is lying on her abdomen. The knees are pulled towards the abdomen, and legs are separated. Arms are pulled up and flexed. The head is turned to one side. In the knee-chest position, the resident will be wearing a gown and possibly socks. The drape should be applied in a diamond shape to cover the back, buttocks, and thighs (Fig. 9-16).

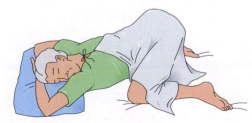

Fig. 9-16. *The knee-chest position.*

More information on different body positions is located in Chapter 11.

Guidelines: Physical Exams

G   Wash your hands before and after the exam.

G   Follow Standard Precautions.

G   Ask the resident to urinate before the exam. Collect any urine needed for a specimen at this time. Gather and label specimens as needed.

G   Provide privacy throughout the exam.

G   Listen to and reassure the resident throughout the exam.

G   Follow any instructions from the doctor or nurse.

G   Protect the resident from falling.

G   Provide enough light for the doctor or nurse.

G   Put instruments in the proper place. Hand instruments to the doctor or nurse as needed.

G   After the exam, help the resident clean up and get dressed. Help the resident safely back to her room. Dispose of any trash and disposable equipment in the exam area. Bring all reusable equipment to the proper cleaning room. Clean and store reusable equipment according to facility policy. Label and bring any specimens to the proper place so that they can go to the lab.

Residents' Rights

Knocking Protects Privacy

Not waiting for permission to enter an examination room may expose the resident not only to the person entering, but also to anyone walking through the hallway. Nursing assistants must always knock on the door and wait to hear "come in" before entering an examination room. Doing this promotes each resident's legal right to privacy and dignity.

Chapter Review

1. What are two resources that families may use to help them choose a care facility for a loved one (LO 2)?

2. Why is it a good idea for nursing assistants to ask family members questions about residents upon admission (LO 4)?

3. Why might a transfer to a new room be difficult for a resident (LO 5)?

4. During discharge of a resident, when does a nursing assistant's responsibility for the resident end (LO 6)?

Multiple Choice

5. If a nursing assistant makes a mistake with resident care, he can demonstrate that he is responsible by (LO 3)
    (A) Coming up with a clever way to distract the resident from his mistake
    (B) Blaming another staff member so that he will not be the only one viewed negatively
    (C) Not documenting the mistake so that there is no legal record of it
    (D) Reporting the mistake to the nurse immediately

6. Which of the following would be the best response by the nursing assistant if a new resident says that he does not want to attend a facility activity (LO 3)?
    (A) "That's okay. I'll ask you again some other time."
    (B) "I think you should go because it will probably make you feel better."
    (C) "It is harder to make friends when you do not attend social events."
    (D) "You will become depressed if you do not participate and socialize."

7. What should the scale be balanced at before measuring a resident's weight (LO 4)?
   (A) 0
   (B) 5
   (C) 50
   (D) -.10

8. How many inches are there in five feet (LO 4)?
   (A) 20
   (B) 30
   (C) 60
   (D) 80

9. In which position is a resident lying flat on her back with her knees flexed and her feet flat on the bed (LO 7)?
   (A) Lithotomy position
   (B) Lateral position
   (C) Dorsal recumbent position
   (D) Knee-chest position

10. In which position is a resident lying on her abdomen with her knees pulled toward the abdomen and her legs separated (LO 7)?
    (A) Lithotomy position
    (B) Lateral position
    (C) Dorsal recumbent position
    (D) Knee-chest position

11. In which position is a resident lying on her back with her feet in padded stirrups (LO 7)?
    (A) Lithotomy position
    (B) Lateral position
    (C) Dorsal recumbent position
    (D) Knee-chest position

10
Bedmaking and Unit Care

Alcmaeon: One Theory about the Nature of Sleep

In the 6th century, medicine was taught in places where teachers, students, and philosophers gathered together. Crotona, in Sicily, south of Italy, was one of these places, or "medical schools." Alcmaeon was one of the teachers at the Crotona school. He believed that harmony in the body maintained health, and that disease was caused by a change in the body's harmony. He also had interesting ideas about sleep. His theory was that sleep was something that occurred when the blood vessels in the brain were filled. When the blood drained out of the brain, the person would awaken.

"Oh it's nice to get up in the mornin'/But it's nicer to lie in bed."

Sir Harry Lauder, 1870–1950

"Egyptian Proverb:
The worst things:
To be in bed and sleep not
To want for one who comes not
To try to please and please not."

F. Scott Fitzgerald, 1896–1940

1. Define important words in this chapter

bariatrics: branch of medicine that deals with the causes, prevention, and treatment of obesity.

biorhythms: natural rhythms or cycles related to bodily functions.

circadian rhythm: the 24-hour day-night cycle.

closed bed: a bed completely made with the bedspread and blankets in place.

depressant: a substance that causes calmness and drowsiness.

disposable: only to be used once and then discarded.

draw sheet: an extra sheet placed on top of the bottom sheet; used for moving residents.

incontinence: the inability to control the bladder or bowels, which leads to an involuntary loss of urine or feces.

insomnia: the inability to fall asleep or remain asleep.

occupied bed: a bed made while a person is in the bed.

open bed: a bed made with linen folded down to the foot of the bed.

parasomnias: sleep disorders.

sleep: natural period of rest for the mind and body during which energy is restored.

stimulant: a drug that increases or quickens actions of the body.

surgical bed: a bed made so that a person can easily move onto it from a stretcher.

unoccupied bed: a bed made while no person is in the bed.

2. Discuss the importance of sleep

Sleep is a natural period of rest for the mind and body during which energy is restored. Sleep and rest are two basic physical needs, as described in Chapter 5. The human body cannot survive long without sleep. Sleep is needed to replace old cells with new ones and provide new energy to organs. It promotes healing and healthy body functioning. Getting enough sleep helps decrease the risk of certain illnesses and disease. Sleep also plays an important part in mental well-being. It helps improve cognitive function and promotes emotional health.

The study of the rhythms of the body is called *biorhythmology*. **Biorhythms** are the natural rhythms or cycles related to body functions that occur due to daily, monthly, or yearly changes. Light and darkness and temperature changes are examples of changes that can affect living organisms.

The most famous biorhythm is the circadian rhythm. The **circadian rhythm** is the 24-hour day-night cycle. It usually appears in infants when they are about three weeks old. The circadian rhythm can affect the body in many ways. In addition to sleep patterns, other changes in the body can occur during the 24-hour cycle. These include variations in blood pressure and body temperature.

3. Describe types of sleep disorders

The inability to fall asleep or to remain asleep is called **insomnia**. A person may have difficulty falling asleep, may not stay asleep through the night, or may wake up too early in the morning. There are many different causes of insomnia. Some of the reasons that people develop sleep disorders, or **parasomnias**, are illness, anxiety, fear, stress, medications, trouble breathing, noise, hunger, or thirst. Some common sleep disorders are described in the following box:

Parasomnias

Somnambulism is sleepwalking. With this sleep disorder, the person performs activities that people normally perform while awake. In most cases, the episodes do not result in injury.

Sleep talking is talking during sleep. This usually occurs without the person being aware of what he is saying, or even that he is talking. Episodes are usually brief and may not happen often.

Bruxism is grinding and clenching the teeth. It can cause headaches, jaw problems and pain, neck aches, and can loosen teeth.

REM behavior disorder (RBD) is talking, often along with violent movements, during REM (dreaming) sleep. The person is acting out his dreams. This disorder is more common among elderly people who have illnesses affecting the nervous system, such as Parkinson's or Alzheimer's disease (Chapter 22).

Sleep apnea is the disruption of breathing while a person is sleeping (breathing stops and starts during sleep). There are different types of sleep apnea, but the most common is obstructive sleep apnea (OSA). People who smoke, are overweight, and are over 60 are at a higher risk for sleep apnea. Males are more likely than females to have sleep apnea.

Signs and symptoms of sleep apnea include loud snoring at night, feeling very tired during the daytime, and having headaches in the morning. NAs should report these signs and symptoms to the nurse. Sleep apnea may be treated with changes in lifestyle, such as quitting smoking or losing weight. Other methods of treatment are oxygen therapy and using a continuous positive airway pressure (CPAP) machine. If left untreated, sleep apnea can result in high blood pressure, stroke, or serious heart problems.

Residents who require surgery will be evaluated for obstructive sleep apnea. Pain management throughout the surgical and postoperative period will be geared toward avoiding respiratory depression and other potential problems. Respiratory depression is a breathing disorder that affects a person's ability to inhale and exhale properly. A CPAP machine may be used for some residents postoperatively after returning to the long-term care facility. Residents may require additional monitoring for respiratory depression and other complications.

4. Identify factors affecting sleep

Many elderly people, especially those living away from their homes, have sleep problems (Fig. 10-1). These problems are caused by many factors, including the following:

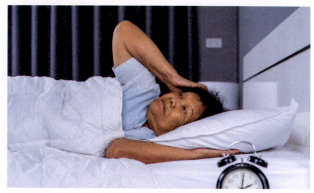

Fig. 10-1. *Living away from home can interfere with quality sleep.*

Environment: Residents may have been used to sleeping with a mate or alone when they lived at home. Adjusting to a new place and possibly a roommate is very difficult. Even if married residents are in the same room at a facility, sleep can be difficult because they are no longer in their home. Ways for NAs to help with environmental issues include the following:

- Listen to residents if they wish to talk. Be compassionate and reassuring.

- Have enough pillows and blankets.

- If a mattress does not fit in the bed frame properly, report it to the nurse or proper department.

Noise level and lighting can affect a resident's ability to sleep. Keeping the room dark is very important to some residents. Other residents prefer to sleep with a light or a night-light on.

Residents who snore may keep roommates awake. Ways for NAs to help address noise level and lighting include the following:

- Keep the noise level low, especially during shift changes, which are often noisy times. Closing doors at night may help.

- Keep voices low.

- Do not bang equipment or meal trays.

- Use blinds or shades to help darken a room for sleep. Keep light controls within residents' reach.

- Report if a resident is snoring excessively or there are complaints from others about snoring.

Problems with odors and inadequate ventilation can cause a person to have difficulty sleeping. Residents may be incontinent (unable to control the bladder or bowels, which leads to an involuntary loss of urine or feces), which can cause odors. Vomit, wound drainage, certain diseases, and body odors are other causes. Ways for NAs to help with odors and ventilation include the following:

- Change incontinence briefs often.

- Keep equipment and supplies clean.

- Give personal care often to help avoid breath and body odors.

- Change soiled bed linens and clothing as soon as possible.

- Weather permitting, open a window to help eliminate odors.

In addition, spray deodorizer may be available to use for persistent odors.

Temperature problems can affect sleep. Some people want the room to be cooler; others like a warmer temperature for sleep. This may be due to normal changes of aging or just personal preference. OBRA requires that long-term care facilities maintain comfortable and safe environments with a temperature range of 71°F–81°F.

Ways for NAs to help with temperature include the following:

- Help find a comfortable temperature for residents, within OBRA's guidelines.

- Report to the nurse if the temperature is a problem.

- Layer clothing and bed covers for warmth.

Anxiety: The resident may be anxious about sleeping alone in a private room. He may have anxiety about sleeping in a new environment with a roommate. He may be worried about illness and a decline in independence. If friends and family have died, he may be sad or depressed. Ways for NAs to help with anxiety include the following:

- Sit with residents and listen if they want to talk. Visits from family, friends, or clergy may also help.

- Use touch and soothing words.

- Offer to give a back rub.

- Report to the nurse if a resident is anxious or depressed. If anxiety is prolonged, the resident may benefit from talking with a mental health professional.

Illness: Some illnesses or diseases cause chronic or occasional pain and discomfort. For example, arthritis can cause chronic pain in different areas of the body. Arthritis is a disease that causes inflammation, or swelling, of the joints, resulting in stiffness, pain, and decreased mobility. (Chapter 21 has more information.) Ways for NAs to help with illness, pain, and discomfort include the following:

- Make sure residents are clean and comfortable before bed.

- Observe and report signs of pain promptly to the nurse. The nurse may give the resident medication. The NA may be asked to help by giving a back rub or a bath. Signs of pain and measures to reduce pain may be found in Chapter 13.

Aging changes: Sleep patterns are different for elderly people than for younger people. They may sleep a similar number of hours, but those hours may be spread out over the 24-hour day. The elderly may take frequent naps during the day, which affects sleep at night. They take longer to fall asleep. Elderly people may get up more often during the night to go the bathroom and have a hard time falling asleep again. Hormonal changes can cause difficulty sleeping. A lack of regular, moderate exercise affects sleep as well. Ways for NAs to help with aging changes include the following:

- Help residents to the bathroom just before bedtime.

- Honor fluid restrictions in the evening if they are ordered.

- Use music or read to residents if it helps with sleep.

- Give residents a chance to nap as needed throughout the day.

- Encourage residents to exercise if it is in their care plan. Exercise often helps people sleep longer and more soundly.

- Encourage residents to wear day clothes instead of nightclothes during the day.

Dietary habits: Drinking or eating products with caffeine, such as soda or chocolate, can prevent sleep (Fig. 10-2). Eating heavy meals before bedtime can cause restlessness or discomfort. This can make it harder to fall asleep or can cause wakefulness during the night. Being hungry can also cause a person to wake during the night. Ways for NAs to help with dietary habits include the following:

- Limit caffeine intake. Offer herbal teas or warm milk instead.

- Avoid serving heavy meals before bedtime. Serve meals earlier in the evening, not late at night. Observe and report if the resident is not eating during meals.

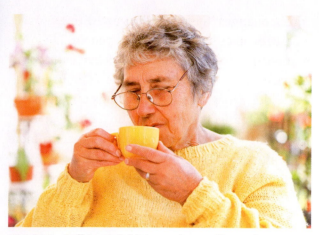

Fig. 10-2. Caffeinated drinks, such as coffee and some teas, can prevent sleep.

Medications, alcohol, and cigarettes: Some medications cause wakefulness and interfere with sleep. For example, antihistamines can either cause a person to become very sleepy or to be unable to fall asleep. Antihistamines are medications used to treat allergic reactions or allergies. Alcoholic drinks, including beer and wine, are depressants and can cause problems with sleep (Fig. 10-3). A **depressant** is a substance that causes calmness and drowsiness. Smoking can also cause problems with sleeping. Nicotine, which is found in cigarettes, is a stimulant. A **stimulant** is a drug that increases or quickens actions of the body. Ways for NAs to help with the effects of medications, alcohol, and cigarettes include the following:

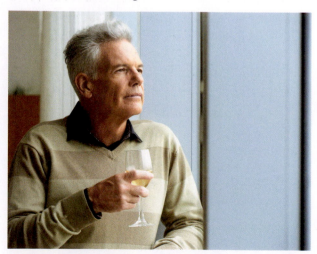

Fig. 10-3. Wine and other alcoholic beverages can prevent a person from sleeping well.

- Report if residents are not taking medications ordered for sleep.

- Report any evidence of unusual sleepiness or sudden inability to fall asleep.

- Discourage smoking and report if residents are drinking alcohol just before bedtime.

Insomnia can cause or contribute to many problems, including decreased mental function, reduced reaction time, irritability, problems with memory, depression, obesity, type 2 diabetes, cardiovascular disease, and decreased immune system function. It is important for NAs to report residents' complaints of sleeping problems.

A care conference may be planned to correct a resident's sleeping problems. Family members may participate. The nurse or doctor will assess the resident's medications to see if they are affecting sleep. NAs can offer any suggestions they have to help improve a resident's ability to sleep.

5. Describe a standard resident unit and equipment

Residents' units are their living spaces. They contain their beds, other furniture, and personal items. These units must be kept clean and neat, while also honoring residents' personal choices. Valuing each resident's choice is part of person-centered care. This room is the resident's home. NAs should always knock and wait for permission before entering.

Residents' belongings are very important to them. NAs must treat residents' personal items with respect and should not move them without permission. Any safety hazards should be reported to the nurse.

Each unit may have slightly different equipment, because residents may bring furniture or other belongings from home. Personal items that make the resident happy should be encouraged. Resident rooms should be personal and home-like.

Standard unit equipment includes the following:

- Bed
- Bedside stand and a dresser
- Overbed table
- Chair
- Bath basin
- Emesis basin (Fig. 10-4)
- Bedpan
- Urinal for males
- Water pitcher and cup
- Privacy screen or curtain
- Call light

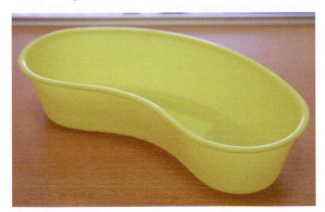

Fig. 10-4. *An emesis basin.*

The bedside stand is used for storing equipment like emesis basins, bath basins, urinals, and bedpans. Soap, toothbrushes, toothpaste, combs and brushes, and other items may also be placed in the bedside stand but have to be kept separate from basins, urinals, and bedpans. Personal articles are usually kept in the top drawer. Basins are generally placed on the top shelf, and bedpans and urinals are on the lower shelf in the section underneath. A telephone, along with personal items, may be placed on the top of the stand.

The overbed table may be used for residents' meals or personal care. It is a clean area and must be kept clean and free of clutter. Bedpans, urinals, and used linen should not be placed on overbed tables because these tables are used

for food. Right before mealtime, the NA should clear this table so that the meal tray can slide smoothly onto it. A water pitcher and cup are routinely kept on the overbed table.

Residents' Rights

Personal Belongings

Making fun of any resident's personal items is inappropriate and cruel. Treat residents' belongings with respect.

6. Explain how to clean a resident unit and equipment

General care of the unit must be done whenever needed throughout the day. Spills should be removed promptly. Bedpans and urinals must be emptied and cleaned immediately after use. Bed linens should be straightened before leaving the resident's room.

NAs will use many different types of equipment and must make sure to use and care for it properly. This prevents infection and injury. Equipment that is used one time and then discarded is called **disposable** equipment. Some types of disposable equipment are cups, tissues, gloves, paper gowns, masks, disposable razors, and absorbent pads. Disposable equipment prevents the spread of microorganisms. NAs should dispose of this equipment in the proper container. Gloves should be worn when using or discarding some types of equipment, such as razors and pads.

Some equipment, such as urinals and bedpans, must be cleaned after each use. NAs must wear gloves when handling these items. This equipment may need to be cleaned and disinfected by the NA or placed in the proper area for cleaning. Reusable equipment should not be used again until it has been properly cleaned.

Guidelines: Resident's Unit

G   Keep residents' units neat and clean. Clean the overbed table after use. Use a paper towel or cloth and facility-approved cleaning fluid. When cleaning, move the damp paper towel or cloth away from you to avoid wiping dirt or dust onto your uniform. Place the table within the resident's reach before leaving.

G   Keep the call light within the resident's reach. Make sure it is within the resident's reach before you leave the room. Report to the nurse immediately if the call light is not working.

G   Straighten bed linens and remove crumbs from the bed after meals and before leaving.

G   Restock all resident supplies daily, including tissues, toilet paper, paper towels, soap, or any other needed items. If this is not your responsibility, write a supply order for the appropriate department.

G   If the bathroom needs to be cleaned, notify the housekeeping department. If the toilet, sink, or tub/shower are not working, report this promptly to the proper department.

G   Check equipment daily to make sure it is working properly and not damaged in any way. Cords may be frayed or cracked; TVs or radios may not work. Wheelchairs, IV poles, canes, crutches, or walkers may be damaged. Report these issues immediately to the proper department.

G   Refill water pitchers regularly unless resident has a fluid restriction. Promptly report to a nurse if a resident is not drinking fluids.

G   Remove anything that might cause odors or safety hazards, like trash, clutter, or spills. Discard any disposable supplies. Clean up spills promptly. If trash needs to be emptied, notify the housekeeping department. Discard any old or spoiled food.

G   Report signs of insects or pests immediately.

G   Leave residents' belongings where you find them. Do not throw away residents' personal items.

G   After providing care, leave the unit neat and tidy. Put away equipment after it has been properly cleaned and disinfected.

Depending on the facility, NAs may be responsible for more thorough unit cleaning. When a resident is transferred, discharged, or dies, the unit will have to be completely cleaned and disinfected. This type of cleaning will require special heavy-duty gloves.

Guidelines: Unit Cleaning After Transfer, Discharge, or Death

G   Wash your hands before doing unit cleaning.

G   Wear the proper PPE as required by your facility.

G   Make sure the area is well ventilated before using strong cleaning solutions.

G   Remove and dispose of equipment and supplies carefully. These may include oxygen tubing, suction canisters, tissue boxes, water pitchers, and cups. Also remove towels, washcloths, and equipment that will be sent for cleaning. If you find any of the resident's personal items, take them to the new unit, or inform the nurse so that they can be sent to the resident or the family.

G   Raise the bed to a safe working level, and remove used linen. Roll dirty linens away from you, checking for personal items. Wash all surfaces of the bed, including both sides of the mattress, with the facility-approved disinfectant. Allow the mattress to dry completely. Remove gloves, wash your hands, and then make a neat, wrinkle-free bed. See Learning Objective 7 for more information on bedmaking guidelines and the procedures for making a bed.

G   Clean all other unit items and equipment as instructed. These may include the telephone, TV and bed controls, bedside stand, overbed table, chairs, bathrooms, windows and window sills, and door handles.

G Report any damaged or broken furniture to the proper department.

G Remove all PPE and wash your hands.

G Place new equipment and supplies in the room for a new resident.

7. Discuss types of beds and demonstrate proper bedmaking

The resident's bed is a place in which he will spend a great deal of time. Neat, well-made beds help residents sleep better each night. In addition, careful bedmaking prevents infection. A clean, neat, dry bed helps prevent skin breakdown and odors and promotes health and comfort. Skin breakdown and pressure injuries are serious problems for the elderly and are covered in detail in Chapter 18.

Many facilities have electric beds for residents. Electric beds can be raised at the head and knee area (Fig. 10-5). Some electric beds have a safety lock that helps prevent the resident or visitor from accidentally moving the bed up or down.

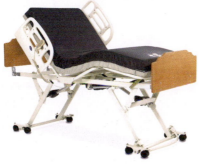

Fig. 10-5. *One type of electric bed.* (© INVACARE CORPORATION. USED WITH PERMISSION. WWW.INVACARE.COM)

The controls on electric beds vary. Generally, a person controls the electric bed by pressing buttons on a control panel. There will be a button to move the entire bed, one for the head of the bed, and another for the bottom of the bed (Fig. 10-6). There may also be controls for the bed to move into special positions. These controls should only be used by the nurses. Residents and families will be taught how to use the bed controls upon admission.

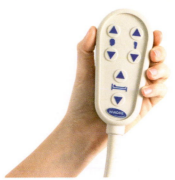

Fig. 10-6. *Controls for an electric bed.* (© INVACARE CORPORATION. USED WITH PERMISSION. WWW.INVACARE.COM)

Beds can be equipped with a variety of functions. Some beds have built-in weight scales for weighing bedridden residents so that they do not have to be transferred to a scale.

Alternating pressure mattresses are used for residents who are at risk for pressure injuries or who have pressure injuries. They are able to alternate the pressure inside the mattress so that one area of the body does not rest on a spot for too long.

There are special beds, called *bariatric beds*, that are used for residents who are obese (Fig. 10-7). **Bariatrics** is the branch of medicine that deals with the causes, prevention, and treatment of obesity. Bariatric equipment may be designated *EC* (expanded capacity), labelled *bariatric*, or be color coded and should have weight limits set by the manufacturer. A bariatric bed is made for people who weigh from 250 to 1,000 pounds. A bariatric bed may be designed to be closer to the floor than regular beds and have reinforced bed rails, as well as a trapeze to aid in movement while in bed. A special step stool can help residents move from the bed to the floor if needed. These stools are wider, longer, and closer to the floor than standard step stools. Chapter 15 contains more information about bariatrics.

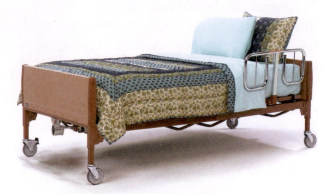

Fig. 10-7. *Bariatric beds are made for people who are obese.* (© INVACARE CORPORATION. USED WITH PERMISSION. WWW.INVACARE.COM)

Beds should remain locked in their lowest positions whenever residents are in them. Special floor cushions or pads may be placed on the floor by the bed to protect residents if they fall.

Guidelines: Bedmaking

G Bed linens must be changed when they are wet, soiled, or too wrinkled for comfort. Residents can develop pressure injuries when left in wet, wrinkled, or soiled linens. Remove and change disposable pads whenever they become soiled or wet (Fig. 10-8).

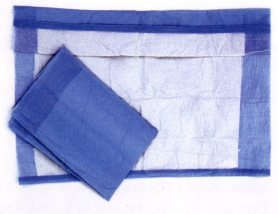

Fig. 10-8. *Disposable absorbent pads help protect sheets from sweat, urine, feces, and other fluids.*

G Before getting clean linen, wash your hands. Always use proper infection prevention procedures. Wear gloves when removing used linens.

G Gather linen in order of placement on the bed. This means first pick up the mattress pad, then all sheets, blankets, bedspreads, and pillowcases.

G Carry clean linen away from your uniform. If it touches your uniform, the linen becomes contaminated (Fig. 10-9).

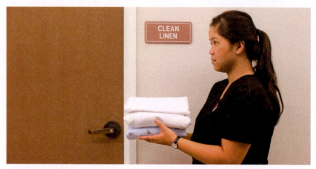

Fig. 10-9. *Carry clean linen away from your uniform.*

G Bring linen into one resident's room at a time. Put it down after flipping the stack of linen so that the first item to be placed on the bed (mattress pad) is now on the top of the stack.

G Never pick up linen from one room and transfer it to another room.

G Place clean linen on a clean surface within reach, such as a bedside stand, overbed table, or chair. Do not place clean linen on the floor or on a contaminated area.

G Use proper body mechanics when making beds. Bend your knees, use a good stance, and raise the bed height to a safe working level.

G Look at linens closely for any personal items, such as dentures, hearing aids and batteries, eyeglasses, rings, watches, and money, before removing them.

G Roll dirty linen away from you as you remove it from the bed. Rolling puts the dirtiest surface of the linen inward, which lessens contamination.

G Do not shake linen, because it may spread airborne contaminants.

G Place used linen in the proper container. Do not place used linen on the floor or on any piece of furniture in the room.

G To save energy, make one side of the bed first. Then go to the other side of the bed to complete bedmaking.

G Keep beds wrinkle-free and free of all crumbs. Remove lumps of any kind in the bed, such as from pads. If a lumpy mattress cannot be smoothed out, inform the nurse. Lumps, crumbs, and wrinkles increase the risk of pressure injuries.

G Wash your hands after handling linen.

Residents' Rights

Compassionate Care for Incontinence

Some residents have episodes of **incontinence** while in bed. When a bed is wet or soiled, the NA should change the sheets, pads, and all clothing immediately. The NA should be compassionate, respectful, and professional; this may help lessen embarrassment or discomfort. The NA should not draw attention to the resident or tell other residents what happened. The NA should check to see that the resident is clean and comfortable. Leaving residents in soiled beds can cause skin breakdown and infection. It is also considered neglectful or abusive behavior.

There are four basic types of beds: closed, open, occupied, and surgical (also called *postoperative, post-op, recovery, gurney,* or *stretcher*). A **closed bed** is usually made for a resident who will be out of bed all day. It is a bed completely made with the bedspread, blankets, and pillows in place. A closed bed is turned into an **open bed** by folding the linen down to the foot of the bed. This makes it easier for a resident to get into the bed in the afternoon for a nap or at bedtime. An NA will also open a bed when a new resident has been assigned to that room.

Making a closed bed

Equipment: clean linen—mattress pad, fitted or flat bottom sheet, disposable absorbent pad (if needed), cotton **draw sheet**, *flat top sheet, blanket(s), bedspread (if used), pillowcase(s), gloves*

1. Wash your hands.

2. If resident is in the room, identify yourself by name. Identify the resident. Greet the resident by name.

3. Explain procedure to the resident. Speak clearly, slowly, and directly. Maintain face-to-face contact whenever possible.

4. Place clean linen on a clean surface within reach (e.g., bedside stand, overbed table, or chair).

5. Adjust the bed to a safe working level, usually waist high. Put the bed in its flattest position. Lock bed wheels.

6. Put on gloves.

7. Loosen the used linen and roll it (soiled side inside) from the head to the foot of the bed. Avoid contact with your skin or clothes. Place it in a hamper or linen bag. Do not place it on the overbed table, chair, or floor. Remove pillows and pillowcases and place pillowcases in a hamper or bag.

8. Remove and discard gloves. Wash your hands.

9. Remake the bed. Place the mattress pad (if used) on the bed, attaching elastic at corners as necessary.

10. Place the bottom sheet on the bed without shaking the linen. If using a flat sheet with seams, this sheet must be placed with the crease in the center of the mattress. The seams on both ends must be placed facing down. If using a fitted bottom sheet, place it right-side up and tightly pull over all four corners of the bed.

11. Make hospital corners to keep the bottom sheet wrinkle-free (Fig. 10-10).

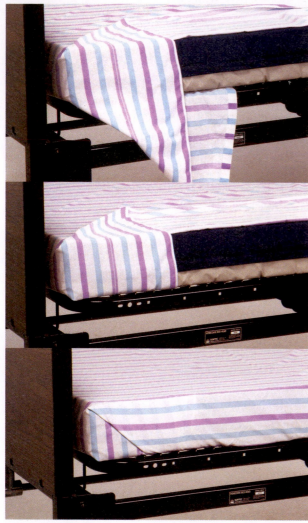

Fig. 10-10. Hospital corners help keep the sheet smooth under the resident.

12. Put on the disposable absorbent pad and then the draw sheet if used. Place them in the center of the bed on the bottom sheet. Smooth and tightly tuck the bottom sheet and draw sheet together under the sides of the bed. Move from the head of the bed to the foot of the bed.

13. Place the top sheet over the bed and center it. The seam must be up.

14. Place the blanket over the bed and center it.

15. Place the bedspread over the bed and center it.

16. Tuck the top sheet and blanket under the foot of the bed and make hospital corners.

17. Fold down the top sheet to make a cuff of about six inches over the blanket.

18. With one hand, grasp the clean pillowcase at the closed end. Turn it inside out over your arm. Next, using the hand that has the pillowcase over it, grasp one narrow edge of the pillow. Pull the pillowcase over it with your free hand (Fig. 10-11). Do the same for any other pillows. Place them at the head of the bed with open ends away from the door. Make sure zippers or tags are on the inside.

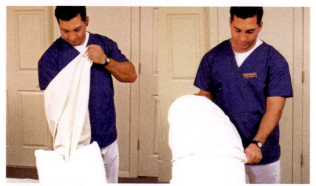

Fig. 10-11. After the pillowcase is turned inside out over your arm, grasp one end of the pillow. Pull the pillowcase over the pillow.

19. Return the bed to its lowest position.

20. Leave call light within the resident's reach.

21. Wash your hands.

22. Take the laundry bag to the proper area.

23. Document procedure using facility guidelines.

Tip

Seams and the Skin

Residents' skin may be very fragile. Seams rubbing against an elderly person's skin can cause the skin to tear or crack. Remember to follow these rules for placing linens properly on beds:

Bottom Sheet: Seam Down = Bottom Down

Top Sheet: Seam Up = Top Up

Making an open bed

Equipment: clean linen—mattress pad, fitted or flat bottom sheet, disposable absorbent pad (if needed), cotton draw sheet, flat top sheet, blanket(s), bedspread (if used), pillowcase(s), gloves

1. Wash your hands.

2. Make a closed bed, as described in previous procedure.

3. Stand at the head of the bed. Grasp the top sheet, blanket, and bedspread, and fold them down to the foot of the bed. Then bring them back up the bed to form a large cuff.

4. Bring the cuff on the top linen to a point where it is one hand-width above the linen underneath. This way, when the resident gets into bed, he will not pull out all the linen at the foot of the bed.

5. Make sure all linen is wrinkle-free.

6. Wash your hands.

7. Document procedure using facility guidelines.

An **occupied bed** is a bed made while the resident is in the bed. A resident may have a doctor's order to stay in bed at all times. These orders are called *absolute bedrest* (*ABR*), *strict bedrest*, or *complete bedrest* (*CBR*). Having two coworkers work together when making this type of bed is safer. Making an occupied bed gives an NA an opportunity to observe a resident's skin for signs of breakdown. Bedbound residents are at great risk for pressure injuries.

An **unoccupied bed** is a bed made while no resident is in the bed. If the resident can be safely moved out of bed, making the bed will be easier.

Making an occupied bed

Equipment: clean linen—mattress pad, fitted or flat bottom sheet, disposable absorbent pad (if needed), cotton draw sheet, flat top sheet, blanket(s), bedspread (if used), bath blanket, pillowcase(s), gloves

1. Wash your hands.

2. Identify yourself by name. Identify the resident. Greet the resident by name.

3. Explain procedure to the resident. Speak clearly, slowly, and directly. Maintain face-to-face contact whenever possible.

4. Provide for the resident's privacy with a curtain, screen, or door.

5. Place clean linen on a clean surface within reach (e.g., bedside stand, overbed table, or chair).

6. Adjust the bed to a safe working level, usually waist high. Lower the head of the bed. Lock bed wheels.

7. Put on gloves.

8. Loosen the top linen from the end of the bed on the working side.

9. Unfold the bath blanket over the top sheet and remove the top sheet. Keep the resident covered at all times with the bath blanket.

10. You will make the bed one side at a time. Raise the bed rail (if bed has them) on the far side of the bed. After raising the bed rail, go to the other side of the bed. Gently help the resident to turn onto her side slowly, moving her away from you, toward the raised bed rail (Fig. 10-12).

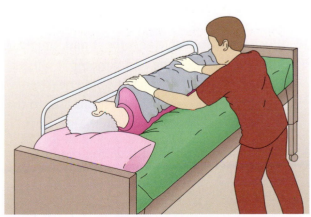

Fig. 10-12. *Turn resident onto her side, toward the raised bed rail.*

11. Loosen the bottom used linen, mattress pad, and absorbent pad, if present, on the working side.

12. Roll the bottom used linen toward the resident and center of bed, soiled side inside. Tuck it snugly against the resident's back.

13. Place the mattress pad (if used) on the bed, attaching elastic at corners on the working side.

14. Place the clean bottom linen or fitted bottom sheet with the center crease in the center. If a flat sheet is used, tuck it in at the top and on the working side. Make hospital corners to keep bottom sheet wrinkle-free. If a fitted sheet is used, tightly pull the two fitted corners on the working side.

15. Smooth the bottom sheet out toward the resident. Be sure there are no wrinkles in the mattress pad. Roll the extra material toward the resident. Tuck it under the resident's body (Fig. 10-13).

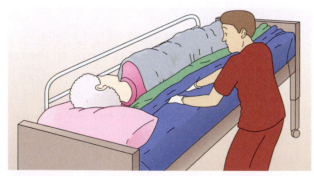

Fig. 10-13. Tuck extra material under the resident's body.

16. If using a disposable absorbent pad, unfold it and center it on the bed. Smooth it out toward the resident. Tuck the side near you under the mattress. Smooth it out toward the resident. Tuck as you did with the sheet.

17. If using a draw sheet, place it on the bed. Tuck it in on your side, smooth, and tuck as you did with the other bedding.

18. Raise the bed rail nearest you. Go to the other side of the bed and lower that bed rail.

Help the resident roll or turn onto the clean bottom sheet, toward the raised bed rail (Fig. 10-14). Explain that she will be moving over a roll of linen. Protect the resident from any soiled matter on the old linens.

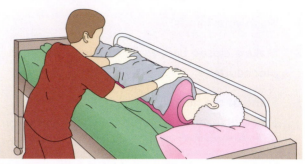

Fig. 10-14. While helping the resident turn onto the clean linen, try to avoid contact with soiled matter on dirty linen.

19. Loosen the used linen. Check for any personal items. Roll the linen from the head to the foot of the bed, avoiding contact with your skin or clothes. Do not shake the used linen. Place it in a hamper or bag. Do not place it on the overbed table, chair, or floor.

20. Pull the clean linen through as quickly as possible. Start with the mattress pad and wrap it around the corners. Pull and tuck in clean bottom linen, just like the other side. Pull and tuck in the disposable absorbent pad and draw sheet if used. Make hospital corners with the bottom sheet. Finish with the bottom sheet free of wrinkles.

21. Ask the resident to turn onto her back, helping as needed. Keep the resident covered and comfortable, with a pillow under her head. Raise the bed rail nearest you.

22. Unfold the top sheet. Place it over the resident and center it. Ask the resident to hold the top sheet and pull the bath blanket out from underneath (Fig. 10-15). Put it in the hamper or bag.

23. Place the blanket over the top sheet and center it. Match the top edges. Place the bedspread over the blanket and center it. Match

the top edges. Tuck the top sheet, blanket, and bedspread under the foot of the bed and make hospital corners on each side. Loosen the top linens over the resident's feet.

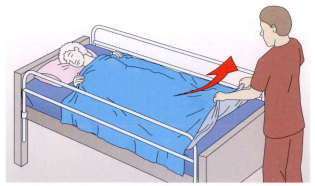

Fig. 10-15. *With the resident holding on to the top sheet, pull the bath blanket out.*

24. At the top of the bed, fold down the top sheet over the blanket about six inches to make a cuff.

25. Gently hold and lift the resident's head and remove the pillow. Do not hold it near your face. Remove the soiled pillowcase by turning it inside out. Place it in the hamper or bag.

26. Remove and discard gloves. Wash your hands.

27. With one hand, grasp the clean pillowcase at the closed end. Turn it inside out over your arm. Next, using the same hand that has the pillowcase over it, grasp the center of the end of the pillow. Pull the pillowcase over it with your free hand. Do the same for any other pillows. Place pillows gently under resident's head with open ends away from the door. Make sure zippers or tags are on the inside.

28. Make sure the bed is wrinkle-free. Make the resident comfortable.

29. Return the bed to its lowest position. Leave the bed rails in the ordered position. Remove privacy measures.

30. Leave call light within the resident's reach.

31. Be courteous and respectful at all times.

32. Wash your hands.

33. Take the laundry bag to the proper area.

34. Report any changes in the resident to the nurse. Document procedure using facility guidelines.

A **surgical bed** is made so that it can easily accept residents who must return to bed on stretchers or gurneys. Residents on stretchers are usually returning from treatment or hospital visits. When transferring residents from stretchers to beds, the bed and stretcher wheels must be locked. The bed and stretcher must be touching during the transfer.

The NA should discuss the preparation for the arrival of a resident on a stretcher with the nurse and should gather any extra equipment/supplies as instructed.

Making a surgical bed

Equipment: clean linen (see Procedure: Making a closed bed), gloves

1. Wash your hands.

2. Place clean linen on a clean surface within reach (e.g., bedside stand, overbed table, or chair).

3. Adjust the bed to a safe working level, usually waist high. Lock bed wheels.

4. Put on gloves.

5. Remove all used linen, rolling it (soiled side inside) from the head to the foot of the bed. Avoid contact with your skin or clothes. Place it in a hamper or linen bag.

6. Remove and discard gloves.

7. Wash your hands.

8. Make a closed bed. Do not tuck the top linens under the mattress.

9. Fold the top linens down from the head of the bed and up from the foot of the bed (Fig. 10-16).

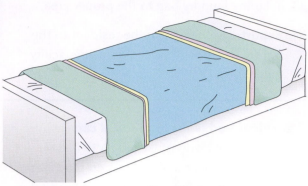

Fig. 10-16. Fold the linens down from the head of the bed and up from the foot of the bed.

10. Form a triangle with the linen. Fanfold the linen triangle into pleated layers and position opposite the stretcher side of the bed (Fig. 10-17). Fanfolding means folding several times into pleats. After fanfolding, form a small tip with the end of the linen triangle. The tip can be grasped quickly and pulled over the returning resident. This step quickly provides much-needed warmth to the resident.

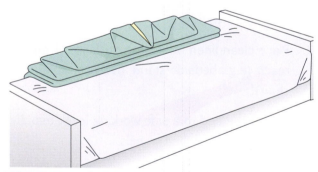

Fig. 10-17. Fanfold the linen so that it is in pleated layers and position the linen opposite the stretcher side of bed.

11. Put on clean pillowcases. Place the clean pillows on a clean surface off the bed, such as on the bedside stand or chair.

12. Leave the bed in its locked position. Leave both bed rails down.

13. Move all furniture to make room for the stretcher.

14. Do not place the call light on the bed. That is placed after the resident returns to bed.

15. Wash your hands.

16. Take the laundry bag or hamper to the proper area.

17. Document procedure using facility guidelines.

Chapter Review

1. List three functions that sleep performs (LO 2).

2. What is usually stored in the bedside stand (LO 5)?

3. What is the overbed table used for? Can a bedpan be placed on it (LO 5)?

4. Where should the call light always be placed (LO 6)?

5. Define *disposable* equipment (LO 6).

6. Why should NAs carry clean linen away from their uniforms (LO 7)?

7. Why should linen never be shaken (LO 7)?

8. Describe the difference between a closed bed and an open bed (LO 7).

9. While making an occupied bed, what should the NA observe (LO 7)?

10. When is a surgical bed made (LO 7)?

Multiple Choice

11. A disruption of breathing while a person is sleeping is known as (LO 3)
    (A) Insomnia
    (B) Sleep apnea
    (C) REM behavior disorder
    (D) Bruxism

12. The inability to fall asleep or stay asleep is known as (LO 3)
    (A) Insomnia
    (B) Sleep apnea
    (C) REM behavior disorder
    (D) Bruxism

13. Which of the following is a type of stimulant that may prevent residents from sleeping (LO 4)?
    (A) Hot water
    (B) Nicotine
    (C) Ibuprofen
    (D) Beer

14. Which of the following is a type of depressant (substance that causes calmness and drowsiness)(LO 4)?
    (A) Caffeine
    (B) Nicotine
    (C) Cigarettes
    (D) Wine

11 Positioning, Moving, and Lifting

A View from the Past

"Having lost the use of my legs during the polio epidemic that swept across the eastern United States during the summer of 1944, I was soon immersed in a process of rehabilitation that was . . . as much spiritual as physical. That was a full decade before the discovery of the Salk vaccine ended polio's reign as the disease most dreaded by America's parents and their children. Treatment of the disease had been standardized by 1944: following the initial onslaught of the virus, patients were kept in isolation for a period of ten days to two weeks. Following that, orthodox medical opinion was content to subject patients to as much heat as they could stand. Stiff paralyzed limbs were swathed in heated, coarse woolen towels known as 'hot packs.' As soon as the hot packs had baked enough pain and stiffness out of a patient's body so that he could be moved on and off a stretcher, the treatment was ended, and the patient faced a series of daily immersions in a heated pool. I would ultimately spend two full years at the appropriately named New York State Reconstruction Home. . . . We would learn during our days in the New York State Reconstruction Home to confront the world that was. My future had arrived."

from *Falling Into Life* by Leonard Kriegel

"Take her up tenderly/Lift her with care."

Thomas Hood, 1798–1845

1. Define important words in this chapter

ambulation: the act of moving or walking, with or without an assistive device.

dangle: to sit up with the legs hanging over the side of the bed in order to regain balance.

ergonomics: the science of designing equipment, areas, and tasks to make them safer and to suit the worker's abilities.

Fowler's: semi-sitting body position in which a person's head and shoulders are elevated 45 to 60 degrees.

lateral: body position in which a person is lying on either side.

logrolling: moving a person as a unit, without disturbing the alignment of the body.

mechanical lift: special equipment used to lift and move or lift and weigh a person; also called *hydraulic lift*.

positioning: the act of helping people into positions that promote comfort and health.

posture: the way a person holds and positions his body.

prone: body position in which a person is lying on his stomach, or front side of the body.

shearing: rubbing or friction resulting from the skin moving one way and the bone underneath it remaining fixed or moving in the opposite direction.

Sims': body position in which a person is lying on his left side with the upper knee flexed and raised toward the chest.

supine: body position in which a person is lying flat on his back.

transfer belt: a belt made of canvas or other heavy material used to help people who are weak, unsteady, or uncoordinated to stand, sit, or walk.

2. Explain body alignment and review the principles of body mechanics

The positioning of the body plays an important part in the proper functioning of the body. Whether standing, sitting, or lying down, the body should be in correct alignment and exhibiting good posture. **Posture** is the way a person holds and positions his body.

Correct body alignment helps the body achieve balance without causing muscle or joint strain. In addition, body alignment allows the body to function at its highest level. The lungs are able to expand and contract, blood circulation is more efficient, digestion is easier, and the kidneys are better able to clean the body of wastes. Body alignment also helps prevent complications of immobility, such as contractures and atrophy. A contracture is the permanent and painful shortening of a muscle, tendon, or ligament. Atrophy is the weakening or wasting of muscles.

Body mechanics was first introduced in Chapter 7. When a nursing assistant does not move and position residents using proper body mechanics, injury can result.

Guidelines: Using Proper Body Mechanics

G   Assess the load. Before lifting, assess the weight of the load to determine if you can safely move the object without help. Know the lift policies at your facility. Never attempt to lift someone you are not sure you can lift.

G   Think ahead, plan, and communicate the move. Check for any objects in your path or any potential risks, such as a wet floor. Make sure the path is clear. Watch for hazards, like high-traffic areas, combative residents, or a loose toilet seat. Decide exactly what you are going to do together and agree on verbal cues you will use before attempting to move the resident.

G   Check your base of support and be sure you have firm footing. Use a wide but balanced stance to increase support, and keep this stance when walking. Have enough room to maintain a wide base of support. Make sure you and the resident are wearing nonskid shoes that are securely fastened.

G   Face what you are lifting. Your feet should always face the direction you are moving. This enables you to move your body as one unit and keeps your back straight. Do not twist; twisting at the waist increases the likelihood of injury. Turn and face the area you are moving the object to, then set the object down.

G   Keep your back straight. Keeping your head up and shoulders back will keep the back in the proper position. Taking a deep breath will help you regain correct posture.

G   Begin in a squatting position and lift with your legs. Bend at the hips and knees, and use the strength of your leg muscles to stand and lift the object. You will need to push your buttocks out to accomplish this. Before you stand with the object you are lifting, remember that your legs, not your back, will enable you to lift. You should be able to feel your leg muscles as they work. Lift with the large leg muscles to decrease stress on the back.

G   Tighten your stomach muscles when beginning the lift. This will help to take weight off the spine and maintain alignment.

G   Keep the object close to your body. This decreases stress on your back. Lift objects only to your waist. Carrying them any higher can affect your balance.

G   Push when possible rather than lifting. When you lift an object, you must overcome gravity to balance the load. When you push an object, you only need to overcome the friction between the surface and the object. Use your body weight to move the object, rather than your lifting muscles. Stay close to the object. Use both arms and tighten your stomach muscles.

3. Explain why position changes are important for bedbound residents and describe basic body positions

Residents who spend a lot of time in bed often need help getting into comfortable positions. They also need to change positions periodically to avoid skin breakdown or pressure injuries. Too much pressure on one area for too long can cause a decrease in circulation, which can lead to the formation of pressure injuries, as well as other problems like muscle contractures. Pressure injuries are a serious condition and are a major problem in long-term care. More information about pressure injuries and prevention may be found in Chapter 18.

Positioning means helping residents into positions that promote comfort and health. Bedbound residents should be repositioned at least every two hours. Residents in wheelchairs or chairs should be repositioned at least every hour. Nursing assistants should follow posted turn schedules and care plans carefully. Each time there is a change of position, NAs should document the position and the time. When positioning residents, NAs must use proper body mechanics to help prevent injury. NAs should also check the skin for whiteness, redness, warm spots, or skin that is a different color than the surrounding area, especially around bony areas, each time they reposition residents. The following are guidelines for positioning residents in the five basic body positions:

Supine: In this position, the resident lies flat on his back. To maintain correct body position, the head and shoulders should be supported with a pillow (Fig. 11-1). Pillows, rolled towels, or washcloths can also be used to support the arms (especially a weak or immobilized arm) or hands. A pillow should be placed under the calves so the heels are elevated ("floating") and do not touch the bed. Pillows or a footboard (padded board placed against the resident's feet) can keep the feet properly positioned.

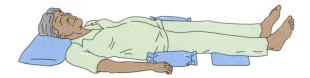

Fig. 11-1. A person in the supine position is lying flat on his back.

Lateral/side: A resident in the lateral position is lying on either side (Fig. 11-2). There are many variations of this position. Pillows can support the arm and leg on the upper side, the back, and the head. Ideally, the knee on the upper side of the body should be flexed. The leg is brought in front of the body and supported on a pillow. There should be a pillow under the bottom foot so that the toes are not touching the bed. If the top leg cannot be brought forward, it should be placed slightly behind the bottom leg, not resting directly on it. Pillows should be used between the two legs and ankles to help relieve pressure and avoid skin breakdown.

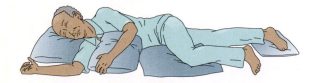

Fig. 11-2. A person in the lateral position is lying on his side.

Prone: A resident in the prone position is lying on the abdomen, or front side of the body (Fig. 11-3). This is not comfortable for many people, especially elderly people. An NA should only place a resident in the prone position as directed. In this position, the arms are either placed at the sides, raised above the head, or one raised and one by the side. The head is turned to one side. A small pillow may be used under the head and legs. This keeps the feet from touching the bed.

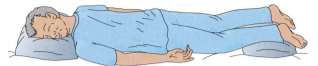

Fig. 11-3. *A person lying in the prone position is lying on his abdomen.*

Fowler's: A resident in the Fowler's position is in a semi-sitting position (45 to 60 degrees) (Fig. 11-4). The head and shoulders are elevated. The resident's knees may be flexed and elevated, using a pillow or rolled blanket as a support. The feet may be supported, using a footboard or other support. The spine should be straight. In a high-Fowler's position, the upper body is sitting nearly straight up (60 to 90 degrees). In a semi-Fowler's position, the upper body is not raised as high (30 to 45 degrees).

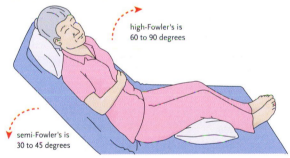

high-Fowler's is 60 to 90 degrees

semi-Fowler's is 30 to 45 degrees

Fig. 11-4. *A person lying in the Fowler's position is partially reclined.*

Sims': The Sims' position is a left side-lying position (Fig. 11-5). The lower arm is behind the back, and the upper knee is flexed and raised toward the chest, using a pillow as support. There should be a pillow under the bottom foot so that the toes and ankle do not touch the bed.

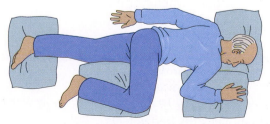

Fig. 11-5. *A person in the Sims' position is lying on his left side with one leg drawn up.*

Many positioning devices are available to help make residents more comfortable in different body positions. Chapter 25 contains a list of these devices.

A draw sheet, turning sheet, transfer sheet, or glide sheet should be used if the resident cannot help with moving. A draw sheet is an extra sheet placed on top of the bottom sheet when the bed is made (Fig. 11-6). Draw sheets help prevent skin damage caused by shearing. **Shearing** is rubbing or friction resulting from the skin moving one way and the bone underneath it remaining fixed or moving in the opposite direction.

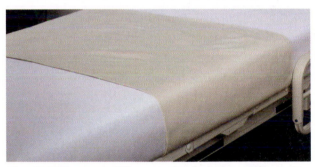

Fig. 11-6. *There are different assist devices used for positioning and transferring. This photo shows a draw sheet that can be left in place after the move or transfer is complete.* (© MEDLINE INDUSTRIES, INC. 2019)

It is always safer when at least two workers can move a resident together. A nursing assistant should always get help if she feels it is not safe to move the resident by herself.

Assisting a resident to move up in bed with assistance (using assist device)

Equipment: draw sheet or other assist device

1. Identify yourself by name. Identify the resident. Greet the resident by name.

2. Wash your hands.

3. Explain procedure to the resident. Speak clearly, slowly, and directly. Maintain face-to-face contact whenever possible. Encourage resident to assist if possible.

4. Provide for the resident's privacy with a curtain, screen, or door.

5. Adjust the bed to a safe level, usually waist high. Lock the bed wheels.

6. Lower the head of bed to make it flat. Move the pillow to the head of bed.

7. Stand on the opposite side of the bed from your helper. Each of you should be turned slightly toward the head of the bed. For each of you, the foot that is closest to the head of the bed should be pointed in that direction. Stand with your feet shoulder-width apart. Bend your knees. Keep your back straight.

8. Roll the assist device up to the resident's side. Have your helper do the same on her side of the bed. Grasp the device with your palms up at the resident's shoulders and hips. Have your helper do the same.

9. Shift your weight to your back foot (the foot closer to the foot of the bed). Have your helper do the same (Fig. 11-7). On the count of three, you and your helper both shift your weight to the forward foot. Slide the assist device and resident toward the head of the bed.

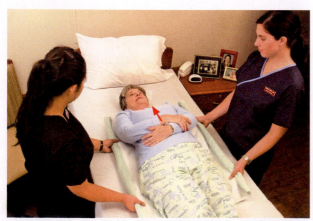

Fig. 11-7. *Both people shift their weight to their back foot and prepare to move.*

10. Place the pillow under the resident's head.

11. Make the resident comfortable. If using a draw sheet, unroll it and leave it in place for the next repositioning (Fig. 11-8). If using another type of assist device, you will need to remove it.

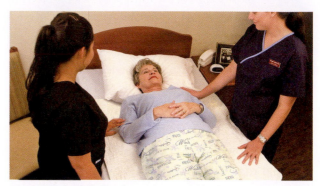

Fig. 11-8. *Unroll the draw sheet and leave it in place.*

12. Return bed to its lowest position. Remove privacy measures.

13. Leave call light within the resident's reach.

14. Wash your hands.

15. Be courteous and respectful at all times.

16. Report any changes in the resident to the nurse. Document procedure using facility guidelines.

Moving a resident to the side of the bed

1. Identify yourself by name. Identify the resident. Greet the resident by name.

2. Wash your hands.

3. Explain procedure to the resident. Speak clearly, slowly, and directly. Maintain face-to-face contact whenever possible. Encourage resident to assist if possible.

4. Provide for the resident's privacy with a curtain, screen, or door.

5. Adjust the bed to a safe level, usually waist high. Lock the bed wheels.

6. Lower the head of the bed.

7. Stand on the side of the bed to which you are moving the resident.

8. Stand with feet shoulder-width apart. Bend your knees. Keep your back straight.

9. Gently slide your hands under the resident's head and shoulders and move them toward you (Fig. 11-9).

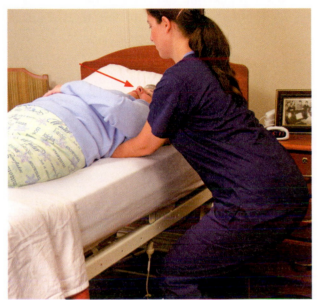

Fig. 11-9. Gently move the resident's head and shoulders toward you.

10. Gently slide your hands under the resident's midsection and move it toward you.

11. Gently slide your hands under the resident's hips and legs and move them toward you (Fig. 11-10).

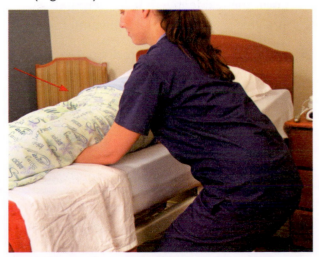

Fig. 11-10. Gently move the hips and legs toward you.

12. Make the resident comfortable.

13. Return bed to its lowest position. Remove privacy measures.

14. Leave call light within the resident's reach.

15. Wash your hands.

16. Be courteous and respectful at all times.

17. Report any changes in the resident to the nurse. Document procedure using facility guidelines.

Moving a resident to the side of the bed with assistance (using assist device)

Equipment: draw sheet or other assist device

1. Identify yourself by name. Identify the resident. Greet the resident by name.

2. Wash your hands.

3. Explain procedure to the resident. Speak clearly, slowly, and directly. Maintain face-to-face contact whenever possible. Encourage resident to assist if possible.

4. Provide for the resident's privacy with a curtain, screen, or door.

5. Adjust the bed to a safe level, usually waist high. Lock the bed wheels.

6. Lower the head of bed. Move the pillow to the head of bed.

7. Stand on the opposite side of the bed from your helper. You should be facing each other. Stand up straight, facing the side of the bed, with feet shoulder-width apart. Point feet toward the side of the bed. Bend your knees.

8. Roll the draw sheet or other assist device up to the resident's side. Have your helper do the same on his side of the bed. Grasp the device with your palms up at the resident's shoulders and hips. Have your helper do the same.

9. On the count of three, slide the resident toward the side of the bed. Your weight should be equal on each foot because you are moving the person to the side of the bed, not to the head of the bed.

10. Place the pillow under the resident's head.

11. Make the resident comfortable. If using a draw sheet, unroll it and leave it in place for the next repositioning. If using another type of assist device, you will need to remove it.

12. Return bed to its lowest position. Remove privacy measures.

13. Leave call light within the resident's reach.

14. Wash your hands.

15. Be courteous and respectful at all times.

16. Report any changes in the resident to the nurse. Document procedure using facility guidelines.

Turning a resident toward you

1. Identify yourself by name. Identify the resident. Greet the resident by name.

2. Wash your hands.

3. Explain procedure to the resident. Speak clearly, slowly, and directly. Maintain face-to-face contact whenever possible.

4. Provide for the resident's privacy with a curtain, screen, or door.

5. Adjust the bed to a safe level, usually waist high. Lock the bed wheels.

6. Lower the head of the bed to make it flat.

7. If the bed has bed rails, raise the far bed rail.

8. Move the resident to the far side of the bed, using previous procedure.

9. Cross the resident's far arm over her chest. Move the arm on the side the resident is being turned to out of the way. Cross the far leg over the near leg.

10. Stand with your feet shoulder-width apart. Bend your knees.

11. Place one hand on the resident's far shoulder. Place the other hand on the far hip.

12. While supporting the body, gently roll the resident onto her side as one unit, toward you. Use your body to block the resident to prevent her from rolling out of bed. Make sure resident's face is not covered by the pillow.

13. Position the resident properly:

- Head supported by a pillow (resident's face should not be obstructed by the pillow)

- Shoulder adjusted so resident is not lying on her arm or hand

- Top arm supported by a pillow

- Back supported by a supportive device

- Hips properly aligned

- Supportive device between the legs with the top knee flexed; knee and ankle supported

- Pillow under the bottom foot so that toes are not touching the bed

14. Cover the resident with top linens and straighten. Make the resident comfortable.

15. Return bed to its lowest position. Leave bed rails in ordered position. Remove privacy measures.

16. Leave call light within the resident's reach.

17. Wash your hands.

18. Be courteous and respectful at all times.

19. Report any changes in the resident to the nurse. Document procedure using facility guidelines.

Logrolling allows a resident to be turned as a unit, without disturbing the alignment of the body. The head, back, and legs must be kept in a straight line. This is necessary in cases of neck or back problems, head or spinal cord injuries, or after neck, back, or hip surgeries. To promote safety, two people or more should perform this procedure together. An assist device, such as a draw sheet, helps with moving.

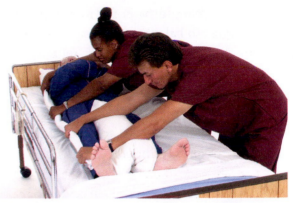

Fig. 11-11. Both workers should grasp the draw sheet on the far side.

Logrolling a resident with assistance

Equipment: draw sheet or other assist device

1. Identify yourself by name. Identify the resident. Greet the resident by name.

2. Wash your hands.

3. Explain procedure to the resident. Speak clearly, slowly, and directly. Maintain face-to-face contact whenever possible.

4. Provide for the resident's privacy with a curtain, screen, or door.

5. Adjust the bed to a safe level, usually waist high. Lock the bed wheels.

6. Lower the head of the bed to make it flat.

7. Both you and your helper stand on the same side of the bed. One person stands at the resident's head and shoulders. The other stands near the resident's midsection.

8. Place a pillow under the resident's head to support the neck during the move.

9. Place the resident's arms across his chest. Place a pillow between the knees.

10. Stand with feet shoulder-width apart. Bend your knees.

11. Grasp the draw sheet or other assist device on the far side (Fig. 11-11).

12. On the count of three, gently roll the resident toward you. Turn the resident as a unit (Fig. 11-12). Use your bodies to block the resident to prevent him from rolling out of bed.

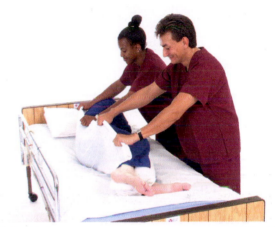

Fig. 11-12. On the count of three, both workers should roll the resident toward them, turning him as a unit.

13. Reposition the resident comfortably in proper alignment. If using a draw sheet, unroll it and leave it in place for the next repositioning. If using another type of assist device, you will need to remove it. Cover the resident with top linens and straighten.

14. Return bed to its lowest position. Remove privacy measures.

15. Leave call light within the resident's reach.

16. Wash your hands.

17. Be courteous and respectful at all times.

18. Report any changes in the resident to the nurse. Document procedure using facility guidelines.

To **dangle** means to sit up on the side of the bed with the legs hanging over the side. This helps residents regain balance before standing up, equalizes blood flow in the body, returns blood flow to the head, and allows blood pressure to stabilize. It helps prevent dizziness and light-headedness that can cause fainting. Residents who cannot walk may have an order to dangle their legs for a few minutes regularly.

Assisting a resident to sit up on the side of the bed: dangling

1. Identify yourself by name. Identify the resident. Greet the resident by name.

2. Wash your hands.

3. Explain procedure to the resident. Speak clearly, slowly, and directly. Maintain face-to-face contact whenever possible.

4. Provide for the resident's privacy with a curtain, screen, or door.

5. Adjust the bed to its lowest position. Lock the bed wheels.

6. Raise the head of bed to sitting position. Fold linens to the foot of the bed.

7. Stand at the side of the bed with your feet shoulder-width apart. Bend your knees. Keep your back straight. Help the resident slowly move toward the side of the bed on which you are standing.

8. Place one arm under the resident's shoulder blades. Place the other arm under the resident's thighs (Fig. 11-13).

9. On the count of three, gently and slowly turn the resident into a sitting position with his legs dangling over the side of bed (Fig. 11-14).

10. Ask the resident to sit up straight and hold onto the edge of the mattress with both hands. Help the resident to put on nonskid shoes if he is going to get out of bed.

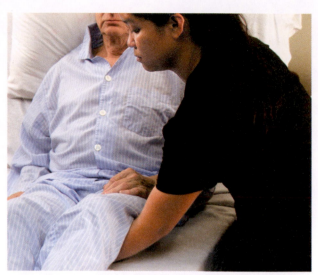

Fig. 11-13. One arm should be under the resident's shoulder blades, and the other arm should be under the thighs.

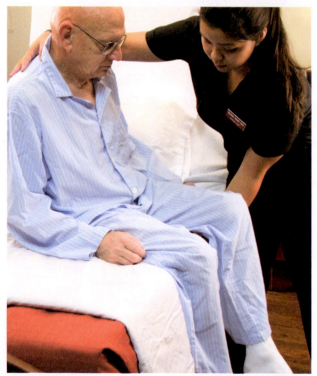

Fig. 11-14. The weight of the resident's legs hanging down from the bed helps the resident sit up.

11. Have the resident dangle as long as ordered. The care plan may direct you to allow the resident to dangle for several minutes and then return him to lying down, or it may direct you to allow the resident to dangle in preparation for walking or a transfer. Follow the care plan. Place a supportive device behind the

resident's back while he is dangling. Do not leave the resident alone. Check for dizziness. If the resident feels dizzy or faint, help him lie down again and report to the nurse.

12. Take vital signs as ordered (Chapter 13).

13. Remove the resident's shoes or slippers.

14. Gently help the resident back into bed. Place one arm around the resident's shoulders. Place the other arm under the resident's knees. Slowly swing the resident's legs onto the bed.

15. Make the resident comfortable. Cover the resident with top linens and straighten. Replace the pillow under the resident's head.

16. Leave bed in its lowest position. Remove privacy measures.

17. Leave call light within the resident's reach.

18. Wash your hands.

19. Be courteous and respectful at all times.

20. Report any changes in the resident to the nurse. Document procedure using facility guidelines.

4. Describe how to safely transfer residents

Transferring a resident means that a nursing assistant is moving him from one place to another. Examples include transferring a resident from a bed to a chair or wheelchair or from a wheelchair to a toilet or portable commode.

Some residents have a stronger side and a weaker side. The weaker side is called the *involved* or *affected* side. Nursing assistants must plan the move so that the stronger side moves first and the weaker side follows. It is difficult for the weaker arm and leg to bear enough weight for the transfer if moved first. More information about transferring residents who are recovering from a hip replacement or stroke may be found in Chapters 21 and 22.

Safety is one of the most important things to consider during transfers. The Occupational Safety and Health Administration (OSHA) has set specific ergonomic guidelines to help avoid injuries during transfers. **Ergonomics** is the science of designing equipment, areas, and work tasks to make them safer and to suit the worker's abilities. One goal of ergonomics is to reduce stress on the body to avoid potential injury.

Certain parts of the body, such as the back, are more prone to injury. OSHA's ergonomic guidelines address ways to help avoid these work-related injuries. OSHA states that manual lifting and transferring of residents should be reduced and eliminated when possible. This means that proper safety and lift equipment should be available in facilities. Staff should be trained how to use this equipment and should use it whenever possible to avoid injury.

To reduce injuries, many facilities have adopted *no-lift*, *zero-lift*, or *lift-free* policies, which set forth strict guidelines for lifting and transferring residents. Manual lifting may be prohibited entirely, and equipment might always be required to lift and move residents. The more restrictions placed on lifting, the less chance there is of injury. Nursing assistants must follow facility policies on lifting, and should always get help when they need it.

When evaluating residents for transfers, staff may determine that residents require a transfer belt for safety. A **transfer belt** is a safety device used to transfer residents who are weak, unsteady, or uncoordinated. The belt is made of canvas or other heavy material, has a strong buckle, and sometimes has handles. It is secured around the resident's waist, outside the clothing. It should never be placed on bare skin. The belt gives NAs something firm to hold on to when helping with transfers. The NA should grasp the belt securely on both sides, with hands in an upward position. Transfer belts cannot be used if a resident has fragile bones, fractures, or has had recent abdominal, chest, or back surgery.

Applying a transfer belt

Equipment: transfer belt, nonskid footwear

1. Identify yourself by name. Identify the resident. Greet the resident by name.

2. Wash your hands.

3. Explain procedure to the resident. Speak clearly, slowly, and directly. Maintain face-to-face contact whenever possible.

4. Provide for the resident's privacy with a curtain, screen, or door.

5. Adjust bed to its lowest position. Lock bed wheels.

6. Supporting the back and hips, help the resident to a sitting position with her feet flat on the floor.

7. Put nonskid footwear on the resident and fasten it securely.

8. Place the belt over the resident's clothing, below the rib cage and above the waist. Do not put it over bare skin.

9. Tighten the buckle until it is snug. Leave enough room to insert flat fingers/hand comfortably under the belt. The belt must not interfere with circulation or breathing.

10. Check to make sure that skin or skin folds (for example, breasts) are not caught under the belt.

11. Position the buckle slightly off-center in the front or back for comfort.

A slide or transfer board may be used to help transfer residents who have weak legs or are unable to bear any weight on their legs. Slide boards can be used for most transfers that involve moving from one sitting position to another (Fig. 11-15). These boards can be used for transferring from wheelchairs or chairs to beds, vehicles, shower chairs, and other areas.

Slide boards are made of sturdy material, such as wood, so they can hold the resident's weight. Slide boards should not be used against bare skin. Before beginning a transfer, the NA should make sure that the resident's fingers are not under the board.

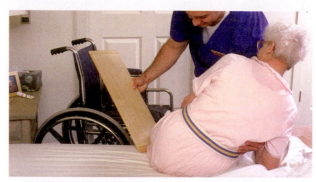

Fig. 11-15. *A slide or transfer board can help with bed-to-chair transfers.*

Other devices can help promote safety with transferring, such as a sliding sheet, a mechanical lift (later in the chapter), and special air-inflated mattresses (Fig. 11-16).

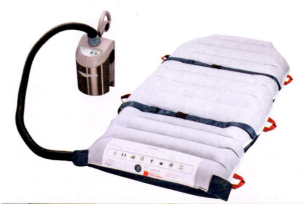

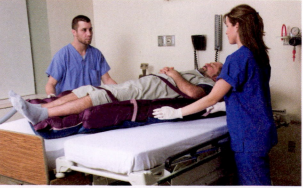

Fig. 11-16. *These are two types of air-filled safety devices used for transferring.* (TOP PHOTO OF THE HOVERMATT® SINGLE-PATIENT USE AIR TRANSFER SYSTEM COURTESY OF HOVERTECH INTERNATIONAL, WWW.HOVERMATT.COM, AND BOTTOM PHOTO OF THE HOVERMATT® AIR TRANSFER SYSTEM COURTESY OF HOVERTECH INTERNATIONAL, WWW.HOVERMATT.COM)

Wheelchairs and Geriatric Chairs

Wheelchairs must always be locked before transferring residents to or from the wheelchair (Fig. 11-17). Here are some general guidelines for wheelchair use:

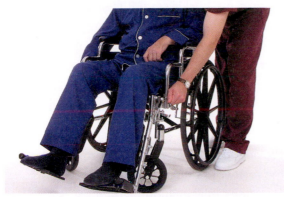

Fig. 11-17. A nursing assistant must always lock the wheelchair before a resident gets into or out of it.

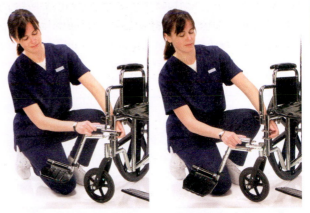

Fig. 11-18. To remove footrests, pull back the lever and pull the footrest off the knobs.

Guidelines: Wheelchairs and Geriatric Chairs

G   To open a standard wheelchair, pull on both sides to make the armrests separate and the seat flatten. To close the wheelchair, lift the center of the seat and pull upward until the sides of the chair fold inward.

G   If a standard wheelchair has a removable armrest, press a button by the armrest, and lift it off. To attach an armrest, line up the button and slip into place until the button clicks.

G   To remove the footrest, locate the lever, pull back, and pull the footrest off the knobs (Fig. 11-18). To reattach the footrest, line up the knobs and slide footrest into place until it clicks.

G   To lift or lower the footrest, support the leg or foot, squeeze lever, and pull up or push down.

G   When moving down a ramp, go down backward, with the resident facing the top of the ramp, also going down backward. You could lose control of the wheelchair if it moves down first.

G   When using an elevator, turn the chair around before entering it, so the resident faces forward in the elevator.

G   When a resident is in a wheelchair or any chair, reposition him at least every hour. This helps reduce pressure, increase circulation, and promote comfort.

G   When positioning a resident in a wheelchair, make sure his hips are at the very back of the chair. To do this, lock the wheelchair wheels. Stand in front of the wheelchair and ask the resident to grasp the armrests while his feet are flat on the floor. Brace one or both knees against the resident's knee(s). On the count of three, ask the resident to push with his feet into the floor and move himself toward the back of the chair. Gently assist as needed. Help him get into a comfortable position.

G   A geriatric chair, or geri-chair, is a special chair that reclines. A tray table can be attached to it. This chair helps residents who are mostly bedbound avoid staying in bed all day. The chair helps keep residents in proper alignment, which reduces pressure on the skin.

G   Lock the wheels on both sides before moving a resident into or out of a geri-chair. The tray tables on geri-chairs can be heavy. Use caution when handling the tray table. Do not catch your fingers or the resident's fingers in the tray when attaching or releasing it. When the tray table is attached, geri-chairs may be considered restraints. See Chapter 7 for more information about restraints.

Transferring a resident from a bed to a chair or wheelchair

Equipment: wheelchair, transfer belt, nonskid footwear

1. Identify yourself by name. Identify the resident. Greet the resident by name.

2. Wash your hands.

3. Explain procedure to the resident. Speak clearly, slowly, and directly. Maintain face-to-face contact whenever possible.

4. Provide for the resident's privacy with a curtain, screen, or door.

5. Place the wheelchair at the head of the bed, facing the foot of the bed, or at the foot of bed, facing the head of bed. The arm of the wheelchair should be almost touching the bed. It should be placed on the resident's stronger, or unaffected, side.

6. Remove or fold up both wheelchair footrests close to the bed.

7. Lock the wheelchair wheels.

8. Raise the head of the bed. Adjust the bed level to its lowest position. Lock bed wheels.

9. Assist the resident into a sitting position with his feet flat on the floor. Adjust the bed height if needed. Let the resident sit for a few minutes to adjust to the change in position.

10. Put nonskid footwear on the resident and fasten it securely.

11. Stand in front of and face the resident. Stand with your feet about shoulder-width apart. Bend your knees. Keep your back straight.

12. Place the transfer belt around the resident's waist over his clothing (not on bare skin). Tighten the buckle until it is snug. Leave enough room to insert flat fingers/hand comfortably under the belt. Check to make sure that skin or skin folds (for example, breasts) are not caught under the belt. Grasp the belt securely on both sides, with hands in an upward position.

13. Provide instructions one at a time to allow the resident to help with the transfer. Instructions may include: "When you start to stand, push with your hands against the bed." "Once standing, if you're able, you can take small steps in the direction of the chair." "Once standing, reach for the chair with your stronger hand."

14. With your legs, brace (support) the resident's lower legs to prevent slipping. This can be done by placing one or both of your knees against the resident's knees. Or you can stand toe to toe with the resident. Bend your knees and keep your back straight.

15. Count to three to alert the resident. On the count of three, with hands still grasping the transfer belt on both sides and moving upward, slowly help the resident to stand.

16. Tell the resident to take small steps in the direction of the chair while turning his back toward it. If more help is needed, help the resident pivot (turn) to stand in front of wheelchair with the back of the resident's legs against the wheelchair (Fig. 11-19).

17. Ask the resident to put his hands on the wheelchair armrests if he is able. When the chair is touching the back of the resident's legs, help him lower himself into the chair.

18. Reposition the resident so that his hips touch the back of the wheelchair seat. See previous guidelines on how to do this.

19. Attach footrests. Place the resident's feet on the footrests. Check that the resident is in proper alignment. Gently remove the transfer belt.

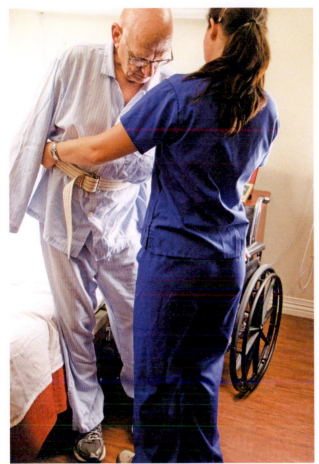

Fig. 11-19. *Help the resident pivot to the front of the wheelchair. Pivoting is safer than twisting.*

20. Make the resident comfortable.

21. Leave the bed in its lowest position. Remove privacy measures.

22. Leave call light within the resident's reach.

23. Wash your hands.

24. Be courteous and respectful at all times.

25. Report any changes in the resident to the nurse. Document procedure using facility guidelines.

To transfer back to bed from a wheelchair, follow these steps:

1. Perform steps 1 through 7 above.

2. Adjust the bed level to a low position. The height of the bed should be equal to or slightly lower than the chair. Lock bed wheels.

3. Perform steps 11 through 15 above.

   The resident should be allowed to stand until he feels stable enough to move toward the bed. Do not let go of the transfer belt.

4. Help resident pivot to the bed with the back of the resident's legs against the bed. When he feels the bed, he should slowly sit down on the side of the bed.

5. Gently remove the transfer belt. Remove footwear. Make the resident comfortable.

6. Return the bed to its lowest position. Remove privacy measures.

7. Leave call light within the resident's reach.

8. Wash your hands.

9. Be courteous and respectful at all times.

10. Report any changes in the resident to the nurse. Document procedure using facility guidelines.

Stretchers

A stretcher, also called a *gurney*, is a medical device used to move injured or ill persons from one place to another. Stretchers may be used for residents who cannot walk or sit in a wheelchair but need to be transported somewhere. A resident who is severely ill and must be transported by ambulance will need to be moved on a stretcher.

Stretchers have safety belts that are used when the resident is on the stretcher. The nursing assistant must secure these safety belts after the resident is on the stretcher, before moving him. The stretcher's brakes should be locked when it is not in motion.

While on a stretcher, the resident should be kept covered for warmth and for privacy. The NA should not leave a resident alone on a stretcher.

If the NA is accompanying a resident who is being transported, she should make sure to hand off care to the nurse at the new facility.

A draw sheet or other assist device is used to transfer a resident to a stretcher. The procedure below shows how to transfer a resident to a stretcher from a bed using four staff members. At least three people are necessary to safely transfer a resident to a stretcher.

Transferring a resident from a bed to a stretcher with assistance

Equipment: stretcher, bath blanket, draw sheet or other assist device

1. Identify yourself by name. Identify the resident. Greet the resident by name.

2. Wash your hands.

3. Explain procedure to the resident. Speak clearly, slowly, and directly. Maintain face-to-face contact whenever possible.

4. Provide for the resident's privacy with a curtain, screen, or door.

5. Lower the head of the bed to make it flat. Lock bed wheels.

6. Fold linens to foot of the bed. Cover the resident with the bath blanket. Do not expose the resident during the procedure.

7. Move the resident to the side of the bed. Have your coworkers help you do this. Refer to the procedure *Moving a resident to the side of the bed* earlier in this chapter.

8. Place the stretcher solidly against the bed. Lock stretcher wheels. Bed height should be equal to or slightly above the height of the stretcher. Move the stretcher safety belts out of the way.

9. Two workers should be on one side of the bed opposite the stretcher. Two more workers should be on the other side of the stretcher.

10. Each worker should roll up the sides of the draw sheet or other assist device and prepare to move the resident (Fig. 11-20). Protect the resident's arms and legs during the transfer.

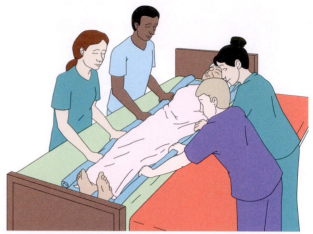

Fig. 11-20. *With two workers on each side, roll up the sides of the assist device and prepare to move the resident.*

11. On the count of three, the workers should lift and move the resident to the stretcher. All should move at once (Fig. 11-21). Make sure the resident is centered on the stretcher.

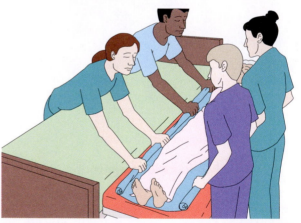

Fig. 11-21. *On the count of three, all workers should lift and move at once.*

12. Raise the head of the stretcher or place a pillow under the resident's head. Make sure the resident is still covered with the bath blanket.

13. Secure the safety belts across the resident. Raise the stretcher's bed rails.

14. Unlock the stretcher's wheels. Take the resident to the proper site, staying with him until

another team member takes over responsibility of the resident.

15. Wash your hands.

16. Be courteous and respectful at all times.

17. Report any changes in the resident to the nurse. Document procedure using facility guidelines.

To return the resident to bed, the bed height should be equal to or slightly below the stretcher.

Mechanical Lifts

Mechanical lifts are types of equipment that are used to lift and move residents. They help prevent injury to staff and residents. There are many different types of mechanical lifts (Fig. 11-22), as well as other names for these lifts, such as *hydraulic, power, standing, heavy duty,* and *pool and bath lifts.*

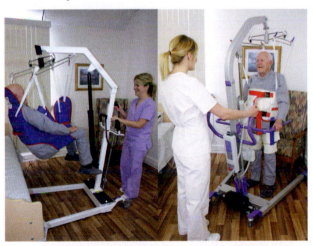

Fig. 11-22. *There are many different types of lifts for transferring both completely dependent residents and residents who can bear some weight.* (PHOTOS COURTESY OF VANCARE INC., VANCARE. COM, 800-694-4525)

Using these lifts requires special training. Nursing assistants should not use equipment they have not been trained to use, as this could cause injury. Once an NA knows how to use a mechanical lift, she can explain how it works to residents to ease any concerns they may have.

This is a basic procedure for transferring a resident using a mechanical lift. Other lifts may have different procedures. NAs should always ask for help if there is anything they do not understand about lift equipment. A lift should not be used if it is broken or does not appear to be functioning properly. Many facilities require two or more people to perform the following procedure. NAs should follow their facility's policy.

Transferring a resident using a mechanical lift with assistance

Equipment: wheelchair or chair, mechanical or hydraulic lift, soft cloth

Before performing this procedure, check to make sure the resident is within the lift's allowable weight limit.

1. Identify yourself by name. Identify the resident. Greet the resident by name.

2. Wash your hands.

3. Explain procedure to the resident. Speak clearly, slowly, and directly. Maintain face-to-face contact whenever possible.

4. Provide for the resident's privacy with a curtain, screen, or door.

5. Adjust the bed to a safe level, usually waist high. Lock the bed wheels.

6. Position the wheelchair or chair next to the bed. Remove the wheelchair footrests close to the bed. Lock the wheelchair wheels.

7. Help the resident turn toward you. Pad the sling where the resident's neck will rest with a soft cloth for comfort. A sheet may be used over the sling to protect it from soiling. Position the sling on the empty side of the bed, on the area where the resident will lie on his back. Fanfold if possible. Make the bottom of the sling even with the resident's knees (some slings stop at the bottom of the buttocks). Help the resident roll onto his back. Spread out the fanfolded edge of the sling.

8. Roll the mechanical lift to the bedside. Make sure the base is opened to its widest point.

Push the base of the lift under the bed. Lock the lift wheels.

9. Place the overhead bar directly over the resident. Be careful so that the bar does not hit anyone.

10. With the resident lying on his back, attach one set of straps to each side of the sling. Attach one set of straps to the overhead bar (Fig. 11-23). Have a coworker support the resident at the head, shoulders, and knees while being lifted. The resident's arms should be folded across his chest. If the device has S hooks, they should face away from resident. Make sure all straps are connected properly and are smooth and straight.

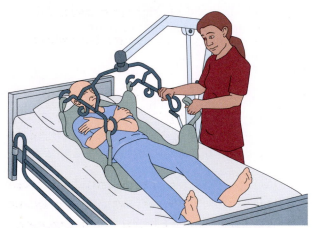

Fig. 11-23. *With the resident's arms folded across his chest, attach the straps to the sling.*

11. Following the manufacturer's instructions, raise the resident two inches above the bed. Pause a moment for the resident to gain balance. Unlock the lift wheels.

12. Have your coworker support and guide the resident's body (Fig. 11-24). You can then move the lift so that the resident is positioned over the chair or wheelchair.

13. Slowly lower the resident into the chair or wheelchair. Push down gently on the resident's knees to help the resident into a sitting, rather than a reclining, position.

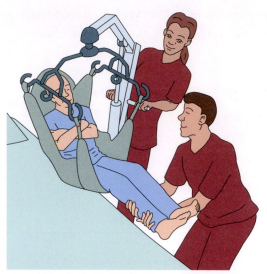

Fig. 11-24. *Make sure that one person supports and guides the resident's body to help prevent injury.*

14. Undo the straps from the overhead bar. Leave the sling in place or remove it, following the nurse's instructions.

15. Be sure the resident is seated comfortably and correctly in the chair or wheelchair. Put nonskid footwear on the resident and fasten it securely. Attach the footrests and place the resident's feet on the footrests. Cover the resident with a lap cover or robe if requested.

16. Return bed to its lowest position. Remove privacy measures.

17. Leave call light within the resident's reach.

18. Wash your hands.

19. Be courteous and respectful at all times.

20. Report any changes in the resident to the nurse. Document procedure using facility guidelines.

A stand-up, or standing lift, is used when a person can bear some weight on his legs, but has poor leg strength and/or balance. The resident must be able to stand and have some arm strength in order to use this lift. There are different types of stand-up lifts, including manual and battery-powered. The stand-up lift consists of both user and operator support bars (the user support bars may consist of two vertical bars or one crossbar), padded swivel swing-out seats (and/or straps, vest, or belt for some models), knee pads, a platform base with foot plate, and four small wheels with locking brakes.

When using a stand-up lift, the nursing assistant must be sure that the brakes are locked before beginning the transfer. The NA should have the resident begin in a sitting position and place his feet firmly on the foot plate of the platform, with his knees pressing against the knee pads. The resident should grasp the support bar(s) and gently pull himself to a standing position, using his own strength. Then the NA can lower both sides of the padded swing-out seat into position. The NA should adjust straps, vest, or belt if these are used. The resident should slowly lower himself onto the seat while holding the support bars and pressing his knees against the knee pads. The NA should unlock the wheel brakes and use the operator bars to transfer the resident to the location desired and then perform these steps in reverse order to release the resident from the lift.

Toilet Transfers

The toilet is better than a bedpan or a urinal for eliminating urine. The bladder empties more completely when a person is able to use a toilet or portable commode. This is due to the person's position over the toilet. In order to use the toilet, residents must be able to bear some weight on their legs.

Falls can occur on the way to the bathroom, while using the toilet, or on the way back to the bed or chair. Nursing assistants should not leave residents alone if residents require assistance. NAs should offer trips to the bathroom often and respond to call lights immediately. Chapter 15 contains more information on bedpans and urinals.

Equipment: 2 pairs of gloves, toilet paper or disposable wipes, transfer belt, wheelchair

1. Identify yourself by name. Identify the resident. Greet the resident by name.

2. Wash your hands.

3. Explain procedure to the resident. Speak clearly, slowly, and directly. Maintain face-to-face contact whenever possible.

4. Provide for the resident's privacy by closing the door.

5. Position the wheelchair at a right angle to the toilet to face the hand bar/wall rail. Place the wheelchair on the resident's stronger side.

6. Remove wheelchair footrests. Lock wheels.

7. Put on gloves.

8. Apply a transfer belt around the resident's waist over clothing (not on bare skin). Grasp the belt securely on both sides, with hands in an upward position.

9. Ask the resident to push against the armrests of the wheelchair and stand, reaching for and grasping the hand bar with her stronger arm (Fig. 11-25). Move the wheelchair out of the way.

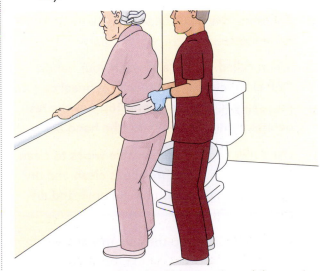

Fig. 11-25. The resident should be standing while grasping the hand bar for support.

10. Ask the resident to pivot her foot and back up until she can feel the front of the toilet with the back of her legs (Fig. 11-26).

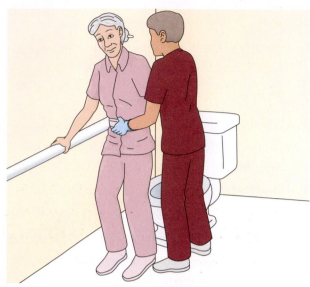

Fig. 11-26. Have the resident pivot and feel the toilet with the back of her legs. Assist as needed.

11. Help the resident to pull down her pants and underwear. You may need to keep one hand on the transfer belt while helping to remove clothing.

12. Help the resident to slowly sit down on the toilet. Give the resident privacy unless she is not supposed to be left alone. Ask her to pull the emergency cord if she needs help. Remove and discard gloves properly. Wash your hands. Leave the bathroom and close the door. Stay near the door until the resident is finished.

13. When called, return and wash your hands. Don clean gloves. Assist with perineal care as necessary (Chapters 12 and 16). Ask the resident to stand and reach for the hand bar.

14. Use toilet paper or disposable wipes to clean the resident. Make sure she is clean and dry before pulling up clothing. Remove and discard gloves properly.

15. Help the resident to the sink to wash her hands.

16. Wash your hands.

17. Help the resident back into the wheelchair. Be sure the resident is seated comfortably and correctly in the wheelchair. Remove the transfer belt. Replace the footrests.

18. Help the resident to leave the bathroom.

19. Leave call light within the resident's reach.

20. Wash your hands again.

21. Be courteous and respectful at all times.

22. Report any changes in the resident to the nurse. Document procedure using facility guidelines.

Vehicle Transfers

When a resident is discharged from a facility, a nursing assistant may need to help him into a vehicle. The front seat of the vehicle is wider and is usually easier to get into. The NA's responsibility does not end until the resident is safely inside the vehicle and the door is closed.

Transferring a resident into a vehicle

Equipment: wheelchair, cart with personal belongings, coworker

1. Identify yourself by name. Identify the resident. Greet the resident by name.

2. Wash your hands.

3. Explain procedure to the resident. Speak clearly, slowly, and directly. Maintain face-to-face contact whenever possible.

4. Place the wheelchair close to the vehicle at a 45-degree angle. Open the door on the resident's stronger side if possible.

5. Lock the wheelchair wheels.

6. Ask the resident to push against the arm rests of the wheelchair to stand, grasp the vehicle or dashboard, and pivot his foot so the side of the seat touches the back of his legs.

7. The resident should then sit in the seat and lift one leg, and then the other, into the vehicle (Fig. 11-27). Assist as needed.

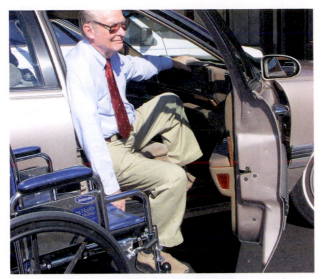

Fig. 11-27. *After the resident sits in the vehicle seat, he should put his legs in one at a time.*

8. Position the resident comfortably in the vehicle. Help fasten the seat belt.

9. Have a coworker place the resident's belongings carefully in the vehicle. Carefully shut the door(s).

10. Return the wheelchair and cart to the appropriate place for cleaning.

11. Wash your hands.

12. Document procedure using facility guidelines.

5. Discuss ambulation

Ambulation means the act of moving or walking, with or without an assistive device. A resident who is ambulatory can get out of bed and move or walk. Residents should ambulate to maintain independence and prevent problems. Regular ambulation and exercise are very important and help to improve the following:

- Quality and health of the skin

- Circulation

- Strength

- Sleep and relaxation

- Appetite

- Elimination

- Oxygen level

If a resident is just starting to ambulate, she should only walk for short distances. Over time, the distance may be increased. Residents may require a transfer belt and/or more than one staff member to ambulate safely. The NA should follow the nurse's instructions and the care plan.

Assisting a resident to ambulate

Equipment: transfer belt, nonskid footwear

1. Identify yourself by name. Identify the resident. Greet the resident by name.

2. Wash your hands.

3. Explain procedure to the resident. Speak clearly, slowly, and directly. Maintain face-to-face contact whenever possible.

4. Provide for the resident's privacy with a curtain, screen, or door.

5. Adjust the bed to its lowest position. Lock bed wheels. Assist the resident into a sitting position with his feet flat on the floor. Adjust the bed height if needed.

6. Before ambulating, put nonskid footwear on the resident and fasten it securely.

7. Stand in front of and face the resident. Stand with feet about shoulder-width apart.

8. Place the transfer belt around the resident's waist over his clothing (not on bare skin). Check to make sure that skin or skin folds (for example, breasts) are not caught under the belt. Grasp the belt securely on both sides, with hands in an upward position.

9. If the resident is unable to stand without help, brace (support) the resident's lower

extremities. This can be done by placing one or both of your knees against the resident's knees (Figs. 11-28 and 11-29). Or you can stand toe to toe with the resident. Bend your knees and keep your back straight.

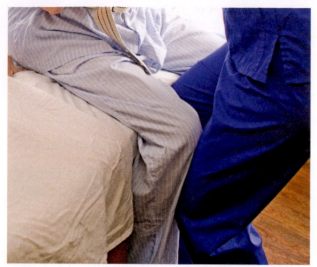

Fig. 11-28. *If resident has a weak knee, brace it against your knee.*

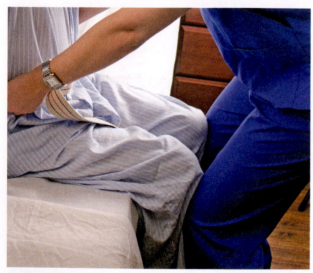

Fig. 11-29. *You can also use both knees to brace the resident's knees.*

10. Hold the resident close to your center of gravity. Provide instructions to allow the resident to help with standing. Tell the resident to lean forward, push down on the bed with his hands, and stand on the count of three. On three, with your hands still grasping the transfer belt on both sides and moving upward, slowly help the resident to stand.

11. Walk slightly behind and to one side of the resident for the full ordered distance, while holding onto the transfer belt (Fig. 11-30). If the resident has a weaker side, stand on the weaker side. Use the hand that is not holding the belt to offer support on the weak side. Ask the resident to look forward, not down at the floor, during ambulation. If the resident becomes dizzy or faint, help him to a nearby seat and call the nurse for help.

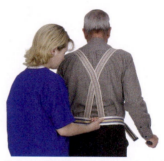

Fig. 11-30. *Walk behind and to one side, while holding onto the transfer belt, when assisting with ambulation.*

12. After ambulation, remove the transfer belt. Make the resident comfortable. Remove footwear. Check that the resident is in proper alignment.

13. Leave bed in its lowest position. Remove privacy measures.

14. Leave call light within the resident's reach.

15. Wash your hands.

16. Be courteous and respectful at all times.

17. Report any changes in the resident to the nurse. Document procedure using facility guidelines.

When helping a resident who has a visual impairment to walk, the NA should let the person walk beside and slightly behind her, as he rests a hand on the NA's elbow. The NA should walk at the resident's normal pace. She should let the resident know when they are about to turn a corner or when a step is approaching. The NA should state whether they will be stepping up or down.

Chapter 25 contains more information on assisting with ambulation for a resident using a walker, cane, or crutches.

Chapter Review

1. How does proper body alignment benefit the human body (LO 2)?

2. Why should a nursing assistant face what she is lifting (LO 2)?

3. In what position should a nursing assistant be before lifting an object (LO 2)?

4. Should objects be lifted by using muscles in the legs or the back (LO 2)?

5. Explain why objects should be kept close to the body when carrying them (LO 2).

6. What is the benefit of using a draw sheet or other assist device when repositioning (LO 3)?

7. For a resident with one weak side and one strong side, which side should move first and why (LO 4)?

8. When moving a resident down a ramp in a wheelchair, in which direction should the resident be facing (LO 4)?

9. What must a resident be able to do in order to use the toilet (LO 4)?

Multiple Choice

10. Which of the following is a description of the supine position (LO 3)?
    (A) Resident is in a semi-sitting position (45 to 60 degrees) with his head and shoulders elevated.
    (B) Resident is lying on either side.
    (C) Resident is lying on his abdomen.
    (D) Resident is lying flat on his back.

11. Which of the following is a description of the lateral position (LO 3)?
    (A) Resident is in a semi-sitting position (45 to 60 degrees) with his head and shoulders elevated.
    (B) Resident is lying on either side.
    (C) Resident is lying on his abdomen.
    (D) Resident is lying flat on his back.

12. Which of the following is a description of the Fowler's position (LO 3)?
    (A) Resident is in a semi-sitting position (45 to 60 degrees) with his head and shoulders elevated.
    (B) Resident is lying on either side.
    (C) Resident is lying on his abdomen.
    (D) Resident is lying flat on his back.

13. Which of the following is a safety device used to help transfer residents who are weak, unsteady, or uncoordinated (LO 4)?
    (A) Compression sleeve
    (B) Transfer belt
    (C) Traction pulley
    (D) Back brace

14. Where should a nursing assistant place a transfer belt before helping a resident to ambulate (LO 5)?
    (A) Underneath the resident's shirt, above his waist
    (B) Around the resident's weaker leg, under his clothing
    (C) Around the resident's waist, over his clothing
    (D) Underneath the resident's armpits, over his shirt

12
Personal Care

1. Define important words in this chapter

additive: a substance added to another substance, changing its effect.

axilla: underarm or armpit area.

bridge: a type of dental appliance that replaces missing or pulled teeth.

dandruff: excessive shedding of dead skin cells from the scalp.

dentures: artificial teeth.

edema: swelling in body tissues caused by excess fluid.

edentulous: lacking teeth; toothless.

gingivitis: an inflammation of the gums.

grooming: practices to care for oneself, such as caring for fingernails and hair.

halitosis: bad breath.

hygiene: practices to keep the body clean.

partial bath: bath that includes washing the face, underarms, hands, and perineal area.

pediculosis: an infestation of lice.

plaque: a substance that accumulates on the teeth from food and bacteria.

tartar: hard deposits on the teeth that are filled with bacteria; may cause gum disease and loose teeth if not removed.

2. Explain personal care of residents

Proper hygiene is important to health. **Hygiene** is the term used to describe practices to keep the body clean. Grooming helps keep a person clean and healthy as well. **Grooming** includes practices like fingernail, foot, and hair care. Hygiene and grooming, along with other personal care tasks, are called *activities of daily living (ADLs)*. ADLs include grooming, dressing, bathing, eating and drinking, transferring, and elimination.

Nursing assistants help residents every day with their ADLs.

The type of daily care provided for residents depends on the shifts nursing assistants work. Care varies according to what time of day it is. Bathing usually happens in the morning; however, it can be done in the evening, depending on residents' preferences and facility policy. Care done in the mornings is referred to as *a.m. care* and care done in the evenings is *p.m. care*. Assisting with a.m. care includes the following:

• Taking the resident to the bathroom, offering a bedpan or urinal, or changing an incontinence brief; helping with perineal care if needed; and assisting with handwashing

• Helping with mouth care or denture care before or after breakfast, as the resident prefers and requires

• Assisting with washing face and hands in bed, in the shower room, or in the bathroom

• Changing the resident's gown, pajamas, or clothing

• Providing breakfast and beverages

• Assisting with bathing

• Helping the resident with shaving, hair care, hand and fingernail care, foot care, and cosmetic application (Fig. 12-1)

• Making the bed and tidying the room

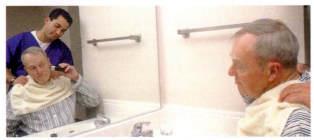

Fig. 12-1. *Assisting residents with grooming, such as shaving, is part of a.m. care.*

Assisting with p.m. care includes the following:

• Taking the resident to the bathroom, offering a bedpan or urinal, or changing an incontinence brief and assisting with handwashing

• Helping with mouth care or denture care after lunch and dinner, as the resident prefers and requires

• Providing lunch, dinner, snacks, and fluids and giving fresh drinking water

• Assisting the resident with bathing

• Giving a back massage

• Changing into a gown or pajamas

• Helping the resident with hair care

• Assisting with washing face and removing makeup as needed

• Changing linens as needed and preparing the bed for the resident's return

• Tidying the resident's room

The personal care nursing assistants provide will depend upon each resident's needs and abilities. The way in which NAs give this care is important for promoting residents' self-esteem and dignity. NAs should encourage residents to perform self-care whenever they can. This may make some tasks, such as getting dressed, take longer. NAs should be patient; residents should do as much as they are able to do, no matter how long it takes. In addition to promoting dignity and independence, doing self-care also helps keep the body functioning well.

It is very difficult for someone to give up all or part of his independence. Many people have never needed help with bathing, dressing, or eating during their adult lives. Being required to accept help with these activities can cause anger, frustration, and sadness. It may be embarrassing for residents to have someone help them with their personal care. Nursing assistants should be empathetic to the emotions residents are experiencing.

Before giving any care, the NA should explain to the resident exactly what she will be doing and answer any questions the resident has. A translator can assist if a language barrier exists. The NA should let the resident make as many choices as possible about the care she will be performing and she should always provide privacy (Fig. 12-2). This is part of providing person-centered care.

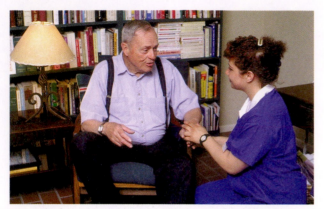

Fig. 12-2. Nursing assistants should let residents make as many decisions as possible about personal care.

Additional ways that nursing assistants can promote dignity and respect when performing personal care tasks include the following:

- Allow residents enough time to use the bathroom without rushing or interrupting them. NAs should ask if residents want to use the bathroom or bedpan before beginning personal care.

- Assist with dressing as needed, but allow as much independence as possible. Residents have the right to choose what they will wear, including jewelry; they can also choose to wear cosmetics. Personal choices should be honored. The NA should be patient while they make these decisions.

- Be patient while residents perform care tasks. NAs should always encourage them to do whatever they can for themselves.

- Be respectful if residents are using the phone or talking with visitors, and leave the room if they want privacy.

- Keep residents covered whenever possible when dressing and bathing.

- Promote residents' safety. Residents should not be left alone during bathing. They should not be rushed during care, as it may cause falls or other injuries. NAs should al-

ways ask for help with performing personal care when needed.

- Take time to talk with residents during personal care. NAs should report any changes, concerns, or problems to the nurse.

3. Describe different types of baths and list observations to make about the skin during bathing

There are four basic types of baths: a partial bath, a shower, a tub bath, and a complete bed bath. The type of bath given is determined first by the resident's needs and abilities and then by the resident's preference.

A **partial bath** includes washing the face, underarms, hands, and the perineal (genital and anal) area. It is best suited to a resident who

- Has drier, fragile, and more sensitive skin

- Should not have daily full baths

- Is unable to get up to take a shower or tub bath

- Wants a quick bath before a meal and plans on taking a shower or bath later in the day

A shower is best suited to a resident who

- Is able to stand during a shower

- Is able to safely sit in a shower chair

A tub bath can take place in a regular bathtub or in a special tub, such as a whirlpool tub. It is best suited to a resident who

- Is able to transfer into and out of a tub

- Has a doctor's order for a special bath using an **additive**—a substance added to another substance, changing its effect—to the tub water; examples of bath additives are bran, oatmeal, sodium bicarbonate, and Epsom salts

A complete bed bath is best suited to a resident who

- Is unable to get out of bed to shower or bathe and requires a full bath

The decision about which bath to give a resident rests first with the doctor or nurse, then with the resident. For example, a doctor may place an order for *no shower* until a wound has healed. Some residents are confined to bed, which prevents them from getting up for a tub bath or a shower. Some residents do not shower for personal reasons; they may simply prefer a tub bath because they have always taken baths at home. Nursing assistants should discuss residents' preferences and decisions regarding bathing with the nurse prior to giving care.

Personal care and bathing gives NAs the opportunity to carefully observe residents' skin for changes. This is especially important in the prevention of pressure injuries, a serious skin wound caused by skin breakdown. There is more information about pressure injury prevention in Chapter 18.

Some residents may discuss health problems and other issues during personal care. They may also bring up personal concerns regarding staff, family, or friends. NAs should listen to residents closely and report concerns or observations to the nurse.

Observing and Reporting: Bathing

- O/R Change in size of one or both pupils
- O/R Difference in appearance from one eye to another
- O/R Yellow or red color in whites of the eyes
- O/R Changes in vision, ability to hear, and sense of smell
- O/R Drooping on one side of the face
- O/R Weight loss
- O/R Drainage coming from any area, including eyes, ears, nipples, or genitals
- O/R Foul odors from any body area
- O/R Pale, blue-tinged (cyanotic), white, reddened, or purple areas on the skin
- O/R Dry, flaky, broken, or cracked skin

- O/R Lumps or bumps on the skin
- O/R Moles or spots on the skin, especially those that are red, white, yellow, dark brown, gray, or black
- O/R Rashes or any skin discoloration
- O/R Bruises
- O/R Blisters
- O/R Cuts, scrapes, or scratches
- O/R Open sores or wounds on any area of the body
- O/R Changes in open sore, wound, or injury, including color, size, drainage, odor, and overall depth of sore
- O/R Swelling/edema of any area, especially the knuckles, fingers, groin, abdomen, legs, ankles, or feet (**edema** is swelling in body tissues caused by excess fluid)
- O/R Poor condition of fingernails or toenails, nails in need of trimming
- O/R Dry, cracked, or broken skin in between toes or toenails
- O/R Itching or scratching
- O/R Change in emotional state
- O/R Change in level of mobility
- O/R Complaints of pain, discomfort, or stiff neck
- O/R Numbness, burning, warmth, or tingling in the extremities or other areas of the body

4. Explain safety guidelines for bathing

Safety is the highest priority when bathing residents. Many accidents happen in bathrooms or shower rooms. Before bathing residents, NAs should assess the area for any risks.

Guidelines: Safety for Bathing

- G Make sure you can perform this procedure alone. If you need help, ask for it. Do not try to bathe a resident alone if you do not believe you can manage the task safely.

G   Know any special orders for bathing. Follow the care plan.

G   Showers, tubs, and all equipment must be cleaned before and after use. You may be responsible for doing this. Follow facility policy and the nurse's instructions.

G   Make sure the floor in the shower or tub room is dry. Wipe up any spills or wet areas.

G   Place nonslip mats in regular tubs. A slippery tub may cause falls.

G   Check to see that hand rails and grab bars are secure and in proper working order. Encourage weak and unsteady residents to use safety bars to get into and out of tubs or showers.

G   Gather all needed supplies and equipment before entering the shower area. Be organized. Place needed items within easy reach.

G   Do not use bath oils, gels, or powders. These items can create slippery surfaces and can put residents at risk of falling.

G   Make sure that the water temperature is not too hot. Water temperature should be no higher than 105°F. Check the water temperature with a water thermometer or against the inside of your wrist. Then have the resident test water himself. Comfortable temperature varies for each person.

G   Put away electrical appliances when they are not in use. Do not use electrical appliances near a water source.

G   Do not leave residents alone while bathing or showering.

5. List the order in which body parts are washed during bathing

When bathing a resident, a specific order must be followed. This reduces the risk of transferring microorganisms from a dirty area to a clean area of the body. The general rule is to wash from cleanest to dirtiest. For example, the face should be washed before the buttocks. The correct order of washing parts of the body is listed below and shown in the illustration (Fig. 12-3):

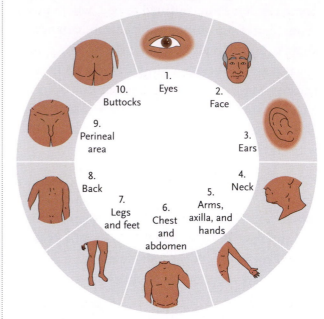

Fig. 12-3. *The numbered parts of the body show the order to follow to give a bed bath. Following this order helps prevent the transfer of microorganisms from a dirty area to a clean area of the body.*

1. Eyes

2. Face

3. Ears

4. Neck

5. Arms, **axilla** (axillae), and hands

6. Chest and abdomen

7. Legs and feet

8. Back

9. Perineal area

10. Buttocks

6. Explain how to assist with bathing

Regular bathing provides many benefits. It promotes health and hygiene. Bathing increases circulation, especially for residents who are bedbound. Bathing also gives NAs an opportunity to observe residents' skin carefully.

The face, underarms, hands, and perineal area should be bathed every day. The perineal area consists of the genitals and the anal area. Residents who have fragile, dry skin may not be bathed every day. Bathing only a couple of times per week will help prevent further dryness. In some facilities, complete baths are done on certain days of the week. NAs should follow bathing schedules and care plans carefully.

Guidelines: Bathing

G If using a tub or shower room for bathing, prepare the room and gather all equipment before moving the resident there.

G Make sure the room is warm enough before starting a bath or shower.

G Wear gloves while bathing a resident and wash hands and change gloves before performing perineal care.

G Make sure all soap residue is removed. This prevents further drying and irritation of the skin.

G During the bath, you will have an opportunity to observe residents closely. Check the skin carefully every time you bathe residents. Review the list of items to observe and report in Learning Objective 3.

Giving a complete bed bath ▶

Equipment: bath blanket, bath basin, soap, water thermometer (if available), 2–4 washcloths, 2–4 bath towels, disposable absorbent pads, clean clothes, 2 pairs of gloves, lotion, deodorant, brush or comb, orangewood stick

When bathing, move the resident's body gently and naturally. Avoid force and overextension of limbs and joints.

1. Identify yourself by name. Identify the resident. Greet the resident by name.

2. Wash your hands.

3. Explain procedure to the resident. Speak clearly, slowly, and directly. Maintain face-to-face contact whenever possible.

4. Provide for the resident's privacy with a curtain, screen, or door. Be sure the room is at a comfortable temperature and there are no drafts.

5. Adjust the bed to a safe level, usually waist high. Lock bed wheels. Lower the bed rail on the working side (if present).

6. Place a bath blanket or towel over the resident. Ask him to hold on to it as you remove or fold back the top bedding to the foot of the bed (Fig. 12-4). Remove top clothing, while keeping the resident covered with the bath blanket. Place clothing in the proper container.

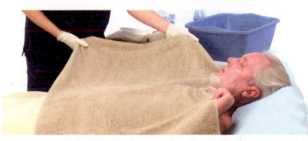

Fig. 12-4. Cover the resident with a bath blanket or towel before removing the top bedding.

7. Fill the basin with warm water. Test the water temperature with a thermometer or against the inside of your wrist. Water temperature should be no higher than 105°F. Have the resident check water temperature to see if it is comfortable. Adjust if necessary. The water will cool quickly. Change the water when it becomes too cool, soapy, or dirty.

8. Put on gloves.

9. Ask the resident to participate in washing. Help him do this when needed.

10. Uncover only one part of the body at a time. Place a towel or absorbent pad under the body part being washed.

11. Wash, rinse, and dry one part of the body at a time. Start at the head. Work down, and

complete the front first. When washing, use a clean area of the washcloth for each stroke.

Eyes, Face, Ears, Neck: With a wet washcloth (no soap), begin with the eye farther away from you. Wash inner to outer area (Fig. 12-5). Use a different area of the washcloth for each stroke. Wash the face from the middle outward. Use firm but gentle strokes. Wash the ears and behind the ears. Wash the neck. Rinse and pat dry with blotting motion.

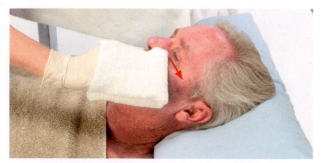

Fig. 12-5. First wash the far eye from the inner to outer area, using a different area of the washcloth for each stroke.

Arms and Axillae: Begin with the arm farther away from you. Remove the arm from under the towel. With a soapy washcloth, wash the upper arm and underarm. Use long strokes from the shoulder down to the wrist (Fig. 12-6). Rinse and pat dry. Repeat for the other arm.

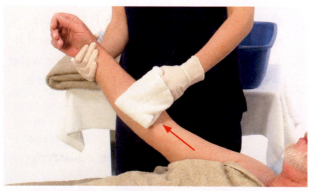

Fig. 12-6. Support the wrist while washing the shoulder, arm, underarm, and elbow.

Hands: Wash the far hand, including the fingers and fingernails. Clean under the nails with an orangewood stick. Rinse and pat dry. Make sure to dry between the fingers. Give

nail care (see procedure later in this chapter). Repeat for the other hand. Put lotion on the resident's elbows and hands.

Chest: Place the towel across the resident's chest. Pull the bath blanket down to the waist. Lift the towel only enough to wash the chest. Rinse it and pat dry. For a female resident, wash, rinse, and dry breasts and under breasts. Check the skin in this area for signs of irritation.

Abdomen: Keep the towel across the chest. Fold the bath blanket down so that it still covers the genital area. Wash the abdomen, rinse, and pat dry. Cover with the towel. Pull the bath blanket up to the resident's chin. Remove the towel.

Legs and Feet: Expose the far leg. Place a towel or absorbent pad under it. Wash the thigh. Use long, downward strokes. Rinse and pat dry. Do the same from the knee to the ankle (Fig. 12-7).

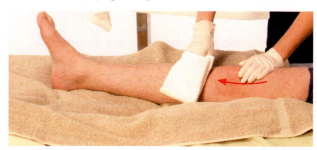

Fig. 12-7. Use long, downward strokes when washing the legs.

Place another towel or absorbent pad under the far foot. Move the basin to the towel. Place the foot into the basin. Wash the foot and between the toes (Fig. 12-8). Rinse the foot and pat dry. Make sure the area between the toes is dry. Give nail care if it has been assigned. Do not give nail care to a resident with diabetes. Do not clip a resident's toenails. Apply lotion to the foot if ordered, especially to the heels. Do not apply lotion between the toes. Remove excess lotion (if any) with a towel. Repeat steps for the other leg and foot.

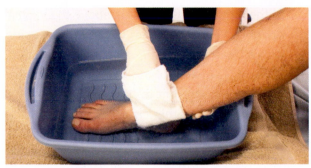

Fig. 12-8. Washing the feet includes cleaning between the toes.

Back: Help the resident move to the center of the bed. Raise the far bed rail (if used) for safety. Help the resident to turn onto his side, toward the raised side rail. Return to the working side of the bed. His back should be facing you. Fold the blanket away from the back. Place a towel lengthwise next to the back. Wash the back and neck with long, downward strokes (Fig. 12-9). Rinse and pat dry. Apply lotion if ordered.

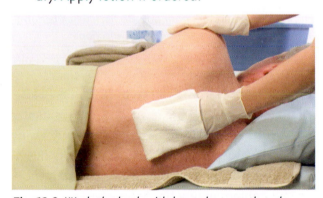

Fig. 12-9. Wash the back with long, downward strokes.

12. Place the towel or absorbent pad under the buttocks and upper thighs. Help the resident turn onto his back. If the resident is able to wash his perineal area, place a basin of clean, warm water, a washcloth, and a towel within reach. Hand items to the resident as needed. If the resident wants you to leave the room, remove and discard your gloves. Wash your hands. Leave the bed rails up (if used). Return the bed to its lowest position. Leave supplies and the call light within reach. If the resident has a urinary catheter in place, remind him not to pull on it.

13. If the resident cannot provide perineal care, you will do it. Remove and discard your gloves. Wash your hands. Put on clean gloves. Provide privacy at all times. Perform perineal care (see following procedure).

14. Cover the resident with the bath blanket. Remove the absorbent pad or towel and place it in the proper container.

15. Empty, rinse, and dry bath basin. Place basin in designated dirty supply area or return to storage, depending on facility policy.

16. Place soiled clothing and linens in proper containers, avoiding contact with your clothing.

17. Remove and discard gloves properly.

18. Wash your hands.

19. Provide deodorant. Place a towel over the pillow and brush or comb the resident's hair (see procedure later in the chapter). Put clean clothing on the resident.

20. Replace bedding, and place the bath blanket in the proper container, avoiding contact with your clothing. Make the resident comfortable.

21. Return the bed to its lowest position. Leave bed rails in the ordered position. Remove privacy measures.

22. Leave call light within the resident's reach.

23. Wash your hands.

24. Be courteous and respectful at all times.

25. Report any changes in the resident to the nurse. Document procedure using facility guidelines.

Providing perineal care

Equipment: bath blanket, bath basin, soap, water thermometer (if available), 2–4 washcloths, 2–4 bath towels, disposable absorbent pads, clean clothes, gloves

1. Identify yourself by name. Identify the resident. Greet the resident by name.

2. Wash your hands.

3. Explain procedure to the resident. Speak clearly, slowly, and directly. Maintain face-to-face contact whenever possible.

4. Provide for the resident's privacy with a curtain, screen, or door. Be sure the room is at a comfortable temperature and there are no drafts.

5. Adjust the bed to a safe level, usually waist high. Lock bed wheels. Lower the bed rail on the working side (if present).

6. Place a bath blanket or towel over the resident. Ask her to hold on to it as you remove or fold back top bedding to the foot of the bed. Remove undergarments, while keeping the resident covered with the bath blanket. Place clothing in the proper container.

7. Fill the basin with warm water (use clean water if you have already been giving a bed bath). Test the water temperature with a thermometer or against the inside of your wrist. Water temperature should be no higher than 105°F. Have the resident check the water temperature to see if it is comfortable. Adjust if necessary.

8. Put on gloves.

9. Place a towel or absorbent pad under the perineal area.

10. Work from front to back (clean to dirty).

    For a female resident: Use water and a small amount of soap, and clean from front to back (Fig. 12-10). Use single strokes. Do not wash from the back to the front, as this may cause infection. Use a clean area of washcloth or clean washcloth for each stroke.

    With your thumb and forefinger, separate the labia majora, the outside folds of perineal skin that protect the urinary meatus and the vaginal opening. The meatus is the opening

of the female urethra that is above the vaginal opening. Wipe from front to back on one side with a clean washcloth, using a single stroke. Using a clean area of the washcloth, wipe the other side from front to back, using a single stroke. Using another clean area of the washcloth, wipe down the center from front to back in one stroke. Clean the perineum (area between vagina and anus) last with a front-to-back motion. Using a clean washcloth, rinse the area thoroughly in the same order. Make sure all soap is removed.

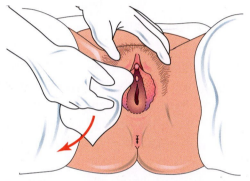

Fig. 12-10. *Always work from front to back when performing perineal care. This helps prevent infection.*

Dry the entire perineal area with a clean towel. Move from front to back, using a blotting motion with the towel. Ask the resident to turn onto her side. Assist as needed. Using a clean washcloth, wash, rinse, and dry buttocks and anal area. Clean the anal area without contaminating the perineal area.

For a male resident: If the resident is uncircumcised, pull back the foreskin first. Gently push skin towards the base of penis. Hold the penis by the shaft. Wash in a circular motion from the tip down to the base (Fig. 12-11). Use a clean area of washcloth or clean washcloth for each stroke.

Thoroughly rinse the penis and pat dry with a clean towel. If resident is uncircumcised, gently return foreskin to normal position. Then wash the scrotum and groin. The groin is the area from the pubis (area around the penis and scrotum) to the upper thighs. Rinse thoroughly and pat dry. Ask the resident to turn on his side. Using a clean washcloth, wash, rinse, and dry buttocks and anal area. Clean the anal area without contaminating the perineal area.

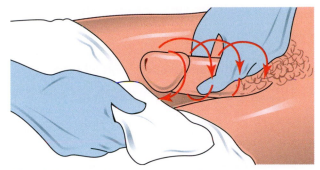

Fig. 12-11. *Wash the penis in a circular motion from the tip down to the base.*

11. Cover the resident with the bath blanket. Remove the absorbent pad or towel and place it in the proper container.

12. Empty, rinse, and dry bath basin. Place basin in designated dirty supply area or return to storage, depending on facility policy.

13. Place soiled clothing and linens in proper containers, avoiding contact with your clothing.

14. Remove and discard gloves properly.

15. Wash your hands.

16. Help resident put on clean undergarments. Replace bedding, and place the bath blanket in the proper container, avoiding contact with your clothing. Make the resident comfortable.

17. Return the bed to its lowest position. Leave bed rails in the ordered position. Remove privacy measures.

18. Leave call light within the resident's reach.

19. Wash your hands.

20. Be courteous and respectful at all times.

21. Report any changes in the resident to the nurse. Document procedure using facility guidelines.

Partial Bath

A partial bath is performed on days when a complete bed bath, tub bath, or shower is not done. It usually includes washing the face, underarms, hands, and perineal area. However, for testing purposes, nursing assistants are often asked to give a partial bath that may be different than what is listed here.

Before shampooing a resident's hair, the nursing assistant should remove any pins, clips, or bands. If the resident's hair is styled in small braids, the NA should leave the braids intact unless the resident requests otherwise.

Shampooing a resident's hair in bed

Equipment: shampoo, hair conditioner (if requested), 2 bath towels, washcloth, water thermometer, pitcher or handheld shower or sink attachment, waterproof pad, bath blanket, shampoo basin, gloves, comb and brush, hair dryer

1. Identify yourself by name. Identify the resident. Greet the resident by name.

2. Wash your hands.

3. Explain procedure to the resident. Speak clearly, slowly, and directly. Maintain face-to-face contact whenever possible.

4. Provide for the resident's privacy with a curtain, screen, or door. Be sure the room is at a comfortable temperature and there are no drafts.

5. Arrange the supplies within reach.

6. Test the water temperature with a thermometer or against the inside of your wrist. Water temperature should be no higher than 105°F. Have the resident check water temperature to see if it is comfortable. Adjust if necessary.

7. Remove all pillows and place the resident in a flat position. Adjust the bed to a safe level, usually waist high. Lock bed wheels.

8. Put on gloves.

9. Place the waterproof pad under the resident's head and shoulders. Cover the resident with the bath blanket. Fold back the top sheet and regular blankets.

10. Place the basin under the resident's head. Place one towel across the resident's shoulders.

11. Protect the resident's eyes with a dry washcloth.

12. Use a pitcher or attachment to wet the hair thoroughly. Apply a small amount of shampoo, about the size of a quarter, to your hands and rub them together.

13. Using both hands, massage the shampoo into a lather in the resident's hair. With your fingertips (not fingernails), massage the scalp in a circular motion, from front to back. Do not scratch the scalp.

14. Rinse the hair until the water runs clear. Use conditioner if the resident wants it. Rinse as directed on the container. Be sure to rinse the hair thoroughly to prevent the scalp from getting dry and itchy.

15. Wrap the resident's hair in a clean towel. Remove the basin and waterproof pad. Dry his face and neck with the washcloth used to protect his eyes.

16. Raise the head of the bed.

17. Gently rub the scalp and hair with the towel.

18. Comb or brush the resident's hair. Dry hair with a hair dryer on a low setting if allowed. Style the hair as the resident prefers.

19. Empty, rinse, and wipe the basin and pitcher. Return to proper storage.

20. Clean the comb or brush. Return hair dryer and comb or brush to proper storage.

21. Place used linen in the proper container.

22. Remove and discard gloves properly. Wash your hands.

23. Make the resident comfortable.

24. Return the bed to its lowest position. Remove privacy measures.

25. Leave call light within the resident's reach.

26. Wash your hands.

27. Be courteous and respectful at all times.

28. Report any changes in the resident to the nurse. Document procedure using facility guidelines.

Shampooing at the Sink

Some residents will have their hair shampooed at a sink. Padding the edge of the sink will help ensure that the resident's neck is comfortable. The resident's head should not be tilted at an angle. The NA should make sure that water and shampoo/conditioner do not get into the resident's eyes. The hair should be rinsed thoroughly.

When assisting a resident on a stretcher with shampooing hair, the height of the stretcher will need to be adjusted to be even with the sink. After the stretcher's wheels are locked and the safety straps are fastened, the side rail on the far side should be raised. Then the NA should follow the same guidelines as listed in the previous procedure.

There are also special types of shampoos and shampoo caps that do not require the use of water (Fig. 12-12). NAs should follow the care plan regarding the type of shampoo to use.

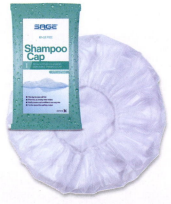

Fig. 12-12. *This is a rinse-free shampoo cap that does not require the use of running water.* (REPRINTED WITH PERMISSION OF SAGE PRODUCTS LLC, WWW.SAGEPRODUCTS.COM, 800-323-2220)

Before giving a tub bath or shower, NAs should check the room and clean it if needed (Fig. 12-13). NAs should prefill the tub with warm water and place all needed clean supplies and equipment in the room. When bathing a resident, the door should remain closed and the resident should be covered whenever possible.

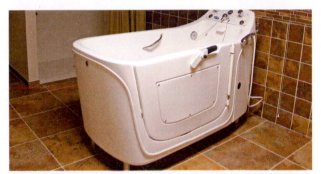

Fig. 12-13. *A common style of tub used in long-term care facilities.*

Giving a shower or tub bath

Equipment: bath blanket, soap, shampoo, water thermometer, 2–4 washcloths, 2–4 bath towels, clean clothes, nonskid footwear, 2 pairs of gloves, lotion, deodorant, hair dryer

1. Wash your hands.

2. Place equipment in the shower or tub room. Put on gloves. The shower or tub area and shower chair must be cleaned before use. Clean them if this is part of your duties. Place the bucket under the shower chair (in case the resident urinates or has a bowel movement). Turn on the heat lamp to warm the room if a heat lamp is available.

3. Remove and discard gloves properly. Wash your hands.

4. Go to the resident's room. Identify yourself by name. Identify the resident. Greet the resident by name.

5. Explain procedure to the resident. Speak clearly, slowly, and directly. Maintain face-to-face contact whenever possible.

6. Provide for the resident's privacy with a curtain, screen, or door.

7. Help the resident put on nonskid footwear. Transport the resident to the shower or tub room. Keep the resident covered during transport.

8. Wash your hands. Put on clean gloves.

9. Help the resident remove clothing and shoes. Cover with a bath blanket.

For a shower:

10. If using a shower chair, place it close to the resident and lock its wheels. Safely transfer the resident into the shower chair (Fig. 12-14).

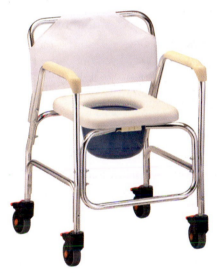

Fig. 12-14. *A shower chair is a sturdy chair designed to be placed in a bathtub or shower. It is water- and slip-resistant. A shower chair must be locked before transferring a resident into it.* (PHOTO COURTESY OF NOVA MEDICAL PRODUCTS, WWW.NOVAMEDICALPRODUCTS.COM)

11. Turn on the water. Test the water temperature with a thermometer or against the inside of your wrist. Water temperature should be no higher than 105°F. Have the resident check water temperature to see if it is comfortable. Adjust if necessary. Check the water temperature frequently throughout the shower.

12. Unlock the shower chair and move it into the shower stall. Lock its wheels.

13. Stay with the resident during the procedure.

14. Let the resident wash as much as possible on her own. Help her to wash as needed. Help her to wash her face.

15. Help resident shampoo and rinse her hair. The resident's head should not be tilted at an angle. Make sure that water and shampoo/conditioner do not get into the resident's eyes. Rinse the hair thoroughly.

16. Using soap, help to wash and rinse the entire body. Move from head to toe (clean to dirty).

17. Turn off water. Unlock shower chair wheels. Roll the resident out of the shower.

For a tub bath:

10. Residents may need help getting into the bath, depending on their level of mobility. Safely transfer the resident onto a chair or tub lift, or help the resident into the bath.

11. Fill the tub halfway with warm water. Test the water temperature with a thermometer or against the inside of your wrist. Water temperature should be no higher than 105°F. Have the resident check water temperature to see if it is comfortable. Adjust if necessary.

12. Stay with the resident during the procedure.

13. Let resident wash as much as possible on her own. Help to wash as needed. Help her to wash her face.

14. Help resident shampoo and rinse her hair.

15. Using soap, help to wash and rinse the entire body. Move from head to toe (clean to dirty).

16. Drain the tub. Cover the resident with the bath blanket while the tub drains.

17. Help the resident out of tub and onto a chair.

Remaining steps for either procedure:

18. Give the resident a towel and help her to pat dry. Remember to pat dry under the breasts, between skin folds, in the perineal area, and between toes.

19. Apply lotion and deodorant as needed.

20. Place soiled clothing and linens in proper containers.

21. Remove and discard gloves properly.

22. Wash your hands.

23. Help the resident dress and comb her hair before leaving the shower or tub room (see procedures later in this chapter). Offer a hair dryer if needed. Put on nonskid footwear. Turn off heat lamp. Return the resident to her room.

24. Make the resident comfortable.

25. Leave call light within the resident's reach.

26. Wash your hands.

27. Be courteous and respectful at all times.

28. Report any changes in the resident to the nurse. Document procedure using facility guidelines.

Some residents will have whirlpool baths. In a whirlpool bath, the water moves around the tub. The water movement helps clean the body, stimulate circulation, and promote wound healing. To take a whirlpool bath, the resident will need to be transported to the whirlpool bath site. The resident is covered, placed in a chair lift, and lowered into the whirlpool bath.

Whirlpool baths can cause a person to become dizzy or feel faint. The NA should not leave a resident alone during this type of bath. If the resident becomes dizzy, the NA should remove him from the bath.

During a whirlpool bath, the NA should help as needed and not rush the resident. Afterwards, she should help the resident get dressed and return him to his room.

7. Describe how to perform a back rub

Back rubs help relax tired, tense muscles and they help improve circulation. Back rubs are often given after bathing or prior to going to bed at night. They may also be given regularly to relieve pain or discomfort. In some cases back rubs should not be given due to certain conditions or illnesses. The NA should follow the care plan. If the resident has broken or open skin on his back, the NA must apply gloves before giving a back rub. Creams, lotions, soaps, or other products should not be used on nonintact skin.

Giving a back rub

Equipment: bath blanket or towel, lotion

1. Identify yourself by name. Identify the resident. Greet the resident by name.

2. Wash your hands.

3. Explain procedure to the resident. Speak clearly, slowly, and directly. Maintain face-to-face contact whenever possible.

4. Provide for the resident's privacy with a curtain, screen, or door.

5. Adjust the bed to a safe level, usually waist high. Lower the head of the bed. Lock bed wheels.

6. Position the resident lying on his side (lateral position) or his stomach (prone position). Many elderly residents find lying on their stomachs uncomfortable. If so, have him lie on his side. Cover the resident with a bath blanket. Fold back the bed covers. Expose the back to the top of the buttocks. Back rubs can also be given with the resident sitting up.

7. Warm lotion by putting the bottle in warm water for five minutes. Run your hands under warm water. Pour lotion on your hands. Rub them together. Always put lotion on your hands first, rather than directly on the resident's skin.

8. Place your hands on each side of upper part of the buttocks. Use the full palm of each hand. Make long, smooth upward strokes with both hands. Move along each side of the spine, up to the shoulders (Figs. 12-15

and 12-16). Circle your hands outward. Move along the outer edges of the back. At the buttocks, make another circle. Move your hands back up to the shoulders. Without taking your hands off the resident's skin, repeat this motion for three to five minutes.

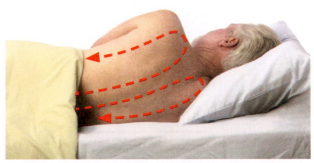

Fig. 12-15. *Move along each side of the spine, up to the shoulders.*

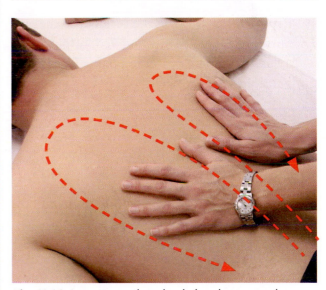

Fig. 12-16. *Long upward strokes help release muscle tension.*

9. Knead with the first two fingers and thumb of each hand. Place them at the base of the spine. Move upward together along each side of the spine. Apply gentle downward pressure with fingers and thumbs. Follow the same direction as with the long smooth strokes, circling at the shoulders and buttocks.

10. Gently massage bony areas (spine, shoulder blades, hip bones). Use circular motions with your fingertips. If any of these areas are pale, white, red, or purple, do not massage them.

11. Let the resident know when you are almost through. Finish with long, smooth strokes.

12. Dry the back if extra lotion remains on it.

13. Remove the bath blanket or towel. Help the resident get dressed. Make the resident comfortable.

14. Return the bed to its lowest position. Remove privacy measures.

15. Store supplies. Place soiled clothing and linens in proper containers.

16. Leave call light within the resident's reach.

17. Wash your hands.

18. Be courteous and respectful at all times.

19. Report any changes in the resident to the nurse, including pale, white, red, or purple areas. Document procedure using facility guidelines.

8. Explain guidelines for performing mouth care

Mouth care, or oral hygiene, is care of the mouth, teeth, and gums. This care must be provided at least twice a day, but some residents will need or want mouth care done more often. Mouth care consists of brushing the teeth, tongue, and gums, flossing teeth, caring for lips, and caring for dentures (Fig. 12-17). Lip care includes applying lip moisturizer and observing and reporting any problems with the lips.

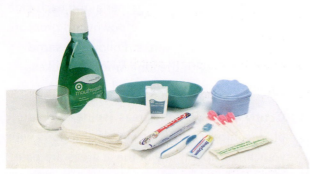

Fig. 12-17. *Some supplies needed for mouth care.*

Regular mouth care helps prevent gum disease and bad breath, or **halitosis**. A healthy mouth also promotes a healthy appetite, which can prevent unintended weight loss, a serious problem with the elderly. Mouth care may also reduce the risk of certain respiratory infections.

Plaque is a substance that accumulates on the teeth from food and bacteria. Plaque can turn into hard deposits, called **tartar**, if left on the teeth too long. Tartar is filled with bacteria and may cause gum disease and loose teeth if not removed by a dentist. **Gingivitis** is an inflammation of the gums. This can lead to periodontal disease when the areas supporting the teeth, such as the gums, become diseased. When giving mouth care, NAs should observe residents' mouths and teeth to help identify problems.

Sometimes an NA's observation signals a problem elsewhere in the body. For example, a person who has fruity breath may have diabetes (Chapter 23). Accurate observing and reporting by the NA is important. These observations may help identify and treat illnesses, as well as prevent the illnesses from getting worse.

Observing and Reporting: Mouth Care

Report any of the following to the nurse:

O/R Dry, cracked, bleeding, or chapped lips

O/R Cold sores on the lips

O/R Raised areas

O/R Swollen, irritated, red, bleeding, or whitish gums

O/R Loose, cracked, chipped, broken, or decayed teeth

O/R Yellow-filled or red sores, such as canker sores inside the mouth

O/R White spots inside the mouth

O/R Pus or drainage

O/R Coated or swollen tongue

O/R Bad breath or fruity-smelling breath

°/R Change in the resident's ability to drink, suck on a straw, or swallow

°/R Gagging or choking

°/R Resident reports of mouth pain

When giving mouth care, NAs must wear gloves. They should follow Standard Precautions. Each resident's toothbrush and toothpaste must be labeled and stored separately from other residents' mouth care items. These items should not be shared among residents.

Tip

Gum Health

Nursing assistants should take care of residents' gums by giving proper, regular mouth care. Studies have shown a link between gum disease and the risk of heart disease, stroke, diabetes, dementia, and Alzheimer's disease.

Providing mouth care

Equipment: toothbrush; toothpaste; emesis basin; gloves; clothing protector, towel, or washcloth; cup of water; lip moisturizer

1. Identify yourself by name. Identify the resident. Greet the resident by name.

2. Wash your hands.

3. Explain procedure to the resident. Speak clearly, slowly, and directly. Maintain face-to-face contact whenever possible.

4. Provide for the resident's privacy with a curtain, screen, or door.

5. If resident is in bed, adjust the bed to a safe level, usually waist high. Raise the head of the bed so the resident is in an upright sitting position (75–90 degrees). Lock bed wheels.

6. Put on gloves.

7. Place a clothing protector, towel, or washcloth across the resident's chest.

8. Wet the toothbrush. Put on a small amount of toothpaste.

9. Clean the entire mouth, including the tongue and all surfaces of the teeth and gumline, using gentle strokes. First brush inner, outer, and chewing surfaces of the upper teeth, then do the same with the lower teeth. Use short strokes. Brush back and forth. Brush the tongue.

10. Give the resident water to rinse the mouth. Place the emesis basin under the resident's chin, with the inward curve under the chin. Have the resident spit water into the basin (Fig. 12-18). Wipe his mouth and remove the protector, towel, or washcloth. Apply lip moisturizer.

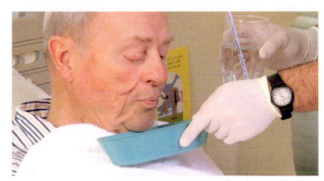

Fig. 12-18. Rinsing and spitting removes food particles and toothpaste.

11. Rinse the toothbrush and place it in the proper container. Empty, rinse, and dry emesis basin. Place the basin in the designated dirty supply area or return to storage, depending on facility policy.

12. Place used linen in the proper container.

13. Remove and discard gloves properly. Wash your hands.

14. Make the resident comfortable.

15. Return the bed to its lowest position. Remove privacy measures.

16. Leave call light within the resident's reach.

17. Wash your hands.

18. Be courteous and respectful at all times.

19. Report any changes in the resident to the nurse. Report any problems with teeth, mouth, tongue, or lips to nurse. These include odor, cracking, sores, bleeding, and any discoloration. Document procedure using facility guidelines.

Edentulous Residents

Edentulous means lacking teeth or being toothless. Giving mouth care to a resident who has no teeth is similar to caring for a resident who has teeth. Using a moistened swab, the NA will clean the outside and inside of the mouth, including the lips and top and bottom gums and gumlines, as well as the tongue. The swab should be changed as needed.

A resident who can brush his own teeth will only need a little assistance. The nursing assistant may need to do the following:

- Collect and set up supplies
- Cover the overbed table
- Raise the head of the bed
- Provide a clothing protector, towel, or washcloth for the chest
- Pour fresh water and mouthwash
- Help with cleaning the face and neck
- Remove the supplies
- Empty, clean, and store supplies

The NA should encourage the resident to do as much self-care as possible and only help the resident with what he cannot do on his own. The NA should discard gloves and wash her hands after assisting with mouth care.

Flossing teeth

Equipment: dental floss, cup of water, emesis basin, gloves, towel

1. Identify yourself by name. Identify the resident. Greet the resident by name.

2. Wash your hands.

3. Explain procedure to the resident. Speak clearly, slowly, and directly. Maintain face-to-face contact whenever possible.

4. Provide for the resident's privacy with a curtain, screen, or door.

5. If resident is in bed, adjust the bed to a safe level, usually waist high. Raise the head of the bed to have the resident in an upright sitting position. Lock bed wheels.

6. Put on gloves.

7. Wrap the ends of the floss securely around each index finger (Fig. 12-19).

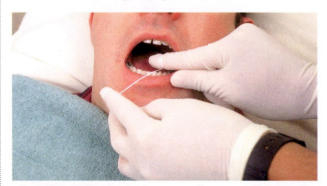

Fig. 12-19. *Before beginning, wrap floss securely around each index finger.*

8. Starting with the back teeth, place the floss between the teeth. Move it down the surface of the tooth. Use a gentle sawing motion (Fig. 12-20).

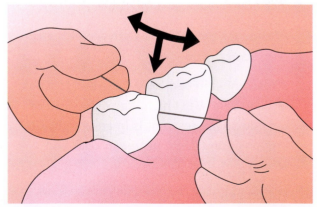

Fig. 12-20. *Floss teeth gently. Being gentle protects the gums.*

Continue to the gumline. At the gumline, curve the floss. Slip it gently into the space between the gum and tooth. Then go back up, scraping that side of the tooth (Fig. 12-21). Repeat on the side of the other tooth.

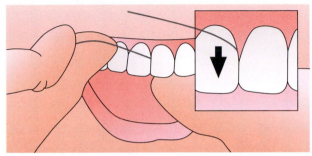

Fig. 12-21. Floss gently in the space between the gum and tooth. This removes food and prevents tooth decay.

9. After every two teeth, unwind the floss from your fingers. Move it so you are using a clean area. Floss all teeth.

10. Offer water so that the resident can rinse debris from his mouth into the basin.

11. Offer the resident a face towel when done flossing all teeth.

12. Discard the floss. Discard the water and empty the basin into the toilet. Rinse and dry the basin. Place the basin in the designated dirty supply area or return it to storage, depending on facility policy. Store supplies.

13. Place used linen in the proper container.

14. Remove and discard gloves properly. Wash your hands.

15. Make the resident comfortable.

16. Return the bed to its lowest position. Remove privacy measures.

17. Leave call light within the resident's reach.

18. Wash your hands.

19. Be courteous and respectful at all times.

20. Report any changes in the resident to the nurse. Report any problems with teeth, mouth, tongue, or lips to nurse. These

include odor, cracking, sores, bleeding, and any discoloration. Document procedure using facility guidelines.

9. Define *dentures* and explain care guidelines

Dentures are artificial teeth. There are different types of dentures. A person may have a full set of dentures, a top or bottom set of dentures, a partial plate, or a bridge. A **bridge** is a type of dental appliance that replaces missing teeth. A bridge may be permanently placed in the mouth or it may be removable for cleaning.

Dentures are very expensive and time-consuming for a specialist to make. They must be handled carefully to avoid breaking or chipping them. If a resident's dentures break, he cannot eat.

Nursing assistants must wear gloves when handling and cleaning dentures. Dentures and denture brushes should not be placed on contaminated surfaces. The type of cleaning product an NA uses will depend on the resident's preference or facility policy. Once dentures are clean, they should either be returned to the resident or stored in a denture cup labeled with the resident's name and room number. They should not be removed from the resident's room.

When in the denture cup, dentures must always be stored in denture solution or in clean, moderate/cool water (not hot water) so that they do not dry out and warp. Dentures may crack if left uncovered.

Residents' Rights

Dentures

Per CMS, if a resident's dentures are damaged or lost, and the facility is determined to be at fault, the facility must replace or repair the dentures at the facility's expense. All referrals for dental services must be made within three days of the damage or loss. The resident must be able to eat and drink while the dentures are being repaired or replaced.

Personal Care

Cleaning and storing dentures

Equipment: denture brush or toothbrush, denture cleanser or tablet, labeled denture cup with cover, 2 towels, gauze squares, gloves, cup of water, emesis basin, denture cream or adhesive (if replacing dentures in mouth)

1. Identify yourself by name. Identify the resident. Greet the resident by name.

2. Wash your hands.

3. Explain procedure to the resident. Speak clearly, slowly, and directly. Maintain face-to-face contact whenever possible. Encourage resident to assist if possible.

4. Provide for the resident's privacy with a curtain, screen, or door.

5. If the resident is in bed, adjust the bed to a safe level, usually waist high. Raise the head of the bed to have the resident in an upright sitting position. Lock bed wheels.

6. Put on gloves.

7. Line the sink or basin with a towel(s) and partially fill the sink with water. This prevents dentures from breaking if dropped. Handle dentures carefully.

8. If a resident cannot remove her dentures, remove them for her (if facility policy).

9. Remove the lower denture first. The lower denture is easier to remove because it floats on the gumline of the lower jaw. Grasp the lower denture with a gauze square (for a good grip) and remove it. The upper denture is sealed by suction. Firmly grasp the upper denture with a gauze square. Give a slight downward pull to break the suction. Turn it at an angle to take it out of the mouth.

10. Hold dentures over the sink. Rinse them in clean, moderate/cool running water before brushing them. Do not use hot water. Hot water may warp or damage dentures.

11. Apply denture cleanser to the brush.

12. Brush the dentures on all surfaces (Fig. 12-22). These include the inner, outer, and chewing surfaces of dentures, as well as the groove that will touch gum surfaces.

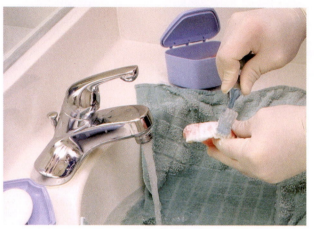

Fig. 12-22. *Brush dentures on all surfaces to properly clean them.*

13. Rinse all surfaces of dentures under clean, moderate/cool running water. Do not use hot water.

14. Offer water so that the resident can rinse her mouth. Ask the resident to spit it into the emesis basin.

15. Rinse the denture cup and lid before placing clean dentures in the cup.

16. Place dentures in the clean, labeled denture cup with solution or moderate/cool water. Dentures should be completely covered with solution. Place the lid on the cup and return the cup to where it is stored.

17. Some residents will want to wear their dentures all of the time. They will only remove them for cleaning. If replacing dentures in the resident's mouth, make sure resident is still sitting upright. If needed, apply denture cream or adhesive to the dentures. When the resident's mouth is open, place the upper denture into the mouth by turning it at an angle. Straighten it. Press it onto the upper gumline firmly and evenly (Fig. 12-23). Insert the lower denture onto the gumline of the lower jaw. Press firmly.

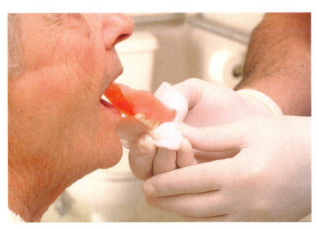

Fig. 12-23. *Press upper denture onto the upper gumline firmly and evenly.*

18. Rinse the brush. Clean, dry, and return equipment to storage. Place basin in the designated dirty supply area or return to storage, depending on facility policy. Drain the sink.

19. Place used linen in the proper container.

20. Remove and discard gloves properly. Wash your hands.

21. Make the resident comfortable.

22. Return bed to its lowest position. Remove privacy measures.

23. Leave call light within the resident's reach.

24. Wash your hands.

25. Be courteous and respectful at all times.

26. Report any changes in the resident or the appearance of dentures to the nurse. Document procedure using facility guidelines.

10. Discuss guidelines for performing mouth care for an unconscious resident

Mouth care must be done at least every two hours when a resident is unconscious. A lack of fluids, breathing through the mouth, and oxygen therapy can all cause the mouth to become dry. Crusts called *sordes* can develop on the lips, gums, and teeth. These contain microorganisms, certain types of cells, mucus, and food.

Regular mouth care keeps the mouth clean and moist and removes sordes.

Residents who are unconscious are at a high risk for aspiration. Aspiration is the inhalation of food, fluid, or foreign material into the lungs; it can cause pneumonia or death. Using as little liquid as possible during mouth care is the best way to prevent aspiration. Turning unconscious residents on their sides before beginning mouth care can also help prevent aspiration. In addition, only swabs soaked in tiny amounts of fluid should be used to clean the mouth. Chapter 14 has more information on aspiration.

Providing mouth care for an unconscious resident

Equipment: sponge swabs, tongue depressor, towel, emesis basin, gloves, cup of water, lip moisturizer, cleaning solution (check the care plan)

1. Identify yourself by name. Identify the resident. Greet the resident by name. Residents who are unconscious may be able to hear you. Speak to them as you would to any resident.

2. Wash your hands.

3. Explain procedure to the resident. Speak clearly, slowly, and directly. Maintain face-to-face contact whenever possible.

4. Provide for the resident's privacy with a curtain, screen, or door.

5. Adjust the bed to a safe level, usually waist high. Lock bed wheels.

6. Put on gloves.

7. Turn resident on his side. Place a towel under his cheek and chin. Place an emesis basin next to the cheek and chin for excess fluid.

8. Hold the mouth open with the tongue depressor. Do not use your fingers to open the mouth or keep it open. You can also use gentle pressure on the chin to open the mouth. Follow the care plan's instructions.

9. Dip the sponge swab in the cleaning solution. Squeeze excess solution to prevent aspiration. Wipe inner, outer, and chewing surfaces of the upper and lower teeth, gums, tongue, and inside surfaces of the mouth. Remove debris with the swab. Change the swab often. Repeat this until the mouth is clean.

10. Rinse with a clean swab dipped in water. Squeeze the swab first to remove excess water.

11. Remove the towel and basin. Pat lips and face dry. Apply lip moisturizer.

12. Discard disposable supplies. Empty, rinse, and dry basin. Place basin in the designated dirty supply area or return to storage, depending on facility policy.

13. Place used linen in proper container.

14. Remove and discard gloves properly. Wash your hands.

15. Make the resident comfortable.

16. Return bed to its lowest position. Remove privacy measures.

17. Leave call light within the resident's reach.

18. Wash your hands.

19. Be courteous and respectful at all times.

20. Report any changes in the resident to the nurse. Report any problems with teeth, mouth, tongue, or lips to nurse. These include odor, cracking, sores, bleeding, and any discoloration. Document procedure using facility guidelines.

When a person is unconscious, his eyes can become dry. An absent blink reflex and the air around the person can contribute to dryness. In addition, eye care must be performed to keep the area around the eyes clean. The nurse may administer eye drops periodically to help keep the eyes moist.

Guidelines: Eye Care for Unconscious Residents

G   Don gloves before bathing the eyes.

G   When cleaning the eye, use a different area of the washcloth for each stroke. Rinse it thoroughly. Use a clean washcloth for the opposite eye.

G   Wipe from the inner area of the eye to the outer area of the eye when cleaning. This helps prevent harmful deposits from being pushed into the tear duct at the inner corner of the eye.

G   Use moist compresses on the eyes as directed.

11. Explain how to assist with grooming

Grooming is a very important part of a person's activities of daily living. Every day, nursing assistants will help some residents with brushing and styling their hair, shaving, dressing, caring for their fingernails, and putting on makeup and jewelry.

Appearance has a great deal to do with the way people feel about themselves. Regular grooming can have a positive effect on self-esteem, attitude, and independence (Fig. 12-24). A well-groomed person is also likely to feel better physically because she is clean and neatly dressed.

When helping with grooming, NAs should always let residents do all they can for themselves. Performing self-care promotes independence. Each resident's personal routines and preferences should be followed. This is part of honoring person-centered care. Residents may be depressed, angry, or embarrassed about the help they need to perform these tasks. NAs should be sensitive and empathetic.

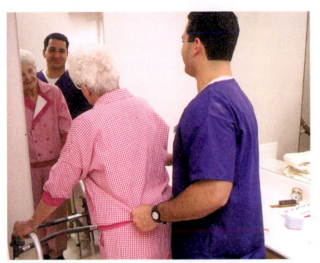

Fig. 12-24. A well-groomed appearance helps a person feel good about herself.

Shaving

Shaving is an important part of the daily grooming routine. NAs must wear gloves when shaving residents due to risk of exposure to blood. This is part of following Standard Precautions.

Guidelines: Shaving

G Some residents will not want to be shaved. Respect personal preferences for shaving.

G Wash and comb beards and mustaches every day after asking the resident how he would like it done. Never trim or shave a beard or mustache without the resident's permission.

G Always wear gloves when shaving.

G When using safety or disposable razors, first soften hair on the face with a warm wet cloth.

G Always shave in the direction of the hair growth.

G Use shaving products, such as aftershave, only with resident's permission.

G Carefully discard any disposable shaving products in the biohazard container for sharps.

G Razors must never be used on more than one resident. Do not share razors.

Types of razors are electric razors, disposable razors, and safety razors. An electric razor is the safest and easiest type of razor to use. It does not require soap or shaving cream and may help prevent nicks and cuts (Fig. 12-25). Residents who are taking anticoagulant medication (medicine that helps prevent clots from forming in the blood; sometimes referred to as *blood thinners*) may be told to only use an electric razor to avoid cuts. An electric razor should not be used near water or any water source or where oxygen is in use.

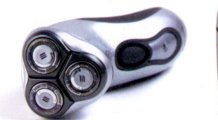
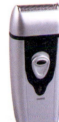

Fig. 12-25. The three-head shaver on the left and foil shaver on the right are two types of electric razors. Electric razors do not require the use of soap or shaving cream.

A safety razor requires the use of shaving cream, lotion, or soap. Safety razors are normally very sharp and have a special safety casing to help prevent cuts. The blades need to be changed periodically. When changing a blade, the NA should handle it carefully and discard the old blade in a biohazard container for sharps.

A disposable razor is used with shaving cream, lotion, or soap. This type of razor can be extremely sharp and must be used carefully. After use, the NA should discard a disposable razor in a biohazard container for sharps and should not try to recap the razor, as it can cause cuts.

Shaving a resident

Equipment: razor, basin filled halfway with warm water (if using a safety or disposable razor), washcloth, 2 towels, mirror, shaving cream or soap (if using a safety or disposable razor), gloves, aftershave lotion (if resident desires it)

1. Identify yourself by name. Identify the resident. Greet the resident by name.

2. Wash your hands.

3. Explain procedure to the resident. Speak clearly, slowly, and directly. Maintain face-to-face contact whenever possible.

4. Provide for the resident's privacy with a curtain, screen, or door.

5. If resident is in bed, adjust the bed to a safe level, usually waist high. Lock bed wheels.

6. Raise the head of the bed so the resident is sitting up. Place a towel across the resident's chest, under his chin.

7. Put on gloves.

Shaving using a safety or disposable razor:

8. Soften the beard with a warm, wet washcloth on the face for a few minutes before shaving. Lather the face with shaving cream or soap and warm water.

9. Hold skin taut. Shave in direction of the hair growth. Shave beard in short, downward, and even strokes on the face and upward strokes on the neck (Fig. 12-26). Rinse the blade often in the basin to keep it clean and wet.

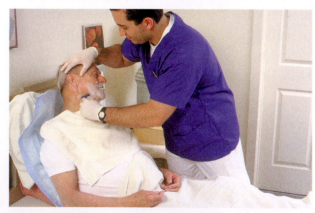

Fig. 12-26. Holding the skin taut, shave in downward strokes on the face and upward strokes on the neck.

10. When you have finished, wash and rinse the resident's face with a warm, wet washcloth. If he is able, let him use the washcloth himself. Use the towel to dry his face. Offer a mirror to the resident.

Shaving using an electric razor:

8. Use a small brush to clean the razor if necessary. Do not use an electric razor near any water source or when oxygen is in use.

9. Turn on the razor and hold skin taut. Shave with smooth, even movements. If using a foil shaver, shave beard with back-and-forth motion in the direction of the beard growth. If using a three-head shaver, shave the beard in a circular motion. Shave the chin and under the chin.

10. Offer a mirror to the resident.

Final steps:

11. Apply aftershave lotion if the resident wishes.

12. Remove the towel and place the towel and washcloth in the proper container.

13. Clean equipment and store it. For a safety razor, rinse the razor and store it. For a disposable razor, dispose of it in a biohazard container for sharps. Do not recap the razor. For an electric razor, clean the head of the razor. Remove whiskers, recap shaving head, and return the razor to its case.

14. Remove and discard gloves properly. Wash your hands.

15. Make sure that the resident and the environment are free from loose hairs. Make the resident comfortable.

16. Return bed to its lowest position. Remove privacy measures.

17. Leave call light within the resident's reach.

18. Wash your hands.

19. Be courteous and respectful at all times.

20. Report any changes in the resident to the nurse. Document procedure using facility guidelines.

When assisting a woman with shaving, the NA should not shave any facial or body hair the resident wants to keep. For example, some women do not shave their underarms or legs. The NA should not judge a resident's personal preferences for shaving. The NA should be gentle to avoid nicks and cuts and should shave in the direction of hair growth.

Nail Care

Proper grooming includes regular nail care. Fingernails can collect and harbor microorganisms. It is important to keep hands and nails clean to help prevent infection. In addition, long and ragged nails can easily scratch residents, visitors, and staff. Cleaning and caring for the nails is a part of the bathing process.

Fingernail care usually requires the use of an orangewood stick. These small sticks are made of wood and help clean under the nails. However, they must be used gently to avoid injury. Emery boards are used for filing the nails. Nail files can tear fragile skin around the nail and must be used carefully.

Some facilities do not allow nursing assistants to cut a resident's fingernails or toenails. Problems with circulation can lead to a serious infection if skin is accidentally cut while caring for the nails. For a resident who has compromised circulation due to a disease such as diabetes (Chapter 23), an infection can lead to a severe wound or even amputation. NAs should follow their facility's policies. The same nail equipment should never be used on more than one resident.

Providing fingernail care

Equipment: orangewood stick, emery board, lotion, basin, soap, washcloth, 2 towels, water thermometer, gloves

1. Identify yourself by name. Identify the resident. Greet the resident by name.

2. Wash your hands.

3. Explain procedure to the resident. Speak clearly, slowly, and directly. Maintain face-to-face contact whenever possible.

4. Provide for the resident's privacy with a curtain, screen, or door.

5. If the resident is in bed, adjust the bed to a safe level, usually waist high. Lock bed wheels.

6. Fill the basin halfway with warm water. Test the water temperature with a thermometer or against the inside of your wrist. Water temperature should be no higher than 105°F. Have the resident the check water temperature to see if it is comfortable. Adjust if necessary. Place the basin at a comfortable level for the resident.

7. Put on gloves.

8. Soak the resident's hands and nails in the basin of water. Soak all 10 fingertips for at least 5–10 minutes.

9. Remove the resident's hands from the water. Wash the hands with a soapy washcloth. Rinse. Pat hands dry with a towel, including between the fingers. Remove the hand basin.

10. Place the resident's hands on the towel. Gently clean under each fingernail with the orangewood stick (Fig. 12-27).

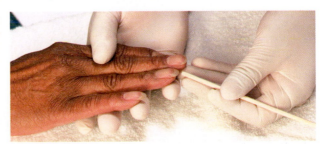

Fig. 12-27. *Be gentle when removing dirt from under the nails with an orangewood stick.*

11. Wipe the orangewood stick on the towel after cleaning under each nail. Wash the resident's hands again. With a clean, dry towel or washcloth, dry them thoroughly, especially between the fingers.

12. Shape nails with an emery board or file, moving in one direction only (not back and forth). File in a curve. Finish with nails smooth and free of rough edges.

13. Apply lotion from fingertips to wrists. Remove excess, if any, with a towel or washcloth.

14. Empty, rinse, and dry basin. Place basin in the designated dirty supply area or return to storage, depending on facility policy.

15. Place used linen in the proper container.

16. Remove and discard gloves properly. Wash your hands.

17. Make the resident comfortable.

18. Return bed to its lowest position. Remove privacy measures.

19. Leave call light within the resident's reach.

20. Wash your hands.

21. Be courteous and respectful at all times.

22. Report any changes in the resident to the nurse. Document procedure using facility guidelines.

Tip

Cosmetics

Cosmetics or makeup are items used to enhance one's appearance or clean the face, skin, hair, and nails. Both women and men use cosmetics. Nursing assistants should help apply cosmetics if needed. The application of makeup, including type and amount, should be based on residents' wishes.

Information about foot care is located in the diabetes section in Chapter 23.

Hair Care

Daily hair care affects the way residents look and feel about themselves. NAs help keep residents' hair clean and styled. It is important that residents be allowed to choose their own hairstyles. Hair ornaments should be used only as requested, and residents' hair should never be combed or brushed into childish styles. Combs and brushes and their containers may need to be labeled with the resident's name and room number.

Because hair thins as people age, pieces of hair can be pulled out of the head while combing or brushing it. The skin on an elderly person's head is fragile. NAs must handle residents' hair very gently.

NAs should never cut residents' hair, even if residents request it or if the hair is extremely matted or tangled. Many facilities have a barber, beautician, and/or professional hairstylist available to residents. NAs can help residents get ready to go to hair appointments.

Dandruff is a skin condition in which dry, white flakes appear on the scalp and hair due to shedding of dead skin from the scalp. Itching can accompany the white flakes. Dandruff may be caused by any of the following:

- Climate, especially dry, cold areas
- Stress
- Excessive sweating
- A type of fungus
- Hormonal changes
- Some types of dermatitis (inflammation of the skin)

NAs should report any white flakes they observe, as well as resident complaints of an itchy scalp. Dandruff can be controlled by using a medicated dandruff shampoo regularly.

Combing or brushing hair

Equipment: comb, brush, towel, mirror, hair care items requested by resident

Use hair care products that the resident prefers for his or her type of hair.

1. Identify yourself by name. Identify the resident. Greet the resident by name.

2. Wash your hands.

3. Explain procedure to the resident. Speak clearly, slowly, and directly. Maintain face-to-face contact whenever possible.

4. Provide for the resident's privacy with a curtain, screen, or door.

5. If resident is in bed, adjust the bed to a safe level, usually waist high. Raise the head of the bed to have the resident in an upright sitting position. Lock bed wheels.

6. Place a towel under the resident's head or around the shoulders.

7. Remove any hair pins, hair ties, or clips.

8. Remove tangles first by dividing hair into small sections. Hold the lock of hair just above the tangle so you do not pull at the scalp. Gently comb or brush through the tangle. Be careful not to break hair or cause any discomfort.

9. After tangles are removed, brush two-inch sections of hair at a time (Fig. 12-28).

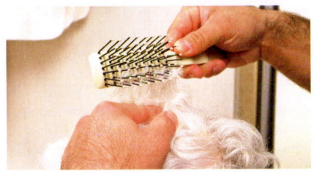

Fig. 12-28. Gently brush hair after tangles are removed.

10. Neatly style hair as the resident prefers. Avoid childish hairstyles. Each resident may prefer different styles and hair products. Offer the mirror to the resident.

11. Make the resident comfortable.

12. Return the bed to its lowest position. Remove privacy measures.

13. Return supplies to proper storage. Clean hair from comb or brush. Clean comb and brush.

14. Place used linen in proper container.

15. Leave call light within the resident's reach.

16. Wash your hands.

17. Be courteous and respectful at all times.

18. Report any changes in the resident to the nurse. Document procedure using facility guidelines.

Pediculosis is the medical term for an infestation of lice. Lice are tiny parasites that attach their eggs to the skin or the hair. Lice are very hard to see with the eye alone. Parts of the body that may have lice infestation include the head, the pubic area (area on and around the genitals), and other areas of the body, such as the underarms.

Signs and symptoms of lice include intense itching, scratching, and scratch marks or rashes on the scalp, neck, or body. Lice eggs can be seen on the hair, behind the ears, and on the neck. The eggs are small and round. They are brown before they hatch and white to light brown after hatching. Lice droppings may be visible on sheets or pillows. They look like a fine black powder.

If an NA notes any of these symptoms, she should report them to the nurse immediately. Lice can spread very quickly. The resident's roommates, spouse, partner, and family and friends may also need to be checked for lice.

Lice can be transmitted through sharing personal items, such as combs, brushes, and clothing. They can also be transmitted by sexual contact or sleeping in the same bed with someone who has lice. To help prevent the spread of lice, residents' combs, brushes, clothes, wigs, hairpieces, caps, hats, and scarves should not be shared with others. Special shampoos, creams, lotions, and sprays may be used to treat lice. Hot water must be used to wash bed linens and clothing to remove lice. Many items that cannot be washed can be put into a large plastic bag that is tightly sealed. After two weeks, the items can be removed, cleaned, and reused.

Another common skin infestation is scabies; Chapter 18 contains more information.

Dressing and Undressing

Dressing and undressing residents is an important part of daily care. When helping with dressing, the NA should know what limitations the resident has. Residents may have one side of the body that is weaker than the other side due to stroke or injury. That side is called the *weaker, affected,* or *involved* side. The NA should not refer to the weaker side as the "bad side" or talk about the "bad" leg or arm.

When dressing residents, the NA should begin with the weaker side of the body to reduce the risk of injury. The acronym *POW* can be used to help remember to put clothing on the weak side first: **P**ut **O**n **W**eak.

When removing clothing, the opposite should be done. The NA should begin with the stronger, or unaffected, side when undressing.

Guidelines: Dressing and Undressing

G   Encourage residents to be as independent as possible when dressing and undressing. Dressing and undressing can increase muscle strength, stimulate circulation, and may help promote self-esteem.

G   Additional time is needed when residents dress themselves. Do not rush them through this process.

G   If required, make sure all residents' clothing is labeled with their names.

G   Be careful when handling residents' clothing. Their clothing may be meaningful to them. Request that clothing be mended when you note rips or tears.

G   Allow residents to choose their own clothing. Encourage use of regular clothing during the day, not nightwear or pajamas.

G   Clothing should fit the resident well. Report if clothing is too tight, too loose, or too long. Clothing that is too long can get caught under a resident's feet and increases the risk of falls.

G   Always provide privacy when dressing or undressing residents. Cover residents at all times. Do not expose any more than is necessary.

G   Put clothing on the weaker, or affected, side first (Fig. 12-29).

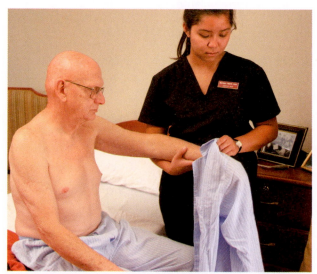

Fig. 12-29. When dressing residents, the NA should start with the affected (weaker) side.

G   Be gentle with the feet and legs when applying socks or stockings. Smooth both socks to remove wrinkles and twists. Report to the nurse if socks are too tight.

G   For a female resident, make sure bra cups fit over the breasts. Help the resident put on the bra if needed. A bra that fastens in the front may be easier for residents to manage by themselves. A bra that fastens in the back can be put around the waist, fastened, and then rotated around and moved up to the proper position. Put arms through the straps last.

G   Pants and skirts that have elastic waists are easier to get on and off. Waistbands should fit comfortably and not be twisted. Belts, if used, should not be too tight.

G   Use special dressing aids, called *assistive devices*, whenever needed. These help residents maintain independence by dressing themselves (Fig. 12-30). Chapter 25 has more information on assistive devices.

G   When undressing, start with the stronger, or unaffected, side.

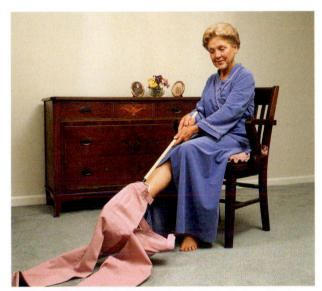

Fig. 12-30. Special dressing aids promote independence by helping residents dress themselves. (PHOTO COURTESY OF NORTH COAST MEDICAL, INC., WWW.NCMEDICAL.COM, 800-821-9319)

Dressing a resident

Equipment: bath blanket, clean clothes of resident's choice, nonskid footwear

When putting on items, move the resident's body gently and naturally. Avoid force and overextension of limbs and joints.

1.   Identify yourself by name. Identify the resident. Greet the resident by name.

2.   Wash your hands.

3.   Explain procedure to the resident. Speak clearly, slowly, and directly. Maintain face-to-face contact whenever possible.

4.   Provide for the resident's privacy with a curtain, screen, or door.

5.   Ask resident what she would like to wear. Dress her in the outfit she chooses.

6.   Place a bath blanket over the resident. Ask her to hold onto it as you remove or fold back the top bedding to the foot of the bed. Remove the gown or top. Keep the resident covered with the bath blanket. Take clothes off the stronger/unaffected side first when undressing. Then remove from the weaker side. Place the gown or top in the proper container for cleaning. Move the bath blanket down to cover the lower body.

7.   Help the resident put on the top. If the top goes over the head, slide the top over the head first. Then place the weaker arm through the sleeve before placing the garment on the stronger arm. Help the resident lean forward and smooth the top down. If the top fastens in the front, slide your hand through one sleeve and grasp the resident's hand on the weaker side, pulling it through. Help the resident lean forward and arrange the top across the back. Pull the second sleeve onto the stronger side as you did with the first one. Fasten the top.

8.   Remove the bath blanket and place it in the proper container. Help the resident to put on skirt or pants. Put the weaker leg through skirt or pants first. Then place the stronger leg through the skirt or pants. Have the resident raise her buttocks or turn the resident from side to side to pull the pants over the buttocks up to the waist. Fasten the pants or skirt if needed and make sure the clothing is comfortable.

9.   Roll one sock over the weaker foot. Make sure the heel of the sock is over the heel of the foot. Make sure there are no wrinkles or twists in the sock after it is on. Repeat for the other foot.

10. Place the bed at its lowest position. Lock bed wheels. Help the resident into a sitting

position, with legs dangling over the side of the bed.

11. Starting with the weaker foot, put on nonskid footwear. Fasten it securely and then put on the other shoe.

12. Finish with the resident dressed appropriately. Make sure the clothing is right-side out and zippers/buttons are fastened. Make sure the pants (or skirt) are not caught under the resident's shoes.

13. Make the resident comfortable. Leave the bed in its lowest position. Remove privacy measures.

14. Leave call light within the resident's reach.

15. Wash your hands.

16. Be courteous and respectful at all times.

17. Report any changes in the resident to the nurse. Document procedure using facility guidelines.

Guidelines: Dressing a Resident with an IV

G Do not pull on or catch the tubing on the clothing. Keep the IV bag above the IV site at all times.

G First remove the clothing, starting with the side without the IV. Slowly pull off clothing, sliding it over the tubing. Lift the IV bag off the hook and pull the garment over the bag (Fig. 12-31). Hang the bag back on the hook.

G Put clothing first on the side with the IV. Lift the bag off of the hook, and slide the clean clothing over the bag. Hang the bag back on the hook.

G Gently pull the clothing over the tubing and the arm. Pull the clothing over the other arm and secure it. Check to make sure that the tubing is not kinked after you are finished.

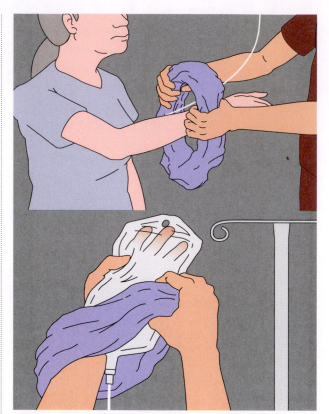

Fig. 12-31. *Pull clothing off slowly, and slide it over the tubing and then the bag.*

G If you notice the IV is not dripping, report to the nurse immediately. Ask the nurse to check the IV if you have concerns.

Chapter Review

1. Define the terms *hygiene* and *grooming* (LO 2).

2. List three ways NAs can help promote residents' dignity when performing personal care (LO 2).

3. Which serious skin wound can NAs help prevent by observing residents' skin closely (LO 3)?

4. In general, what should the water temperature be for bathing residents (LO 4)?

5. Why should residents be involved in choosing a comfortable water temperature (LO 4)?

6. Why should bath oils, gels, and powders be avoided when bathing residents (LO 4)?

7. How often should the perineal area be bathed (LO 6)?

8. What are two benefits of back rubs (LO 7)?

9. What is the best way to prevent aspiration when performing mouth care on residents who are unconscious (LO 10)?

10. Why should NAs explain what they are doing when working with residents who are unconscious (LO 10)?

11. Should NAs wear gloves when shaving residents? Why or why not (LO 11)?

12. Under what circumstances should an electric razor not be used (LO 11)?

13. When dressing and undressing residents, how should NAs refer to the weaker side (LO 11)?

Multiple Choice

14. Which of the following should be washed before the axillae (underarms) (LO 5)?
(A) Legs
(B) Face
(C) Perineal area
(D) Buttocks

15. When bathing a resident, which body part should be washed first (LO 5)?
(A) Eyes
(B) Face
(C) Neck
(D) Arms

16. At a minimum, how often should mouth care be performed (LO 8)?
(A) Once a day
(B) Two times a day
(C) Three times a day
(D) Four times a day

17. How should dentures be stored after they are cleaned if the resident does not want to wear them (LO 9)?
(A) Dentures should be stored in a denture cup filled with icy water.
(B) Dentures should be stored in a denture cup filled with hot water.
(C) Dentures should be stored in a denture cup filled with boiling water.
(D) Dentures should be stored in a denture cup filled with cool water.

18. When dressing a resident, on which side should an NA start (LO 11)?
(A) On the resident's weaker side
(B) On the resident's unaffected side
(C) On the resident's stronger side
(D) On the resident's left side

13
Vital Signs

The Invention of the Stethoscope

In 1816, René Théophile Hyacinthe Laënnec had difficulty hearing the heartbeat of a woman who was overweight. He solved the problem creatively. Using a rolled-up piece of paper, he placed his ear to one end of the paper and placed the other end over the heart. He realized he could clearly hear her heartbeat. This revelation led to the invention of the stethoscope.

"The same heart beats in every human breast."

Matthew Arnold, 1822–1888

"Once Antigonus was told his son was ill, and went to see him. At the door he met some young beauty. Going in, he sat down by the bed and took his pulse. 'The fever,' said Demetrius, 'has just left me.' 'Oh, Yes,' replied the father, 'I met it going out at the door.'"

Plutarch, 46–120 AD

1. Define important words in this chapter

apical pulse: the pulse on the left side of the chest, just below the nipple.

apnea: the absence of breathing.

BPM: the medical abbreviation for *beats per minute.*

brachial pulse: the pulse located inside the elbow, about 1 to 1½ inches above the elbow.

bradycardia: slow heart rate, under 60 beats per minute.

Celsius: the centigrade temperature scale in which the boiling point of water is 100 degrees and the freezing point of water is 0 degrees.

Cheyne-Stokes respiration: alternating periods of slow, irregular respirations and rapid, shallow respirations, possibly along with periods of apnea.

diastolic: the second measurement of blood pressure; phase when the heart relaxes or rests.

dilate: to widen.

dyspnea: difficulty breathing.

eupnea: normal respirations.

expiration: the process of exhaling air out of the lungs.

Fahrenheit: a temperature scale in which the boiling point of water is 212 degrees and the freezing point of water is 32 degrees.

hypertension: high blood pressure, regularly measuring 130/80 mm Hg or higher.

hypotension: low blood pressure, below 90/60 mm Hg.

hypothermia: severe subnormal body temperature; body temperature drops below the level required for normal functioning.

inspiration: the process of inhaling air into the lungs.

Kussmaul breathing: very deep, rapid breathing that is associated with diabetic ketoacidosis and kidney failure; also known as *air hunger.*

orthopnea: shortness of breath when lying down that is relieved by sitting up.

orthostatic hypotension: a sudden drop in blood pressure that occurs when a person stands or sits up; also called *postural hypotension*.

radial pulse: the pulse located on the inside of the wrist, where the radial artery runs just beneath the skin.

respiration: the process of inhaling air into the lungs (inspiration) and exhaling air out of the lungs (expiration).

sphygmomanometer: a device that measures blood pressure.

stethoscope: an instrument used to hear sounds in the human body, such as the heartbeat or pulse, breathing sounds, or bowel sounds.

systolic: first measurement of blood pressure; phase when the heart is at work, contracting and pushing blood out of the left ventricle.

tachycardia: rapid heart rate, over 100 beats per minute.

tachypnea: rapid respirations, over 20 breaths per minute.

thermometer: a device used for measuring the degree of heat or cold.

vital signs: measurements—body temperature, pulse, respirations, and blood pressure—that monitor the functioning of the vital organs of the body.

2. Discuss the relationship of vital signs to health and well-being

The **vital signs** consist of body temperature, pulse, respirations, and blood pressure. Vital signs are important readings that monitor the functioning of the vital organs of the body. They can indicate whether a person is healthy or ill.

Checking residents' vital signs periodically during the day is an important nursing assistant task. The first sign that a person is ill may be a change in her vital signs. When one or more of the vital signs is too high or too low, it signals a potential health problem. This is why it is so important for NAs to accurately report changes in vital signs to the nurse. The box below contains a list of ranges for adult vital signs.

Ranges for Adult Vital Signs

Temp. Site	Fahrenheit	Celsius
Mouth (oral)	97.6°–99.6°	36.4°–37.6°
Rectum (rectal)	98.6°–100.6°	37.0°–38.1°
Armpit (axillary)	96.6°–98.6°	35.9°–37.0°
Ear (tympanic)	96.6°–99.7°	35.9°–37.6°
Forehead (temporal artery)	97.2°–100.1°	36.2°–37.8°

Normal Pulse Rate: 60–100 beats per minute
Normal Respiratory Rate: 12–20 respirations per minute

Blood Pressure

Normal	Systolic 90–119 mm Hg *and* Diastolic 60–79 mm Hg
Low (hypotensive)	Below 90 mm Hg *or* Below 60 mm Hg
Elevated	Systolic 120–129 mm Hg *and* Diastolic less than 80 mm Hg
Stage 1 hypertension	Systolic 130–139 mm Hg *or* Diastolic 80–89 mm Hg
Stage 2 hypertension	Systolic 140 mm Hg or higher *or* Diastolic 90 mm Hg or higher
Hypertensive crisis	Systolic 180 mm Hg or higher *and/or* Diastolic 120 mm Hg or higher

Residents' Rights

Vital Signs

Vital sign measurements may be difficult to obtain. If an NA cannot get a measurement, he should not guess. Recording a guess is not only illegal, but it may put a resident's life in danger. Nurses and doctors make decisions about care based on the reporting done by NAs. If an NA cannot obtain a proper reading, he should tell the nurse. Reports must be accurate.

3. Identify factors that affect body temperature

Body temperature is controlled by the hypothalamus in the brain. The hypothalamus regulates body temperature by balancing the amount of heat the body makes with the amount of heat the body loses.

Body temperature averages 98.6°F (Fahrenheit) or 37°C (Celsius). A normal temperature is a sign of well-being, while a high or low temperature may indicate a problem or an illness. There are many factors that affect body temperature, including the following:

- **The person's age**: As a person ages, protective fatty tissue is lost. Elderly people are less able to prevent heat loss and may feel colder. Reduced blood circulation may also cause changes in body temperature (Fig. 13-1).

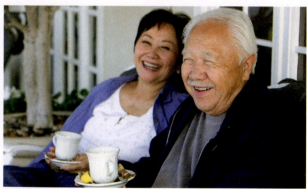

Fig. 13-1. *Elderly people usually have less fat and decreased circulation, which may make them feel colder.*

- **Amount of exercise**: Exercise helps increase body temperature due to the contraction of muscles, which produces heat.

- **The circadian rhythm**: As discussed in Chapter 10, the circadian rhythm is the 24-hour day-night cycle. Average temperature readings change during a 24-hour day. People may have lower average temperatures in the morning and higher temperatures in the late afternoon and evening.

- **Stress**: When a person is experiencing stress, certain hormones, such as adrenaline and cortisol, are released into the body. This hormonal shift may increase body temperature.

- **Illnesses**: Infections, such as meningitis and *Salmonella*, can increase body temperature. Some infections also cause dehydration, which is a serious condition in which a person does not have enough fluid in the body. When fluid levels are too low, body temperature may increase in response.

- **Environment**: The temperature inside and outside influences body temperature. The elderly may become chilled or overheated easily. Adjusting the room temperature, layering clothing, and using blankets can help.

People may have body temperatures that are below normal. Body temperature may be classified as subnormal when it measures below 97°F. Some causes of subnormal body temperature are infection, alcohol usage, diabetes, problems with the thyroid gland, or exposure to extreme cold. Severe subnormal body temperature is called **hypothermia**. With hypothermia, the body temperature drops below the level required for normal functioning. It is a dangerous condition and can lead to death if not treated. NAs must report these signs and symptoms to the nurse immediately:

- Temperature below 97°F

- Pale and/or bluish (cyanotic) skin

- Shivering

- Numbness

- Quick and shallow breathing

- Slow movements

- Changes in mental status

- Mild confusion

An increase in body temperature may indicate an infection or disease. In addition to an elevated temperature reading, signs and symptoms of a fever include headache, fatigue, muscle aches, and chills. Skin may feel warm and look flushed. Residents with darker skin tones may exhibit more subtle skin color changes.

When an NA suspects a fever, she should take a temperature reading. Fevers can develop quickly. It is possible to detect an infection early and prevent complications from occurring. Fevers should be reported to the nurse immediately.

4. List guidelines for measuring body temperature

Thermometers measure temperature in either degrees **Fahrenheit** (F) or **Celsius** (C). Fahrenheit and Celsius are two different scales that are used to measure temperature. The Fahrenheit scale is more common in the United States. In degrees Fahrenheit (F), each long line on the thermometer represents one degree and each short line represents two-tenths of a degree. In degrees Celsius (C), the long lines represent one degree and the short lines represent one-tenth of a degree (Fig. 13-2). In most other countries, the Celsius scale is used, along with the metric system of measurement.

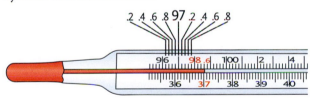

Fig. 13-2. This shows a normal temperature reading: 98.6°F and 37°C.

There are different sites on the body for measuring a temperature: the mouth (oral), the rectum (rectal), the armpit (axillary), the ear (tympanic), and the temporal artery (the artery under the skin of the forehead). A rectal temperature is considered to be the most accurate, while an axillary temperature is considered to be the least accurate.

Common types of thermometers are as follows:

- Digital

- Electronic

- Tympanic

- Temporal artery

- Mercury-free

Digital thermometers can be used to take an oral, rectal, or axillary temperature. This thermometer displays results digitally (Fig. 13-3). A digital thermometer usually takes 2 to 60 seconds to show the temperature. The thermometer will usually flash or beep when the temperature has registered. These models are battery-operated and require battery replacement periodically. A digital thermometer requires the use of a disposable plastic sheath to cover the probe, which helps prevent infection. The sheath is used once and then discarded in a facility-approved container.

Fig. 13-3. A digital thermometer.

The electronic thermometer is battery-operated and is stored in a wall unit for recharging when not in use (Fig. 13-4). It can be used to take an oral, rectal, or axillary temperature. An electronic thermometer registers the temperature digitally in 2 to 60 seconds. The thermometer flashes or makes a sound when the temperature is displayed. The probe on an electronic thermometer must have a disposable probe cover applied before use. The probe cover is used once and then discarded properly. The probe cover cannot be used on more than one resident.

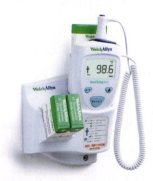

Fig. 13-4. An electronic thermometer. (PHOTO COURTESY OF WELCH ALLYN, WWW.WELCHALLYN.COM, 800-535-6663)

A tympanic thermometer is used to measure the temperature reading in the ear (Fig. 13-5). It registers the temperature in seconds. When using this thermometer, it is important for NAs to follow instructions to get as accurate a reading as possible. Earwax may cause an inaccurate reading. Ear injury is possible with this thermometer. Hearing aids may need to be removed before measuring a tympanic temperature.

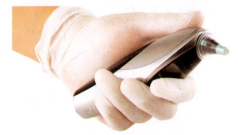

Fig. 13-5. *A tympanic thermometer.*

The temporal artery thermometer is an infrared thermometer that measures the temperature of the temporal artery, the artery under the skin of the forehead, in about three seconds (Fig. 13-6). The probe on the thermometer is moved straight across the forehead to obtain a reading. It is noninvasive, meaning it does not require the thermometer to be inserted into the ear, the mouth, under the arm, or in the rectum. Clothing does not need to be removed in order to take this temperature.

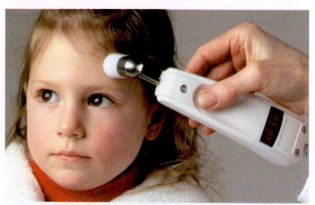

Fig. 13-6. *A temporal artery thermometer.* (PHOTO COURTESY OF EXERGEN CORPORATION, WWW.EXERGEN.COM, 800-422-3006)

The mercury-free thermometer can be used to take an oral, rectal, or axillary temperature. Thermometers are usually color-coded to differentiate between oral and rectal thermometers.

Oral thermometers are usually green or blue. Rectal thermometers are usually red (Fig. 13-7).

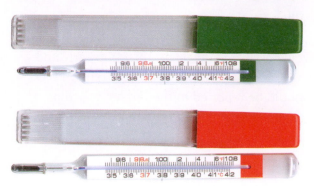

Fig. 13-7. *A mercury-free oral thermometer and a mercury-free rectal thermometer. Oral thermometers are usually green or blue; rectal thermometers are usually red.* (PHOTOS COURTESY OF RG MEDICAL DIAGNOSTICS OF WIXOM, MI, RGMD.COM)

An NA should not take an oral temperature on a person who:

- Is unconscious
- Is using oxygen
- Is confused or disoriented
- Is paralyzed from stroke
- Has facial trauma
- Is likely to have a seizure
- Has a nasogastric tube (Chapter 26)
- Is younger than five years old
- Has sores, redness, swelling, or pain in the mouth
- Has an injury to the face or neck

Any time an NA is measuring a resident's temperature, she should remain with the resident until the temperature reading has been obtained.

Measuring and recording oral temperature

Equipment: clean digital, electronic, or mercury-free thermometer, gloves, disposable sheath/cover for thermometer, tissues, pen and paper

Do not take an oral temperature if the resident has smoked, eaten or drunk fluids, chewed gum, or exercised within the last 10 to 20 minutes.

1. Identify yourself by name. Identify the resident. Greet the resident by name.

2. Wash your hands.

3. Explain procedure to the resident. Speak clearly, slowly, and directly. Maintain face-to-face contact whenever possible.

4. Provide for the resident's privacy with a curtain, screen, or door.

5. Put on gloves.

6. **Digital thermometer**: Put on the disposable sheath. Turn on the thermometer and wait until the *ready* sign appears.

   Electronic thermometer: Remove the probe from the base unit. Put on the probe cover.

   Mercury-free thermometer: Hold the thermometer by the stem. Before inserting it in the resident's mouth, shake the thermometer down to below the lowest number (at least below 96°F or 35°C). To shake the thermometer down, hold it at the end opposite the bulb with the thumb and two fingers. With a snapping motion of the wrist, shake the thermometer (Fig. 13-8). Stand away from furniture and walls while doing so.

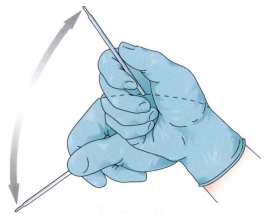

Fig. 13-8. *Shake the thermometer down to below the lowest number before inserting into a resident's mouth.*

7. **Digital thermometer**: Insert the end of the thermometer into the resident's mouth, under the tongue and to one side.

   Electronic thermometer: Insert the end of the thermometer into the resident's mouth, under the tongue and to one side.

   Mercury-free thermometer: Put on the disposable sheath if available. Gently insert the bulb end of the thermometer into the resident's mouth, under the tongue and to one side.

8. **For all thermometers**: Tell the resident to hold the thermometer in his mouth with his lips closed. Assist as necessary. The resident should breathe through his nose. Ask the resident not to bite down or talk.

   Digital thermometer: Hold in place until the thermometer blinks or beeps.

   Electronic thermometer: Hold in place until you hear a tone or see a flashing or steady light.

   Mercury-free thermometer: Hold in place for at least three minutes.

9. **Digital thermometer**: Remove the thermometer. Read the temperature on the display screen. Remember the temperature reading.

   Electronic thermometer: Read the temperature on the display screen. Remember the temperature reading. Remove the probe.

   Mercury-free thermometer: Remove the thermometer. Wipe with a tissue from stem to bulb or remove the sheath. Discard the tissue or sheath. Hold the thermometer at eye level. Rotate until the line appears, rolling the thermometer between your thumb and forefinger. Read the temperature. Remember the temperature reading.

10. **Digital thermometer**: Using a tissue, remove and discard the sheath. Clean the thermometer according to facility policy. Replace the thermometer in the case.

    Electronic thermometer: Press the eject button to discard the cover. Return the probe to the holder.

Mercury-free thermometer: Clean the thermometer according to facility policy. Rinse with clean water and dry. Return it to the case or container.

11. Remove and discard gloves properly.

12. Wash your hands.

13. Immediately record the temperature, date, time, and method used (oral).

14. Make the resident comfortable. Remove privacy measures.

15. Leave call light within the resident's reach.

16. Wash your hands.

17. Be courteous and respectful at all times.

18. Report any changes in the resident to the nurse.

Rectal temperatures may be necessary for residents who are unconscious, have missing teeth or dentures that do not fit properly, have difficulty breathing through the nose, have a seizure disorder, or have been vomiting. Rectal temperatures should not be taken when a resident has recently had rectal surgery or has a colostomy (Chapter 15). Rectal thermometers should be lubricated and inserted carefully ½ inch to 1 inch for adults. NAs must always explain what they will do before starting this procedure. The NA needs the resident's cooperation to take a rectal temperature. She should ask the resident to hold still and reassure him that the procedure will only take a few minutes. It is important to hold onto the thermometer at all times while the thermometer is in the rectum.

Measuring and recording rectal temperature

Equipment: clean digital, electronic, or mercury-free rectal thermometer, lubricant, gloves, tissue, disposable sheath/cover, pen and paper

1. Identify yourself by name. Identify the resident. Greet the resident by name.

2. Wash your hands.

3. Explain procedure to the resident. Speak clearly, slowly, and directly. Maintain face-to-face contact whenever possible. Remind resident that the procedure will take only a few minutes.

4. Provide for the resident's privacy with a curtain, screen, or door.

5. Adjust the bed to a safe level, usually waist high. Lock bed wheels.

6. Help the resident to the left-lying (Sims') position (Fig. 13-9).

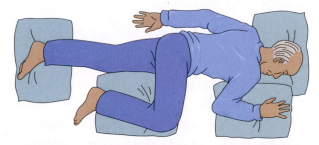

Fig. 13-9. *The resident must be in the left-lying (Sims') position.*

7. Fold back the linens to expose only the rectal area.

8. Put on gloves.

9. *Digital thermometer*: Put on the disposable sheath. Turn on the thermometer and wait until the *ready* sign appears.

   Electronic thermometer: Remove the probe from the base unit. Put on the probe cover.

   Mercury-free thermometer: Hold the thermometer by the stem. Shake the thermometer down to below the lowest number. Put on the disposable sheath.

10. Apply a small amount of lubricant to the tip of the bulb or probe cover (or apply a prelubricated cover).

11. Separate the buttocks. Gently insert the thermometer into the rectum ½ to 1 inch (Fig. 13-10). Stop if you meet resistance. Do not force the thermometer into the rectum.

12. Replace the sheet over the buttocks while holding on to the thermometer at all times.

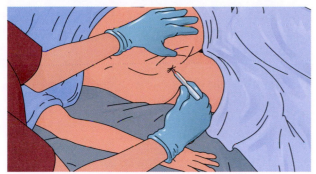

Fig. 13-10. *Gently insert a rectal thermometer ½ to 1 inch into the rectum. Do not force it into the rectum.*

13. **Digital thermometer**: Hold the thermometer in place until it blinks or beeps.

    Electronic thermometer: Hold in place until you hear a tone or see a flashing or steady light.

    Mercury-free thermometer: Hold the thermometer in place for at least three minutes.

14. Gently remove the thermometer. Wipe with tissue from stem to bulb or remove the sheath. Discard the tissue or sheath.

15. Read the thermometer at eye level as you would for an oral temperature. Remember the temperature reading.

16. **Digital thermometer**: Clean the thermometer according to facility policy. Replace the thermometer in the case.

    Electronic thermometer: Press the eject button to discard the cover. Return the probe to the holder.

    Mercury-free thermometer: Clean the thermometer according to facility policy. Rinse with clean water and dry. Return it to the case or container.

17. Remove and discard gloves properly.

18. Wash your hands.

19. Make the resident comfortable.

20. Immediately record the temperature, date, time, and method used (rectal).

21. Return the bed to its lowest position. Remove privacy measures.

22. Leave call light within the resident's reach.

23. Wash your hands.

24. Be courteous and respectful at all times.

25. Report any changes in the resident to the nurse.

Tympanic thermometers measure temperature quickly. The NA should tell the resident that she will be placing the thermometer in the ear canal. She should reassure the resident that this is painless. The short tip of the thermometer will only go into the ear ¼ to ½ inch.

Measuring and recording tympanic temperature

Equipment: tympanic thermometer, gloves, disposable sheath/cover, pen and paper

1. Identify yourself by name. Identify the resident. Greet the resident by name.

2. Wash your hands.

3. Explain procedure to the resident. Speak clearly, slowly, and directly. Maintain face-to-face contact whenever possible.

4. Provide for the resident's privacy with a curtain, screen, or door.

5. Put on gloves.

6. Put a disposable sheath over the earpiece of the thermometer.

7. Position the resident's head so that the ear is in front of you. Straighten the ear canal by gently pulling up and back on the outside edge of the ear (Fig. 13-11). Insert the covered probe into the ear canal. Press the button.

Vital Signs

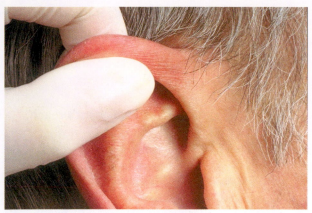

Fig. 13-11. Straighten the ear canal by gently pulling up and back on the outside edge of the ear.

8. Hold the thermometer in place until it blinks or beeps.

9. Read the temperature. Remember the temperature reading.

10. Discard the sheath. Return the thermometer to storage or to the battery charger if the thermometer is rechargeable.

11. Remove and discard gloves properly.

12. Wash your hands.

13. Immediately record the temperature, date, time, and method used (tympanic).

14. Make the resident comfortable. Remove privacy measures.

15. Leave call light within the resident's reach.

16. Wash your hands.

17. Be courteous and respectful at all times.

18. Report any changes in the resident to the nurse.

Axillary temperatures are not as accurate as temperatures taken at other sites. However, they can be safer if a resident is confused, disoriented, uncooperative, or has dementia. The axillary area must be clean and dry before measuring the temperature. The arm should be placed over the chest to hold the thermometer in place.

Measuring and recording axillary temperature

Equipment: clean digital, electronic, or mercury-free thermometer, gloves, tissues, disposable sheath/cover, pen and paper

1. Identify yourself by name. Identify the resident. Greet the resident by name.

2. Wash your hands.

3. Explain procedure to the resident. Speak clearly, slowly, and directly. Maintain face-to-face contact whenever possible.

4. Provide for the resident's privacy with a curtain, screen, or door.

5. Adjust the bed to a safe level, usually waist high. Lock bed wheels.

6. Put on gloves.

7. Remove the resident's arm from the sleeve of the gown or shirt to allow skin contact with the end of the thermometer. Wipe the axillary area with tissues before placing the thermometer.

8. **Digital thermometer**: Put on the disposable sheath. Turn on the thermometer and wait until the *ready* sign appears.

   Electronic thermometer: Remove the probe from the base unit. Put on the probe cover.

   Mercury-free thermometer: Hold the thermometer by the stem. Shake the thermometer down to below the lowest number. Put on a disposable sheath.

9. Position the thermometer (bulb end for mercury-free) in the center of the armpit. Fold the resident's arm over his chest.

10. **Digital thermometer**: Hold the thermometer in place until it blinks or beeps.

    Electronic thermometer: Hold in place until you hear a tone or see a flashing or steady light.

Mercury-free thermometer: Hold the thermometer in place, with the arm close against the side, for 8 to 10 minutes (Fig. 13-12).

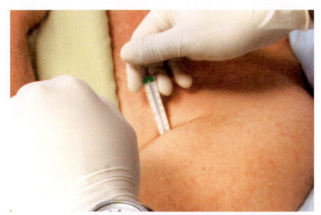

Fig. 13-12. After placing the thermometer, fold the resident's arm over his chest and hold it in place for 8 to 10 minutes.

11. *Digital thermometer*: Remove the thermometer. Read the temperature on the display screen. Remember the temperature reading.

Electronic thermometer: Read the temperature on the display screen. Remember the temperature reading. Remove the probe.

Mercury-free thermometer: Gently remove the thermometer. Wipe with a tissue from stem to bulb or remove the sheath. Discard the tissue or sheath. Read the thermometer at eye level as you would for an oral temperature. Remember the temperature reading.

12. *Digital thermometer*: Using a tissue, remove and discard the sheath. Clean the thermometer according to facility policy. Replace the thermometer in the case.

Electronic thermometer: Press the eject button to discard the cover. Return the probe to the holder.

Mercury-free thermometer: Clean the thermometer according to facility policy. Rinse with clean water and dry. Return it to the case or container.

13. Remove and discard gloves properly.

14. Wash your hands.

15. Put the resident's arm back into the sleeve of the gown. Make the resident comfortable.

16. Immediately record the temperature, date, time, and method used (axillary).

17. Return the bed to its lowest position. Remove privacy measures.

18. Leave call light within the resident's reach.

19. Wash your hands.

20. Be courteous and respectful at all times.

21. Report any changes in the resident to the nurse.

5. Explain pulse and respirations

When the left ventricle of the heart contracts, it causes a wave of blood to move through an artery. This pulse is what is felt at the wrist or other pulse site. The pulse count is the number of times the heart beats per minute. Sometimes the abbreviation **BPM** (beats per minute) is used after a pulse count. The heartbeat or pulse is measured with the fingers or by electronic devices that automatically measure the pulse. There are many areas on the body where a pulse can be felt. Common pulse sites are shown in Figure 13-13.

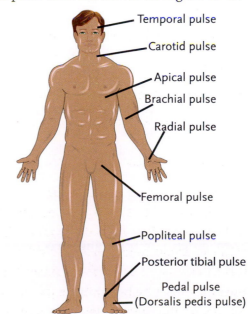

Fig. 13-13. Common pulse sites.

For adults, the normal pulse rate is 60 to 100 beats per minute. When a pulse is high, over 100 beats per minute, a person has **tachycardia**. If it is low, under 60 beats per minute, a person has **bradycardia**. The pulse rate is affected by different factors, including the following:

- **Age**: Pulse rate decreases with advanced age.

- **Sex**: Males may have a slightly lower pulse rate than females.

- **Exercise**: Pulse rate increases with exercise. However, someone who has exercised regularly for years may have a lower pulse, which can be normal for that person.

- **Stress**: Fear, anxiety, and pain can cause the pulse to increase.

- **Hemorrhage**: The pulse rate increases when blood is first lost due to the heart trying to work harder to circulate the blood. If bleeding continues, the pulse rate could decrease.

- **Medications**: Medications can increase or decrease the heart rate.

- **Fever and illness**: When a person is ill and has a fever, blood vessels may **dilate**, or widen, due to the rise in temperature. A decrease in blood pressure then occurs due to the dilated blood vessels. The heart responds by working harder, increasing the pulse rate.

Respiration is the process of **inspiration** (inhaling air into the lungs) and **expiration** (exhaling air out of the lungs). One respiration consists of an inspiration and an expiration. The chest rises during inspiration and falls during expiration. The normal respiration rate for adults ranges from 12 to 20 breaths per minute.

Different types of respirations include the following:

- **Apnea**: absence of breathing; may be temporary

- **Dyspnea**: difficulty breathing

- **Eupnea**: normal respirations

- **Orthopnea**: shortness of breath when lying down that is relieved by sitting up

- **Tachypnea**: rapid respirations

- **Cheyne-Stokes respiration** (agonal respiration): alternating periods of slow, irregular respirations and rapid, shallow respirations, possibly along with periods of apnea. (Many times this type of respiration precedes death; Chapter 27 contains more information)

- **Kussmaul breathing**: very deep, rapid breathing that is associated with diabetic ketoacidosis and kidney failure; also known as *air hunger*.

6. List guidelines for counting pulse and respirations

The **radial pulse** is the most common site for counting pulse beats. This pulse is found on the inside of the wrist on the thumb-side of the body. A pulse may be regular, having the same amount of time between the beats, or irregular, having varying amounts of time between the beats. When checking a resident's pulse, the NA should observe for the following:

- The pulse rate (the number of beats in one minute—normal range is 60 to 100 beats per minute)

- The overall pattern of the pulse: is the pulse regular or irregular?

- The quality or type of pulse: is the pulse strong or weak?

The respiratory rate is usually counted directly after taking the pulse because people tend to breathe more quickly if they know they are being observed. The NA should keep his fingers on the resident's wrist or on the stethoscope over the heart. He should not make it obvious that he is watching the resident's breathing and should not mention that he is counting respirations (Fig. 13-14). When counting respirations, the NA should observe for the following:

- The respiratory rate (the number of times the resident breathes in one minute—normal range is 12 to 20)

- The overall pattern of respirations: is breathing regular or irregular?

- The quality or type of breathing: is shortness of breath or difficulty breathing (dyspnea) noted? Does the resident have noisy breathing? Normal breathing is quiet. Is the breathing deep or shallow?

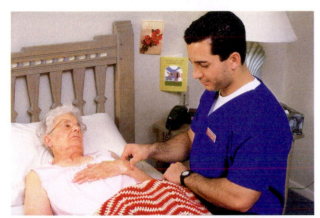

Fig. 13-14. *The respiratory rate should be counted immediately after measuring the radial pulse. Keeping fingers on the resident's wrist makes it less obvious that her breathing is being monitored.*

Counting and recording radial pulse and counting and recording respirations ▶

Equipment: watch with second hand, pen and paper

1. Identify yourself by name. Identify the resident. Greet the resident by name.

2. Wash your hands.

3. Explain procedure to the resident. Speak clearly, slowly, and directly. Maintain face-to-face contact whenever possible.

4. Provide for the resident's privacy with a curtain, screen, or door.

5. Place the tips of your index finger and middle finger on the thumb side of the resident's wrist to locate the radial pulse (Fig. 13-15). Do not use your thumb.

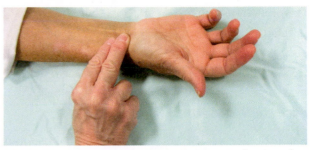

Fig. 13-15. *Count the radial pulse by placing the tips of your index finger and middle finger on the thumb side of the wrist.*

6. Count the beats for one full minute.

7. Keep your fingertips on the resident's wrist. Count respirations for one full minute. Remember that one respiration consists of an inspiration and an expiration. Observe for the pattern and character of the resident's breathing. Normal breathing is smooth and quiet. If you see signs of troubled, shallow, or noisy breathing, such as wheezing, report it to the nurse.

8. Wash your hands.

9. Immediately record the pulse rate, date, time, and method used (radial). Record the respiratory rate and the pattern or character of breathing.

10. Remove privacy measures. Make the resident comfortable.

11. Leave call light within the resident's reach.

12. Wash your hands.

13. Be courteous and respectful at all times.

14. Report any changes in the resident to the nurse. Report to the nurse if the pulse is less than 60 beats per minute or over 100 beats per minute, if the pulse rhythm is irregular, or if breathing is irregular.

A **stethoscope** is an instrument used for listening to sounds within the body, such as the heartbeat or air in the lungs. The *diaphragm* is the larger, round side of the stethoscope; this side is used to hear a pulse (Fig. 13-16). The smaller round side of the stethoscope is referred to as the *bell* side. The NA should clean the earpieces and diaphragm of the stethoscope with alcohol wipes before and after each use.

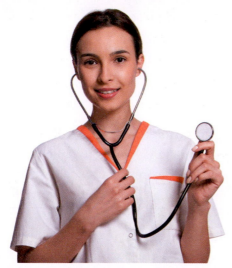

Fig. 13-16. *The diaphragm (the larger side) of the stethoscope is used to hear a pulse and to measure blood pressure.*

A stethoscope will be used to count apical pulse rate. The **apical pulse** is heard by listening directly over the heart with a stethoscope. The apical pulse is on the left side of the chest, just below the nipple. This type of pulse may be checked when residents have a weak radial pulse or an irregular pulse. It may also be checked on infants and people who have heart disease.

Counting and recording apical pulse

Equipment: stethoscope, watch with second hand, alcohol wipes, pen and paper

1. Identify yourself by name. Identify the resident. Greet the resident by name.

2. Wash your hands.

3. Explain procedure to the resident. Speak clearly, slowly, and directly. Maintain face-to-face contact whenever possible.

4. Provide for the resident's privacy with a curtain, screen, or door.

5. Before using the stethoscope, wipe the diaphragm and earpieces with alcohol wipes.

6. Fit the earpieces of the stethoscope snugly into your ears. Place the flat metal diaphragm on the left side of the chest, just below the nipple. Listen for the heartbeat.

7. Use the second hand of your watch. Count beats for one full minute (Fig. 13-17). Each "lubdub" you hear is counted as one beat. A normal heartbeat is rhythmical. Leave the stethoscope in place while counting respirations.

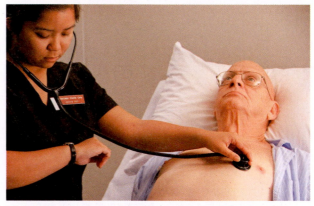

Fig. 13-17. *Count the heartbeats for one full minute to measure the apical pulse.*

8. Immediately record the pulse rate, date, time, and method used (apical). Note any irregularities in the rhythm.

9. Clean the earpieces and diaphragm of the stethoscope with alcohol wipes.

10. Make the resident comfortable. Remove privacy measures.

11. Leave call light within the resident's reach.

12. Wash your hands.

13. Be courteous and respectful at all times.

14. Report any changes in the resident to the nurse.

The apical pulse rate may also be checked to compare it to a pulse rate elsewhere in the body, such as the wrist (radial). In some cases, the apical and radial pulse rates differ. This is significant when a doctor evaluates circulation or a heart problem.

An apical pulse is normally about the same as a radial pulse. The apical pulse will always be the same or higher than any other pulse in the body. It will never be lower than another pulse. When the radial pulse is less than the apical pulse, it may indicate poor circulation to an extremity.

The pulse deficit is the difference between an apical pulse and another pulse. For example, if the apical pulse is 80 beats in one minute, and the radial pulse is 68 beats in one minute, the pulse deficit is 12 (80 - 68 = 12).

Counting and recording apical-radial pulse

Equipment: stethoscope, watch with second hand, alcohol wipes, pen and paper

Find a coworker to assist you.

1. Identify yourself by name. Identify the resident. Greet the resident by name.

2. Wash your hands.

3. Explain procedure to the resident. Speak clearly, slowly, and directly. Maintain face-to-face contact whenever possible.

4. Provide for the resident's privacy with a curtain, screen, or door.

5. Before using the stethoscope, wipe the diaphragm and earpieces with alcohol wipes.

6. Fit the earpieces of the stethoscope snugly into your ears. Place the flat metal diaphragm on the left side of the chest, just below the nipple. Listen for the heartbeat.

7. Your coworker should place her fingertips on the thumb side of resident's wrist to locate the radial pulse.

8. After both pulses have been located, look at the second hand of your watch. When the second hand reaches the 12 or 6, say "Start," and both people will count beats for one full minute. Say "Stop" after one minute.

9. Record both pulse rates, date, time, and method used (apical-radial). Record pulse deficit if the pulse rates are not the same (subtract radial pulse measurement from apical pulse to get pulse deficit). Note any irregularities in the pulse rhythm.

10. Clean the earpieces and the diaphragm of the stethoscope with alcohol wipes.

11. Make the resident comfortable. Remove privacy measures.

12. Leave call light within the resident's reach.

13. Wash your hands.

14. Be courteous and respectful at all times.

15. Report any changes in the resident to the nurse.

7. Identify factors that affect blood pressure

Blood pressure is the measurement of the force of the blood against the walls of certain blood vessels, called *arteries*. Arteries carry blood away from the heart. The left ventricle of the heart causes the blood to surge out of the heart and travel through the body. The force of this movement of blood is the blood pressure. Blood pressure is measured in millimeters of mercury (mm Hg). A blood pressure reading is recorded as a fraction—for example, 110/70.

The top, larger number in a blood pressure reading is the **systolic** blood pressure. This reading measures the pressure of the blood on the walls of the arteries when the heart is contracting to pump blood out from the left ventricle into the body. The normal range for systolic blood pressure for adults is 119 mm Hg or below.

The bottom, lower number is the **diastolic** blood pressure. This reading measures the pressure of the blood in the arteries when the heart is relaxed. This relaxation happens when the heart is not contracting, between the heartbeats. The normal range for diastolic blood pressure for adults is 79 mm Hg or below. The diastolic measurement is always lower than the systolic measurement.

When blood pressure is consistently high, it may be categorized as elevated, stage 1 hypertensive, stage 2 hypertensive, or hypertensive crisis. People with high blood pressure **(hypertension)** have elevated systolic and/or diastolic blood pressures. The ranges for the different categories of hypertension are listed in the orange box on page 227.

When blood pressure is low (below 90 mm Hg or below 60 mm Hg) it is called **hypotension**. Loss of blood or slowed blood flow can cause hypotension, which can be life-threatening. More information on these disorders can be found in Chapter 19. **Orthostatic hypotension**, which is also called *postural hypotension*, is a sudden drop in blood pressure that occurs when a person stands or sits up. Dizziness, lightheadedness, or fainting may accompany orthostatic hypotension.

Blood pressure is affected by different factors, including the following:

- **Age**: Elderly people with circulatory disorders (Chapter 19) may have higher blood pressure readings.

- **Exercise**: Regular exercise and being active decreases blood pressure. However, exercising just before a reading is obtained may cause a higher reading.

- **Stress**: Long-term, chronic stress can raise blood pressure.

- **Race**: African Americans are more likely to have high blood pressure than Caucasians.

- **Heredity**: People whose parents have or had high blood pressure are more likely to develop it than others.

- **Obesity/unhealthy diet**: Being overweight and eating unhealthy diets increase blood pressure.

- **Alcohol**: Regular, high alcohol intake can raise blood pressure.

- **Tobacco products**: Smoking or chewing tobacco products can increase blood pressure.

- **Time of day**: Blood pressure may be lower in the morning and higher later in the day.

- **Illness**: People who have certain diseases, such as diabetes and kidney disease, have a higher frequency of high blood pressure.

8. List guidelines for measuring blood pressure

Blood pressure is measured with a device called a **sphygmomanometer**. The NA will need to gather alcohol wipes, a stethoscope, a blood pressure cuff, and a sphygmomanometer when preparing to take blood pressure. It is important for the NA to choose the correct cuff size for each resident. Available cuff sizes for adults include small adult, adult, large adult, and thigh. There are also sizes available for infants and children. If the NA has questions about which size blood pressure cuff to use, she should talk to the nurse. The cuff must be the proper size and must be placed on the arm (or other extremity) correctly so the amount of pressure on the artery is correct. If not, the reading will be falsely high or low.

Two common types of sphygmomanometers are manual and digital. An aneroid sphygmomanometer is a type of manual sphygmomanometer. This device has a round gauge that is portable or is attached to the wall (Fig. 13-18). It may also hook onto clothing. Manual sphygmomanometers require the use of a stethoscope.

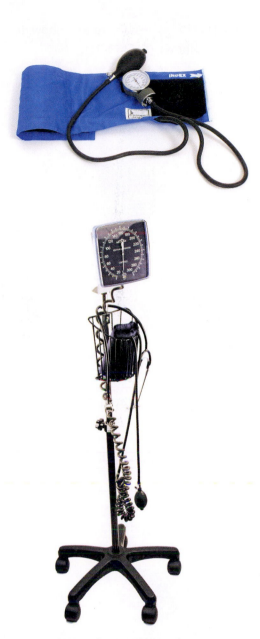

Fig. 13-18. *Two types of aneroid sphygmomanometers.*

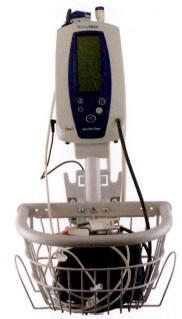

Fig. 13-19. *This type of digital sphygmomanometer measures blood pressure, as well as other vital signs.*

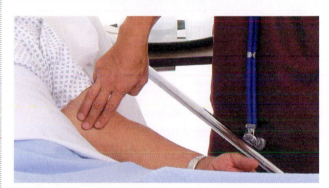

Fig. 13-20. *The brachial pulse is located on the inside of the elbow, about 1 to 1½ inches above the elbow.*

Digital sphygmomanometers display readings digitally. They may also measure other vital signs, such as temperature, pulse rate, and respiratory rate, as well as checking blood oxygen levels (Fig. 13-19). The use of a stethoscope is not required with digital sphygmomanometers.

The **brachial pulse** is used to obtain a blood pressure reading. This is the pulse inside of the elbow, about 1 to 1½ inches above the elbow (Fig. 13-20). Both the radial and the brachial pulse are used in measuring blood pressure. Other pulse sites may be used if necessary.

An NA should not take blood pressure on an arm or a side of the body when these situations exist:

- An intravenous line (IV) is present

- The cuff does not fit the arm properly

- The arm has a cast

- Burns or injuries are present

- The arm is being used for dialysis

- The arm or side has had recent trauma

- The arm or side is paralyzed due to stroke

- An amputation has been performed

- The side has had a mastectomy (or any other surgery or incision)

When measuring blood pressure, the NA should observe for the following:

- The blood pressure reading: A normal reading should be 119/79 or below (elevated readings that differ from the person's regular measurement should be reported).

- The quality or type of sounds: Are the sounds you hear when listening with your stethoscope strong or weak?

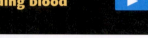

Measuring and recording blood pressure manually

Equipment: sphygmomanometer, stethoscope, alcohol wipes, pen and paper

Do not check blood pressure if the resident has had tobacco, alcohol, caffeine, or food, or has exercised within the last 30 minutes.

1. Identify yourself by name. Identify the resident. Greet the resident by name.

2. Wash your hands.

3. Explain procedure to the resident. Speak clearly, slowly, and directly. Maintain face-to-face contact whenever possible.

4. Provide for the resident's privacy with a curtain, screen, or door.

5. Before using the stethoscope, wipe the diaphragm and earpieces with alcohol wipes.

6. Make sure the resident is positioned comfortably. Ask the resident to roll up his sleeve so that his upper arm is exposed (approximately five inches above the elbow). Do not measure blood pressure over clothing.

7. Position the resident's arm with his palm up. The arm should be level with the heart.

8. With the valve open, squeeze the cuff. Make sure it is completely deflated.

9. Place the properly-sized cuff snugly on the resident's upper arm. The center of the cuff with sensor/arrow is placed over the brachial

artery (1–1½ inches above the elbow, toward inside of elbow) (Fig. 13-21).

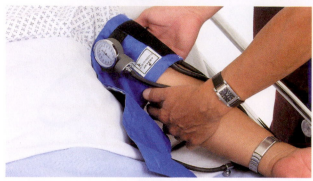

Fig. 13-21. *Place the center of the cuff over the brachial artery.*

10. Ask the resident to remain still and quiet during the measurement.

11. Locate the brachial artery pulse with your fingertips.

12. Place the earpieces of the stethoscope in your ears.

13. Place the diaphragm of the stethoscope over the brachial artery.

14. Close the valve (clockwise) until it stops. Do not overtighten it (Fig. 13-22).

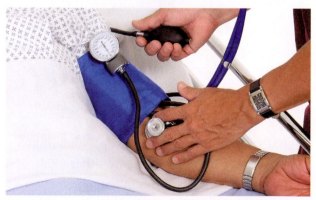

Fig. 13-22. *Close the valve by turning it clockwise until it stops. Do not overtighten it.*

15. Inflate the cuff to between 160 mm Hg–180 mm Hg. If a beat is heard immediately upon cuff deflation, completely deflate the cuff. Re-inflate the cuff to no more than 200 mm Hg.

16. Open the valve slightly with your thumb and index finger. Deflate the cuff slowly.

17. Watch the gauge. Listen for the sound of the pulse.

18. Remember the reading at which the first clear pulse sound is heard. This is the systolic blood pressure.

19. Continue listening for a change or muffling of the pulse sound. The moment you hear a change or the point at which the sound disappears is the diastolic pressure. Remember this reading.

20. Open the valve. Deflate the cuff completely. Remove the cuff.

21. Wash your hands.

22. Immediately record both the systolic and diastolic pressures. Record the numbers like a fraction, with the systolic reading on top and the diastolic reading on the bottom (for example: 110/70). Note which arm was used. Use *RA* for right arm and *LA* for left arm.

23. Wipe the diaphragm and earpieces of the stethoscope with alcohol wipes. Store equipment.

24. Make the resident comfortable. Remove privacy measures.

25. Leave call light within the resident's reach.

26. Wash your hands.

27. Be courteous and respectful at all times.

28. Report the blood pressure to a nurse if the reading is abnormal or significantly different from a previous reading.

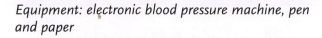

Measuring and recording blood pressure electronically

Equipment: electronic blood pressure machine, pen and paper

1. Identify yourself by name. Identify the resident. Greet the resident by name.

2. Wash your hands.

3. Explain procedure to the resident. Speak clearly, slowly, and directly. Maintain face-to-face contact whenever possible.

4. Provide for the resident's privacy with a curtain, screen, or door.

5. Make sure the resident is positioned comfortably. Ask the resident to roll up his sleeve so that his upper arm is exposed (approximately five inches above the elbow). Do not measure blood pressure over clothing.

6. Position the resident's arm with his palm up. The arm should be level with the heart.

7. Make sure the cuff is completely deflated. Place the properly-sized cuff snugly on the resident's upper arm. The center of the cuff with the sensor/arrow should be placed directly over the brachial artery (1–1½ inches above the elbow, toward inside of elbow).

8. Ask the resident to remain still and quiet during the measurement.

9. Turn on the blood pressure machine. If needed, choose the proper setting for an adult. Press the start button.

10. When the measurement is complete, the reading will be displayed on the screen and the machine may beep. The cuff should deflate.

11. Remove the cuff.

12. Wash your hands.

13. Immediately record both the systolic and diastolic pressures that are displayed on the screen. Note which arm was used.

14. Make the resident comfortable. Remove privacy measures.

15. Leave call light within the resident's reach.

16. Wash your hands.

17. Be courteous and respectful at all times.

18. Report the blood pressure to a nurse if the reading is abnormal or significantly different from a previous reading. Clean and store the equipment according to the manufacturer's recommendations.

Orthostatic Hypotension

Some people have a decrease in blood pressure when they move from a lying to a sitting or a standing position. A resident who has orthostatic hypotension may need to have his blood pressure measured three times. The first measurement will be taken after the resident has been lying down for five minutes. The second will be taken while the resident is sitting up, and the third will be taken when the resident is standing and has been standing for one to five minutes. All three readings will need to be documented, as in this example: Lying down=130/80, Sitting=110/76, and Standing=90/66.

9. Describe guidelines for pain management

Although pain is not a vital sign, it seriously affects a person's well-being and is important to monitor and manage. It can be very difficult to cope with pain. It is uncomfortable and can greatly affect residents' daily lives and their ability to perform ADLs.

Pain is a subjective experience (something reported by a person) and vital signs are objective measurements (information collected by using the senses). Pain is also a personal experience, which means it is different for each person. This means pain can be challenging to understand.

All caregivers are responsible for recognizing pain and taking appropriate action to provide pain management. Because NAs are with residents the most, they play a significant role in pain monitoring, management, and prevention. Care plans are developed using NAs' observations and reports.

NAs must treat residents' complaints of pain seriously and take action to help them (Fig. 13-23). The following are questions that nurses may ask residents to assess their pain. A nurse may ask an NA to ask these questions and then immediately report the information to the nurse, using the resident's words:

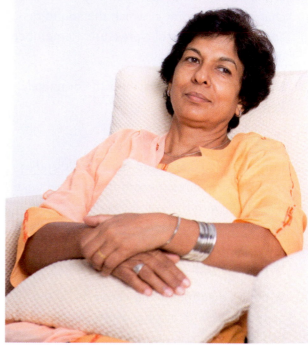

Fig. 13-23. NAs should believe residents when they say they are in pain and take quick action to help them. Being in pain is unpleasant. NAs should be empathetic and responsive.

- Where is the pain? Please point to the exact site or area to show me.

- When did the pain start? Please describe the pain.

- How long does the pain last? Minutes? Seconds? How often does it occur?

- How severe is the pain? To help assess this, the NA can ask the resident to rate the pain on a scale of 0 to 10, with 0 being no pain and 10 being the worst pain the resident can imagine. In some facilities a visual pain scale is used. The scale has drawings of faces with different expressions, and the NA must ask the resident to pick the face that most closely resembles the intensity of pain he is experiencing.

- What makes the pain better? What makes the pain worse?

- Have you experienced this pain before?

- Do you remember what you were doing when the pain started?

Types of Pain

Acute pain: sudden onset pain that generally lasts less than 6 months.

Chronic pain: pain lasting over a long period of time, usually over 6 months.

Visceral pain: pain from damage to internal organs; occurs in the trunk area of the body (appendicitis is an example).

Neuropathic pain: pain indicating damage to the nervous system (diabetes is one cause).

Radiating pain: pain felt in one area of the body that originated in another area of the body.

Phantom limb pain: pain felt in a body part that is not present anymore, such as an arm that has been amputated.

Breakthrough pain: severe pain that happens unexpectedly (often associated with cancer; Chapter 24 has more information).

Culture plays a role in determining whether or not a resident expresses her pain. Due to background or beliefs, some residents believe in expressing pain freely, while others are not comfortable saying that they are in pain.

Residents may be hesitant to express their pain due to concerns about addiction to pain medication, resulting constipation, or fatigue from the pain medication. Some residents may believe that pain is a normal part of aging, although it is not. Other residents may think that staff members are too busy to deal with their pain.

It is important that NAs watch for body language or other messages that indicate that residents may be in pain. Signs and symptoms of pain are important to observe and report.

Observing and Reporting: Pain

- O/R Increased pulse, respirations, or blood pressure
- O/R Sweating
- O/R Nausea
- O/R Vomiting
- O/R Tightening the jaw
- O/R Squeezing eyes shut
- O/R Holding or guarding a body part
- O/R Frowning
- O/R Grinding teeth
- O/R Increased restlessness
- O/R Agitation or tension
- O/R Change in behavior
- O/R Crying
- O/R Sighing
- O/R Groaning
- O/R Breathing heavily
- O/R Difficulty moving or walking

Guidelines: Measures to Reduce Pain

- G Report complaints of pain or unrelieved pain promptly to the nurse.
- G Check on the resident often and ask if the pain has been relieved.
- G Give back rubs frequently if allowed.
- G Assist in frequent changes of position. Use pillows to properly support the body. Be careful when moving, lifting, or transferring the resident.
- G Offer warm baths or showers.
- G Assist the resident to the bathroom or commode or offer the bedpan or urinal.
- G Encourage slow, deep breathing.
- G Be patient, caring, gentle, empathetic, and responsive to residents who are in pain.

Chapter Review

1. What are the four vital signs that are regularly monitored (LO 2)?

2. List two reasons an NA should never document a guess of a resident's vital signs (LO 2).

3. What are four symptoms of a fever (LO 3)?

4. If a resident has recently eaten or had something to drink, how long must an NA wait before she can measure his oral temperature (LO 4)?

5. Generally, how far should the tip of a tympanic thermometer be inserted into the ear (LO 4)?

6. What is the most common site for taking the pulse (LO 6)?

7. Why is the respiratory rate usually counted directly after taking the pulse, while the fingers are still on the person's wrist (LO 6)?

8. Where is the apical pulse located (LO 6)?

9. Why must a blood pressure cuff be the proper size and put on the arm correctly (LO 8)?

10. What pulse point is commonly used to measure blood pressure (LO 8)?

11. What are five ways an NA can help reduce a resident's pain (LO 9)?

Multiple Choice

12. Which body site is generally considered to be the most accurate for obtaining temperatures (LO 4)?
    (A) The mouth
    (B) The rectum
    (C) The armpit
    (D) The ear

13. What color is a rectal thermometer (LO 4)?
    (A) Blue
    (B) Green
    (C) Red
    (D) White

14. What is the normal pulse rate for adults (LO 5)?
    (A) 40 to 90 beats per minute
    (B) 60 to 100 beats per minute
    (C) 25 to 50 beats per minute
    (D) 80 to 120 beats per minute

15. Which of the following falls within the normal respiration rate for adults (LO 5)?
    (A) 14 breaths per minute
    (B) 22 breaths per minute
    (C) 5 breaths per minute
    (D) 9 breaths per minute

16. Which side of a stethoscope is used for measuring pulse rate (LO 6)?
    (A) The left side
    (B) The classic side
    (C) The dome side
    (D) The diaphragm side

17. Which blood pressure measurement reflects the phase when the heart relaxes and is always lower than the other measurement (LO 7)?
    (A) Systolic
    (B) Radial
    (C) Apical
    (D) Diastolic

18. When a resident complains of pain, which of the following would be the best response by the NA (LO 9)?
    (A) The NA should give the resident pain medication.
    (B) The NA should ask questions to find out more information about the pain.
    (C) The NA should ignore the complaint unless the resident repeats it.
    (D) The NA should contact the resident's family to find out what course of action they would like to take.

14
Nutrition and Fluid Balance

Pernicious Anemia

A Nobel Prize was awarded to George R. Minot, William P. Murphy, and George H. Whipple for discovering that a serious and fatal disease called pernicious anemia could actually be cured. Minot worked for many years and finally discovered that with a simple change in diet, adding large amounts of liver, the disease could be cured. The three men eventually proved the disease was caused by a lack of vitamin B12. Today many people live long lives with this disease by simply increasing their vitamin B12 intake.

"In general, mankind, since the improvement of cookery, eats twice as much as it requires."
Benjamin Franklin, 1706–1790

"Every tooth in a man's head is more valuable than a diamond."
Miguel de Cervantes, 1547–1616

1. Define important words in this chapter

apathy: a lack of interest.

diet cards: cards that list residents' names and information about special diets, allergies, likes and dislikes, and any other dietary instructions.

diuretics: substances that increase urine formation and cause the body to excrete sodium, potassium, and water through the kidneys.

fasting: a period of time during which food is given up voluntarily.

fluid balance: maintaining equal input and output.

fluid overload: a condition in which the body cannot eliminate the fluid consumed.

glucose: natural sugar.

graduate: container for measuring fluid volume.

input: the fluid a person consumes; also called *intake*.

intake: the fluid a person consumes; also called *input*.

lactose intolerance: inability of the body to digest lactose, a type of sugar found in milk and other dairy products.

malnutrition: the lack of proper nutrition that results from insufficient food intake or an improper diet.

metabolism: the process of breaking down and transforming all nutrients that enter the body to provide energy and growth.

nutrient: a necessary substance that provides energy, promotes growth and health, and helps regulate metabolism.

nutrition: the process by which the body uses food to maintain health.

output: fluid that is eliminated each day through urine, feces, vomitus, and perspiration; also includes suctioned material and wound drainage.

puree: to blend or grind food into a thick paste.

restrict fluids (RF): a medical order to limit the amount of fluids a person drinks to the level set by a doctor.

special diet: a diet for people who have certain illnesses or conditions; also called *therapeutic* or *modified diet*.

vegans: people who do not eat any animals or animal products, including milk, cheese, other dairy items, or eggs; vegans may also choose not to use or wear any animal products.

vegetarians: people who do not eat meat, fish, or poultry and may or may not eat eggs and dairy products.

2. Describe common nutritional problems of the elderly and the chronically ill

Aging and illness affect **nutrition**, or the process by which the body uses food to maintain health. Malnutrition, unhealthy weight loss, and dehydration are serious problems among the elderly. **Malnutrition** is the lack of proper nutrition that results from insufficient food intake or an improper diet. Difficulty swallowing, called *dysphagia*, and the inability to chew can contribute to a lack of appetite. Fatigue, nausea, and pain often accompany certain illnesses, decreasing appetite. Other problems that affect nutritional intake include the following:

- Older people produce less saliva, which affects eating and swallowing. Swallowing problems put people at a high risk for aspiration, which is the inhalation of food, fluid, or foreign material into the lungs. There is more information about aspiration later in this chapter.

- Medications can have side effects on the digestive system, such as diarrhea and constipation, both of which can interfere with appetite.

- A decrease in physical activity and mobility can cause constipation and a lack of appetite.

- The ability to smell and taste food and drink decreases as people age. Medication can also interfere with the senses of smell and taste. This affects the appetite and the ability to eat (Fig. 14-1).

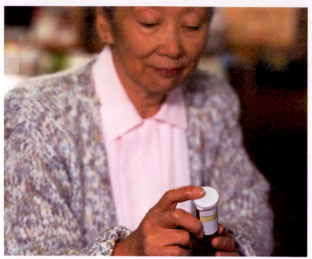

Fig. 14-1. *Many elderly people take a variety of medications, which can affect the way food smells and tastes.*

- The inability to see well can affect the way food looks, decreasing interest in food.

- Problems with teeth, dentures, or poor oral hygiene make chewing difficult.

- Depression and lack of social interaction can decrease appetite.

- Older people may be prescribed special diets that restrict certain foods and drinks, which can lead to poor food and fluid intake. More information about special diets is located later in this chapter.

- Many illnesses affect nutritional intake. Some make eating and swallowing difficult, such as stroke, which can result in paralysis; cancers of the head, neck, or mouth; Parkinson's disease; multiple sclerosis; and Alzheimer's disease. Other illnesses affect appetite, such as cancer or liver disease. The body's ability to digest food or absorb nutrients may be compromised, such as with celiac disease. More information about these diseases may be found later in the chapter and in Chapters 15, 22, and 24 of the textbook.

3. Describe cultural factors that influence food preferences

Cultural and ethnic background has a significant impact on a person's food preferences. Family traditions also influence food choices (Fig. 14-2). Where a person comes from affects his food choices as well. For example, people from the southwestern United States may eat spicy foods. People from Asia may prefer rice with their meals, rather than potatoes or bread.

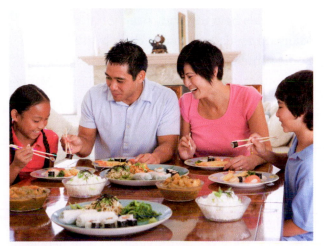

Fig. 14-2. Family traditions influence food likes and dislikes.

Some people do not eat certain foods due to religious reasons. For example, many Jewish people follow a kosher diet. Pork and shellfish are not allowed in a kosher diet, and meat and dairy products cannot be eaten together. Some Catholics do not eat meat on Fridays. Muslims may follow a halal diet and do not drink alcohol or eat pork. People from many religious traditions may occasionally fast. **Fasting** is a practice during which food is voluntarily given up for a period of time.

Some people are vegetarians or vegans. **Vegetarians** do not eat meat, fish, or poultry. They may or may not eat eggs and dairy products. **Vegans** are vegetarians who do not eat any animals or animal products, including milk, cheese, other dairy items, or eggs. Vegans may also choose not to use or wear any animal products, including wool, silk, and leather.

A resident's food preferences are first discussed upon admission to a facility. These evaluations may need to be redone periodically as the resident's likes and dislikes, as well as nutritional needs, change.

Residents have the legal right to choose food options that reflect their preferences, culture, religion, and ethnicity. Honoring food preferences is also part of promoting person-centered care. NAs must report requests for diet substitutions to the nurse right away.

4. Identify six basic nutrients

The human body cannot survive without food and water. Every day the body needs each of the main nutrients for cells, tissues, organs, and systems to continue to function properly. A **nutrient** is a necessary substance that provides energy, promotes growth and health, and helps regulate metabolism. **Metabolism** is the process of breaking down and transforming all nutrients that enter the body in order to provide energy and growth. There are six main nutrients required by the body for healthy growth and development:

1. **Water** is the most essential nutrient for life; it is needed by every cell in the body. Water helps move oxygen and other nutrients into the cells and removes the waste products from each of the cells. Without water, a person can only live a few days. Water helps with digestion and absorption of food. It helps to maintain a normal body temperature through perspiration. Keeping enough fluid in the body is necessary for health.

2. **Fats** are a good source of energy. Fat also gives flavor to foods (Fig. 14-3). Fat falls into four categories: saturated, trans, monounsaturated, and polyunsaturated. Saturated and trans fats can increase cholesterol levels and the risk of some diseases, like cardiovascular disease. Mono-unsaturated and polyunsaturated fats can be helpful in the diet, and can decrease the risk of cardiovascular disease and type 2 diabetes.

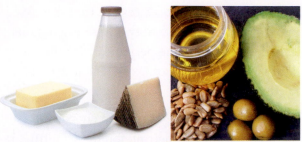

Fig. 14-3. Some fats come from animal sources, such as butter, beef, pork, fowl, fish, and dairy products. Some fats come from plant sources, such as olives, nuts, and seeds.

3. **Carbohydrates** supply the body with energy and help the body use fat efficiently. Carbohydrates also add needed fiber to diets, which helps with solid waste elimination (Fig. 14-4).

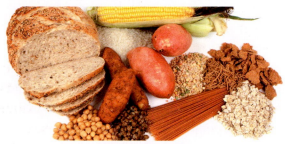

Fig. 14-4. Some sources of carbohydrates.

4. **Proteins** are needed by every cell in the body. They help the body grow new tissue, enable tissue repair, and provide additional energy (Fig. 14-5).

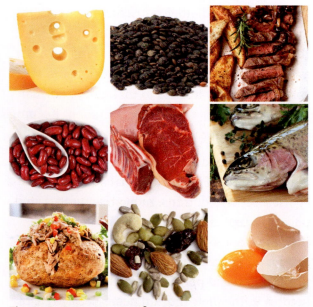

Fig. 14-5. Some sources of protein.

5. **Vitamins** are substances that are needed by the body to function. The body does not make most vitamins; they can only be obtained by eating certain foods. Some vitamins are fat-soluble, meaning they are carried and stored in body fat. Vitamins A, D, E, and K are examples. Others are water-soluble vitamins, meaning they are broken down by water in the body and cannot be stored. They are eliminated through urine and feces. Vitamins B and C are examples of water-soluble vitamins.

6. **Minerals** help the body function normally. Many minerals are needed daily by the body. Some minerals keep bones and teeth strong, while others help maintain fluid balance. Minerals give the body energy and control body processes. They are found in many foods.

5. Explain the USDA's MyPlate

In 2011, in response to increasing rates of obesity, the United States Department of Agriculture (USDA) developed MyPlate to help people build a healthy plate at meal times (Fig. 14-6). The MyPlate icon emphasizes vegetables, fruits, grains, protein, and low-fat dairy products.

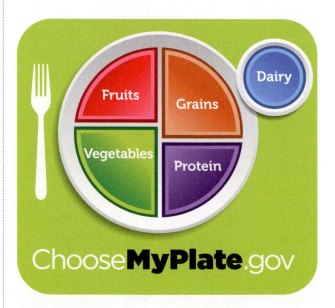

Fig. 14-6. The US Department of Agriculture developed the MyPlate icon and website (ChooseMyPlate.gov) to help promote healthy eating practices.

The goal of MyPlate is to guide people in making healthy food choices. The icon is based on scientific information about nutrition and health. It shows the amounts of each food group that should be on a person's plate. MyPlate gives suggestions and tools for making healthy choices; however, it does not provide specific messages about what a person should eat. The MyPlate icon includes the following food groups:

Vegetables and fruits: Fruits and vegetables should make up half of a person's plate. Vegetables include all fresh, frozen, canned, and dried vegetables, and vegetable juices. There are five subgroups within the vegetable group, organized by their nutritional content. These are dark green vegetables, red and orange vegetables, beans and peas, starchy vegetables, and other vegetables. A variety of vegetables from these subgroups should be eaten every day. Dark green, red, and orange vegetables have the best nutritional content (Fig. 14-7).

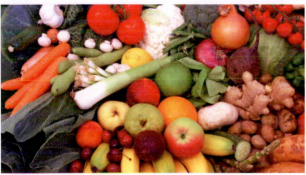

Fig. 14-7. Eating a variety of vegetables, especially dark green, red, and orange vegetables, every day helps promote health.

Vegetables are low in fat and calories and have no cholesterol (although sauces and seasonings may add fat, calories, and cholesterol). They are good sources of dietary fiber, potassium, vitamin A, vitamin E, vitamin C, and vitamin B.

Fruits include all fresh, frozen, canned, and dried fruits, and 100% fruit juices. Most choices should be whole, cut-up, or pureed fruit, rather than juice, for the additional dietary fiber provided. Fruit can be added as a main dish, side dish, or a dessert.

Fruits, like vegetables, are naturally low in fat, sodium, and calories and have no cholesterol. They are important sources of dietary fiber and many nutrients, including folic acid, potassium, and vitamin C. Foods containing dietary fiber help provide a feeling of fullness with fewer calories. Folic acid helps the body form red blood cells. Vitamin C is important for growth and repair of body tissues.

Grains: A person should make half his grain intake whole grains. There are many different grains. Some common ones are wheat, rice, oats, cornmeal, and barley. Foods made from grains include bread, pasta, oatmeal, breakfast cereals, tortillas, and grits. Grains can be divided into two groups: whole grains and refined grains. Whole grains contain bran and germ, as well as the endosperm. Refined grains retain only the endosperm. The endosperm is the tissue within flowering plants. It surrounds and nourishes the plant embryo. Examples of whole grains include brown rice, wild rice, bulgur, oatmeal, whole-grain corn, whole oats, whole wheat, and whole rye. Consuming foods rich in fiber reduces the risk of heart disease and other diseases and may reduce constipation.

Protein: MyPlate guidelines emphasize the importance of eating a variety of protein foods every week. Meat, poultry, seafood, and eggs are animal sources of proteins. Beans, peas, soy products, vegetarian meat substitutes, nuts, and seeds are plant sources of proteins. Protein shakes and bars are other forms of protein.

Seafood should be eaten twice a week in place of meat or poultry. Seafood that is higher in oils and low in mercury, such as salmon or trout, is a better choice (Fig. 14-8). Lean meats and poultry, as well as eggs and egg whites, can be eaten on a regular basis. A person should eat plant-based protein foods more often. Beans and peas, soy products (tofu, tempeh, many vegetarian products), vegetarian meat substitutes, nuts, and seeds are low in saturated fat and high in fiber. Some nuts and seeds (flax, walnuts) are excellent sources of essential fatty acids. These fatty acids may reduce the risk of cardiovascular disease. Sunflower seeds and almonds are good sources of vitamin E.

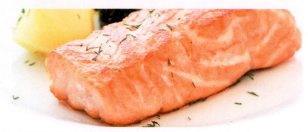

Fig. 14-8. Fish, like this salmon, contains healthy oils and is a good source of protein.

Dairy: All milk products and foods made from milk that retain their calcium content, such as yogurt and cheese, are part of the dairy category. Most dairy group choices should be fat-free (0%) or low-fat (1%). Fat-free or low-fat milk or yogurt should be chosen more often than cheese. Milk and yogurt contain less sodium than most cheeses.

Milk provides nutrients that are vital for the health and maintenance of the body. These nutrients include calcium, potassium, vitamin D, and protein. Fat-free or low-fat milk provides these nutrients without the extra calories and saturated fat. Soy and almond products enriched with calcium are an alternative to dairy foods.

The following guidelines provide additional tips for making healthy food choices:

Guidelines: Healthy Food Choices

G Balance calories. Calorie balance is the relationship between the calories obtained from food and fluids consumed and the calories used during normal body functions and physical activity. Proper calorie intake varies from person to person. To find the proper calorie intake, the USDA suggests visiting ChooseMyPlate.gov.

G Enjoy your food, but eat less. Eating too fast or eating without paying attention to your food can lead to overeating. Recognize when you feel hungry and when you are full. Notice what you are eating. Stop eating when you feel satisfied.

G Avoid oversized portions. Choose smaller-sized portions when eating. Portion out food before you eat it, and use smaller bowls and plates for meals. When eating out, split food with others or take part of your meal home.

G Eat these foods more often: vegetables, fruits, whole grains, fat-free or 1% milk, and low-fat dairy products. These foods have better nutrients for health.

G Eat these foods less often: foods high in solid fats, added sugars, and salt. These foods include fatty meats (like bacon and hot dogs), cheese, fried foods, ice cream, and cookies.

G Check sodium content in foods. Read product labels to determine if they contain salt or sodium. Foods high in sodium include the following:

- Cured meats, including ham, bacon, lunch meat, sausage, and hot dogs

- Salty or smoked fish, including herring, sardines, anchovies, and smoked salmon

- Processed cheese and other cheeses

- Salted foods, including nuts, pretzels, potato chips, dips, and spreads, such as salted butter and margarine

- Vegetables preserved in brine, such as pickles, sauerkraut, olives, and relishes

- Sauces with high concentrations of salt, including steak and soy sauces, ketchup, mustard, and mayonnaise

- Commercially prepared foods such as breads, canned soups and vegetables, and certain breakfast cereals

Select canned foods that are labeled *sodium-free, very low sodium, low-sodium,* or *reduced sodium.*

G Drink water instead of sugary drinks. Drinking water or unsweetened beverages reduces sugar and calorie intake. Sweetened beverages, such as soda, fruit punch, and sports drinks, are a major source of sugar and calories in diets.

6. Explain the role of the dietary department

The dietary department is responsible for providing nutritious meals and snacks for all residents. Each resident is evaluated upon admission in order to create his diet plan. The dietary department creates food to match the diet ordered by the doctor, while also taking into consideration the resident's preferences and nutritional needs.

In addition to planning and making meals, the dietary department prepares food so that it looks appetizing and that residents are able to manage it. The dietary department also prepares diet cards. **Diet cards** list the resident's name and information about special diets, allergies, likes and dislikes, and other dietary instructions.

For residents who are unable to eat in the dining room, meals arrive in a warming cart. Each meal comes with a diet card. The NA must verify that each resident has received the correct meal by checking the resident's identification against the diet card.

Dietary staff must follow strict infection prevention guidelines in food preparation. Food must be stored and cooked properly to avoid foodborne illness. Surveys are performed by health departments to check for cleanliness and to observe infection prevention practices.

Menus

Menus are prepared for different diets and are often completed each day. NAs may need to help residents complete their menu choices. If asked to help with a menu, the NA should make sure the menu offered matches the correct resident. When reading the menu options, the NA should speak slowly and clearly and make the food choices sound appetizing. He should answer any questions or concerns the resident has, and should mark the selection that the resident wants. After completing each category, he should submit the menu promptly. When the food arrives, it must be checked to see that the resident received what she ordered.

7. Explain the importance of following diet orders and identify special diets

Special diets are often ordered for residents who have certain illnesses or conditions (Fig. 14-9). Sometimes they are ordered to help a resident gain or lose weight. Some diets are ordered for a short time before a medical test or surgery. Doctors prescribe the special diet, also called a *therapeutic* or *modified* diet, and then the dietitian plans the diet, along with input from the resident.

Residents who have orders for specific diets require additional care and supervision. Special diets may restrict or eliminate certain foods or fluids. As stated earlier, it is very important for an NA to check resident identification against the diet card before serving meal trays. The food on the tray should be checked to see if it matches the diet ordered. Serving a resident the wrong food can cause serious problems, such as allergic reactions and possibly death.

Some types of special diets are listed below:

Liquid Diet. Liquid diets are made up of foods that are in a liquid state at room temperature. Liquid diets are usually ordered as *clear* or *full*. A clear liquid diet consists of fluids that a person can see through, such as clear soups and juices. A full liquid diet includes all of the liquids served on a clear liquid diet, with the addition of cream soups, milk, and ice cream. A liquid diet may be ordered for a short time due to a medical condition or before or after surgery or a diagnostic test.

Soft Diet and Mechanical Soft Diet. The soft diet is soft in texture and consists of soft foods that are easier to chew and swallow. Foods that are hard to chew and swallow, such as raw fruits and vegetables and some meats, are restricted. High-fiber foods, fried foods, and spicy foods may also be limited to help with digestion. The soft diet is often used for people who are making the transition from a liquid diet to a regular diet. It is also used for people who are recovering from surgery or a long illness, or who have dental problems or have had dental surgery.

The mechanical soft diet gets its name from how foods are prepared, such as with blenders, food processors, meat grinders, or cutting utensils. These items are used to chop or blend foods to make them easier to chew and swallow. Unlike the soft diet, the mechanical soft diet does not limit spices, fat, and fiber. Only the texture of foods is changed. For example, meats can be ground and moistened with sauces or water to ease swallowing. This diet is used for people who are recovering from surgery, who have difficulty swallowing, or who have dental problems.

Pureed Diet. To **puree** food means to blend or grind it into a thick paste. This consistency means the food should be thick enough to hold its form in the mouth, but it does not need to be chewed. The pureed diet is used for people who have trouble chewing and swallowing and who cannot tolerate regular or mechanical soft diets.

Bland Diet. In the bland diet, foods that irritate the stomach and digestive tract are eliminated. These include spicy foods, citrus juices, caffeinated beverages, and alcohol. This diet is used for people who have intestinal problems or conditions, such as Crohn's disease (Chapter 15) or gastric ulcers.

Lactose-Free Diet. **Lactose intolerance** is the inability of the body to digest lactose, a type of sugar found in milk and other dairy products. A lactose-free diet means that all products with lactose must be eliminated. These include milk and all foods or beverages made with milk. Other types of milk may be allowed, such as lactose-free, soy, almond, or rice milk.

High-Residue or High-Fiber Diet. High-residue or high-fiber diets increase the intake of fiber and whole grains, such as whole grain cereals, bread, and raw fruits and vegetables (Fig. 14-9). This diet helps with problems such as bowel disorders, constipation, and other gastrointestinal illnesses (Chapter 15).

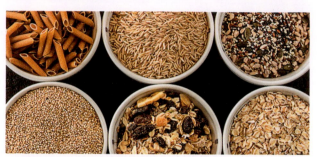

Fig. 14-9. *Intake of fiber and whole grains will be ordered for a high-residue diet.*

Low-Residue or Low-Fiber Diet. This diet decreases the intake of fiber, grains, seeds, raw fruits and vegetables, and other foods, such as dairy and coffee. This diet is used for people with bowel disorders such as diverticulitis (Chapter 15).

Modified Calorie Diets. A high-calorie diet increases the amount of calories to help a person gain weight. This may be necessary due to malnutrition, surgery, or illness. In order to lose weight, a person may need to eat a calorie-controlled diet, which decreases calorie intake. Common abbreviations for these diets are *High-Cal* or *Low-Cal*.

Residents' Rights

Obesity and Bias

Residents, their families and friends, and staff members may be overweight or obese. Studies have shown that people who are overweight or obese often experience prejudice because of their weight. NAs should not judge anyone who is overweight. They should not make negative or judgmental comments or show disgust or distaste. More information about obesity may be found in Chapter 15.

Low-Sodium. With a low-sodium diet, salt is restricted. For residents on these diets, salt shakers or salt packets should not be on a meal tray.

Condiments with high concentrations of salt, including Worcestershire, barbecue, steak, and soy sauces; ketchup; and mustard, may be restricted as well. This type of diet is often used for people who have heart disease or kidney disease. Common abbreviations for this diet are *Low Na*, which means low sodium, or *NAS*, which stands for *No Added Salt*.

High-Protein Diet. A high-protein diet increases high-protein foods, such as lean meats, seafood, eggs, beans, nuts, and foods with added protein, such as protein shakes. This diet is used for people recovering from surgery and for healing serious wounds, such as burns.

Renal Diet. With a renal diet, protein may be decreased. Foods like vegetables and starches, such as breads, cereals, and pasta, are encouraged. This diet is often used for people who have kidney or liver disease. Protein is restricted because the body cannot use the protein properly, and it may lead to further damage of these organs. Protein is never completely eliminated from the diet, though, because the body needs protein to function.

Low-Fat Diet. This diet consists of foods that are low in saturated fats, such as fresh fruits and vegetables, low-fat or fat-free dairy products, and white meats of chicken and turkey. Foods high in saturated fat include fatty meats, high-fat dairy products (especially cheese), hydrogenated oils, and desserts and baked goods. Saturated fats can put a person at risk for heart disease and artery problems. However, eating unsaturated fat can reduce the risk of heart disease and improve HDL (good) cholesterol levels. Foods that contain healthier fats include olive oil, nuts, avocado, and fatty fish such as salmon. The low-fat diet is also used for people who have gallbladder or liver disease. A common abbreviation for this diet is *Low-Fat*.

High-Potassium Diet. This diet increases foods that are high in potassium, such as bananas, grapefruit, oranges, orange juice, prune juice, prunes, dried apricots, figs, raisins, dates, cantaloupes, tomatoes, potatoes with skins, sweet potatoes and yams, winter squash, legumes, avocados, and unsalted nuts. People who take diuretics or blood pressure medications may be placed on this diet. **Diuretics** are substances that increase urine formation and cause the body to excrete sodium, potassium, and water through the kidneys. Because diuretics increase urine output, a person may have a low potassium level.

Fluid-Restricted Diet. People with severe heart disease and kidney disease may have trouble processing fluid. To prevent further damage, doctors may restrict fluid intake. For residents on fluid restrictions, the NA will need to measure and document the amount of fluid consumed and eliminated. *Intake*, or *input*, is the fluid a person consumes, while *output* is the fluid that is eliminated. More information about fluid restrictions and intake and output may be found later in the chapter. Additional fluids or foods that count as fluids, such as soups, ice cream, etc., should not be offered to a resident on a fluid-restricted diet. The abbreviation for this diet is *RF*, which stands for *Restrict Fluids*.

High-Iron Diet. With this diet, the intake of iron is increased. Examples of iron-rich foods are green, leafy vegetables such as spinach and kale; legumes; lean meats; some nuts; and breads and cereals that are enriched with iron. The high-iron diet is ordered for people who have anemia (Chapter 19), which may be due to blood loss.

Diabetic Diet. Diabetes is a condition in which the pancreas does not produce insulin or does not produce enough insulin. Insulin converts **glucose**, or natural sugar, into energy for the body. Without insulin to process glucose, these sugars collect in the blood. This causes problems with circulation and can damage vital organs.

People with diabetes must be very careful about what they eat (Fig. 14-10). Calories and carbohydrates are carefully controlled, and protein and fats are also regulated. The foods and the amounts are determined by nutritional and energy needs. A registered dietitian and the resident will make up a meal plan, including snacks, that will include all of the right types and amounts of food for each day.

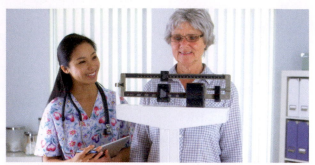

Fig. 14-10. People who have diabetes must be very careful about what they eat and must keep their weight in a healthy range.

The meal plan may use a carbohydrate-counting approach (often called *carb counting*). After the proper amount of carbohydrates is determined by the dietitian, they need to be counted in each meal or snack. Nutrition labels need to be read, paying attention to serving size and carbohydrate content. Food portions may need to be measured.

Residents who have diabetes must eat the right amount of the right type of food at the right time, and they must eat everything that is served. This is necessary to maintain blood sugar. NAs should encourage them to eat all of their meals and snacks. Other foods should not be offered without the nurse's approval. If a resident is not following the diet, does not finish meals and snacks, or throws food away, the NA should notify the nurse immediately.

People who have diabetes should avoid foods that are high in sugar. Sugary foods can cause problems with insulin balance. A meal tray for a resident with diabetes may have artificial sweetener, low-calorie jelly, and/or low-calorie maple syrup. Artificial sweeteners, rather than sugar, may be used in coffee or tea. The American Diabetes Association's (ADA) website, diabetes.org, has more information. Additional information on diabetes may be found in Chapter 23.

Gluten-Free Diet. This diet is free of a protein called *gluten*, which is found in wheat, rye, and barley. It is used for people with celiac disease, which is an autoimmune disease that can cause damage to the lining of the small intestine if gluten is consumed. A blood test can diagnose this disease. Foods containing wheat flour are eliminated from the diet. Examples of food normally containing wheat include tortillas, crackers, breads, cakes, pasta, and cereals. Some sauces and dressings also have wheat in them. Other items that may contain gluten include beer, hot dogs, candy, broths, and medications. In addition, vitamins, lipsticks, and lip balms may have gluten in them.

Unlike celiac disease, gluten intolerance is a condition that does not cause damage to the intestine. It does, however, cause unpleasant symptoms such as abdominal pain, gas, and diarrhea when products containing gluten are consumed. If a person has a gluten intolerance, eliminating gluten from the diet will usually stop these symptoms.

Vegetarian Diet. A vegetarian diet may be needed due to a medical condition or health problem, such as diabetes or obesity, or it simply may be a person's choice not to eat meat due to cultural, ethical, personal, or religious reasons. Some types of vegetarian diets follow:

- A lacto-ovo vegetarian diet excludes all meats, fish, and poultry, but allows eggs and dairy products.

- A lacto-vegetarian diet eliminates poultry, meats, fish, and eggs, but allows dairy products.

- An ovo-vegetarian diet omits all meats, fish, poultry, and dairy products, but allows eggs.

Vegan Diet. A vegan diet consists of only plant-based foods. It eliminates all poultry, meats, fish, eggs, and dairy products, along with all foods that are derived from animals, such as gelatin. Honey may also be eliminated. There are different types of vegan diets. The whole-food vegan diet includes whole plants like nuts, seed, and legumes. The raw-food diet includes raw fruits, nuts, and seeds. A vegan diet may be ordered for people who have heart disease, diabetes, or other diseases, or it may be a personal choice. Both vegetarians and vegans may require extra supplements, such as iron supplements, B-complex vitamins, especially vitamin B-12, and calcium and zinc supplements.

Limited Animal-Based Diets. Some people follow a pescatarian diet. This diet eliminates all meats and poultry but allows fish and other seafood. Eggs and dairy products may also be consumed.

A flexitarian diet is a diet some people follow in which plant-based foods are eaten primarily, but meats and other animal products are eaten occasionally.

Tip

NPO

The abbreviation *NPO* stands for *nothing by mouth*. It comes from the Latin *nil per os*. This means that a resident is not allowed to have anything to eat or drink. Some residents have a serious problem with swallowing, and it is unsafe to give them anything by mouth. These residents will receive nutrition another way, either through a feeding tube or intravenously (Chapter 26). Some residents may not be able to drink for a short time before a medical test or surgery. If this abbreviation is listed on a resident's diet card or in the care plan, NAs must not offer the resident any food or drink, including water or ice chips.

8. Explain thickened liquids and identify three basic thickening consistencies

Residents with dysphagia (difficulty swallowing) are evaluated by speech-language pathologists to determine if they should consume thickened liquids to help with swallowing. Thickened liquids have a thickening powder or agent added to them, which improves the ability to control fluid in the mouth and throat. Residents with swallowing problems may require thickened fluids because thinner fluids, such as water or tea, can increase the risk of choking. Thickened liquids move down the throat more slowly, reducing coughing and limiting the risk of choking.

After the speech-language pathologist assesses a resident, the doctor writes the order for the type of thickening agent the resident needs. Thickening agents may come in powder or gel form. Some beverages are pre-thickened; pre-thickened mixes just need water added.

Either the dietary department prepares the liquid (if it is not pre-thickened) or the thickening agent is added at the nursing unit before serving. If the thickened liquid needs to be prepared at the nursing unit, the thickener must be mixed thoroughly with the liquid. The liquid may require a waiting period to reach the proper consistency.

NAs should follow instructions for residents who have orders for thickened liquids. These residents should not drink any fluid that is not thickened. This means drinks such as soda, water, tea, and coffee are not allowed. A water pitcher should not be left at the resident's bedside. Before serving any fluids to a resident with this restriction, the NA should talk to the nurse. It may take a resident a long time to drink a thickened drink. The NA should be patient and encouraging.

These are three types of thickened consistencies generally used by facilities:

1. **Nectar Thick.** This consistency is similar to a fruit nectar or other thicker juices, such as tomato juice. A resident can drink this from a cup with or without a straw.

2. **Honey Thick.** This consistency is similar to that of honey. It will pour very slowly, and spoons are usually used to consume these types of liquids.

3. **Pudding Thick.** This consistency is semi-solid, much like the consistency of pudding. A spoon will stand up straight when put into this thickened liquid. Spoons are used to consume these liquids.

9. List ways to identify and prevent unintended weight loss

Sometimes residents unintentionally lose weight, which may be due to a medical condition, such as cancer, HIV, diabetes, or other diseases. It can also be due to an unappetizing diet. Unintended weight loss is a serious problem for the elderly. It increases a person's risk for malnutrition and can contribute to skin breakdown, which may lead to pressure injuries. This is why it is very important for NAs to report any weight loss they notice, no matter how small.

When weight loss occurs, staff will evaluate potential causes and may change special diet orders to encourage the resident to eat more. It may be better for the resident to eat a less restricted diet. If an NA notices food going uneaten or if a resident complains about the food, she should report it to the nurse.

Observing and Reporting: Unintended Weight Loss and Malnourishment

- Resident needs help eating or drinking
- Resident eats less than 75% of meals/snacks served
- Resident has mouth pain
- Resident has dentures that do not fit properly
- Resident has difficulty chewing or swallowing
- Resident coughs or chokes while eating
- Resident is sad, cries, or withdraws from others
- Resident is confused, wanders, or paces

If you notice any of these signs, report it immediately to the nurse. Also report if the resident has any of the following signs or symptoms, which could indicate malnourishment:

- Feeling of coldness throughout the body
- Weight loss

- Abdominal distention
- Abdominal pain
- Constipation
- Edema (swelling in body tissues caused by excess fluid)
- Cracks or splits at the corners of the mouth
- Inflammation of the mucous membranes of the mouth
- Dry or peeling skin
- Brittle, easily cracked nails
- Rapidly thinning hair that breaks off easily; hair that changes or loses color
- Frequent infections
- Muscle weakness
- Fainting
- Fatigue
- Withdrawal or **apathy** (lack of interest)
- Anxiety and irritability
- Problems with sleeping
- Low body temperature
- Slow pulse
- Low blood pressure

Guidelines: Preventing Unintended Weight Loss

- Report observations and warning signs to the nurse immediately.
- Report any decrease in appetite to the nurse. If a resident has a loss of appetite, ask her about it.
- Encourage residents to eat by talking about eating and the food being served in a positive way (Fig. 14-11).
- Check diet cards and meal trays to make sure residents are receiving the correct food.

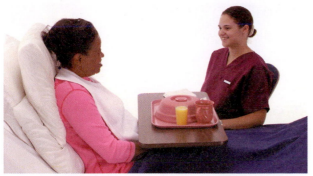

Fig. 14-11. Being friendly and positive during mealtime can promote appetite and prevent unintended weight loss.

G   Respond promptly to resident complaints about foods. Serve favorite foods.

G   Season food to the resident's preferences.

G   Use special assistive equipment as needed to increase independence with eating.

G   Record the meal/snack intake as ordered.

G   Ask the nurse for a dietitian, occupational therapist, or speech-language pathologist consultation if necessary.

Tip

Making the Most of Snacks and Nourishments

Residents are usually fed three meals a day, along with additional snacks or nourishments. Supplemental snacks or nourishments include liquids such as milk, juice, and specially formulated nutritional drinks that may contain added protein, vitamins, or other ingredients. Solid snacks include foods like cheese and crackers, peanut butter, sherbet, gelatin, or small sandwiches. These items may be served once or twice or more often per day, and facilities are required to offer snack options that reflect each resident's personal preferences.

Sometimes snacks or nourishments are required for special diets. For example, a resident with diabetes needs all of her snacks to maintain her blood sugar while taking insulin injections. Another resident who is losing too much weight will need to drink all of his nutritional supplements to maintain a healthy weight. NAs should encourage residents to eat all of their snacks or supplements. If a resident does not finish a snack, a family member eats it, or the NA finds it in the trash, he should notify the nurse.

Family and friends may bring food or drinks into the facility for residents. Staff members must ensure that food and drinks are handled and stored properly.

Any needed assistance should be provided by staff to ensure residents can consume the item. If an NA has any concerns about food or drink brought into the facility, she should report this to the nurse.

10. Describe how to make dining enjoyable for residents

Breakfast, lunch, and dinner are often the times of the day that residents anticipate the most. Meals give residents the opportunity to see friends, to socialize, and to be independent. Mealtimes are also important for getting proper nourishment. Due to serious problems of weight loss and dehydration, NAs are responsible for encouraging eating and promoting appetites.

Guidelines: Dining

G   Follow a routine for dining. This encourages structure. Generally facilities have regular mealtimes, three times a day.

G   Residents may want to look their best for meals. Assist them with their grooming requests. All residents should be neat and clean for meals. Dress residents appropriately for dining.

G   Make sure that residents have their eyeglasses, hearing aids, dentures, and any other equipment required for eating comfortably.

G   Give residents the opportunity to perform oral care or help them perform oral care before meals.

G   Assist residents with washing their hands before eating as needed.

G   Help them with elimination needs or help them to the bathroom before eating.

G   Honor requests to seat residents by their friends. Seat residents with common interests together. Encourage conversation.

G   Position residents properly for eating. Usually this position is upright, at a 90-degree angle, which helps prevent swallowing and choking problems.

G Place residents in appropriate chairs. Wheelchairs should be positioned at the right height for the table. Many tables at facilities are adjustable. These tables should be adjusted to the right height for wheelchairs. Make sure special seats, such as geriatric chairs (geri-chairs, Chapter 11), are available if needed. Residents who use geri-chairs must be sitting upright, not reclining, while eating.

G Serve food promptly to maintain the correct temperature. Keep food covered until ready to serve. If food appears undercooked, do not serve it; report this to the nurse.

G Give residents the proper eating tools. If they need assistive devices, such as special utensils or cups, make sure they are available (Fig. 14-12). Staff must provide assistance if residents require help using these devices.

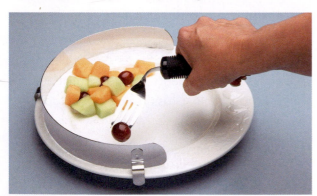

Fig. 14-12. This special utensil and plate are examples of assistive devices that can help with eating. (PHOTO COURTESY OF NORTH COAST MEDICAL, INC., WWW.NCMEDICAL.COM, 800-821-9319)

G Cut food into small portions when necessary. Do this before bringing food to the table if possible. This promotes dignity.

G Do not share a resident's food with others.

G Allow enough time for eating. Do not rush residents through their meals.

G Keep the noise level low. Do not shout or bang trays or plates (Fig. 14-13).

G Remain positive during mealtime. Make conversation when residents wish to talk.

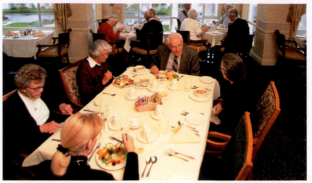

Fig. 14-13. An appealing environment is important for promoting appetites. Keep the noise level low.

G Honor requests regarding food. Residents have the legal right to ask for and receive different food. They can also request additional food. Check diet orders first before getting any extra food or additive, such as sugar or salt.

11. Describe how to serve meal trays and assist with eating

Meals are usually served on trays and are delivered from the kitchen. NAs must work quickly to make sure that food is served at the proper temperature and that residents do not have to wait long for their meals.

Guidelines: Serving Meal Trays

G Wash your hands before serving any meal trays. Wear gloves if required.

G Check the diet card for special diet orders, and identify each resident before serving a meal tray. Make sure the food looks correct for each person. Serving a resident the wrong food can cause serious health problems, even death.

G Serve all residents sitting at one table before serving other tables, so the residents will be able to eat together.

G If a resident needs your help to eat, leave the tray on the cart until you are able to do this task. Keep the door to the food cart closed after removing each tray. Maintaining the proper temperature of food helps prevent foodborne illnesses.

G Wearing gloves, prepare the food before helping residents eat. Only do what residents cannot do for themselves. Open juice or milk cartons if residents need help. If a resident is able to use a straw and wants one, place it in the container using the wrapper; do not touch straws with your fingers. Pour beverages into cups if residents do not want to use cartons. Get coffee, tea, or other drinks when residents request them. Butter rolls, bread, and vegetables as residents prefer.

G Season food according to the resident's preference, including pureed food. Making sure each resident's individual choices are honored is part of person-centered care. Remember not to use salt if a resident is on a low-sodium diet.

G When serving additional snacks or nourishments, follow the same guidelines as for serving regular meal trays. Provide needed help with snacks and nourishments. Report to the nurse if residents do not finish their supplemental snacks or nourishments.

Trivia

The Discovery of Coffee

It is commonly believed that coffee was first used by the Ethiopians in 800 AD, although various legends surround its discovery. One popular legend says that an Ethiopian goatherder named Kaldi found his goats dancing by a shrub with red berries (coffee beans). Legend has it that Kaldi tried the beans and found them to have the same energizing effect on him as they had on his goats. He shared the berries with some monks who realized that it helped them stay awake for evening prayers. And so the appreciation for coffee was born.

NAs may be required to serve meal trays to residents in isolation. Transmission-Based Precautions should be followed as ordered, in addition to Standard Precautions. Personal protective equipment may need to be donned before entering an isolation room.

For residents in isolation, disposable equipment may be used for food. It will be discarded properly after use. However, food may also be served on regular dishes with standard utensils. These items are washed and disinfected after use. Food inside an isolation room must never be shared with visitors, other residents, or staff. NAs should discard uneaten food in the proper container inside the isolation room.

Residents' Rights

Meal Trays

Before serving meal trays on a unit, the NA should check with the nurse about any special diet orders and names of residents who are not allowed to have anything to eat or drink (NPO). Diet cards should be checked carefully.

Helping residents meet their basic needs, such as eating and drinking, is part of honoring their legal rights. When food is delivered to residents' rooms, trays must be set up in a timely manner. Their trays must be prepared so they can eat as easily as possible. Not opening a milk carton or not cutting up food when needed can prevent a resident from maintaining a healthy diet. This can be considered neglectful or abusive behavior. NAs should be attentive to residents and help them meet their needs.

Residents will need different levels of assistance with eating. Being organized will help make the dining experience run smoothly. Residents who require the least amount of assistance should be helped first. The NA should make sure that everything is ready, such as opening cartons and cutting and seasoning food. When the resident is ready to feed himself, the NA can move on to the next resident. This process is continued until all residents who can eat on their own are set up and eating. The NA should check back with these residents from time to time to see if they need anything else.

Some residents will be completely unable to feed themselves. Even though the NA will help these residents eat, she should encourage them to do whatever they can for themselves. For example, if a resident can hold and use a napkin, she should. If she can hold and eat finger foods, the NA should offer them. Special assistive devices for eating can be helpful too.

Promoting independence with eating positively affects self-esteem. It is very difficult when a person has to depend on another person for assistance with a basic need such as eating. NAs should be sensitive to this and give privacy while residents are eating.

Guidelines: Helping Residents at Mealtime

G   Treat the resident with respect. Do not make fun of or judge any food choices.

G   Follow all infection prevention precautions.

G   Offer a clothing protector to the resident before assisting with eating. Do not refer to the clothing protector as a "bib." If she refuses to wear one, respect her wishes. Residents have the right to choose whether or not to use a clothing protector.

G   Sit at the resident's eye level and make eye contact. Give the resident your full attention.

G   Identify foods and fluids in front of the resident. Call pureed foods and soft foods by their correct names. For example, ask, "Would you like some steak?" rather than asking if they want "some of this brown stuff."

G   Ask the resident which foods she wants to eat first and honor her choices.

G   Do not mix foods unless the resident requests it.

G   If you are concerned that food is too hot, do not touch it to test its temperature. Put your hand over the food to sense the heat. Do not blow on it to cool it if it feels too hot. Offer other foods first to give it time to cool down.

G   Eating is a social time, and even residents who must be fed or who get their nutrition via tubes (Chapter 26) may still enjoy being social with others. Make conversation if the resident wishes, discussing appropriate

topics, such as the news, weather, the resident's life, things the resident enjoys, etc. Say positive things about the food being served. For example, "This smells really good," and, "This looks really fresh." Meal time should be a pleasant experience, and cheerful company can actually increase how much a resident eats and drinks. Do not rush residents through their meals.

G   Pay attention to the person you are helping; do not talk to other staff members while assisting residents with eating.

G   Alternate between food and drink. Offer fluids to the resident throughout the meal.

G   If a resident wants different food than what is being served, tell the dietitian or the nurse right away. Residents have the right to food and drink choices that meet their needs and preferences.

G   If a resident refuses to eat, respect this. Do not insist that she eat the food, but report it to the nurse immediately.

Feeding a resident

Equipment: meal; beverage; eating utensils; clothing protector; washcloths, wipes, towel, or paper towels

1.   Identify yourself by name. Identify the resident. Greet the resident by name.

2.   Wash your hands.

3.   Explain procedure to the resident. Speak clearly, slowly, and directly. Maintain face-to-face contact whenever possible.

4.   Provide for the resident's privacy with a curtain, screen, or door.

5.   Look at the diet card or menu. Ask the resident to state her name. If the resident is unable to state her name, check identification another way, such as looking at a photo ID or an armband. Verify that the resident has received the right tray.

6. Raise the head of the bed. Make sure the resident is in an upright sitting position (at a 90-degree angle).

7. Adjust the bed height so you will be able to sit at the resident's eye level. Lock bed wheels.

8. Place the tray where it can be easily seen by the resident, such as on the overbed table.

9. Help the resident clean her hands with a wet washcloth, hand wipe, towel, or paper towel if the resident cannot do it herself.

10. Help the resident to put on a clothing protector if desired.

11. Sit facing the resident at the resident's eye level (Fig. 14-14). Sit on the stronger side if the resident has one-sided weakness. Do not sit on the resident's bed.

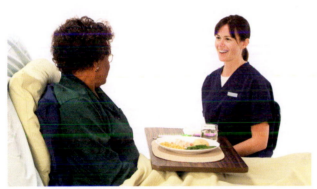

Fig. 14-14. The resident should be sitting upright, and the NA should be sitting at her eye level.

12. Tell the resident what foods and beverages are on the tray. Offer a drink and ask what the resident would like to eat first.

13. Check the temperature of the food (see previous guidelines). Using utensils, offer the food in bite-sized pieces, telling the resident the content of each bite of food offered (Fig. 14-15). Alternate types of food, allowing for the resident's preferences. Do not feed all of one type before offering another type. Make sure the resident's mouth is empty before the next bite or sip is offered. Report any swallowing problems to the nurse immediately. If

the resident has one-sided weakness, direct food to the unaffected, or stronger, side.

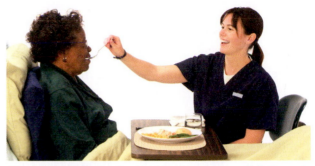

Fig. 14-15. Offer the food in bite-sized pieces. Tell the resident the content of each bite of food.

14. Ask the resident if she is ready for the next sip of the beverage. Offer sips of beverage to the resident throughout the meal. If you are holding the cup, touch it to the resident's lips before you tip it. Give small, frequent sips.

15. Talk with the resident during the meal (Fig. 14-16).

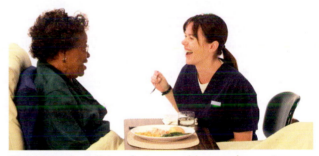

Fig. 14-16. Socializing during mealtime makes eating more enjoyable. It may help promote a healthy appetite.

16. Use a washcloth, wipe, towel, or paper towel to wipe food from the resident's mouth and hands as needed during the meal. Wipe again at the end of the meal (Fig. 14-17).

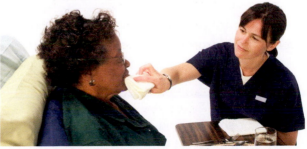

Fig. 14-17. Wiping food from the mouth during the meal helps to maintain the resident's dignity.

17. Remove the clothing protector if used. Place it and used washcloths or wipes in the proper containers.

18. Remove the food tray. Check for eyeglasses, dentures, hearing aids, or any personal items before removing the tray. Place the tray in the proper area to be picked up.

19. Make the resident comfortable. Keep the resident in the upright position for at least 30 minutes after eating and drinking. Make sure the bed is free from crumbs.

20. Return the bed to its lowest position. Remove privacy measures.

21. Leave call light within the resident's reach.

22. Wash your hands.

23. Be courteous and respectful at all times.

24. Report any changes in the resident to the nurse. Document procedure using facility guidelines. Record intake of solid food and fluids properly (see Learning Objective 14 for more information).

Residents' Rights

Residents' Rights and Eating

Residents have the legal right to refuse food and drink. Residents also have the right to ask for and receive different kinds of food. Report any refusals or requests for different food or drink right away.

12. Describe how to assist residents with special needs

Residents with certain diseases or conditions, such as Parkinson's disease, stroke, dementia, head trauma, blindness, or confusion, may need special assistance when eating. For example, a resident who has Parkinson's disease may have tremors or shaking and stiffness, which make it very difficult to eat without help. These techniques can be helpful when residents have special needs.

Guidelines: Dining Techniques

G Use assistive devices for eating when necessary. They help people feed themselves. Utensils with padded handles and plates with high edges to prevent food from sliding off are two examples of assistive devices for eating. These devices are ordered for specific residents and should be included on the meal tray.

G To help maintain independence with eating, residents may benefit from physical and verbal cues. A *cue* is something that signals that a person should do something. The hand-over-hand approach is an example of a physical cue. The resident lifts a utensil if he is able, and you put your hand over his to help with eating (Fig. 14-18). With your hand placed over the resident's hand, assist in getting food on the utensil. Steer the utensil from the plate to the mouth and back. Repeat this until the resident is finished with his meal.

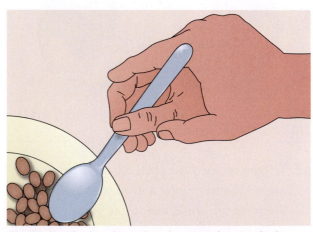

Fig. 14-18. *The hand-over-hand approach is used when a resident can help by lifting utensils. It helps promote independence.*

G Verbal cues must be short and clear so that they are easily understood. After each task is done, give additional prompts one at a time, such as, "Pick up your spoon." "Put some potatoes on your spoon." "Lift the spoon to your mouth." Wait until the resident has finished one task before asking him to do another. The cues are repeated until the resident has finished eating.

G For residents who have had a stroke and have a paralyzed or weaker side, always put food into the stronger, or unaffected, side of the mouth. This helps prevent choking. Make sure food is swallowed before offering more bites.

G For residents who have Parkinson's disease, dementia, confusion, or trauma, use physical and verbal cues if needed. Allow enough time to chew and swallow. Place food and drinks within the resident's reach.

G For residents who are visually impaired or blind, read menus aloud if needed. Allow enough time for making a decision about menu items. When assisting with eating, face them when speaking and use a normal tone of voice. Place the plate or tray directly in front of residents. Use the face of an imaginary clock to explain the position of items in front of them (Fig. 14-19). If necessary, let residents know when to open their mouths and what food they are eating.

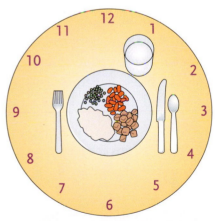

Fig. 14-19. *Use the face of an imaginary clock to explain the position of food to resident with a visual impairment.*

G If residents eat too quickly, remind them to chew, and set the utensils down between bites. Use smaller cups and plates and put less food on plates.

G If residents bite down on utensils, ask them to open their mouths. Wait until the jaw relaxes to pull the utensil out of the mouth. Offer finger foods instead. Use smaller utensils, but do not use plastic utensils. Avoid using forks.

G If residents cannot or will not chew, lightly press on the edge of the lips or on the chin to stimulate chewing. You can also show residents how to chew by doing it yourself. Serve softer foods that require less chewing; dip meats and other foods in sauce or gravy.

G If residents will not stop chewing, ask them to stop chewing. Offer smaller bites of food and feed softer foods that do not need as much chewing.

G If residents hold food in their mouths, remind them to chew and swallow the food. After feeding a bite of food, lightly press an empty teaspoon against the lips to encourage swallowing. This may help stimulate saliva production, along with the swallowing reflex.

G If residents pocket food in their cheeks, ask them to chew and swallow the food. Touch the outside of the cheek and ask them to use their tongue to get the food. Using your fingers on the cheek near the lower jaw, gently push food toward the teeth. Avoid offering food such as rice that can stick inside the mouth or on dentures. Give sips of fluid often. Check the mouth for food often before offering more food, but do not place your fingers inside the mouth. Ask the resident to open his mouth so that you can check for food. Ask residents not to stand up with food in their mouths.

G If residents have poor lip closure, remind them to close their lips. Show them how to do this if necessary. A speech-language pathologist or a nurse may teach residents to practice blowing a whistle to help close their lips.

G If residents have no teeth or are missing teeth, thickened liquids or soft or pureed diets may be ordered.

G   If residents have dentures that do not fit properly, report it to the nurse immediately. A dentist will evaluate the resident as soon as possible for denture replacement. Thickened liquids or soft or pureed diets may be ordered until dentures are replaced. Residents must be able to eat while waiting for denture repair.

G   If residents have a change in vision, it can cause problems with seeing food clearly, which may reduce appetite. Make sure eyeglasses are clean and are worn if needed. Report to the nurse if eyeglasses are damaged or broken. Read menus out loud and describe food in front of residents, using the imaginary clock if necessary.

G   If residents have a protruding tongue or tongue thrust, use special straws and cups to help. A *tongue thrust* is a forceful protrusion of the tongue, often during eating and drinking. The jaw will need to be encouraged to move upward so that the tongue will retract and the lips will close on the eating utensil. A speech-language pathologist or a nurse may teach residents to practice blowing a whistle to help close their lips.

G   If residents will not open their mouths, touch the lower lip. This may encourage the mouth to open. Identify each bite of food you offer. Do not feed sticky food such as peanut butter.

G   If residents fall asleep while eating, seat them with residents who talk a lot and are very social. Make appropriate conversation while residents are eating.

G   If residents choke when drinking, remind them to lift their chins before taking a sip of fluid. Offer fluids when residents have no food in their mouths. Residents should be seated, not standing, while drinking.

G   If residents are susceptible to choking when eating, avoid foods like cake, hot dogs, peanut butter, nuts, popcorn, raw vegetables, and certain fruits, like grapes.

G   If residents forget to eat, remind them to take another bite. Offer praise and encouragement. Do not rush them.

G   If residents drool excessively, make sure they are in an upright eating position, using proper posture. A consultation with a speech-language pathologist may be ordered to help residents learn better swallowing techniques. If drooling interferes with basic safety, medications may be ordered to decrease drooling. Clothing protectors, towels, or pads can be used to protect clothing.

G   If residents have poor sitting balance, seat them in regular dining chairs with armrests, not wheelchairs. Position them upright at a 90-degree angle. Knees should be flexed, and feet and arms should be fully supported. Push chairs under tables and place forearms on the table.

G   If residents tend to lean to one side, ask them to keep their elbows on the table. Using a wheelchair wedge cushion may help.

G   If residents tend to fall forward, using a geriatric chair may help. A wheelchair wedge cushion may also help.

G   If residents have poor neck control, a soft neck brace may be used to stabilize the head. For residents are in geriatric chairs, a wedge cushion behind the head and shoulders may be used.

Chapter 22 contains tips for feeding residents who are cognitively impaired.

13. Discuss dysphagia and list guidelines for preventing aspiration

Difficulty swallowing, or dysphagia, can be a serious problem for elderly residents. Illnesses (such as stroke), certain medications, problems with the mouth and throat muscles, weakness, and food choices are some causes of dysphagia. Problems with teeth or dentures also put a person at risk for swallowing problems. The lack of proper oral hygiene can affect the ability to eat or drink safely.

NAs must report signs and symptoms of swallowing problems to the nurse immediately. Nurses, doctors, and other care team members, such as the speech-language pathologist, will determine what steps to take to reduce dysphagia.

Observing and Reporting: Dysphagia

O/R Eating very slowly

O/R Avoidance of eating

O/R Spitting out pieces of food

O/R Difficulty chewing food

O/R Difficulty swallowing small bites of food or pills (signs of this include uneaten food, pills not being taken when directed, pills being hidden or pocketed in the mouth or cheek)

O/R Swallowing several times when eating a single bite

O/R Dribbling saliva, food or fluid from the mouth

O/R Keeping food inside the mouth or cheeks during and after meals

O/R Vomiting while eating or drinking

O/R Frequent throat clearing

O/R Food or fluid coming up into or out of the nose

O/R Coughing during or after meals

O/R Choking during meals or while drinking

O/R Gurgling sound in voice during or after meals

O/R Problems breathing when eating or drinking

O/R Visible effort to swallow

O/R Watering eyes when eating or drinking

In addition, observing and reporting the following may help the care team assess a resident who has dysphagia:

O/R Type of food or drink that caused the problem

O/R Time of day the problem occurred

O/R Whether or not the resident had dentures in place when the problem happened

O/R Whether or not the resident was talking or laughing when the choking occurred

O/R How the resident was positioned while eating or drinking

O/R Whether or not the resident was ambulating (walking) while eating or drinking

Swallowing problems greatly increase a person's risk for choking on food or drink. When a person chokes, mucus, food or fluids, or emesis (vomitus) may move into the lungs. Inhaling food, drink, or foreign material into the lungs is called *aspiration*, which can cause pneumonia or death. It is very important to prevent aspiration.

Guidelines: Preventing Aspiration

G Place residents in proper position for eating and drinking. They must sit upright at a 90-degree angle (Fig. 14-20). Do not feed residents in a reclining position.

G Feed residents slowly.

G Avoid distractions while eating.

G Offer small pieces of food or small spoonfuls of pureed food.

G Offer food, then a liquid. Repeat this.

G Place food in the nonparalyzed or unaffected (stronger) side of the mouth.

G Make sure food is actually swallowed after each bite before offering more food or fluids. However, do not put your fingers inside a resident's mouth.

G Keep residents sitting upright for at least 30 minutes after eating and drinking.

G Provide careful mouth care after eating.

G Closely observe residents who choke easily during eating and drinking. Report signs of aspiration, such as gagging, vomiting, clutching throat, cyanosis (bluish skin color), darkening skin, unconsciousness, shortness of breath, difficulty breathing, or the resident complaints of chest pain or tightness in the chest to the nurse immediately.

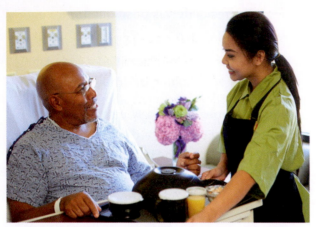

Fig. 14-20. *Sitting as upright as possible when eating and drinking helps prevent aspiration.*

More information on swallowing difficulties and alternative methods of feeding is located in Chapter 26.

Residents' Rights

Patience When Feeding Residents

Feeding residents quickly is dangerous. It increases the risk of choking and aspiration. When helping residents eat, the NA should take her time and not rush residents through the dining process. Being patient and positive helps promote each resident's safety, and may increase the amount the resident eats and drinks.

14. Describe intake and output (I&O)

The fluid a person consumes is called **intake**, or **input**. **Output** is the fluid that is eliminated from the body each day. Output includes urine, feces, and vomitus, as well as perspiration and moisture in the air that a person exhales. It also includes suctioned material and wound drainage. When a person maintains equal intake and output, or consumes and eliminates equal amounts of fluid, it is called **fluid balance**.

Most people maintain fluid balance naturally. However, residents on special diets or who have certain illnesses may need to have their intake and output (I&O) measured. Measuring I&O means that staff record and add together all of the amounts of food and fluids the resident takes in and eliminates within 24 hours. This is recorded on an Intake/Output (I&O) sheet (Fig. 14-21).

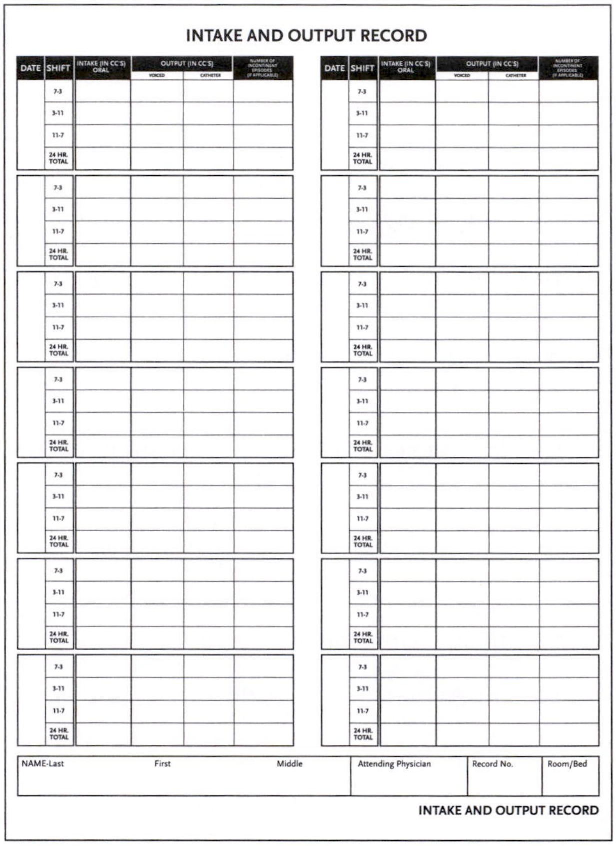

INTAKE AND OUTPUT RECORD

DATE	SHIFT	INTAKE (IN CC'S) ORAL	OUTPUT (IN CC'S) VOIDED	CATHETER	NUMBER OF INCONTINENT EPISODES (IF APPLICABLE)	DATE	SHIFT	INTAKE (IN CC'S) ORAL	OUTPUT (IN CC'S) VOIDED	CATHETER	NUMBER OF INCONTINENT EPISODES (IF APPLICABLE)
	7-3						7-3				
	3-11						3-11				
	11-7						11-7				
	24 HR. TOTAL						24 HR. TOTAL				

NAME-Last   First   Middle   Attending Physician   Record No.   Room/Bed

INTAKE AND OUTPUT RECORD

Fig. 14-21. *A sample intake and output (I&O) record.*

Fluids are usually measured in milliliters (mL). Milliliters are units of measurement in the metric system. One milliliter is 1/1000 of a liter. Ounces (oz) are converted to milliliters. One ounce equals 30 milliliters, so to convert ounces to milliliters, the number of ounces must be multiplied by 30. **Graduates** are containers that measure fluid in milliliters and may also measure in ounces (Fig. 14-22). Some common conversions are listed in the box below.

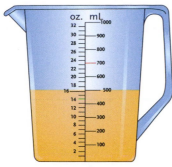

Fig. 14-22. A graduate is a container for measuring fluid volume.

Conversions

One ounce equals 30 milliliters (mL). To convert ounces to milliliters, the number of ounces must be multiplied by 30.

1 oz. = 30 mL

2 oz. = 60 mL

3 oz. = 90 mL

4 oz. = 120 mL

5 oz. = 150 mL

6 oz. = 180 mL

7 oz. = 210 mL

8 oz. = 240 mL

¼ cup = 2 oz. = 60 mL

½ cup = 4 oz. = 120 mL

¾ cup = 6 oz. = 180 mL

1 cup = 8 oz. = 240 mL

2 cups = 16 oz. = 480 mL

4 cups = 32 oz. = 960 mL

For example, an NA serves a resident an eight-ounce glass of juice. The resident consumes about half of the juice, or four ounces. To determine her intake, the ounces must be converted to milliliters. Four ounces multiplied by 30 equals 120 milliliters. The NA would document 120 mL of juice consumed on the intake sheet.

Measuring and recording intake and output

Equipment: I&O sheet, pen and paper

Measure intake first.

1. Identify yourself by name. Identify the resident. Greet the resident by name.

2. Wash your hands.

3. Explain procedure to resident. Speak clearly, slowly, and directly. Maintain face-to-face contact whenever possible.

4. Provide for the resident's privacy with a curtain, screen, or door.

5. A list of container sizes should be available to help with measuring. For example, a water cup equals 240 mL, a cereal bowl equals 150 mL, and a milk carton equals 240 mL. Note the amount of fluid the resident is served on paper.

6. When the resident has finished a meal or snack, measure any leftover fluids. Note this amount on paper. (If the amount is between measurement lines, you may need to round up to the nearest 25 mL. Follow policy.)

7. Subtract the leftover amount from the amount served. If you have measured in ounces, convert to milliliters (mL) by multiplying by 30.

8. Record the amount of fluid consumed (in mL) in the input column on the I&O sheet. Record the time and type of fluid consumed.

9. Wash your hands.

Measuring output is the other half of monitoring fluid balance.

Chapter 16 contains information about emptying and measuring urine from a catheter drainage bag.

Equipment: I&O sheet, graduate, gloves, additional PPE if required

1. Wash your hands.

2. Put on gloves before handling bedpan/urinal.

3. Pour the contents of the bedpan or urinal into the graduate. Do not spill or splash any of the urine.

4. Place the graduate on a flat surface. Measure the amount of urine at eye level. Keep the

container level (Fig. 14-23). (If the amount is between measurement lines, you may need to round up to the nearest 25 mL. Follow policy.)

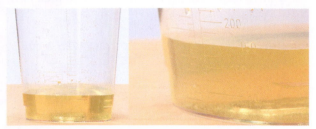

Fig. 14-23. *Keep the container on a flat surface while measuring output.*

5. After measuring urine, empty the contents of the graduate into the toilet without splashing.

6. Rinse the graduate and pour the rinse water into the toilet.

7. Rinse the bedpan/urinal and pour the rinse water into the toilet. Flush the toilet.

8. Place the graduate and bedpan in the area for cleaning or clean and store them according to policy.

9. Remove and discard gloves properly.

10. Wash hands before recording output.

11. Immediately document the time and amount of urine in the output column on the sheet. Report any changes to the nurse.

All facilities keep track of how much food and liquid a resident consumes. Percentages are often used to document food intake, but the specific method can vary (Fig. 14-24). The dietitian calculates the percentages for meals. The NA may be asked to document how much of the meal a resident ate. For example, if the resident ate the entire meal served, the NA would document that 100% was eaten. If the resident ate about half of the meal, the NA would document 50% was eaten, and so on.

It is very important for NAs to document food intake accurately. When documenting intake, NAs must document the food that was eaten, not the food that remains on the plate or tray. If a resident eats less than 75% of his or her meal, the NA should report it to the nurse.

15. List ways to identify and prevent dehydration

Water is one of the most essential nutrients for life. Drinking enough water or other fluids each day can help prevent constipation, urinary incontinence, and dehydration. Dehydration is a serious condition that occurs when a person does not have enough fluid in the body. Proper fluid intake also helps to dilute wastes and flush out the urinary system, which lessens the risk of infection.

A general recommendation for daily fluid intake is 64 ounces (or eight 8-ounce glasses) for a healthy person. However, that is not necessarily a firm guideline for health. Some people may need more than 64 ounces, while others may need less. The amount needed depends on factors such as activity, heat, age, weight, and overall health.

Because the sense of thirst decreases as people age, fluids should be offered to residents often. A doctor may prescribe an order to encourage fluids (sometimes called *force fluids*) for a resident who is at risk of dehydration.

Observing and Reporting: Dehydration

- °/R Resident drinks fewer than six 8-ounce glasses of liquid per day

- °/R Resident drinks little or no fluids at meals

- °/R Resident needs help drinking from a cup or glass

- °/R Resident has trouble swallowing liquids

- °/R Resident has frequent vomiting, diarrhea, or fever

- °/R Resident is easily confused or tired

- °/R Resident is thirsty

Nutrition and Fluid Balance

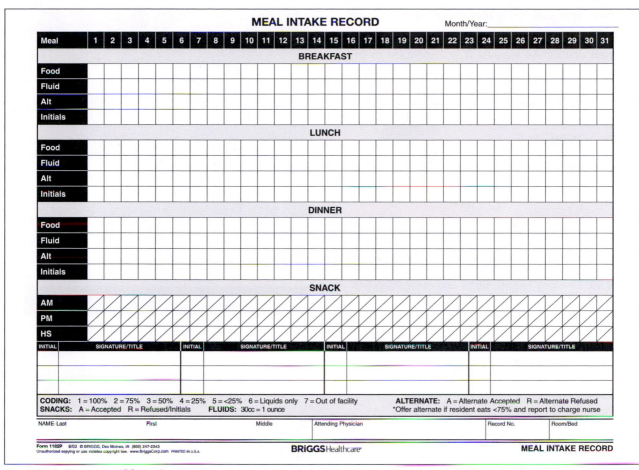

Meal	1	2	3	4	5	6	7	8	9	10	11	12	13	14	15	16	17	18	19	20	21	22	23	24	25	26	27	28	29	30	31
BREAKFAST																															
Food																															
Fluid																															
Alt																															
Initials																															
LUNCH																															
Food																															
Fluid																															
Alt																															
Initials																															
DINNER																															
Food																															
Fluid																															
Alt																															
Initials																															
SNACK																															
AM																															
PM																															
HS																															

MEAL INTAKE RECORD   Month/Year: _____

INITIAL	SIGNATURE/TITLE	INITIAL	SIGNATURE/TITLE	INITIAL	SIGNATURE/TITLE	INITIAL	SIGNATURE/TITLE

CODING: 1 = 100% 2 = 75% 3 = 50% 4 = 25% 5 = <25% 6 = Liquids only 7 = Out of facility   **ALTERNATE:** A = Alternate Accepted R = Alternate Refused
SNACKS: A = Accepted R = Refused/Initials   **FLUIDS:** 30cc = 1 ounce   *Offer alternate if resident eats <75% and report to charge nurse

NAME-Last	First	Middle	Attending Physician	Record No.	Room/Bed

Form 1182P   8/02 © BRIGGS, Des Moines, IA (800) 247-2343
Unauthorized copying or use violates copyright law. www.BriggsCorp.com PRINTED IN U.S.A.   **BRiGGS** Healthcare·   **MEAL INTAKE RECORD**

Fig. 14-24. *One type of form for documenting meal intake.* (REPRINTED WITH PERMISSION OF BRIGGS HEALTHCARE®, 800.247.2343, BRIGGSHEALTHCARE.COM)

O/R Resident has a dry mouth

O/R Resident has a decrease in urinary output

Also report if the resident has any of these signs or symptoms:

O/R Severe thirst

O/R Dry mouth and mucous membranes

O/R Cracked lips

O/R Dry, warm, wrinkled, or clammy skin

O/R Sunken eyes

O/R Flushed face

O/R Dark urine

O/R Strong-smelling urine

O/R Constipation or weight loss

O/R Weakness, dizziness, lightheadedness, or confusion

O/R Headache

O/R Irritability

O/R Rapid or weakened pulse

O/R Irregular heartbeat

O/R Low blood pressure

Guidelines: Preventing Dehydration

G Report observations and warning signs to the nurse immediately.

G Encourage residents to drink fluids every time you see them. As long as the resident does not have a fluid restriction, offer fresh water or other fluids often (Fig. 14-25).

G Offer drinks that residents enjoy. Some may prefer water or sparkling water (seltzer water). Some may not like water and prefer other types of beverages, such as juice, milk, or tea. Some residents will not want ice in their drinks. As always, it is important to provide person-centered care. Honor personal preferences.

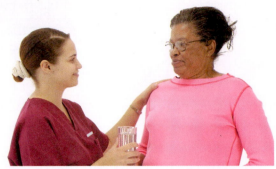

Fig. 14-25. Drinking enough water and other fluids promotes health. Encouraging residents to drink often can help prevent dehydration.

G   Make sure you know if the resident requires thickened liquids and which thickening consistency is needed.

G   Make sure water pitcher and cup are close enough to the resident and light enough for the resident to lift, approximately half full.

G   Offer assistance if the resident cannot drink without help. Use assistive devices as needed.

G   Offer ice chips, flavored ice sticks, and gelatin often. These items are considered liquids. Do not offer ice chips or sticks if resident has a swallowing problem.

G   Keep accurate intake and output (I&O) records.

G   Follow posted schedules for offering fluids.

In order to encourage fluid intake, NAs can remember the acronym POURR:

Post a regular schedule for offering fluids to residents.

Observe residents carefully for signs and symptoms of dehydration.

Use other kinds of fluids, such as flavored frozen ice sticks, to improve fluid balance and increase fluid intake.

Remind all staff, visitors, and volunteers as necessary of the importance of following the schedule.

Report changes in fluid balance or any signs and symptoms of dehydration promptly.

Serving fresh water

Equipment: water pitcher, ice scoop, cup, straw, gloves

1. Identify yourself by name. Identify the resident. Greet the resident by name.

2. Wash your hands.

3. Put on gloves.

4. Scoop ice into the water pitcher without touching the ice scoop to the pitcher. Add fresh water without allowing the pitcher to touch the faucet.

5. Use and store the ice scoop properly. Do not allow the ice to touch your gloved hand and fall back into the container. Place the scoop into the proper receptacle after each use.

6. Take the pitcher to the resident.

7. Pour water into the cup for the resident. Offer the resident a drink of water. Leave the pitcher and cup at the bedside.

8. Make sure the pitcher and cup are light enough for the resident to lift. Leave a straw if the resident desires it and is allowed to use one (if he does not have swallowing problems).

9. Make the resident comfortable.

10. Leave call light within the resident's reach.

11. Remove and discard gloves properly.

12. Wash your hands.

13. Be courteous and respectful at all times.

16. List signs and symptoms of fluid overload and describe conditions that may require fluid restrictions

Fluid overload is a condition that occurs when more fluid enters the body than is eliminated from the body. The body cannot eliminate the additional fluid, and fluid gathers in certain areas of the body, such as the ankles. Fluid overload can occur when the heart, kidneys, or lungs are not working properly. People can also have this problem after having surgery.

Observing and Reporting: Fluid Overload

O/R Weight gain (daily weight gain of one to two pounds)

O/R Fatigue

O/R Lung congestion, difficulty breathing, or shortness of breath, especially if lying down

O/R Swelling of the ankles, feet, fingers, or hands (edema)

O/R Coughing

O/R Decreased urine output

O/R Increased heart rate

O/R Skin that appears tight, smooth, and shiny

O/R Swollen abdomen due to excess fluid, called *ascites*

Fluid overload is usually treated with medicine to eliminate the excessive fluid, increasing the number of pillows used for sleep, and careful monitoring of weight gain and edema.

Fluid restrictions are ordered when the amount of fluid must be carefully measured and limited due to certain disorders. Examples are congestive heart failure (CHF) (Chapter 19), or chronic renal failure (Chapter 16). Some residents will have a **restrict fluids (RF)** order, which means the person is allowed to drink, but must limit the daily amount to a level set by the doctor. This is different from an NPO order, which means the resident should not have any fluids. When a resident has a restrict fluids order, the NA should not give the resident extra fluids or a water pitcher unless the nurse approves it. Other reasons for fluid restrictions include the following:

• Recent surgery

• Illness, such as a gastrointestinal (GI) illness

• Special medical test

• Having a feeding tube (Chapter 26)

Chapter Review

1. List five common nutritional problems that elderly people may experience (LO 2).

2. According to MyPlate's suggestions, what should half of a person's plate be made up of (LO 5)?

3. List some examples of plant sources of protein foods (LO 5).

4. According to MyPlate, what fat percentages should a person choose most often from the dairy group (LO 5)?

5. List the information contained on diet cards (LO 6).

6. What is one common abbreviation for a sodium-controlled diet (LO 7)?

7. What is the difference between a clear liquid diet and a full liquid diet (LO 7)?

8. What is the benefit of thickening liquids (LO 8)?

9. What is the proper position in which to place a resident for eating (LO 10)?

10. If a resident refuses to wear a clothing protector, what should the NA do (LO 11)?

11. How should an NA properly test the temperature of food if she feels it might be too hot (LO 11)?

12. To which side of the mouth should food be directed if a resident has a weaker side—the weaker (affected) or stronger (unaffected) side (LO 12)?

13. When assisting a resident who is visually impaired, how should the NA describe the position of food and objects in front of the resident (LO 12)?

14. List four examples of output (LO 14).

15. How many milliliters (mL) equal one ounce (oz.) (LO 14)?

16. What are three ways that proper fluid intake benefits the body (LO 15)?

17. What is a restrict fluids (RF) order (LO 16)?

Multiple Choice

18. Which of the following is the correct term for a person who does not eat any animals or animal products (LO 3)?
    (A) Omnivore
    (B) Vegan
    (C) Carnivore
    (D) Pescetarian

19. Which of the following is the most essential nutrient for life (LO 4)?
    (A) Water
    (B) Protein
    (C) Vegetables
    (D) Grains

20. Which of the following abbreviations means that a resident should not have anything to eat or drink (LO 7)?
    (A) RR
    (B) RF
    (C) NPO
    (D) ADA

21. Which of the following puts a resident at an increased risk of unintended weight loss (LO 9)?
    (A) The resident is a vegetarian.
    (B) The resident has difficulty swallowing.
    (C) The resident enjoys socializing during mealtime.
    (D) The resident eats snacks between meals.

22. One way for an NA to help prevent aspiration is to (LO 13)
    (A) Place food in the resident's weaker side of the mouth
    (B) Not offer the resident a drink until the meal has been eaten
    (C) Make sure the resident is sitting upright for eating and drinking
    (D) Feed the resident quickly

15
The Gastrointestinal System

Privies Over the Centuries

"Sewage disposal was not unprovided for in the 14th century, though far from adequate. Privies . . . and public latrines existed, though they did not replace open street sewers. Castles and wealthy townhouses had privies built . . . with a hole in the bottom allowing the deposit to fall into a river or a ditch. . . . Town houses away from the riverbank had cesspools in the backyard. They frequently seeped into wells and other water sources. . . . The 15th and later centuries preferred to ignore human elimination."

From *A Distant Mirror* by Barbara Tuchman

"One should eat to live, not live to eat."

Moliere, 1622–1673

"Give no more to every guest Than he's able to digest."

Jonathan Swift, 1667–1745

1. Define important words in this chapter

absorption: the transfer of nutrients from the intestines to the cells.

anatomy: the study of body structure.

biology: the study of all life forms.

body systems: groups of organs that perform specific functions in the human body.

bowel elimination: the physical process of releasing or emptying the colon or large intestine of solid waste, called *stool* or *feces*.

cells: the basic structural units of all organisms.

chyme: semiliquid substance made as a result of the chemical breakdown of food in the stomach.

colon: the large intestine.

colostomy: surgically created opening through the abdominal wall into the large intestine to allow feces to be expelled.

constipation: the inability to eliminate stool, or the infrequent, difficult, and often painful elimination of hard, dry stool.

Crohn's disease: a disease that causes the lining of the digestive tract to become inflamed (red, sore, and swollen).

defecation: the process of eliminating feces from the rectum through the anus.

diarrhea: frequent elimination of liquid or semiliquid feces.

digestion: the process of converting food so that it can be absorbed into the blood and used by body tissues.

diverticulitis: inflammation of sacs that develop in the wall of the large intestine due to diverticulosis.

diverticulosis: a disorder in which sac-like pouchings develop in weakened areas of the wall of the large intestine (colon).

duodenum: the first part of the small intestine, where the common bile duct enters the small intestine.

electrolytes: chemical substances that are essential to maintaining fluid balance and homeostasis in the body.

elimination: the process of expelling wastes.

enema: a specific amount of water or other fluid, with or without an additive, introduced into the colon to stimulate the elimination of stool.

fecal impaction: a mass of dry, hard stool that remains packed in the rectum and cannot be expelled.

fecal incontinence: an inability to control the muscles of the bowels, which leads to an involuntary passage of stool or gas.

feces: solid body waste excreted through the anus from the large intestine; also called *stool*.

flatulence: air in the intestine that is passed through the rectum; also called *gas* or *flatus*.

fracture pan: a bedpan that is flatter than a regular bedpan; used for small or thin people or those who cannot lift their buttocks onto a standard bedpan.

gastroesophageal reflux disease (GERD): a chronic condition in which the liquid contents of the stomach back up into the esophagus.

gastrointestinal tract: a continuous tube from the opening of the mouth all the way to the anus, where solid wastes are eliminated from the body.

heartburn: a condition that results from a weakening of the sphincter muscle that joins the esophagus and the stomach; also known as *acid reflux*.

hemorrhoids: enlarged veins in the rectum that can cause itching, burning, pain, and bleeding.

homeostasis: the condition in which all of the body's systems are balanced and are working at their best.

ileostomy: surgically created opening into the end of the small intestine, the ileum, to allow feces to be expelled.

ingestion: the process of taking food or fluids into the body.

irritable bowel syndrome (IBS): a chronic condition of the large intestine that is worsened by stress.

malabsorption: a condition in which the body cannot absorb or digest a particular nutrient properly.

occult: hidden.

organ: a structural unit in the human body that performs a specific function.

ostomy: surgical creation of an opening from an area inside the body to the outside.

pathophysiology: the study of the disorders that occur in the body.

peristalsis: muscular contractions that push food through the gastrointestinal tract.

physiology: the study of how body parts function.

portable commode: a chair with a toilet seat and a removable container underneath that is used for elimination; also called *bedside commode*.

rectal suppository: a medication in a cylindrical shape that is given rectally to cause a bowel movement.

specimen: a sample, such as tissue, blood, urine, stool, or sputum, used for analysis and diagnosis.

stoma: an artificial opening in the body.

stool: solid body waste excreted through the anus from the large intestine; also called *feces*.

tissues: a group of cells that performs similar tasks.

ulcerative colitis: a chronic inflammatory disease of the large intestine.

urostomy: surgical creation of an opening for the passage of urine.

2. Explain key terms related to the body

Biology is the study of all life forms. Anatomy and physiology are a part of the science of biology. **Anatomy** is the study of body structure, while **physiology** looks at how body parts function.

The human body is made up of many different kinds of cells. **Cells** are the basic structural units of all organisms. Living cells divide, grow, and die, renewing the tissues and organs of the body. There are different types of cells, but most are made up of the same components. Examples of cells are blood, nerve, and muscle cells.

Tissues are made up of groups of cells. Together, these groups of cells perform specific body functions. Examples of tissues are epithelial, connective, muscle, and nervous tissues.

Groups of tissues come together to form **organs**. Each organ has a specific function to perform to keep the body healthy. The heart is an example of an organ.

Organs in the human body are organized into body systems. **Body systems** are made up of different organs that perform specific functions in the body. Each system in the body has its own unique function. The circulatory system, consisting of the heart, blood vessels, and blood, is one example of a body system. The urinary system, consisting of the kidneys, ureters, bladder, and urethra, is another body system. Chapters 15 through 24 discuss body systems and related care. This textbook has organized the human body into these ten systems:

1. Gastrointestinal, or Digestive
2. Urinary
3. Reproductive
4. Integumentary (skin)
5. Circulatory or Cardiovascular
6. Respiratory
7. Musculoskeletal
8. Nervous
9. Endocrine
10. Immune and Lymphatic

Staying healthy and functioning normally are very important. In order to do this, the body must keep certain internal conditions stable, regardless of external factors. This is called *homeostasis*. **Homeostasis** is the condition in which all of the body's systems are balanced and are working at their best. The body maintaining its temperature around 98.6° Fahrenheit, regardless of how cold or hot it is outside, is an example of homeostasis.

Pathophysiology is the study of the disorders (conditions or diseases) that occur in the body. All body systems chapters (Chapters 15 through 24) contain information about diseases, along with normal, age-related changes for each body system listed above. Knowing what normal changes of aging are for each body system will help nursing assistants recognize any abnormal changes in residents.

3. Explain the structure and function of the gastrointestinal system

The gastrointestinal (GI) system, also called the *digestive system*, is made up of two sections: the gastrointestinal tract and the accessory organs (Fig. 15-1). The **gastrointestinal tract** is a continuous tube from the opening of the mouth all the way to the anus, where solid wastes are eliminated from the body.

Food enters the mouth when a person eats, and the tongue moves food around in the mouth. The salivary glands secrete a fluid called *saliva*, which begins lubricating and dissolving the food. The teeth break up food during a process called *mastication* (chewing). Food forms into a bolus, a mass of food that is easier to swallow. The bolus moves into the pharynx or throat, where it travels down to the esophagus, a tube about ten inches in length. This occurs as part of the swallowing reflex. Breathing pauses during swallowing because breathing and swallowing cannot occur at the same time. The epiglottis acts like a lid, shutting off the larynx during the swallowing process. This blocks food from entering the trachea and causing choking. Food moves into the stomach from the esophagus because of muscular contractions, called **peristalsis**, that push it toward the stomach.

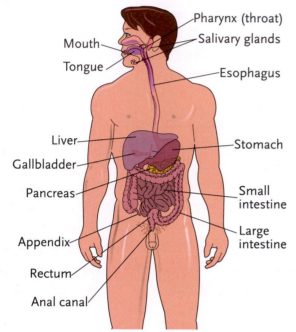

Pharynx (throat)
Mouth
Salivary glands
Tongue
Esophagus
Liver
Stomach
Gallbladder
Pancreas
Small intestine
Large intestine
Appendix
Rectum
Anal canal

Fig. 15-1. The GI system consists of all the organs needed to digest food and process waste.

When the food reaches the stomach, it mixes with gastric juice. This fluid is capable of killing most microorganisms that enter the stomach. The stomach changes the food into a substance called **chyme**. Food usually stays in the stomach for about two to six hours after eating. From there, the chyme passes into the first part of the small intestine, called the **duodenum**. The small intestine is about 20 feet long and is approximately one inch in diameter.

The small intestine receives secretions from the liver and the pancreas. The small intestine also secretes intestinal digestive juice from its walls. The liver produces bile, which is stored in the gallbladder. Bile is a substance that breaks down fats. When needed, the gallbladder sends the bile to the small intestine through the common bile duct. The pancreas produces juices that digest carbohydrates, proteins, and fats. These juices are sent to the small intestine through the pancreatic duct, which joins the common bile duct.

The small intestine is lined with villi, tiny finger-like projections that absorb food and fluids. **Absorption** takes place because nutrients from food are broken down into tiny molecules that move into the blood. Approximately 90% of food and fluids is absorbed in the small intestine.

The rest of absorption occurs in the large intestine. It is about two and one-half inches in diameter and about five feet long. The large intestine helps regulate water balance by absorbing water and electrolytes and eliminating solid waste products as **feces**. **Electrolytes** are chemical substances that are essential to maintaining fluid balance and homeostasis within the body.

The first part of the large intestine, the cecum, has a valve that prevents the feces from moving backward into the small intestine. The appendix is attached to the cecum. The exact function of the appendix is not known. The rest of the large intestine consists of the ascending, transverse, descending, and sigmoid **colon**, along with the rectum and anus. The chyme takes three to ten hours to become feces within the colon. Feces is made up of water, solid waste material, bacteria, and mucus. Feces is eliminated from the body by peristalsis through the anus, the rectal opening. This process is called **defecation**.

The functions of the gastrointestinal system are the

- **Ingestion** of food (taking food or fluids into the body)

- **Digestion** of food (converting food so that it can be absorbed into the blood and used by body tissues)

- Absorption of nutrients

- **Elimination** of waste products from food/fluids

Destination: Homeostasis

Fluid balance is a vital part of the body's ability to maintain homeostasis. A person becomes dehydrated when his output is greater than his intake. The body reacts quickly to try to correct dehydration. One of the primary responses is to stimulate thirst. If the intake of water and other fluids is not increased, the body responds by decreasing sweating and urination. If fluid balance is not restored, other more severe symptoms occur, such as kidney failure. Eliminating dehydration can be as simple as drinking a glass of water. When adequate fluids are reintroduced into the body, fluid balance and homeostasis are restored.

Trivia

Process of Digestion

Lazzaro Spallanzani (1729–1799), an Italian scientist, studied the process of digestion. He performed experiments with turkeys, owls, and kites (a type of bird), along with many other animals. His studies revealed that gastric juice is a primary factor in digestion.

4. Discuss changes in the gastrointestinal system due to aging

For each system in the body, there are normal changes of aging. Knowing these normal changes for each body system will help NAs better recognize and understand what is abnormal for the body as a person ages.

Normal age-related changes for the gastrointestinal system include the following:

- Ability to taste decreases.

- Process of digestion takes longer and is less efficient.

- Body waste moves more slowly through the intestines, causing more frequent constipation.

- Difficulty chewing and swallowing may occur.

- Absorption of vitamins and minerals decreases.

- Production of saliva and digestive fluids decreases.

In addition to normal changes of aging, there are signs and symptoms related to each body system that need to be reported to the nurse. This information is contained in all body systems chapters.

5. List normal qualities of stool and identify signs and symptoms to report about stool

Bowel elimination is the physical process of releasing or emptying the colon or large intestine of stool or feces. Feces, or **stool**, are solid waste products eliminated by the colon. The frequency of bowel movements varies; they can occur as often as one to three times per day or as infrequently as several times a week. Regular bowel movements help keep the gastrointestinal system healthy. It is especially important for elderly people to have regular bowel movements because this helps prevent serious problems, such as fecal impactions.

Stool is normally brown in color, and its consistency is soft, moist, and formed (not loose). Certain foods can change its color. For example, red gelatin or beets can make stool appear red. Green, leafy vegetables can make stool look green. Iron supplements can cause stool to turn black. Stool is tubular in shape, which is due to its passage through the colon. The amount of stool produced per day depends upon the food eaten.

Normal bowel elimination means not having any pain when passing stool. A change in stool's appearance, such as blood, pus, mucus, or worms in stool, can signal a health problem.

Observing and Reporting: Stool

O/R Bloody or abnormally colored stool (whitish, black [tarry])

O/R Hard, dry stools

O/R Liquid stools (diarrhea)

°/R Constipation (inability to have a bowel movement)

°/R Pain when having a bowel movement

°/R Blood, pus, mucus, or discharge in stool

°/R Fecal incontinence (involuntary loss of stool)

6. List factors affecting bowel elimination and describe how to promote normal bowel elimination

There are many factors that may affect normal bowel elimination:

Growth and Development: Aging affects the regularity of bowel elimination. Peristalsis slows due to a decrease in muscle tone. Tooth loss and less saliva may make eating less appealing and more challenging. Nutrients are not absorbed as well, making digestion more difficult.

To promote normal elimination, the NA should encourage fluids and nutritious meals, as well as regular exercise and activity if allowed. Regular oral care may help. Dentures should be clean, in place, and should fit properly.

Psychological Factors: The lack of privacy may affect bowel elimination. Having a roommate for the first time, being in a place that is not home, and needing help with elimination can disrupt normal elimination patterns. Anxiety, stress, fear, or anger can increase the frequency of bowel movements, causing watery, loose stools, and may even cause incontinence. Depression can decrease the frequency of elimination.

To promote normal elimination, it is very important for the NA to always provide privacy and allow plenty of time for elimination. Call lights should be left within reach, and the NA should respond to call lights and requests for help with elimination immediately. Any concerns that residents express should be reported to the nurse.

Diet: A diet low in fiber may decrease elimination and cause constipation. Foods high in

animal fats, such as dairy products, red meat, and eggs, may also cause constipation. Products containing caffeine may cause or aggravate diarrhea. Some foods cause gas, which can increase elimination but may also cause discomfort. Beans, whole grains, apples, cabbage, onions, dairy products, and carbonated drinks are examples of foods that can cause gas.

To promote normal elimination, the NA should encourage nutritious meals. Fiber intake may be increased and fatty, sugary foods may need to be decreased if constipation is a problem. A doctor may add probiotics to the resident's diet as well. A probiotic contains live bacteria and may be prescribed to increase the amount of beneficial bacteria in the gastrointestinal tract. Probiotics may come in the form of food (for example, yogurt or yogurt drinks) or pills. Probiotics may also be used for other conditions. However, probiotics are not safe for everyone, so they should not be used without a doctor's order.

Fluid Intake: The sense of thirst decreases as a person ages. A decrease in fluids may cause constipation. A lack of strength or coordination can also lower fluid intake. Some beverages, such as orange or prune juice, can increase bowel elimination.

To promote normal elimination, the NA should encourage the resident to drink fluids as long as he does not have a fluid restriction. A pitcher and cup should be left within the resident's reach and they should be light enough for the resident to lift.

Physical Activity and Exercise: A lack of exercise and mobility can weaken muscles and slow elimination. Regular physical activity helps bowel elimination by strengthening abdominal and pelvic muscles. This helps peristalsis.

To promote normal elimination, the NA should encourage exercise and regular movement. Walking, stretching, lifting light weights, and other types of approved exercise can help (Fig. 15-2).

Medications: Some medications affect bowel elimination. Antibiotics can cause diarrhea; pain relievers may cause constipation.

To promote normal elimination, laxatives may be ordered. Laxatives can help with elimination, but may cause diarrhea. The NA should report diarrhea or constipation to the nurse promptly.

Assisting with Elimination

Residents who are unable to get out of bed to use the toilet may be given a bedpan or a urinal. There are two kinds of bedpans: a standard bedpan and a fracture bedpan (Fig. 15-3). A **fracture pan** is a bedpan that is flatter than the regular bedpan. It is used for small or thin people or those who cannot lift their buttocks onto a standard bedpan. It is also used when a person has a hip fracture. Women generally use a bedpan for urination and bowel movements. Men generally use a urinal for urination and a bedpan for bowel movements.

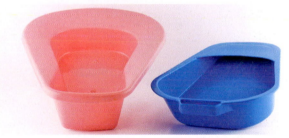

Fig. 15-3. *A standard bedpan is on the left side, and a fracture pan is on the right.*

Feces and urine are considered infectious wastes. NAs must always wear gloves when handling bedpans, urinals, or basins that contain wastes. Additional personal protective equipment (PPE) may be needed as well. NAs should be careful not to spill wastes when removing bedpans or waste containers from beds. Elimination equipment should never be placed on an overbed table or on top of a side table. A bedpan cover or disposable pad should be used to transfer bedpans to the bathroom. The NA should discard wastes in the toilet (unless a nurse needs to check the contents) and immediately place

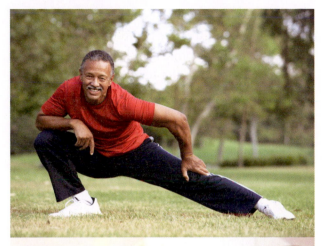
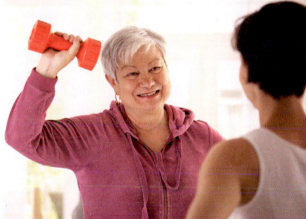

Fig. 15-2. *Regular exercise is important for promoting normal elimination, and it has many other health benefits as well. Nursing assistants should encourage approved exercise.*

Personal Habits: For many people, bowel elimination occurs not long after eating. Drinking warm fluids may also trigger bowel elimination because they stimulate peristalsis. Positioning in bed also affects elimination. A resident who is lying flat on his back (supine) will have difficulty with elimination because it is difficult to contract the muscles in this position.

To promote normal elimination, the NA should make sure each resident is helped to the bathroom at the time of day that is best for the resident. Using a familiar bathroom may help. For a resident who cannot make it to the bathroom, the NA should get a portable commode. If the resident uses a bedpan, the head of the bed should be raised. The best position for elimination is squatting and leaning forward.

the containers in the proper area for cleaning or clean and store them according to policy. Cleaning them right away helps avoid odors.

A standard bedpan should be placed so that the wider end is aligned with a resident's buttocks. A fracture pan should be placed with the handle toward the foot of the bed. Warm water may be used to warm a cold bedpan, but the bedpan then must be completely dried before being placed under a resident.

Assisting a resident with use of a bedpan

Equipment: bedpan, bedpan cover, disposable bed protector, bath blanket, toilet paper, disposable wipes, 2 towels, supplies for perineal care, 2 pairs of gloves

1. Identify yourself by name. Identify the resident. Greet the resident by name.

2. Wash your hands.

3. Explain procedure to the resident. Speak clearly, slowly, and directly. Maintain face-to-face contact whenever possible.

4. Provide for the resident's privacy with a curtain, screen, or door.

5. Adjust the bed to a safe level, usually waist high. Raise the far bed rail (if used). Before placing the bedpan, lower the head of the bed. Lock bed wheels.

6. Put on gloves.

7. Cover the resident with the bath blanket. Ask him to hold it while you pull down the top covers underneath. Do not expose more of the resident than you need to. Keep the resident covered from the chest down except when placing or removing the bedpan.

8. Place the bed protector under the resident's buttocks and hips. To do this, have the resident turn toward the raised bed rail. If the resident cannot do this, you must turn him (see Chapter 11). Be sure the resident cannot

roll off the bed. Place bed protector on the empty side of the bed, on the area where the resident will lie on his back. The side of the protector nearest the resident should be fanfolded (folded several times into pleats) and tucked under the resident (Fig. 15-4).

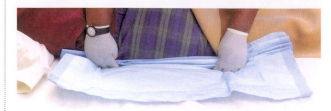

Fig. 15-4. *Fanfold the bed protector near the resident's back.*

Ask the resident to turn onto his back, or turn him as you did before. Unfold the rest of bed protector so it completely covers the area under and around the resident's buttocks and hips.

9. Keeping him covered, ask the resident to remove his undergarments or help him do so.

10. Place the bedpan near his hips in the correct position. A **standard bedpan** should be positioned with the wider end aligned with the resident's buttocks. A **fracture pan** should be positioned with handle toward the foot of the bed.

11. If the resident is able, ask him to raise his hips by pushing with his feet and hands on the count of three (Fig. 15-5). Slide the bedpan under his hips.

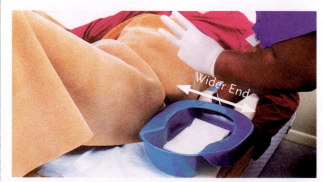

Fig. 15-5. *On the count of three, slide the bedpan under the resident's hips. The wider end of bedpan should be aligned with resident's buttocks.*

If a resident cannot do this himself, keep the bed flat and turn the resident away from you toward the raised bed rail. Slip the bedpan under his hips and gently roll him back onto the bedpan. Keep the bedpan centered underneath.

12. Remove and discard gloves properly. Wash your hands.

13. Raise the head of the bed. Prop the resident into a semi-sitting position using pillows. Make sure both bed rails are up, and return the bed to its lowest position.

14. Make sure the bath blanket is still covering the resident. Place toilet paper and wipes within the resident's reach. Ask the resident to clean his hands with a wipe when finished if he is able.

15. Leave the call light within the resident's reach. Wash your hands. Ask the resident to signal when finished. Leave the room and close the door.

16. When called by the resident, return and wash your hands. Put on clean gloves.

17. Raise the bed to a safe level. Lower the head of the bed. Make sure the resident is still covered. Do not overexpose the resident. Lower the bed rail on the near/working side.

18. Remove the bedpan carefully and gently. Cover the bedpan.

19. Give perineal care if help is needed. Wipe from front to back. Dry the perineal area with a towel. Remove and discard the bed protector. Help the resident put on undergarments. Cover the resident and remove the bath blanket.

20. Place the towel and bath blanket in a hamper or bag, and discard disposable supplies.

21. Take the bedpan to the bathroom. Note color, odor, amount, and consistency of contents. Empty contents into the toilet unless a specimen is needed, urine is being measured for intake/output monitoring, or the nurse needs to check the contents. If you notice anything unusual about the stool or urine (for example, the presence of blood), do not discard it. You will need to inform the nurse.

22. Turn the faucet on with a paper towel. Rinse the bedpan with cold water and empty it into the toilet. Flush the toilet. Place the bedpan in the proper area for cleaning or clean and store it according to policy.

23. Remove and discard gloves properly. Wash your hands.

24. Make the resident comfortable.

25. Return bed to its lowest position. Remove privacy measures.

26. Leave call light within the resident's reach.

27. Wash your hands.

28. Be courteous and respectful at all times.

29. Report any changes in the resident to the nurse. Document procedure using facility guidelines.

Bedpans and urinals are usually kept in the bathroom when they are not being used (Fig. 15-6). If the bathroom is shared, this equipment has to be labeled.

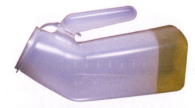

Fig. 15-6. *One type of urinal.*

Assisting a male resident with a urinal

Equipment: urinal, disposable bed protector, disposable wipes, 2 pairs of gloves

1. Identify yourself by name. Identify the resident. Greet the resident by name.

2. Wash your hands.

3. Explain procedure to the resident. Speak clearly, slowly, and directly. Maintain face-to-face contact whenever possible.

4. Provide for the resident's privacy with a curtain, screen, or door.

5. Adjust the bed to a safe level, usually waist high. Lock bed wheels.

6. Put on gloves.

7. Place the bed protector under the resident's buttocks and hips.

8. Hand the urinal to the resident. If the resident is not able to help himself, place the urinal between his legs and position the penis inside the urinal (Fig. 15-7). Replace the covers.

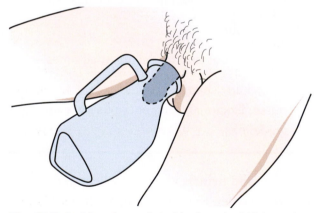

Fig. 15-7. Position the penis inside the urinal if the resident cannot do this himself.

9. Remove and discard gloves properly. Wash your hands.

10. Raise the head of the bed. Make sure both bed rails are up, and return the bed to its lowest position. Place wipes within the resident's reach. Ask the resident to clean his hands with a wipe when finished if he is able. Leave the call light within reach. Wash your hands. Ask resident to signal when done. Leave the room and close the door.

11. When called by the resident, return and wash your hands. Put on clean gloves.

12. Have resident hand urinal to you, or gently remove urinal. Remove the bed protector. Discard disposable supplies.

13. Take the urinal to the bathroom. Note color, odor, amount, and qualities (for example, cloudiness) of contents. Empty contents into the toilet unless a specimen is needed, urine is being measured for intake/output monitoring, or the nurse needs to check the contents.

14. Turn the faucet on with a paper towel. Rinse the urinal with cold water and empty rinse water into the toilet. Flush the toilet. Place urinal in proper area for cleaning or clean and store it according to policy.

15. Remove and discard gloves properly. Wash your hands.

16. Leave the bed in its lowest position. Remove privacy measures.

17. Make the resident comfortable.

18. Leave call light within the resident's reach.

19. Wash your hands.

20. Be courteous and respectful at all times.

21. Report any changes in the resident to the nurse. Document procedure using facility guidelines.

Portable, or bedside, commodes are used for people who can get out of bed but who find it difficult to walk to the bathroom. A **portable commode** is a chair with a toilet seat and a removable container underneath (Fig. 15-8). The removable container must be in place before the resident uses the commode and it must be cleaned after each use. Commodes may have wheels. The wheels must be locked before helping residents onto commodes. If the commode does not have wheels, make sure it is stable. Once the resident is seated, she can be left alone to use the commode if it is safe to do so.

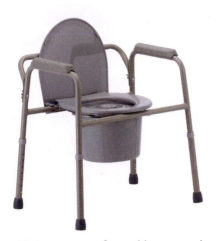

Fig. 15-8. This is one type of portable commode. (PHOTO COURTESY OF NOVA MEDICAL PRODUCTS, WWW.NOVAMEDICALPRODUCTS.COM)

Helping a resident use a portable commode

Equipment: portable commode with basin, toilet paper, disposable wipes, nonskid footwear, towel, bath blanket, supplies for perineal care, 3 pairs of gloves

1. Identify yourself by name. Identify the resident. Greet the resident by name.

2. Wash your hands.

3. Explain procedure to the resident. Speak clearly, slowly, and directly. Maintain face-to-face contact whenever possible.

4. Provide for the resident's privacy with a curtain, screen, or door.

5. Lock commode wheels. Adjust the bed to its lowest position. Lock bed wheels.

6. Put on gloves.

7. Make sure the resident is wearing nonskid footwear that is securely fastened. Help the resident out of bed and to the portable commode.

8. If needed, help the resident remove clothing and sit comfortably on the toilet seat. Place the bath blanket over the resident's legs. Place toilet paper and wipes within resident's reach. Ask the resident to clean his hands with a wipe when finished if he is able.

9. Leave the call light within reach. Remove and discard gloves properly. Wash your hands. Ask the resident to signal when finished. Leave the room and close the door.

10. When called by the resident, return and wash your hands. Put on clean gloves.

11. Give perineal care if help is needed. Wipe from front to back. Dry the perineal area with a towel. Help the resident put on undergarments. Place the towel and bath blanket in a hamper or bag, and discard disposable supplies.

12. Remove and discard gloves properly. Wash your hands.

13. Help the resident back to bed. Leave the bed in its lowest position. Remove privacy measures.

14. Make the resident comfortable.

15. Put on clean gloves.

16. Remove the waste basin. Note color, odor, amount, and consistency of contents. Empty contents into the toilet unless a specimen is needed, urine is being measured for intake/output monitoring, or the nurse needs to check the contents.

17. Turn the faucet on with a paper towel. Rinse the container with cold water and empty it into the toilet. Flush the toilet. Place the commode in the proper area for cleaning or clean and store it according to policy.

18. Remove and discard gloves properly. Wash your hands.

19. Leave call light within the resident's reach.

20. Wash your hands.

21. Be courteous and respectful at all times.

22. Report any changes in the resident to the nurse. Document procedure using facility guidelines.

7. Discuss common disorders of the gastrointestinal system

Heartburn

Heartburn, also known as *acid reflux*, occurs when the sphincter muscle that joins the esophagus and the stomach weakens. Normally this muscle works to prevent return, or reflux, of stomach contents back into the esophagus. If this is not done, stomach juices will move into the esophagus and cause burning and pain. The esophagus has a delicate lining that can be damaged by these stomach juices. Symptoms include a burning feeling in the esophagus and pain in the chest, around the breastbone (sternum) or in the rib area. The pain may also move into the neck area. Pain usually occurs directly after eating a meal. Heartburn often causes a bitter taste in the mouth or the feeling of food coming back up into the throat or the mouth. This may worsen when a person is lying down. Treatment includes medication—antacids are one example—as well as a change in diet and/or sleep position.

Gastroesophageal Reflux Disease (GERD)

Gastroesophageal reflux disease (GERD) is a chronic condition in which the liquid contents of the stomach back up into the esophagus. The liquid can inflame and damage the lining of the esophagus, which can cause bleeding, ulcers, or difficulty swallowing. Frequent heartburn is a common symptom of GERD. Other symptoms are chest pain, hoarseness in the morning, difficulty swallowing, or a tightness in the throat. Coughing and bad breath are other signs. Possible causes are obesity, hiatal hernia, a weak lower esophageal sphincter, and slow digestion. Other causes are diets high in acidic and spicy foods, smoking, and alcohol use.

Treatment includes medication, losing weight, stopping smoking, not drinking alcohol, and avoiding spicy and acidic foods. Wearing loose-fitting clothing may help. Bending over to lift objects can push acid up into the esophagus and make GERD worse; it should be avoided. Serving frequent, small meals throughout the day is advised, as well as serving the last meal of the day three to four hours before bedtime. Sitting up for at least two to three hours after eating may help. Elevating the head of the bed and using extra pillows to keep the body upright may help reduce acid reflux while in bed (Fig. 15-9).

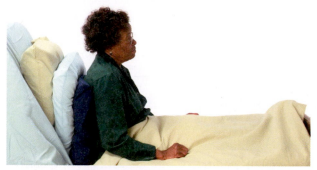

Fig. 15-9. *Sitting upright, elevating the head of the bed, and using extra pillows may help reduce acid reflux.*

Ulcers

Ulcers are raw sores in the stomach (peptic or gastric ulcers) and the small intestine (duodenal ulcers). Dull or burning pain occurs one to three or more hours after eating, accompanied by belching or vomiting. Peptic ulcers can cause bleeding, and stool may appear black (tarry). Ulcers are caused by excessive acid secretion. Infection of the stomach by a bacteria called *Helicobacter pylori* may also cause ulcers. Long-term use of aspirin or ibuprofen may also contribute to the development of ulcers. Treatment includes antacids and other medications, including antibiotics in certain cases, as well as a change in diet. Alcohol, caffeine, and cigarette use should be avoided, as they increase the production of gastric acid.

Gallbladder Disorders

The gallbladder's function is to store bile, which is manufactured by the liver. Bile helps with the digestion of fats, cholesterol, and fat-soluble vitamins. Bile is released by the gallbladder through the bile ducts into the small intestine. If a bile duct is blocked, bile flow will decrease or stop. Disorders that can block the flow of bile include gallstones, gallbladder surgical procedures, and pancreatic disorders and tumors. Gallstones form when the substances in the bile solidify. Blockage of the bile ducts can cause inflammation of the gallbladder called *cholecystitis*.

Treatments for gallbladder disorders include medications and dietary changes. The surgical removal of the gallbladder, or *cholecystectomy*, may be necessary. If this surgery is performed, bile flows to the small intestine directly from the liver. A person does not need a gallbladder to live.

Cirrhosis

Cirrhosis is a liver disease that occurs in response to liver damage. Some causes of liver damage are alcohol abuse, hepatitis, and fatty liver syndrome. When cirrhosis occurs, the liver's functioning decreases. Symptoms of cirrhosis include fatigue, bruising easily, itchy skin, jaundice (yellowing of the whites of the eyes and the skin), ascites in the abdomen, and edema in the legs. Treatment is dependent upon the cause. Alcohol must be eliminated, and the person will need to maintain a healthy weight. Medications and liver transplants are treatments for hepatitis.

Hernia

A hernia occurs when pressure pushes a part of a body cavity out through a weakened area of muscle or connective tissue. Causes of this type of pressure include heavy lifting and constipation. There are many types of hernias; inguinal, incisional, and femoral are a few examples. Symptoms of a hernia include a swollen area in the abdomen or the groin and discomfort in the abdominal area or groin when lifting. A hernia may become strangulated, blocking blood supply. A bowel obstruction can also occur with a hernia. Both of these situations are considered medical emergencies, generally requiring surgery.

Crohn's Disease and Ulcerative Colitis

Crohn's disease is a form of inflammatory bowel disease (IBD). Crohn's disease causes the lining of the digestive tract to become inflamed (red, sore, and swollen). This inflammation occurs in both the small and large intestines. Symptoms include diarrhea, rectal bleeding, abdominal cramping and pain, fever, and weight loss. Treatment depends on the severity of the symptoms and may include medications, dietary changes, and stopping smoking. With severe symptoms, hospitalization may be necessary and the person may need total parenteral nutrition (Chapter 26). Surgery may be required.

Ulcerative colitis is a disorder that causes inflammation of and sores in the lining of the large intestine (colon). It is a form of inflammatory bowel disease (IBD). Symptoms include diarrhea, abdominal pain, cramping, rectal bleeding, poor appetite, fever, and weight loss. Treatment includes medications, dietary changes, and surgery.

Diverticulosis and Diverticulitis

Diverticulosis is a disorder of the intestinal wall of the large intestine (colon). Sac-like pouchings of the intestinal wall develop in weakened areas of this wall. Signs and symptoms of diverticulosis include abdominal pain or tenderness, nausea and vomiting, fever, and constipation. Risk factors for getting this disorder include advancing age, a sedentary lifestyle, certain medications, a low-fiber diet, obesity, smoking, or genetics.

Some people with diverticulosis develop **diverticulitis**. Diverticulitis occurs when inflammation develops inside one or more of the sac-like pouchings. Stool and bacteria can become trapped inside the sacs, resulting in mild to severe abdominal pain, generally on the left side. Fever, nausea, and vomiting can also occur, along with stool changes such as severe constipation or diarrhea, and potentially a bowel obstruction. If the condition worsens, it can be life-threatening. The intestine can tear, causing stool and bacteria to enter the abdominal cavity. Peritonitis, the inflammation of the lining of the abdominal cavity due to microorganisms, results.

Treatment for this disorder includes rest, medications to reduce inflammation and treat infection, exercise, and more fluids to prevent constipation. During bouts of diverticulitis, a low-fiber diet may be ordered. A colostomy may be needed, which allows the intestine to heal. Total parenteral nutrition (TPN, Chapter 26) may be ordered, which helps reduce the bulk that moves through the intestine. The person may be unable to eat or drink while having TPN, which may last weeks or months.

Flatulence

Flatulence, also called *gas* or *flatus*, is excessive air in the digestive tract that is passed through the rectum. Cramping or abdominal pain may result. Causes include eating foods high in fiber, as well as foods that a person cannot tolerate, such as lactose in dairy products. The inability to digest lactose, a type of sugar in milk and other dairy products, is called *lactose intolerance*. Other causes of gas include the following:

- Swallowing air when eating

- Antibiotics

- **Malabsorption**, which means that nutrients from the intestinal tract are not properly absorbed; this can also be accompanied by diarrhea.

- **Irritable bowel syndrome (IBS)**, which is a chronic condition of the large intestine that is worsened by stress. IBS causes abdominal pain and discomfort, bloating, constipation, and diarrhea. Irritable bowel syndrome (IBS) is not the same as inflammatory bowel disease (IBD). With IBS, there are no changes in the bowel tissue, such as with Crohn's

disease. Treatment includes increased fluids; reducing stress; avoiding food that causes gas; increasing exercise, sleep, and rest; certain medications; and a high-fiber diet, gluten-free diet, or low FODMAP (fermentable oligo-, di-, and monosaccharides and polyols) diet. FODMAP diets are used for people who are sensitive to certain carbs. These carbs, such as some fruits, dairy, legumes, and foods with pits or seeds, are eliminated from the diet. A person with IBS should try to eat at regular times and should not skip meals.

Two body positions are used to help reduce gas: the left side-lying (Sims') position, and the flat on the back (supine) position. Lying on the left side allows gas to escape due to gravity. Placing a resident in this position for at least 20 minutes usually helps eliminate gas. Gas that remains in the abdominal cavity following surgery can cause severe pain in the abdomen, chest, shoulder, or ribs. The supine position can be used to allow gas inside the abdomen to escape more quickly.

Constipation

Constipation is the inability to eliminate stool, or the infrequent, difficult, and often painful elimination of hard, dry stool. It occurs when body waste moves slowly through the intestines. Constipation is a common problem for elderly people. As people age, digestion takes longer and is less efficient. Constipation can also result from poor diet, lack of exercise, a decrease in fluid intake, medications, disease, or ignoring the urge to eliminate. Signs of constipation include abdominal swelling, gas, irritability, and no recent bowel movement.

Treating constipation often involves increasing intake of fiber and fluids, as well as physical activity if possible. Medications may be ordered, such as laxatives, enemas, or suppositories. An **enema** is a specific amount of water or other fluid, with or without an additive, introduced into the colon to stimulate the elimination of stool. A **rectal suppository** is a medication in a cylindrical shape that is given rectally to cause a bowel movement. Some states allow NAs to give rectal suppositories. A procedure on how to give a suppository is included in the instructor's material. More information on enemas may be found in the next learning objective.

Diarrhea

Diarrhea is the frequent elimination of liquid or semiliquid feces. Abdominal cramps, urgency, nausea, and vomiting can accompany diarrhea, depending on the cause. Infections, microorganisms, irritating foods, and medications can cause diarrhea. Treatment is usually medication and a change of diet. A change in diet or a diet of bananas, rice, applesauce, and tea/toast (BRAT diet) is often prescribed for short-term use. Treatment for diarrhea associated with *C. difficile* (*C. diff*) may include fecal transplantation (fecal microbiota therapy, FMT). This involves transplanting the stool from a healthy person to the colon of the affected person. It is used for people who have not responded to antibiotic therapy. The donor stool is tested to try to prevent any potential disease transmission.

Fecal Incontinence

Fecal incontinence is an inability to control the muscles of the bowels, which leads to an involuntary passage of stool or gas. Causes of fecal incontinence include muscle and nerve damage, disorders of the spinal cord or anus, injuries to the anal muscles during childbirth, injuries due to anal operations, trauma, fecal impaction, constipation, and tumors. Treatment often includes changes in diet, medication, bowel training, and surgery. CMS requires that the goal of care for fecal incontinence is to restore as much normal bowel function as possible. More information about bowel training is located in Learning Objective 12 of this chapter.

Fecal Impaction

A **fecal impaction** is a buildup of dry, hardened feces in the rectum that results from unrelieved constipation. A person cannot remove an impaction on his own. Signs and symptoms of a fecal impaction include no stool for several days, cramping, abdominal or rectal pain, abdominal swelling (distention), nausea, and vomiting. Another sign is the seeping or oozing of liquid stool, which can be mistaken for diarrhea. Other signs are an increase in urination or the inability to urinate, fever, confusion, or disorientation. When an impaction occurs, the nurse or doctor will insert one or two gloved fingers into the rectum to break the mass into fragments. Usually the stool can then be passed. A fecal impaction can be a serious, even fatal, condition if a complete bowel obstruction occurs and is not immediately treated. Report signs and symptoms promptly to the nurse. Ways to prevent fecal impactions include drinking plenty of fluids, eating a high-fiber diet, following an elimination schedule, and exercising regularly.

Hemorrhoids

Hemorrhoids are enlarged veins in the rectum. They may also be visible outside the anus. Untreated constipation, obesity, pregnancy, chronic diarrhea, overuse of enemas or laxatives, and straining during bowel movements are common causes of hemorrhoids. Rectal itching, burning, pain, and bleeding during bowel elimination are symptoms of hemorrhoids. Treatment includes dietary changes, such as increasing fiber and water intake, medications, compresses, and sitz baths (Chapter 18). Surgery may be necessary. Excessive cleaning and wiping of the area should be avoided. When cleaning the anal area, the NA should be very gentle. Scented soaps should not be used, as these may further irritate the anal area.

Information on hepatitis, a gastrointestinal system disorder, may be found in Chapter 6. Here are a few additional resources for information relating to gastrointestinal disorders:

- Crohn's & Colitis Foundation, ccfa.org

- National Institute of Diabetes and Digestive and Kidney Diseases, niddk.nih.gov

Obesity and Disorders of the Gastrointestinal System

Obesity increases the risk for certain gastrointestinal diseases or disorders, including the following:

- Gastroesophageal reflux disease (GERD)

- Gallbladder disease

- Fatty liver syndrome

- Cancers of the gastrointestinal system, such as colorectal cancer, pancreatic cancer, and esophageal cancer

Boxes about obesity will be located in all body systems chapters; there is more information about obesity in Learning Objective 13 of this chapter.

8. Discuss how enemas are given

An enema is given when a person needs help eliminating stool from the colon. A specific amount of water or other fluid flows inside the colon in order to stimulate the elimination of stool. Some facilities allow NAs to give enemas. If allowed, the NA should follow facility policy and make sure he is trained to give enemas. He should talk to the nurse if he has any questions.

Enemas are ordered for these reasons:

- Preparation for a diagnostic test

- Preparation for surgery

- To remove stool that a resident cannot eliminate on his own

A doctor will write an enema order. There are four different types of enemas:

- Tap water enema (TWE): 500–1000 mL water from a faucet (nothing added to the water)

- Soapsuds enema (SSE): 500–1000 mL water with 5 mL of mild castile soap added

- Saline enema: 500–1000 mL water with two teaspoons of salt added

- Commercial enema (also called *pre-packaged enema*): 120 mL solution that may have oil or other additive

Tap water, soapsuds, and saline enemas are all considered *cleansing enemas*. They all require more fluid than commercially prepared enemas do. Equipment needed for a cleansing enema includes an IV pole, the enema solution, and tubing and a clamp. For best results, the NA should encourage the resident to hold in the enema solution as long as possible—at least 10 to 20 minutes.

Guidelines: Enemas

G   Provide plenty of privacy for the resident. Make sure others cannot see the resident and that he is not unnecessarily exposed in any way.

G   Place the resident in the Sims' position (Fig. 15-10). If positioned on the left side, water does not have to flow against gravity. Water temperature should not be over 105°F to avoid internal burning. Water that is too cold can cause intense cramping.

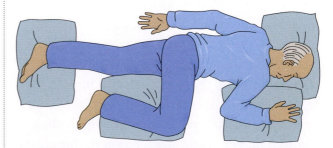

Fig. 15-10. The Sims' position (left side-lying position) is the proper position for an enema.

G   When giving a cleansing enema, remove the air from the enema tubing before inserting the tube into the rectum. Allowing a small amount of water to flow into a bedpan will allow the air to escape.

G Give the enema slowly, holding the enema tubing in place. Enemas are given gradually to avoid cramping. Stop immediately if the resident has pain or if you feel resistance.

G Be reassuring and gentle during the procedure. Observe for cramping, pain or discomfort, bleeding, the ability to retain the fluid, and any change in the resident's condition during and following the enema.

Giving a cleansing enema

Equipment: bath blanket, IV pole, enema solution, additive (if needed), tubing and clamp, disposable bed protector, bedpan, bedpan cover, lubricating jelly, water thermometer, tape measure, toilet paper, disposable wipes, towel, robe, nonskid footwear, paper towel, supplies for perineal care, 2 pairs of gloves

1. Identify yourself by name. Identify the resident. Greet the resident by name.

2. Wash your hands.

3. Explain procedure to the resident. Speak clearly, slowly, and directly. Maintain face-to-face contact whenever possible.

4. Provide for the resident's privacy with a curtain, screen, or door.

5. Adjust the bed to a safe level, usually waist high. Lock bed wheels.

6. Put on gloves.

7. Place the bed protector under the resident. Ask the resident to remove his undergarments or help him do so.

8. Help the resident into a left-sided Sims' position. Place the bedpan close to the resident's body. Cover with a bath blanket.

9. Place the IV pole beside the bed.

10. Clamp the enema tube. Prepare the enema solution. Add specific additive if ordered. Fill the bag with 500–1000 mL of warm water (105°F) and swish the fluid to mix well. Check the water temperature with the water thermometer.

11. Unclamp the tube. Let a small amount of solution run through the tubing to release the air. Reclamp the tube.

12. Hang the bag on the IV pole. Using the tape measure, make sure the bottom of enema bag is not more than 12 inches above the resident's anus (Fig. 15-11).

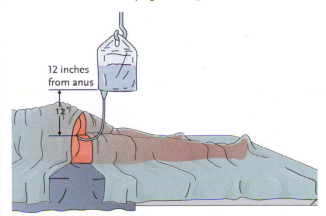

12 inches from anus

Fig. 15-11. The bottom of the bag should not be more than 12 inches above the anus.

13. Uncover the resident enough to expose the anus only.

14. Lubricate 2–4 inches of the tip of the tubing with lubricating jelly.

15. Ask the resident to breathe deeply to relieve cramps during the procedure.

16. Place one hand on the upper buttock. Lift to expose the anus. Ask the resident to take a deep breath and exhale (Fig. 15-12). Using the other hand, gently insert the tip of the tubing 2–4 inches into the rectum. Stop

immediately if you feel resistance or if the resident complains of pain. If this happens, clamp the tubing. Tell the nurse immediately.

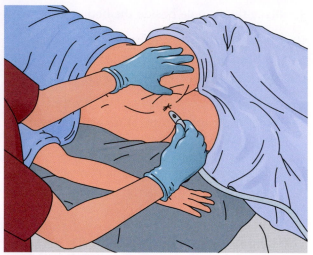

Fig. 15-12. Lift the upper buttock to expose the anus. Ask the resident to take a deep breath before inserting the tubing.

17. Unclamp the tubing. Allow the solution to flow slowly into the rectum. Ask the resident to take slow, deep breaths. If the resident complains of cramping, clamp the tubing and stop for a couple of minutes. Encourage him to take as much of the solution as possible. The resident should let you know when he cannot take any more fluid.

18. Clamp the tubing before the bag is empty, when the solution is almost gone. Gently remove the tip from the rectum. Place the tip into the enema bag. Do not contaminate yourself, the resident, or the bed linens.

19. Ask the resident to hold the solution inside for as long as possible.

20. Help the resident to use the bedpan or commode or to get to the bathroom. If the resident is using the bedpan, raise the head of the bed. Make sure both bed rails are up, and return the bed to its lowest position before you leave the room. If the resident uses a commode or toilet, help him put on a robe and nonskid footwear. Lower the bed to its lowest position before the resident gets up.

21. Remove and discard gloves properly. Wash your hands.

22. Place toilet paper and wipes within the resident's reach. Ask the resident to clean his hands with a wipe when finished if he is able. If the resident is using the toilet, ask him not to flush it when finished.

23. Leave the call light within the resident's reach. Wash your hands. Ask the resident to signal when finished. Leave the room and close the door.

24. When called by the resident, return and wash your hands. Put on clean gloves.

25. Raise the bed to a safe level. Lower the head of the bed. Make sure the resident is still covered. Do not overexpose the resident. Lower the bed rail on the near/working side if you raised it for the resident to use a bedpan.

26. Remove the bedpan carefully and gently. Cover the bedpan.

27. Give perineal care if help is needed. Wipe from front to back. Dry the perineal area with a towel. Remove and discard the bed protector. Help the resident put on undergarments. Cover the resident and remove the bath blanket.

28. Place the towel and bath blanket in a hamper or bag, and discard disposable supplies.

29. Take the bedpan to the bathroom. Call the nurse to observe enema results, whether in the bedpan or toilet. Empty the contents into the toilet.

30. Turn the faucet on with a paper towel. Rinse the bedpan with cold water and empty it into the toilet. Flush the toilet. Place the bedpan in the proper area for cleaning or clean and store it according to policy.

31. Remove and discard gloves properly. Wash your hands.

32. Make the resident comfortable.

33. Return bed to its lowest position. Remove privacy measures.

34. Leave call light within the resident's reach.

35. Wash your hands.

36. Be courteous and respectful at all times.

37. Report any changes in the resident to the nurse. Document procedure using facility guidelines.

A commercially prepared enema usually has 120 mL of solution and may have additives (Fig 15-13). An oil-retention enema has a type of oil in it, such as mineral oil. An oil-retention enema is given for the following reasons: to lubricate the intestine to make stool pass more easily, to soften stool for ease of elimination, to reduce straining with bowel movements, and to eliminate a fecal impaction.

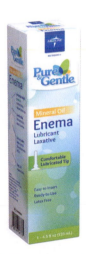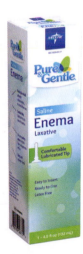

Fig. 15-13. *Commercially prepared enemas may come with additives, such as saline or mineral oil.* (© MEDLINE INDUSTRIES, INC. 2019)

Commercially prepared enemas do not require an IV pole, tubing, or clamp because they are prepackaged and premixed. The tip of the enema is usually prelubricated and should be inserted only about 1½ inches into the rectum. Commercially prepared enemas generally take longer to work than cleansing enemas. The NA should encourage the resident to hold in the enema

solution as long as possible—for at least 20 minutes. Oil-retention enemas should be retained for 30 to 60 minutes.

Giving a commercial enema

Equipment: bath blanket, standard or oil-retention commercial enema kit, disposable bed protector, bedpan, bedpan cover, lubricating jelly, toilet paper, disposable wipes, towel, robe, nonskid footwear, supplies for perineal care, 2 pairs of gloves

1. Identify yourself by name. Identify the resident. Greet the resident by name.

2. Wash your hands.

3. Explain procedure to the resident. Speak clearly, slowly, and directly. Maintain face-to-face contact whenever possible.

4. Provide for the resident's privacy with a curtain, screen, or door.

5. Adjust the bed to a safe level, usually waist high. Lock bed wheels.

6. Put on gloves.

7. Place the bed protector under the resident. Ask the resident to remove his undergarments or help him do so.

8. Help the resident into a left-sided Sims' position. Place the bedpan close to the resident's body. Cover with a bath blanket.

9. Uncover the resident enough to expose the anus only.

10. Add extra lubricating jelly to the tip of the bottle if needed.

11. Ask the resident to breathe deeply to relieve cramps during the procedure.

12. Place one hand on the upper buttock. Lift to expose the anus. Ask the resident to take a deep breath and exhale. Using other hand, gently insert the tip of the tubing about 1½ inches into the rectum. Stop immediately if you feel resistance or if the resident

complains of pain. If this happens, tell the nurse immediately.

13. Slowly squeeze and roll the enema container so that the solution runs inside the resident. Stop when the container is almost empty.

14. Gently remove the tip from the rectum, continuing to keep pressure on the container until you place the bottle inside the box upside down (Fig. 15-14).

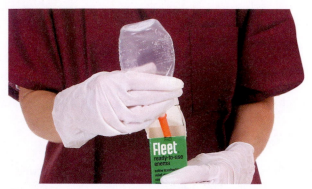

Fig. 15-14. Place enema bottle upside down in the box.

15. Ask the resident to hold the solution inside for as long as possible.

16. Help the resident to use the bedpan or commode or to get to the bathroom. If the resident is using the bedpan, raise the head of the bed. Make sure both bed rails are up, and return the bed to its lowest position before you leave the room. If the resident uses a commode or toilet, put on a robe and nonskid footwear. Lower the bed to its lowest position before the resident gets up.

17. Remove and discard gloves properly. Wash your hands.

18. Place toilet paper and wipes within the resident's reach. Ask the resident to clean his hands with a hand wipe when finished if he is able. If the resident is using the toilet, ask him not to flush it when finished.

19. Leave the call light within the resident's reach. Wash your hands. Ask the resident to signal when finished. Leave the room and close the door.

20. When called by the resident, return and wash your hands. Put on clean gloves.

21. Raise the bed to a safe level. Lower the head of the bed. Make sure the resident is still covered. Do not overexpose the resident. Lower the bed rail on the near/working side if you raised it for the resident to use a bedpan.

22. Remove the bedpan carefully and gently. Cover the bedpan.

23. Give perineal care if help is needed. Wipe from front to back. Dry the perineal area with a towel. Help the resident put on undergarments. Cover the resident and remove the bath blanket.

24. Place the towel and bath blanket in a hamper or bag, and discard disposable supplies.

25. Take the bedpan to the bathroom. Call the nurse to observe enema results, whether in the bedpan or toilet. Empty the contents into the toilet.

26. Turn the faucet on with a paper towel. Rinse the bedpan with cold water and empty it into the toilet. Flush the toilet. Place the bedpan in the proper area for cleaning or clean and store it according to policy.

27. Remove and discard gloves properly. Wash your hands.

28. Make the resident comfortable.

29. Return bed to its lowest position. Remove privacy measures.

30. Leave call light within the resident's reach.

31. Wash your hands.

32. Be courteous and respectful at all times.

33. Report any changes in the resident to the nurse. Document procedure using facility guidelines.

A follow-up cleansing enema may be ordered after an oil-retention enema. This helps clean the bowels more thoroughly and eliminate remaining oil in the intestine. The resident may want to bathe after this procedure and the bowel movements that follow. The NA should help as needed.

9. Demonstrate how to collect a stool specimen

A **specimen** is a sample, such as tissue, blood, urine, stool, or sputum, that is used for analysis and diagnosis. Specimens are used for different types of tests. A stool specimen may be needed to test for blood, pathogens, and other things. Stool may be collected and tested for ova and parasites (O&P) to detect worms or amoebas. If the specimen is being examined for ova and parasites, it must be taken to the lab immediately. This examination must be done while the stool is still warm. Stool that cannot be sent to the lab immediately may need to be placed in a special refrigerator used strictly for specimens. Specimens should never be placed in a refrigerator that is used for food or drinks.

When collecting a stool specimen, the NA should first show the resident the correct container to use. She should explain that urine or toilet paper should not be included in the sample because they can ruin the sample, creating the need for a new specimen.

A plastic collection container called a *hat* is sometimes inserted into a toilet to collect and measure urine or stool (Fig. 15-15). Hats should be labeled with the resident's name and room number and must be cleaned after each use.

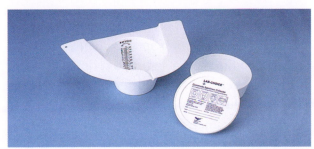

Fig. 15-15. *A "hat" is placed under the toilet seat to collect a specimen.*

When a specimen is collected, it is put into a specimen container and a label is applied before it is taken to the lab. The label must include this information: the resident's name, date of birth, doctor's name, room number, and the date and time. A specimen may need to be placed in a clean specimen bag before it is transported (Fig. 15-16).

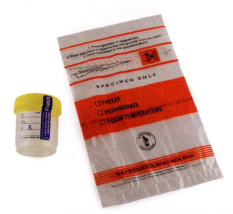

Fig. 15-16. *A specimen may need to be placed inside a clean specimen bag before it is taken to the lab.*

The NA should ask the resident to let her know when he is ready to have a bowel movement, and she should be ready to collect the specimen.

Collecting a stool specimen

Equipment: specimen container and lid, completed label (labeled with resident's name, date of birth, doctor's name, room number, date, and time), biohazard specimen bag, 2 tongue blades, 2 pairs of gloves, bedpan (if resident cannot use portable commode or toilet), hat for toilet (if resident uses portable commode or toilet), plastic bag, toilet paper, disposable wipes, supplies for perineal care, lab slip

1. Identify yourself by name. Identify the resident. Greet the resident by name.

2. Wash your hands.

3. Explain procedure to the resident. Speak clearly, slowly, and directly. Maintain face-to-face contact whenever possible.

4. Provide for the resident's privacy with a curtain, screen, or door.

5. Put on gloves.

6. Fit the hat to the toilet or commode, or provide the resident with a bedpan.

7. When the resident is ready to move his bowels, ask him not to urinate at the same time and not to put toilet paper in with the sample. Provide a plastic bag to discard toilet paper separately.

8. Make sure both bed rails are up, and the bed is in its lowest position. Place toilet paper and wipes within the resident's reach. Ask the resident to clean his hands with a wipe when finished if he is able.

9. Ask the resident to signal when he is finished with the bowel movement. Make sure the call light is within reach.

10. Remove and discard gloves properly. Wash your hands. Leave the room and close the door.

11. When called by the resident, return and wash your hands. Put on clean gloves.

12. Give perineal care if help is needed.

13. Using the two tongue blades, take about two tablespoons of stool and put it in the container. Without touching the inside of the container, cover it tightly. Apply the label and place the specimen in a clean biohazard specimen bag. Seal the bag.

14. Wrap the tongue blades in toilet paper and place them in the plastic bag with the used toilet paper. Discard the bag in the proper container.

15. Turn the faucet on with a paper towel. Rinse the bedpan with cold water and empty it into the toilet. Flush the toilet. Place bedpan in area for cleaning or clean and store it according to policy.

16. Remove and discard gloves properly. Wash your hands.

17. Make the resident comfortable.

18. Return bed to its lowest position. Remove privacy measures.

19. Leave call light within the resident's reach.

20. Wash your hands.

21. Be courteous and respectful at all times.

22. Report any changes in the resident to the nurse. Document procedure using facility guidelines. Take specimen and lab slip to designated place promptly.

If collecting a specimen from a resident in isolation, special steps are required. Some steps are performed before entering the isolation room. Two labels are completed, leaving one label outside the room on a biohazard specimen bag. Proper personal protective equipment (PPE) is donned before entering the room. After collecting the specimen and covering the container, the NA should place one completed label on the container. Before leaving the isolation room, gloves must be removed and discarded and hands should be washed.

Using a clean paper towel, the NA should carefully pick up the specimen container and leave the room. The specimen container must immediately be put into the biohazard specimen bag on the isolation cart. Then the NA discards the paper towel, seals the bag, and takes the specimen to the proper site. Handwashing is performed as a final step.

10. Explain occult blood testing

Hidden, or **occult**, blood is detected in stool by use of a microscope or a special chemical test. Occult blood may be a sign of a serious problem, such as cancer. There are different types of tests to detect occult blood in stool. In some facilities, stool specimens are sent to laboratories for testing. In other facilities, staff members do it onsite. NAs may be asked to perform this test if they are trained and allowed to do so. Specific dietary orders or medications may be necessary prior to occult blood testing. The date on the testing card should be checked before use to make sure it has not expired.

Testing a stool specimen for occult blood

Equipment: labeled stool specimen, occult blood test kit (Fig. 15-17), 2 tongue blades, plastic bag, gloves

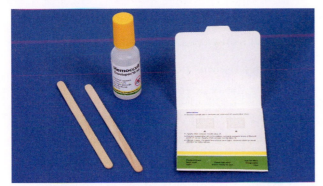

Fig. 15-17. *This is one type of occult blood test kit.*

1. Wash your hands.

2. Put on gloves.

3. Open the test card.

4. Pick up a tongue blade. Get a small amount of stool from the specimen container.

5. Using a tongue blade, smear a small amount of stool onto Box A of the test card (Fig. 15-18).

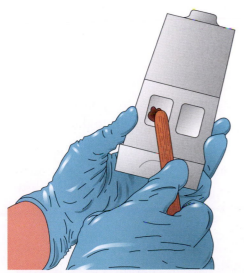

Fig. 15-18. *Smear a small amount of stool onto Box A.*

6. Flip the tongue blade (or use a new tongue blade). Get some stool from another part of the specimen. Smear a small amount of stool onto Box B of the test card.

7. Close the test card. Turn it over to the other side.

8. Open the flap.

9. Open the developer. Apply developer to each box. Follow the manufacturer's instructions.

10. Wait the amount of time listed in the instructions, usually 10–60 seconds.

11. Watch the squares for any color changes. Record color changes. Follow instructions.

12. Place the tongue blade(s) and test packet in the plastic bag.

13. Dispose of the plastic bag properly in a bio-hazard container.

14. Remove and discard gloves properly.

15. Wash your hands.

16. Document procedure using facility guidelines. Report results to the nurse.

11. Define *ostomy* and identify the difference between ileostomy and colostomy

An **ostomy** is the surgical creation of an opening from an area inside the body to the outside. The terms *ileostomy* and *colostomy* refer to the surgical removal of a portion of the intestines. In a resident with one of these ostomies, the end of the intestine is brought out of the body through an artificial opening in the abdomen. This opening is called a **stoma**. Stool, or feces, is eliminated through the ostomy rather than through the anus.

An ostomy may be necessary due to bowel disease, such as diverticulitis, Crohn's disease, or colon cancer. An ostomy can be either permanent or temporary; a temporary ostomy allows the colon to heal from a specific condition.

The terms *ileostomy* and *colostomy* indicate what section of the intestine was removed and the type of stool that will be eliminated. An **ileostomy** is a surgically created opening into the end of the small intestine, the ileum, to allow stool to be expelled. Stool will be liquid and may be irritating to the skin. A **colostomy** is a surgically created opening into the large intestine to allow stool to be expelled. With a colostomy, stool will generally be semisolid.

Residents who have had an ostomy wear a disposable pouching system that fits over the stoma to collect the feces. The pouching system is custom fitted over the stoma to collect the stool (Fig. 15-19). The pouching system is attached to the skin by adhesive, and a belt may also be used to secure it. Looser clothing should be worn, as tight clothing may interfere with the ability of the pouch to fill.

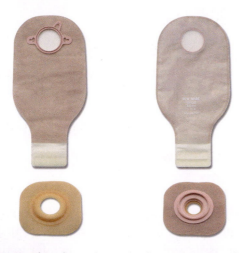

Fig. 15-19. This photo shows the front and back of a two-piece system. The top is an ostomy pouch, and the bottom is a skin barrier. (PHOTOS COURTESY OF HOLLISTER INCORPORATED, LIBERTYVILLE, ILLINOIS, HOLLISTER.COM)

Some people with ostomies feel embarrassed or angry. They often feel they have lost control of a basic bodily function. Ostomies can cause odor, discomfort, and worry that the pouching system will fall off. NAs should be sensitive and supportive and should always provide privacy for ostomy care.

Guidelines: Ostomy Care

G If providing ostomy care is part of your allowed responsibilities, follow your facility's policies.

G Follow Standard and/or Transmission-Based Precautions, including wearing gloves and any additional personal protective equipment when needed. Wash your hands carefully.

G Make sure residents with ostomies receive careful skin care and proper hygiene.

G Remove ostomy pouches carefully to avoid tearing the resident's skin.

G Before removing the pouch, let a little air out of the pouch to relieve any built-up pressure. This can prevent the pouch from exploding.

G Observe the contents of the ostomy pouch before discarding the used pouch. If anything unusual is noted, such as blood or a change in the stool quality or amount, notify the nurse.

G Replace the ostomy pouch whenever stool is eliminated, if a leak occurs, and as directed.

G Assist residents with ostomies to wash their hands properly.

G During ostomy care, observe for signs of skin irritation, rashes, swelling, or bleeding around the stoma. Report these signs, along with complaints of pain or discomfort, immediately.

G Use skin barriers as ordered.

G Make sure the bottom of the pouch is securely clamped before applying it to the stoma.

G Make sure the pouch is attached securely to the resident before completing ostomy care.

G Make sure the pouch is secure before the resident goes to activities or appointments or receives visitors.

G Be supportive, empathetic, and caring. Do not act uncomfortable with any aspect of ostomy care (odor, changing of the pouch, etc.). Your support will help the resident adapt to this important change in lifestyle.

Caring for an ostomy

Equipment: disposable bed protector, bath blanket, clean ostomy pouching system, belt (if needed), disposable wipes (made for ostomy care), basin of warm water, washcloth, 2 towels, plastic disposable bag, gloves, special deodorant (if used)

1. Identify yourself by name. Identify the resident. Greet the resident by name.

2. Wash your hands.

3. Explain procedure to the resident. Speak clearly, slowly, and directly. Maintain face-to-face contact whenever possible.

4. Provide for the resident's privacy with a curtain, screen, or door.

5. Adjust the bed to a safe level, usually waist high. Lock bed wheels.

6. Put on gloves.

7. Place the bed protector under the resident. Cover the resident with a bath blanket. Pull down the top sheet and blankets. Expose only the ostomy site. Offer the resident a towel to keep clothing dry.

8. Undo the ostomy belt if used. Pull gently on one edge of the ostomy pouch to release air.

9. Remove the ostomy pouch carefully. Place it in the plastic bag. Note the color, odor, consistency, and amount of stool in the pouch.

10. Wipe the area around the stoma with disposable wipes for ostomy care. Discard wipes in the plastic bag.

11. Using a washcloth and warm water, wash the area gently in one direction, away from the stoma (Fig. 15-20). Rinse. Pat dry with another towel. Temporarily cover stoma opening with a wipe.

12. Apply deodorant to the pouch (if used). Remove the wipe and place it in the plastic bag. Put the clean ostomy pouch on the resident. Hold it in place and seal it securely. Make sure the bottom of the pouch is clamped. Attach to the ostomy belt (if used).

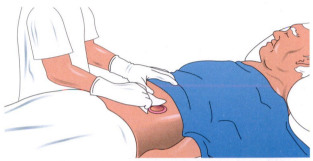

Fig. 15-20. *Wash the area gently, moving in one direction, away from the stoma.*

13. Remove and discard the bed protector. Place soiled linens in the proper container. Discard the plastic bag in the proper container.

14. Remove and discard gloves properly.

15. Wash your hands.

16. Make the resident comfortable.

17. Return bed to its lowest position. Remove privacy measures.

18. Leave call light within the resident's reach.

19. Wash your hands.

20. Be courteous and respectful at all times.

21. Report any changes in the resident to the nurse. Document procedure using facility guidelines.

Other Type of Ostomy

A **urostomy** is the surgical creation of an opening for the passage of urine. The urine is eliminated through a stoma into an external collection pouch. A urostomy might be necessary due to a birth defect, disease, injury, or nerve damage.

12. Explain guidelines for assisting with bowel retraining

Residents who have had an illness, injury, or a period of inactivity may need assistance in re-establishing a regular routine and normal bowel function. Retraining is the process of assisting residents to regain control of their bowels.

Taking regular trips to the bathroom at specific times each day will help with bowel retraining. Doctors may order suppositories, enemas, laxatives, or stool softeners to assist. Most care team members will be involved with implementing and charting bowel retraining. NAs should follow the care plan for each resident.

Guidelines: Bowel Retraining

G Follow the care plan consistently. Explain the training schedule to the resident. Direct any questions the resident has to the nurse.

G Follow Standard Precautions. Wear gloves when handling body wastes. For residents in isolation, additional personal protective equipment may be needed. Follow the care plan.

G Observe the resident's elimination habits. This helps predict when a trip to the bathroom or a bedpan will be necessary.

G Keep a record of elimination, including episodes of incontinence. Keeping accurate records will help establish a routine.

G Offer a bedpan or a trip to the bathroom at specific times each day.

G Answer call lights promptly.

G Provide privacy for elimination, and do not rush the resident.

G Help with perineal care as needed. This promotes proper hygiene. Watch for skin changes and report them.

G Encourage fluids throughout the day if allowed.

G Encourage the proper diet.

G Dispose of wastes promptly and properly.

G Praise attempts and successes in controlling the bowels. However, do not talk to residents as if they are children. Keep your voice low. Do not draw attention to any aspect of retraining.

G Each resident has different needs and may respond to different types of encouragement. Finding out each resident's needs and preferences is part of giving person-centered care.

G Never show frustration or anger toward residents who are incontinent. That is abusive behavior. Negative reactions will only make the problem worse. Be positive and patient with retraining efforts.

Residents' Rights

Handling Incontinence

NAs must always act professionally when handling incontinence or helping to reestablish routines. Residents who are struggling with bowel elimination do not need the added worry of a caregiver's negative reactions. NAs should be patient when setbacks occur.

13. Discuss bariatrics and related care

Bariatrics was first discussed in Chapter 10. This branch of medicine deals with the causes, prevention, and treatment of obesity. Healthcare facilities must be able to accommodate residents who require bariatric care.

Specialized equipment may be used for residents who are obese. This includes larger beds that are lower to the floor, stronger bed rails, oversized chairs for dining areas and lobbies, extra-capacity wheelchairs, and bariatric stretchers. Larger gowns may be needed. Bariatric equipment also includes mechanical lifts, slings, trapezes, other types of support and transfer equipment, and extra-capacity scales. Bariatric elimination equipment includes sturdier bedpans, portable commodes, and toilets mounted to the floor of the room (Fig. 15-21). Oversized shower areas and shower chairs with heavy-duty hand bars may be available. Adjustments may need to be made to the facility as well. Doorways and spaces between toilets and walls may need to be widened.

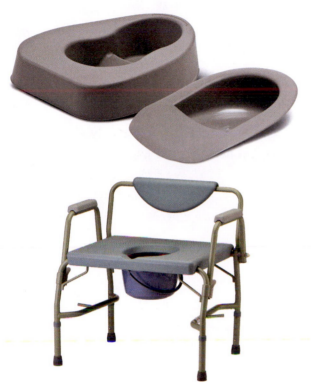

Fig. 15-21. *In the top photo, a bariatric standard bedpan is in back, and a bariatric fracture pan is in front. The bottom photo shows a bariatric portable commode.* (TOP PHOTO © MEDLINE INDUSTRIES, INC. 2019 AND BOTTOM PHOTO COURTESY OF NOVA MEDICAL PRODUCTS, WWW.NOVAMEDICALPRODUCTS.COM)

At least two caregivers, and possibly more, will be needed to safely transfer a resident using a bariatric mechanical lift. NAs should always check equipment weight limits and know a resident's weight before transferring him. Transfer belts are available in larger sizes for residents who require them. Ambulation may require a bariatric walker.

People who are obese tend to have more fragile skin. The doctor may order the use of special lotions, and soap may be used in limited amounts or not at all. (Prescription medicated lotions must be applied by the nurse.) Careful skin care should be a priority. During bathing, the skin should be observed closely and should always be thoroughly rinsed and dried. Caregivers must pay special attention to drying between skin folds, including on the neck, under the breasts, on the stomach, and in the perineal area, as well as between the toes. Signs of skin irritation or other problems should be reported to the nurse.

Monitoring vital signs on people who are obese may require special equipment or other adjustments. Blood pressure may be measured using a thigh cuff on the patient's arm. A blood pressure device designed for the wrist may be used if accurate readings cannot be obtained otherwise. If the pulse rate cannot be determined using the radial pulse, the apical pulse may be counted instead.

Residents who are obese may encounter different health risks than other people. Obesity is a risk factor for obstructive sleep apnea (OSA). Residents who are obese should be evaluated for OSA. A CPAP machine will be prescribed to address OSA if necessary (Chapter 10). Surgery may present complications for people who are obese. During surgery a tube may be inserted in a patient's airway to assist with breathing under anesthesia. This is called *intubation*, and it is usually removed immediately after surgery (Chapter 26). The ability to intubate a patient who is obese may be compromised, and the patient may need intubation for a longer period of time following surgery. The patient may be more prone to respiratory depression (a decrease in the ability to inhale and exhale normally) postoperatively and may require supplemental oxygen, along with pulse oximetry. This may require an extended hospital stay and careful monitoring.

Chapter Review

1. What are four functions of the gastrointestinal system (LO 3)?

2. List five normal age-related changes of the gastrointestinal system (LO 4).

The Gastrointestinal System

3. List three normal qualities of stool (LO 5).

4. When is a fracture pan, rather than a standard bedpan, used for elimination (LO 6)?

5. How should a standard bedpan be positioned? How should a fracture pan be positioned (LO 6)?

6. List three possible treatments for constipation (LO 7).

7. What action should be avoided when providing perineal care for a resident who has hemorrhoids (LO 7)?

8. What position must the resident be in for an enema (LO 8)?

9. If a resident feels pain while receiving an enema, what should the NA do (LO 8)?

10. Why does a stool specimen need to be delivered to the lab immediately when testing for ova and parasites (LO 9)?

11. What items should not be included in a stool specimen (LO 9)?

12. How is occult blood found in stool (LO 10)?

13. When may an ostomy be necessary (LO 11)?

14. How do colostomies and ileostomies differ (LO 11)?

15. List ten guidelines for bowel retraining (LO 12).

16. How many people are needed to use a bariatric mechanical lift to safely transfer a resident who is obese (LO 13)?

Multiple Choice

17. The basic structural units of all organisms are called (LO 2)
(A) Tissues
(B) Body systems
(C) Organs
(D) Cells

18. _____ is the condition in which all of the body's systems are balanced and are working at their best (LO 2).
(A) Homeostasis
(B) Physiology
(C) Circulatory
(D) Pathophysiology

19. How should a resident who has gastroesophageal reflux disease (GERD) be positioned after eating (LO 7)?
(A) Lying flat on her back
(B) Sitting upright
(C) Reclining at approximately 45 degrees
(D) On her stomach

16
The Urinary System

Watching the Kidneys

Galen, 130–200 A.D., wrote a 17-book set entitled *On the Uses of the Parts of the Body of Man*. One portion of the work dealt with the function of the kidneys. To help determine how the kidneys produced urine, Galen tied the ureters of living animals and watched the kidneys swell with urine.

"A human being: an ingenious assembly of portable plumbing."
Christopher Morley, 1890–1957

*"Now is this golden crown like a deep well
That owes two buckets filling one another;
The emptier ever dancing in the air,
The other down, unseen and full of water."*
William Shakespeare, from *Richard II*

1. Define important words in this chapter

24-hour urine specimen: a urine specimen consisting of all urine voided in a 24-hour period.

catheter-associated urinary tract infection (CAUTI): an infection that occurs in the urethra, bladder, ureter, or kidney when bacteria travels up a catheter.

chronic renal failure (CRF): a progressive condition in which the kidneys cannot filter certain waste products; also called *chronic kidney failure*.

clean-catch specimen: a urine specimen that does not include the first and last urine voided; also called *midstream specimen*.

condom catheter: a catheter that has an attachment on the end that fits onto the penis; also called *external* or *Texas catheter*.

dialysis: a process that cleans the body of wastes that the kidneys cannot remove due to kidney failure.

end-stage renal disease (ESRD): condition in which kidneys have failed and dialysis or transplantation is required to sustain life.

indwelling catheter: a catheter that remains inside the bladder for a period of time, with urine draining into a bag.

ketones: chemical substances that the body produces when it does not have enough insulin in the blood.

micturition: the process of emptying the bladder of urine; also called *urination* or *voiding*.

renal calculi: kidney stones.

routine urine specimen: a urine specimen that can be collected any time a person voids.

specific gravity: a test performed to measure the density of urine.

sphincter: a ring-like muscle that opens and closes an opening in the body.

straight catheter: a catheter that does not remain inside the person; it is removed immediately after urine is drained or collected.

urinary incontinence: the inability to control the bladder, which leads to an involuntary loss of urine.

urinary tract infection (UTI): an infection of the urethra, bladder, ureter, or kidney.

voiding: the process of emptying the bladder of urine; also called *urination* or *micturition*.

2. Explain the structure and function of the urinary system

The urinary system consists of two kidneys, two ureters, the urinary bladder, the urethra, and the meatus (Fig. 16-1). The kidneys are bean-shaped organs. They lie slightly above the waist against the rear wall of the abdominal cavity and on either side of the spine. Each kidney is about four to five inches in length, one inch thick, and weighs between four and six ounces. The kidneys are partially protected by the back muscles and the lower ribs. The kidneys clean and filter waste products and toxic materials from the blood. They regulate the amount of electrolytes within the body. They also help to regulate blood pressure and water balance.

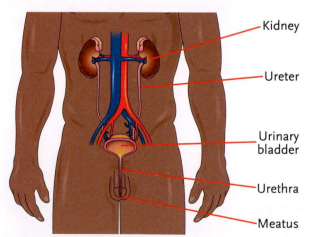

Fig. 16-1. The urinary system consists of two kidneys and two ureters, the bladder, the urethra, and the meatus.

Substances needed by the body are reabsorbed; the substances not needed—toxins and waste products—stay in the kidney and form urine. The urine is then transferred to the bladder through tubes called *ureters*. The ureters are

narrow tubes about one foot in length. When a person urinates, the ureters also prevent the backflow of urine into the kidneys.

The urinary bladder temporarily stores the urine. When the bladder has collected about 200 to 400 milliliters (mL) of urine, nerve impulses are transmitted to the lower portion of the spinal cord. The spinal cord sends nerve impulses back, causing the muscles of the bladder to contract. This relaxes the internal sphincter. The urine moves into the urethra, the tube that carries the urine out of the body. In males, the urethra is approximately seven to eight inches long. In females, it is approximately three to four inches long (Fig. 16-2).

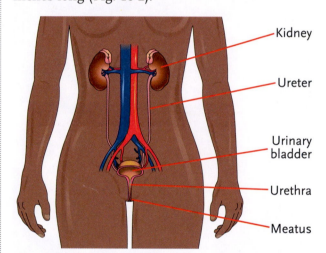

Fig. 16-2. The female urethra is shorter than the male urethra. This is one reason that the female bladder is more likely to become infected by bacteria.

There is an external sphincter in the body that needs to voluntarily relax in order to pass urine. A **sphincter** is a ring-like muscle that opens and closes an opening in the body. Urine then passes out of the body through the meatus, the opening at the end of the urethra. This is the process of urinating, which is also called **micturition** or **voiding**. When this sphincter is damaged, weakened, or loses contact with the nervous system, it can cause urinary incontinence. **Urinary incontinence** is the inability to control the bladder, which leads to an involuntary loss of urine. There is more information about urinary incontinence later in this chapter.

The functions of the urinary system are to:

- Eliminate waste products from the blood

- Maintain water balance in the body

- Regulate the levels of electrolytes in the body

- Assist in regulation of blood pressure

Destination: Homeostasis

When the body's fluid balance is disturbed, the kidneys work hard to continue to remove waste products from the blood. When water intake decreases, the body adjusts by retaining or saving more water. To do this, the kidneys increase the amount of water returned to the bloodstream. This causes less water to be moved into the urine, which temporarily produces a more concentrated form of urine. This helps the body's water balance remain stable and helps restore homeostasis.

Tip

Tiny Stones, Big Pain

A kidney stone is a hard mass developed from crystals that separate from the urine and build up on the inner surface of the kidney. Kidney stones (also called **renal calculi**) can block a ureter, which causes extreme pain. During a blockage, urine production decreases due to a reflex that causes tiny vessels in the kidney to constrict, or become smaller. The nursing assistant should report symptoms such as blood in the urine, painful urination, a frequent urge to urinate, back pain, flank pain, or lower abdominal pain to the nurse.

---

3. Discuss changes in the urinary system due to aging

Normal age-related changes for the urinary system include the following:

- The kidneys do not filter the blood as efficiently.

- Bladder muscle tone weakens.

- Bladder holds less urine, which causes more frequent urination.

- Bladder may not empty completely, causing an increased chance of infection.

4. List normal qualities of urine and identify signs and symptoms to report about urine

Urination is the physical process of releasing or emptying the bladder of urine. Urine consists of water and waste products removed from the blood by the kidneys. Humans must urinate several times daily in order to remain healthy. Regular urination is vital to keep the urinary system healthy.

Urine is normally light, pale yellow or amber in color (Fig. 16-3). However, certain medications and some foods change the color of urine. For example, beets, berries, and some food dyes can make urine appear pink or red. Urine should be clear or transparent and have a faint smell, although some conditions, medications, and foods can alter the odor of urine. For example, asparagus can cause urine to have a strong odor (it has been likened to cooked cabbage), and uncontrolled diabetes can cause urine to have a sweet or fruity smell. Urine can become cloudy as it stands, but if it is cloudy when freshly voided, it can be a sign of infection. Normal urine output varies with age and the amount and type of liquids consumed. Adults usually produce approximately 1200 to 1500 mL of urine per day. Elderly adults may produce less urine.

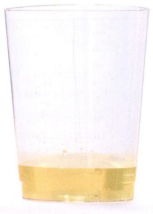

Fig. 16-3. *Urine is normally light or pale yellow in color. It should be clear, not cloudy.*

Normal urination should not be painful. Blood, pus, mucus, protein, bacteria, glucose, or other abnormal matter should not be present in urine. (There is more information about glucose later in the chapter.) A change in the appearance of urine can signal a health problem.

Observing and Reporting: Urine

O/R Cloudy urine

O/R Dark or rust-colored urine

O/R Strong-, offensive-, or fruity-smelling urine

O/R Pain, burning, or pressure when urinating

O/R Blood, pus, mucus, or discharge in urine

O/R Episodes of incontinence

O/R Frequent voiding, voiding in small amounts

5. List factors affecting urination and describe how to promote normal urination

There are many factors that may affect normal urination:

Growth and Development: Aging affects the bladder's ability to hold urine. The bladder is not able to hold the same amount of urine as it did when a person was younger. Older people may have to urinate more often. Urination during the night occurs more frequently with the elderly. The bladder may not empty completely, causing a higher risk of infection. In males, an enlargement of the prostate gland may result in the inability to urinate properly.

To promote normal urination, the NA should encourage fluids and provide water and other beverages often. Offering frequent trips to the bathroom and following a toileting schedule may help. The NA should always respond to call lights and bathroom requests promptly. The best position for women to urinate is sitting; for men, it is standing. The flat-on-back (supine) position should be avoided if possible, as it does not put pressure on the bladder and works against gravity. Exercise and activity should be encouraged. When helping with perineal care, the NA

should wipe from front to back. Careful perineal care will help reduce the risk of infection. Residents, as well as NAs, should wash their hands frequently.

Psychological Factors: A lack of privacy can affect urination. Having a roommate for the first time, being in a place that is not home, and needing help with elimination can disrupt normal elimination patterns. Stress and fear can affect urination. They can cause a person to void frequent, small amounts of urine. Depression can alter urination patterns. A person may not be motivated to change exercise habits and increase fluid intake. This can make urinary elimination more difficult.

To promote normal urination, it is very important for the NA to always provide privacy and allow plenty of time for urination. Call lights should be left within reach, and the NA should respond to call lights and requests for help with toileting immediately.

Fluid Intake: The sense of thirst generally decreases as a person ages. Reduced fluid intake decreases urine production. The body's ability to remove wastes in the urine may be affected. When wastes build up, infections and other problems can occur. Drinking alcoholic beverages and caffeinated beverages generally increases urine production.

To promote normal urination, the NA should encourage the resident to drink fluids. The NA should report to the nurse if she thinks the resident is consuming excessive amounts of caffeine, sodium, or alcohol. The pitcher and cup should be left within the resident's reach and they should be light enough for the resident to lift.

Physical Activity and Exercise: A lack of exercise lessens sphincter control, which can increase episodes of urinary incontinence. Childbirth can weaken a woman's muscle tone. Indwelling catheters (Learning Objective 8) and trauma can weaken muscle tone and increase the risk of infection.

To promote normal urination, the NA should encourage regular walks and other types of exercise that are allowed. Kegel exercises strengthen the pelvic floor muscles and should be encouraged. To locate the Kegel muscles, a person can stop the flow of urine once or twice while urinating. To do Kegel exercises, she should squeeze the muscles for five to ten seconds and relax for ten seconds. These can be done many times per day and can be done anywhere in any position.

Personal Habits: If a resident is confined to bed, urination may be more difficult due to his body position. The sitting position for women and standing position for men are the best positions for urination. Complete emptying of the bladder may be difficult when having to use a bedpan or urinal.

To promote normal urination, the NA should raise the head of the bed. Running water in the bathroom sink or placing the resident's hand under warm running water may encourage urination.

Medications: Some medications affect urination. Residents who have high blood pressure may be taking diuretics, which are medications that increase urine output by causing the body to excrete sodium, potassium, and water through the kidneys.

To promote normal urination, the NA should offer a trip to the bathroom or bedpan or urinal often. Fluid intake should be encouraged if fluids are allowed, even if the increase in fluids causes more frequent urination.

Disorders: Certain disorders affect urination. Fevers cause increased sweating and may decrease urine production. Diabetes, diseases of the bladder or urethra, and infection can increase urination. More information about these diseases may be found later in this chapter and in Chapter 23 of the textbook.

Chapter 15 contains information about how to assist residents with bedpans and urinals.

6. Discuss common disorders of the urinary system

Urinary Tract Infection (UTI)

A **urinary tract infection (UTI)** is an infection of the urethra, bladder, ureter, or kidney. The most common cause of this bacterial infection is *E. coli* bacteria, which is a form of bacteria commonly found in the gastrointestinal tract. If it moves from the anus into the urethra and then the bladder, it can cause a urinary tract infection.

Women are more susceptible to UTIs than men. This is due, in part, to the female urethra being shorter than the male urethra. In addition, because the female urethra is located directly in front of the vagina and the anus, it is closer to potential sources of bacteria. Bacteria can reach a woman's bladder more easily. Women often develop urinary tract infections after having sexual intercourse. Urinating immediately after sexual intercourse helps prevent these infections.

Symptoms of UTIs include burning or pain with urination, blood in the urine, frequent or urgent urination, and confusion.

Drinking plenty of water and other fluids can help prevent UTIs. Wiping from front to back after elimination helps to prevent infection (Fig. 16-4). Taking showers, rather than baths, can also help prevent UTIs. Antibiotics are usually prescribed to treat UTIs. Medication with phenazopyridine may also be prescribed to reduce the pain and burning associated with UTIs. Phenazopyridine normally causes urine to turn orange or red, which is not harmful. It may also cause permanent stains to underwear and contact lenses. The NA should report if a resident has cloudy, dark, or foul-smelling urine, if the resident urinates often and in small amounts, or if the resident complains of burning or discomfort during urination.

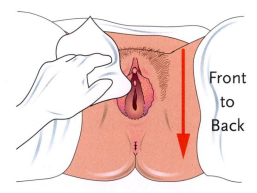

Front to Back

Fig. 16-4. *After elimination, wiping from front to back helps prevent infection.*

Chronic Renal Failure

Chronic renal failure (CRF), also called *chronic kidney failure*, is a condition in which the kidneys cannot effectively filter waste products from the blood, nor can they perform other life-sustaining duties. Chronic renal failure worsens over time. Slowly the kidneys become damaged, and waste products and fluid accumulate in the body.

This disease can result from diabetes, high blood pressure (hypertension), chronic urinary tract infections, inflammation of the kidneys (nephritis), or some medications, especially certain analgesics. Symptoms may appear only after damage to the kidneys has been done. Initial signs and symptoms of this disorder include the following:

• Unintended weight loss

• Nausea and vomiting

• Fatigue

• Headache

• Frequent hiccups

• Itching due to excessive waste products in the blood

If kidney function is seriously impaired, dialysis may be necessary. Kidney **dialysis** is an artificial means of removing the body's waste products. It is done when the person's kidneys are no longer able to perform this function. It can improve and extend life for several years. Dialysis is done regularly and continuously until a kidney transplant is performed or until the person dies. While a resident is undergoing dialysis, he will have some type of fluid restriction.

End-stage renal disease (ESRD) occurs when the kidneys have failed and dialysis or transplantation is required to sustain life. Diabetes is the most common cause of end-stage renal disease. Dialysis is necessary for anyone who has ESRD.

Urine Retention

Urine retention is an inability to adequately or completely empty the bladder. Retention can be short-term or long-term. Surgical procedures, obstruction, infection, and some disorders, such as multiple sclerosis and diabetes, are common causes of urine retention (these diseases are discussed in Chapters 22 and 23 of the textbook). In men, the most common cause of urine retention is enlargement of the prostate gland. Symptoms include the following:

• Difficulty in starting to urinate

• Weak flow of urine

• Frequent urge to urinate

• A painful urge, but inability, to urinate

• Dribbling at the end of urinating and in between urinating

• Swollen (distended) bladder

• Abdominal swelling

• Lower abdominal pain

If an NA observes any of the symptoms listed above, he should report to the nurse. If the condition is not treated, it can lead to a urinary tract infection or damage to the urinary tract and kidneys. Urine retention is usually treated with medications and catheterization (use of a tube to drain urine from the bladder).

Here are a few additional resources for information relating to urinary disorders:

- National Kidney Foundation, kidney.org

- Prostate Cancer Foundation, pcf.org

Obesity and Disorders of the Urinary System

Obesity increases the risk for certain urinary diseases or disorders, including the following:

- Stress incontinence

- Urinary tract infections (UTIs)

- Cancers of the kidney and prostate

7. Discuss reasons for incontinence

Urinary incontinence is the inability to control the muscles of the bladder, which leads to an involuntary loss of urine. Urinary incontinence can occur in residents who are confined to bed, ill, or paralyzed. Other physical reasons for urinary incontinence include circulatory or nervous system diseases or injuries, such as stroke, dementia, or multiple sclerosis; prostate problems; or childbirth.

Incontinence is not a normal part of aging. Whatever the reason for incontinence, it is important for the NA to act professionally when handling this problem. He should never show anger or frustration toward residents who are incontinent. Residents who are incontinent need reassurance and understanding.

There are different types of urinary incontinence:

- Stress incontinence is a loss of urine due to an increase in intra-abdominal pressure; it may be caused by sneezing, laughing, or coughing.

- Urge incontinence is involuntary voiding due to an abrupt urge to void.

- Mixed incontinence means symptoms of both urge and stress incontinence are present.

- Functional incontinence is urine loss caused by environmental, cognitive, or physical reasons.

- Overflow incontinence is due to overflow or overdistention of the bladder.

Incontinence can be very difficult for residents to handle emotionally. Residents may avoid discussing the problem due to embarrassment. It may cause frustration and anger. Family and friends may share these feelings as well. NAs can help by always being professional and positive when dealing with episodes of incontinence.

Guidelines: Urinary Incontinence

G   Know residents' routines and urinary habits. Recognize their physical signs, such as holding the lower abdomen, which might indicate the need to urinate.

G   Follow elimination schedules and the care plan carefully.

G   Leave call lights within reach. Answer call lights promptly to prevent accidents.

G   Offer a bedpan or take residents to the bathroom often.

G   Encourage plenty of fluids unless residents have fluid restrictions.

G   Walking can stimulate circulation and the need to void. Take daily walks close to a bathroom.

G   Some residents will wear disposable incontinence pads or briefs for adults. They help keep body wastes away from the skin

(Fig. 16-5). Always refer to incontinence products as briefs or pads; never call them *diapers*. Residents are not infants, and using that term is disrespectful.

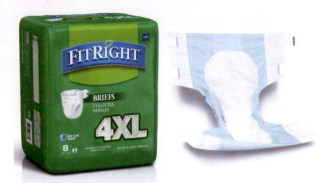

Fig. 16-5. *A type of incontinence brief.* (© MEDLINE INDUSTRIES, INC. 2019)

G   When residents wear incontinence briefs, check them at least every two hours. Change wet or soiled briefs immediately (see procedure in this learning objective). Before changing an incontinence brief, wash your hands and don gloves.

G   Change wet or soiled clothing immediately.

G   Change bed linens any time they are wet or soiled. Leaving residents in wet linens puts them at risk for pressure injuries (Chapter 18). It is also abusive or neglectful behavior.

G   Use disposable absorbent pads under bed linen for residents who are incontinent.

G   Give careful skin care and perineal care. This helps prevent skin breakdown. Urine is irritating to the skin. Bathe residents often.

G   Provide privacy for episodes of incontinence. Keep your voice low to keep incontinence a private matter. Never expose more of the resident than is necessary.

G   Be calm, patient, and professional.

G   Family and friends may watch how you behave to see how they should react to the problem. Be reassuring and remain positive.

Changing an incontinence brief

Equipment: incontinence brief in the correct size, bath blanket, disposable bed protector, plastic bag, supplies for perineal care, gloves

1.   Identify yourself by name. Identify the resident. Greet the resident by name.

2.   Wash your hands.

3.   Explain procedure to the resident. Speak clearly, slowly, and directly. Maintain face-to-face contact whenever possible.

4.   Provide for the resident's privacy with a curtain, screen, or door.

5.   Adjust the bed to a safe level, usually waist high. Raise the far bed rail (if used). Lock bed wheels.

6.   Lower the head of the bed. Position the resident lying flat on her back.

7.   Place a bath blanket over the resident. Ask her to hold on to it as you remove or fold back top bedding to the foot of the bed.

8.   Put on gloves.

9.   Place the bed protector under the resident's buttocks and hips.

10.   Turn the resident away from you toward the raised bed rail.

11. Remove the used incontinence brief and place it in the plastic bag. When removing the soiled brief, roll it inward, soiled side inside, without spilling its contents.

12. Gently roll the resident back onto the bed protector. Give perineal care if help is needed. Wipe from front to back. Dry the perineal area with a towel.

13. Remove gloves and discard. Wash your hands. Don clean gloves.

14. Open all tabs on the clean incontinence brief. Place the brief under the resident, centering the back of the pad. Turn the resident from side to side as needed.

15. Wrap the brief around the resident, making sure the front and back of the brief covers the resident.

16. Pull all tabs to secure the brief. For a male resident, make sure the penis is placed in a comfortable position.

17. Remove and discard the bed protector. Cover the resident and remove the bath blanket, placing it in the proper container while avoiding contact with your clothing.

18. Remove and discard gloves properly.

19. Wash your hands.

20. Make the resident comfortable.

21. Return bed to its lowest position. Leave bed rails in the ordered position. Remove privacy measures.

22. Leave call light within the resident's reach.

23. Wash your hands.

24. Be courteous and respectful at all times.

25. Report any changes in the resident to the nurse. Show the used incontinence brief to the nurse if requested. Document procedure using facility guidelines.

8. Describe catheters and related care

Residents who are unable to pass urine normally may need a urinary catheter. A catheter is a tube used to add or drain fluid that is inserted through the skin or into a body opening. Some residents need intermittent catheterization. A **straight catheter** is a type of catheter that is inserted to drain urine from the bladder several times a day and is removed each time after the urine is drained.

For other residents, a catheter may need to remain inside the bladder for a period of time. This type of a catheter is called an **indwelling catheter** (Fig. 16-6). This catheter is held in place by a balloon filled with sterile water and the urine drains into a bag.

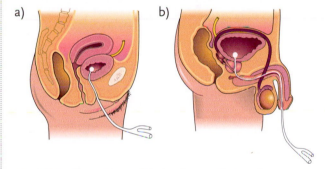

a)   b)

Fig. 16-6. *Illustrations of indwelling catheters for a) female and b) male residents.*

Another type of catheter that is used for males is an external catheter, or **condom catheter** (also called a *Texas catheter*). It has an attachment on the end that fits onto the penis and is fastened with special tape. The urine drains through the condom catheter into the tubing, then into the drainage bag. A smaller bag, called a *leg bag*, collects the urine. It attaches to the resident's leg. A condom catheter is changed daily or as needed.

Nurses or doctors insert urinary catheters. NAs do not insert, irrigate, or remove catheters. NAs may be asked to give daily catheter care, clean the area around the urethral opening, and empty the drainage bag. The bag is emptied into a measuring container (a graduate). Measuring urinary output was discussed in Chapter 14.

Serious complications, such as infections, can occur from poor catheter care. If bacteria travel up the catheter, they can cause infection in the urethra, bladder, ureter, or kidney. When that occurs, it is called a **catheter-associated urinary tract infection (CAUTI)**. These infections can be life-threatening. It is very important for NAs to follow proper guidelines for urinary catheters.

Residents' Rights

Catheters

According to CMS requirements, residents who are not catheterized at the time of admission should not be catheterized unless their medical situation warrants it. A resident who enters the facility with a catheter should be assessed for removal of the catheter as soon as possible. This ensures that residents receive treatment appropriate for their conditions and are not exposed to unnecessary risk of infection.

Guidelines: Catheters

G   Thoroughly wash your hands before performing catheter care.

G   Don gloves before performing any part of catheter care.

G   Keep the genital area clean to prevent infection. Pathogens can enter the bladder more easily with catheters. Daily care of the genital area is extremely important.

G   When cleaning the urinary meatus, move in one direction, away from the meatus. Use a clean area of the cloth for each stroke.

G   Secure the tubing properly to either the inner thigh or the abdomen (for a male) with a catheter strap.

G   Make sure the drainage bag always hangs lower than the level of the hips or bladder, including when the resident is ambulating or in a wheelchair. Urine must never flow back into the bladder from the tubing or bag. This can cause infection.

G   Do not hang the drainage bag from a bedrail; the drainage bag should be secured to a non-movable part of the bed frame that is opposite the door to the hallway. When the resident is in a wheelchair, the bag may fit into a special pouch located on the side or back of the wheelchair, or it may have a special cover that is used to conceal it. Keeping the bag covered promotes the resident's dignity.

G   To help keep urine draining properly, keep tubing as straight as possible. Make sure there are no kinks in the tube and that the resident is not lying on the tubing. The tubing should be over the leg, not underneath it. Do not allow the tubing to loop below the drainage bag.

G   Keep the drainage bag off the floor. Make sure the catheter tubing does not touch the floor.

G   When draining the bag, open and close the tubing clamp without touching the tip of the clamp to any other object. If the tip touches other objects, it can transfer pathogens to the inside of the tubing, which can move up into the bladder and cause infection.

G   Do not let the catheter drainage spout touch the graduate when draining the catheter bag.

G   Be careful not to disconnect the catheter when positioning or transferring residents with catheters. Do not try to reattach a catheter tube that has disconnected. Inform the nurse immediately so that she can reattach the tube. This is a sterile procedure.

G   Report any of the following to the nurse: blood in the urine, urine leaking from the catheter, or the catheter bag filling suddenly or not filling for several hours. Also report complaints of pain, pressure, or odor.

Providing catheter care

Equipment: bath blanket, disposable bed protector, bath basin with warm water, soap, water thermometer, 2–4 washcloths or disposable wipes, towel, gloves

1.   Identify yourself by name. Identify the resident. Greet the resident by name.

2. Wash your hands.

3. Explain procedure to the resident. Speak clearly, slowly, and directly. Maintain face-to-face contact whenever possible.

4. Provide for the resident's privacy with a curtain, screen, or door.

5. Adjust the bed to a safe level, usually waist high. Lock bed wheels.

6. Lower the head of the bed. Position the resident lying flat on her back.

7. Remove or fold back top bedding. Keep the resident covered with the bath blanket.

8. Test water temperature with a thermometer or against the inside of your wrist to ensure it is safe. Water temperature should be no higher than 105°F. Have the resident check the water temperature. Adjust if necessary.

9. Put on gloves.

10. Ask the resident to flex her knees and raise her buttocks off the bed by pushing against the mattress with her feet. Place a clean bed protector under her perineal area, including her buttocks.

11. Expose only the area necessary to clean the catheter. Avoid overexposing the resident.

12. Place a towel under the catheter tubing before washing.

13. Wet a washcloth in the basin. Apply soap to the washcloth. If a male resident is uncircumcised, gently pull back the foreskin first. Clean the area around the meatus. Use a clean area of the washcloth for each stroke.

14. Hold the catheter near the meatus. Avoid tugging the catheter throughout the procedure.

15. Clean at least four inches of the catheter nearest the meatus. Move in only one direction, away from the meatus (Fig. 16-7). Use a clean area of the washcloth for each stroke.

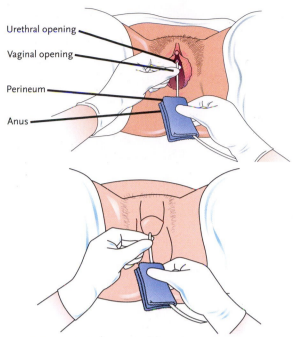

Urethral opening
Vaginal opening
Perineum
Anus

Fig. 16-7. *Hold the catheter near the meatus to avoid tugging the catheter. Moving in only one direction, away from the meatus, helps prevent infection. Use a clean area of the washcloth for each stroke.*

16. Dip a clean washcloth in the water. Rinse the area around the meatus, using a clean area of washcloth for each stroke. With a clean, dry towel, dry the area around the meatus.

17. Dip a clean washcloth in the water. Rinse at least four inches of the catheter nearest the meatus. Move in only one direction, away from the meatus. Use a clean area of the cloth for each stroke.

18. With a clean, dry towel, dry at least four inches of the catheter nearest the meatus. Move in only one direction, away from the meatus. Do not tug the catheter.

19. Remove and discard the bed protector. Remove the towel from under the catheter tubing, and place towel and washcloths in proper containers.

20. Empty the basin into the toilet and flush the toilet. Place basin in the proper area for cleaning or clean and store it according to facility policy.

21. Remove and discard gloves properly. Wash your hands.

22. Replace top covers. Remove bath blanket and place it in the proper container. Make the resident comfortable.

23. Return bed to its lowest position. Remove privacy measures.

24. Leave call light within the resident's reach.

25. Wash your hands.

26. Be courteous and respectful at all times.

27. Report any changes in the resident to the nurse. Document procedure using facility guidelines.

Emptying a catheter drainage bag

Equipment: graduate (measuring container), alcohol wipes, paper towels, gloves

1. Identify yourself by name. Identify the resident. Greet the resident by name.

2. Wash your hands.

3. Explain procedure to the resident. Speak clearly, slowly, and directly. Maintain face-to-face contact whenever possible.

4. Provide for the resident's privacy with a curtain, screen, or door.

5. Put on gloves.

6. Place a paper towel on the floor under the drainage bag. Place the graduate on the paper towel.

7. Open the clamp on the drainage bag so that the urine flows out of the bag and into the graduate (Fig. 16-8). Do not let the spout or clamp touch the graduate.

8. When urine has drained out of the bag, close the clamp. Using alcohol wipes, clean the drain spout. Return the drain spout to its holder on the catheter bag.

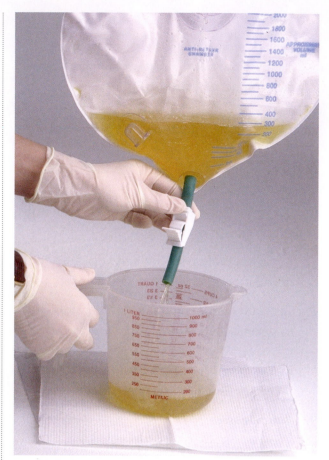

Fig. 16-8. *Keep the drain spout and clamp from touching the graduate while draining urine.*

9. Go into the bathroom. Place the graduate on a flat surface and measure at eye level. Note the amount and appearance of the urine. Empty urine into the toilet and flush the toilet.

10. Place the container in the area for cleaning or clean and store it according to facility policy. Discard the paper towel.

11. Remove and discard gloves properly. Wash your hands.

12. Leave call light within the resident's reach.

13. Wash your hands.

14. Be courteous and respectful at all times.

15. Report any changes in the resident to the nurse. Document procedure and amount of urine (output) using facility guidelines.

Changing a condom catheter

Equipment: condom catheter and collection bag, catheter tape, plastic bag, bath blanket, disposable bed protector, supplies for perineal care, gloves

1. Identify yourself by name. Identify the resident. Greet the resident by name.

2. Wash your hands.

3. Explain procedure to the resident. Speak clearly, slowly, and directly. Maintain face-to-face contact whenever possible.

4. Provide for the resident's privacy with a curtain, screen, or door.

5. Adjust the bed to a safe level, usually waist high. Lock bed wheels.

6. Lower the head of the bed. Position the resident lying flat on his back.

7. Remove or fold back the top bedding, keeping the resident covered with the bath blanket.

8. Put on gloves.

9. Place a clean bed protector under the resident's buttocks.

10. Adjust the bath blanket to expose only the genital area.

11. Gently remove the condom catheter. Disconnect the condom from the tube and immediately cap the tube. Do not allow the tube to touch anything. Place the condom and tape in the plastic bag.

12. Help as necessary with perineal care.

13. Move pubic hair away from the penis so it does not get rolled into the condom.

14. Hold the penis firmly. Place the condom at the tip of the penis and roll toward the base of the penis. Leave space (at least one inch) between the drainage tip and glans of penis to prevent irritation. If the resident is not circumcised, be sure that foreskin is in a normal position.

15. Gently secure the condom to the penis with the special tape provided (Fig. 16-9). Apply the tape in a spiral manner. Never wrap the tape all the way around the penis because it can impair circulation.

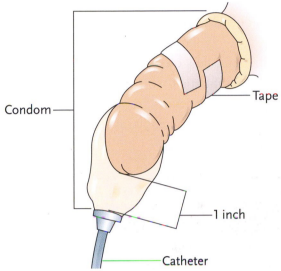

Fig. 16-9. *Gently secure the condom to the penis with provided tape, applying it in a spiral.*

16. Connect the catheter tip to the drainage tubing. Do not touch the tip to any object but the drainage tubing. Make sure the tubing is not twisted or kinked.

17. Check to see if the collection bag is secured to the leg. Make sure the drain is closed.

18. Remove and discard the bed protector. Discard the plastic bag properly. Place soiled clothing and linens in proper containers. Clean and store supplies.

19. Remove and discard gloves properly.

20. Wash your hands.

21. Replace the top covers. Remove the bath blanket. Make the resident comfortable.

22. Return bed to its lowest position. Remove privacy measures.

23. Leave call light within the resident's reach.

24. Wash your hands.

25. Be courteous and respectful at all times.

26. Report any changes in the resident to the nurse. Document procedure using facility guidelines.

After a condom catheter is applied, the NA should check it often to make sure urine is draining freely. The condom catheter should be reapplied if it falls off. The NA should report signs or symptoms that the catheter is interfering with circulation in the penis: pale, gray, or blue-tinged skin or complaints of numbness, tingling, or pain.

9. Explain how to collect different types of urine specimens

Urine specimens are collected for various types of tests. The NA should be sure to verify that he has the correct resident when collecting a urine specimen. The specimen must be put in the proper container and labeled with the resident's name, date of birth, doctor's name, room number, date, and time. Some urine specimens require special containers.

Urine that cannot be sent to the lab immediately may need to be placed in a special refrigerator used strictly for specimens. Specimens should never be placed in a refrigerator that is used for food or drinks.

When collecting a urine specimen, the NA should first show the resident the correct container to use. The resident should be prepared to give a specimen the next time he has to urinate. The NA should explain that stool or toilet paper should not be included in the container because they can ruin the sample. After obtaining the specimen, it should be taken to the lab or proper place promptly.

There are many tests that can be performed on urine. A **routine urine specimen** can be collected any time the resident voids. The resident will void into a bedpan, urinal, commode, or hat (collection container).

Collecting a routine urine specimen

Equipment: specimen container and lid, completed label (labeled with resident's name, date of birth, doctor's name, room number, date, and time), biohazard specimen bag, 2 pairs of gloves, bedpan or urinal (if resident cannot use portable commode or toilet), hat for toilet (if resident uses portable commode or toilet), plastic bag, disposable wipes, toilet paper, paper towels, supplies for perineal care, lab slip

1. Identify yourself by name. Identify the resident. Greet the resident by name.

2. Wash your hands.

3. Explain procedure to the resident. Speak clearly, slowly, and directly. Maintain face-to-face contact whenever possible.

4. Provide for the resident's privacy with a curtain, screen, or door.

5. Put on gloves.

6. Fit the hat to the toilet or commode, or provide the resident with a bedpan or urinal.

7. Have resident void into the hat, urinal, or bedpan. Ask the resident not to put toilet paper or stool in with the sample. Provide a plastic bag to discard the toilet paper separately.

8. Make sure both bed rails are up, and the bed is in its lowest position. Place toilet paper and wipes within the resident's reach. Ask the resident to clean his hands with a wipe when finished if he is able.

9. Ask the resident to signal when he is finished. Make sure call light is within reach.

10. Remove and discard gloves properly. Wash your hands. Leave the room and close the door.

11. When called by the resident, return and wash your hands. Put on clean gloves.

12. Give perineal care if help is needed.

13. Take the bedpan, urinal, or hat to the bathroom.

14. Pour urine into the specimen container. The specimen container should be at least half full.

15. Cover the urine container with its lid. Do not touch the inside of the container. Wipe off the outside with a paper towel and discard the paper towel. Apply the label and place the specimen in a clean biohazard specimen bag.

16. Discard extra urine in the toilet. Turn the faucet on with a paper towel. Rinse the bedpan, urinal, or hat with cold water and empty it into the toilet. Flush the toilet. Place equipment in the proper area for cleaning or clean and store it according to policy.

17. Remove and discard gloves properly. Wash your hands.

18. Make the resident comfortable.

19. Return bed to its lowest position. Remove privacy measures.

20. Leave call light within the resident's reach.

21. Wash your hands.

22. Be courteous and respectful at all times.

23. Report any changes in the resident to the nurse. Document procedure using facility guidelines. Take specimen and lab slip to designated place promptly.

Urine Straining

Urine is strained to detect the presence of renal calculi, or kidney stones, that can develop in the urinary tract. Urine straining is the process of pouring all urine through a fine filter to catch any particles. Kidney stones can be as small as grains of sand or as large as golf balls. If any stones are found, they are saved and then sent to a laboratory for examination.

A routine urine specimen is collected first in order to strain urine. In the bathroom, the NA will pour urine through a strainer or a 4x4-inch piece of gauze into a specimen container. Any stones are trapped in the filter. The filter is placed in the specimen container and then into a clean specimen bag for transport to the lab.

A **clean-catch specimen**, or midstream specimen (CCMS), does not include the first and last urine voided in the sample. The perineal area is cleaned and then the resident urinates a small amount into the toilet to clear the urethra. The resident then urinates midstream in a clean or sterile container. The resident stops urinating while the NA removes the container, then the resident finishes voiding into the toilet. This specimen is collected to detect bacteria in the urine.

Collecting a clean-catch (midstream) urine specimen

Equipment: specimen kit with container and lid, completed label (labeled with resident's name, date of birth, doctor's name, room number, date, and time), biohazard specimen bag, cleansing wipes, gloves, bedpan or urinal (if resident cannot use portable commode or toilet), plastic bag, toilet paper, disposable wipes, paper towels, supplies for perineal care, lab slip

1. Identify yourself by name. Identify the resident. Greet the resident by name.

2. Wash your hands.

3. Explain procedure to the resident. Speak clearly, slowly, and directly. Maintain face-to-face contact whenever possible.

4. Provide for the resident's privacy with a curtain, screen, or door.

5. Put on gloves.

6. Open the specimen kit. Do not touch the inside of the container or lid.

7. If the resident cannot clean her perineal area, you will do it. Use the cleansing wipes to do this. Use a clean area of the wipe or a clean

wipe for each stroke. Refer to the perineal care procedure in Chapter 12 if needed.

8. Ask the resident to urinate a small amount into the bedpan, urinal, or toilet, and to stop before urination is complete.

9. Place the container under the urine stream. Do not touch the resident's body with the container. Have the resident start urinating again. Fill the container at least half full. Ask the resident to stop urinating and remove the container. Have the resident finish urinating in the bedpan, urinal, or toilet.

10. After urination, provide a plastic bag so the resident can discard the toilet paper. Give perineal care if help is needed. Ask the resident to clean her hands with a wipe if she is able.

11. Cover the urine container with its lid. Do not touch the inside of the container. Wipe off the outside with a paper towel and discard the paper towel. Apply the label and place the specimen in a clean biohazard specimen bag.

12. Discard extra urine in the toilet. Turn the faucet on with a paper towel. Rinse the bedpan, urinal, or hat with cold water and empty it into the toilet. Flush the toilet. Place equipment in the proper area for cleaning or clean and store it according to policy.

13. Remove and discard gloves properly. Wash your hands.

14. Make the resident comfortable.

15. Return bed to its lowest position. Remove privacy measures.

16. Leave call light within the resident's reach.

17. Wash your hands.

18. Be courteous and respectful at all times.

19. Report any changes in the resident to the nurse. Document procedure using facility guidelines. Take specimen and lab slip to designated place promptly.

A **24-hour urine specimen** collects all the urine voided by a resident in a 24-hour period. It is used to test for certain chemicals and hormones. Usually the collection begins at 7 a.m. and continues until 7 a.m. the next day. When beginning a 24-hour urine specimen collection, the resident must void and discard the first urine so that the collection begins with an empty bladder. All urine must be collected and stored properly. If any is accidentally thrown away, spilled, or improperly stored, the collection will need to be started over.

Collecting a 24-hour urine specimen

Equipment: 24-hour specimen container with lid, completed label (labeled with resident's name, date of birth, doctor's name, room number, date, and time), bedpan or urinal (for residents confined to bed), hat for toilet (if resident can use portable commode or toilet), gloves, toilet paper, disposable wipes, supplies for perineal care, sign to alert other team members that a 24-hour urine specimen is being collected, form to record output, lab slip with date and time of first void

1. Identify yourself by name. Identify the resident. Greet the resident by name.

2. Wash your hands.

3. Explain procedure to the resident. Speak clearly, slowly, and directly. Maintain face-to-face contact whenever possible. Emphasize that all urine must be saved. Ask the resident not to put toilet paper or stool in with the sample.

4. Provide for the resident's privacy with a curtain, screen, or door.

5. Place a sign near the resident's bed to let all care team members know that a 24-hour specimen is being collected. Sign may read *Save all urine for 24-hour specimen.*

6. When starting the collection, have the resident completely empty her bladder. Measure and note amount of urine if the resident's

intake and output is being monitored. Discard the urine. Note the exact time of this voiding. The collection will run until the same time the next day (Fig. 16-10).

7. Wash hands and put on gloves each time the resident voids.

8. Pour urine from the bedpan, urinal, or hat into the container. The container may be stored at room temperature, in a special refrigerator, or on ice. Follow instructions.

9. After each voiding, help as necessary with perineal care. Ask the resident to clean her hands with a wipe after each voiding if she is able.

10. After each voiding, place equipment in the proper area for cleaning or clean and store it according to policy.

11. Remove and discard gloves properly.

12. Wash your hands.

13. After the last void of the 24-hour period, add the urine to the specimen container. Remove the sign.

14. Make the resident comfortable.

15. Return bed to its lowest position. Remove privacy measures.

16. Leave call light within the resident's reach.

17. Wash your hands.

18. Be courteous and respectful at all times.

19. Report any changes in the resident to the nurse. Document procedure using facility guidelines. Take specimen containers and lab slip to designated place promptly.

INTAKE-OUTPUT RECORD

Resident/Patient Name ___ Room No. ___

FLUID INTAKE	URINE	EMESIS or DRAINAGE

7:00 A.M. to 3:00 P.M.
8-Hour Total

3:00 P.M. to 11:00 P.M.
8-Hour Total

11:00 P.M. to 7 A.M.
8-Hour Total

Form 3039 © Briggs, Des Moines, IA 50306 PRINTED IN U.S.A. R404
DON'T BREAK THE LAW Save 13%* 1-800-247-2343 www.BriggsCorp.com
MAKE THE CALL
*savings on buying vs. copying

Fig. 16-10. *One type of form to record urine output over 24 hours.* (REPRINTED WITH PERMISSION OF BRIGGS HEALTHCARE®, 800.247.2343, BRIGGSHEALTHCARE.COM)

A catheterized urine specimen is obtained when a resident cannot urinate on his own, when an infection in the urinary tract may be present, or if the resident is retaining urine. A nurse will collect this type of specimen. To collect this urine specimen, the nurse will insert a straight catheter through the urethra into the bladder using sterile technique. The urine is obtained this way to avoid contamination.

A specimen may have to be collected from a resident who has a urostomy. The nurse will remove the urostomy appliance and collect this specimen directly from the stoma. The appliance is then resealed over the stoma.

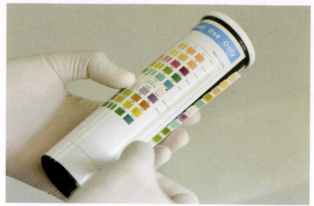

Fig. 16-11. *Reagent strips change color when they react with urine. The color is then compared to a color chart to determine levels of each chemical factor.*

> **Tip**
>
> **Five "Rights" of Specimen Collection**
>
> Knowing and remembering the five "rights" of specimen collection will help prevent mistakes and ensure that specimens are collected properly:
>
> 1. The Right Resident
> 2. The Right Specimen
> 3. The Right Container
> 4. The Right Date/Time
> 5. The Right Storage/Delivery
>
> Properly collecting a specimen helps to ensure prompt laboratory results. It also means that an additional specimen will not need to be collected, which promotes the resident's dignity.

10. Explain types of tests that are performed on urine

Facilities use different methods to test urine. Dip strips can be used to test for such things as pH level, glucose, ketones, blood, and specific gravity. These strips, called *reagent strips*, have different sections that change color when they react with urine (Fig. 16-11).

Testing pH levels: pH stands for potential hydrogen. The pH scale ranges from 0 to 14. The lower the number, the more acidic the fluid. The higher the number, the more alkaline the fluid. The normal pH range for urine is 4.6–8.0. A pH imbalance may be due to medication, food, or illness.

Testing for glucose and ketones: In diabetes, the pancreas does not produce enough insulin or does not produce any insulin (Chapter 23). Insulin is the substance the body needs to convert glucose, or natural sugar, into energy. Without insulin to process glucose, these sugars collect in the blood. Some sugar appears in the urine.

People who have diabetes may also have ketones in the urine. **Ketones** are chemical substances produced when the body burns fat for energy or fuel. They are produced when there is not enough insulin to help the body use sugar for energy. Without enough insulin, glucose builds up in the blood. Since the body cannot use glucose for energy, it breaks down fat instead. When this occurs, ketones build up in the blood and spill into the urine.

Testing for blood: In normal urine, blood should not be present. Illness and disease can cause blood to appear in urine. Some blood is hidden, or occult. This blood can be detected by testing the urine.

Testing specific gravity: A **specific gravity** (also called *urine density*) test is performed to measure the concentration of chemical particles in the urine. The test evaluates the body's water balance and urine concentration by showing how the density of urine compares with water. Normal values range from 1.002 to 1.028. Certain disorders increase or decrease specific gravity.

For example, heart failure can increase specific gravity, while kidney failure can decrease it.

If performing urine testing with testing strips, the NA should check the expiration date to make sure that the strips have not expired. Testing strips that have expired may give inaccurate results, which can prolong the resident's discomfort or problem. The NA should inform the nurse and obtain a new bottle if the strips have expired. Testing strips are usually stored in a light-resistant bottle. When testing a urine specimen, the strips should be removed one at a time and the bottle should be capped tightly before storing.

The doctor will order the specific type of specimen to be collected and how often urine tests should be performed.

Testing urine with reagent strips

Equipment: urine specimen as ordered, reagent strip, gloves, paper towel

1. Wash your hands.

2. Put on gloves.

3. Place paper towel on surface before setting down the urine specimen.

4. Take a strip from the bottle and recap the bottle. Close it tightly.

5. Dip the strip into the specimen.

6. Follow the manufacturer's instructions for when to remove the strip from the specimen. Remove the strip at the correct time.

7. Follow the manufacturer's instructions for how long to wait after removing the strip. After the proper time has passed, compare the strip with the color chart on the bottle. Do not touch the bottle with the strip.

8. Read the results.

9. Store the strips. Discard used items. Discard the specimen in the toilet. Flush the toilet.

10. Remove and discard gloves properly.

11. Wash your hands.

12. Record and report results. Document procedure using facility guidelines.

11. Explain guidelines for assisting with bladder retraining

Illness, injury, or inactivity can cause a loss of normal bladder function. Residents may need help in reestablishing a regular routine and normal bladder function. Urinary incontinence may be a problem when retraining the bladder. Because incontinence can be embarrassing or difficult for a resident to discuss, the NA should be professional, sensitive, and empathetic when incontinence occurs.

Most of the resident's care team members will be involved with charting and implementing bladder retraining. NAs should understand and follow the care plan for each resident.

Guidelines: Bladder Retraining

G Follow the plan consistently. Explain the training schedule to the resident. Direct any questions the resident has to the nurse.

G Follow Standard Precautions. Wear gloves when handling body wastes. For residents in isolation, additional personal protective equipment (PPE) may be needed. Follow the care plan.

G Observe the resident's elimination habits. This helps predict when a trip to the bathroom or a bedpan or urinal will be necessary.

G Encourage plenty of fluids throughout the day if allowed, even if incontinence is a problem. About 30 minutes after fluids are consumed, offer a bedpan, urinal, or trip to the bathroom.

G Offer a bedpan or urinal or a trip to the bathroom before beginning long procedures and after the procedures have been completed (Fig. 16-12).

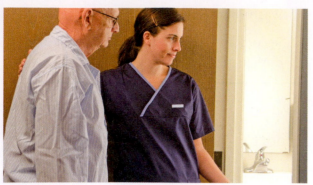

Fig. 16-12. *Offer regular trips to the bathroom, especially before and after performing care.*

G   Answer call lights promptly. Residents should never have to wait to go to the bathroom.

G   Provide privacy with elimination, and do not rush the resident.

G   Have the resident lean forward slightly to put pressure on the bladder. If she is having trouble urinating, try running water in the sink.

G   Help with perineal care as needed. This promotes proper hygiene and helps prevent skin breakdown. Watch for skin changes and report them.

G   Keep accurate intake and output (I&O) records. Output includes episodes of incontinence. Keeping accurate records will help establish a routine.

G   Dispose of wastes properly.

G   Praise attempts and successes in controlling the bladder.

G   Never show frustration or anger toward residents who are incontinent. The problem is out of their control. Be positive and patient with the retraining efforts.

Residents' Rights

Bladder Retraining

Residents have the right to assistance with their elimination needs as often as necessary. It is important that they not feel afraid to request help as frequently as they need it. NAs should let residents know that they are willing to help whenever they are needed.

Chapter Review

1. What are four functions of the urinary system (LO 2)?

2. List four normal age-related changes of the urinary system (LO 3).

3. List three normal qualities of urine (LO 4).

4. What is the best position for women to urinate? What is the best position for men to urinate (LO 5)?

5. Why are women more susceptible to urinary tract infections (UTIs) than men (LO 6)?

6. How should residents wipe after elimination in order to prevent infection (LO 6)?

7. What is dialysis (LO 6)?

8. Define five different types of incontinence (LO 7).

9. Why should a catheter drainage bag always hang lower than the level of the hips or bladder (LO 8)?

10. What items should not be included in a urine specimen (LO 9)?

11. List four things reagent strips can detect in urine (LO 10).

Multiple Choice

12. What type of catheter is removed immediately after urine is drained and does not remain inside the bladder (LO 8)?
    (A) Indwelling catheter
    (B) Straight catheter
    (C) Drainage catheter
    (D) Condom catheter

13. Approximately how long after fluids are consumed should an NA offer a resident a bedpan, urinal, or trip to the bathroom (LO 11)?
    (A) One hour
    (B) Ten minutes
    (C) Thirty minutes
    (D) Two hours

17
The Reproductive System

An Amazing Recovery

Ephraim McDowell, 1771–1830, a doctor of the Kentucky frontier, was visited in 1809 by a woman with a large ovarian cyst. He asked her to travel 60 miles to his office for an operation which she would probably not survive. She decided to travel the distance on horseback. The physician opened her abdomen without anesthesia while she read from the Bible. He cut out an ovary weighing nearly 20 pounds. After a 25-day recovery, she left the area and returned home. The woman lived another 31 years. McDowell gained international fame for his removal of cysts.

*"In the dark womb where I
began
My mother's life made me.
Through all the months of
human birth
Her beauty fed my common
earth."*

John Masefield, 1878–1967

*"Little creature, formed of joy
and mirth,
Go, love without the help of any
thing on earth."*

William Blake, 1757–1827

1. Define important words in this chapter

benign prostatic hypertrophy: a disorder that can occur in men as they age, in which the prostate becomes enlarged and causes problems with urination and/or emptying the bladder.

cervical cancer: a form of female reproductive cancer that begins in the cervix.

chlamydia: a sexually transmitted infection caused by bacteria.

endometrial cancer: a form of female reproductive cancer that begins in the uterus.

erectile dysfunction (ED): the inability to have or maintain a penile erection.

genital herpes: a sexually transmitted, incurable infection caused by herpes simplex viruses type 1 (HSV-1) or type 2 (HSV-2).

genital HPV infection: a sexually transmitted infection caused by human papillomavirus.

glands: organs that produce and secrete chemicals called *hormones.*

gonads: the male and female sexual reproductive glands.

gonorrhea: a sexually transmitted infection caused by bacteria.

hormones: chemical substances produced by the body that control numerous body functions.

menopause: the end of menstruation; occurs when a woman has not had a menstrual period for 12 months.

menstruation: the shedding of the lining of the uterus that occurs approximately every 28 days; also known as a *period.*

ovarian cancer: a form of female reproductive cancer that begins in the ovaries.

ovum: female sex cell or egg.

prostate cancer: a form of male reproductive cancer that begins in the prostate gland.

sexually transmitted infections (STIs): infections caused by sexual contact with infected people; signs and symptoms are not always apparent.

sperm: male sex cells.

syphilis: a sexually transmitted infection caused by bacteria.

testicular cancer: a form of male reproductive cancer that begins in the testes.

trichomoniasis: a sexually transmitted infection caused by protozoa (single-celled animals).

vaginitis: an inflammation of the vagina.

2. Explain the structure and function of the reproductive system

The reproductive system consists of the reproductive organs, which are different in men and women. This system allows human beings to reproduce, or create new human life. Reproduction begins when male and female sex cells, **sperm** and **ovum**, join. These sex cells are formed in the male and female sexual reproductive glands, called the **gonads**. **Glands** are organs that produce and secrete chemicals called *hormones*. **Hormones** are chemical substances produced by the body that control numerous body functions, including the body's ability to reproduce. More information about glands and hormones is located in Chapter 23.

The Male Reproductive System

The male reproductive system consists of the penis, testes, scrotum, epididymis, vas deferens, erectile tissue, seminal vesicle, ejaculatory duct, and prostate gland (Fig. 17-1). The testes are found within the sac of skin known as the *scrotum*. The scrotum supports the testes and regulates the temperature of the testes. The testes produce testosterone, the male hormone needed for the reproductive organs to function properly, as well as sperm.

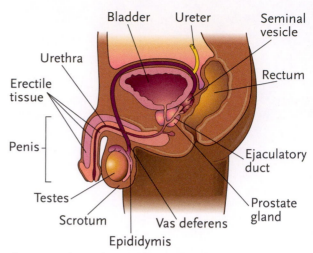

Fig. 17-1. *The male reproductive system.*

Sperm travel from the testes to the epididymis, a coiled tube that can be as long as 20 feet. The epididymis receives and stores sperm. After maturing in the epididymis, sperm move into the vas deferens, the tube that sperm travel through in order to reach the ejaculatory duct. During their trip, the sperm mix with fluid produced in three glands: the seminal vesicles, the prostate gland, and Cowper's glands.

From the ejaculatory duct, sperm empty into the urethra, where they are released from the body through the penis. The penis is the sex organ located outside the body, in front of the scrotum. The penis is composed of erectile tissue that becomes filled with blood during sexual excitement. As the penis fills with blood, it becomes enlarged and erect and is able to release semen. Semen is released in small amounts during ejaculation, from about two to five milliliters at a time. Every milliliter of semen contains 20 to 150 million sperm.

The Female Reproductive System

The female reproductive system is made up of the ovaries, fallopian tubes, uterus, vagina, the external genitals—the vulva—and the mammary glands or breasts (Fig. 17-2). The ovaries produce the female sex cells or eggs (ova) and they produce the female hormones, estrogen and progesterone. Each month from puberty to menopause, ova are released from ovaries (usually alternating ovaries) during the process called *ovulation*. This monthly cycle is maintained by estrogen and progesterone. The ovum or egg cell then travels into the respective fallopian tube, one of two tubes that open into the uterus.

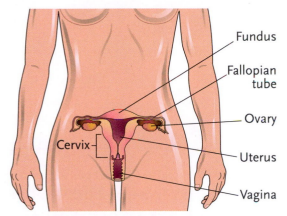

Fig. 17-2. *The female reproductive system.*

As the ovum reaches the fallopian tube, it may be fertilized by a sperm that will swim its way up into the tube. If it is not fertilized, the ovum will die within about 24 to 48 hours. Sperm usually die within five days. If an ovum is fertilized, it moves into the uterus, or womb. The uterus is a hollow, pear-shaped, muscular organ located within the pelvis. It lies behind the bladder and in front of the rectum.

A fertilized ovum will implant into the lining of the uterus, or the endometrium. This is where the fetus develops. If an ovum is not fertilized, the secretion of female hormones decreases. The endometrium then breaks up and is expelled in a process called **menstruation**.

The vagina is the muscular canal that opens to the outside of the body. It serves as the outlet for the blood during a woman's menstrual cycle. It acts as the receiver of sperm during sexual intercourse and is the birth canal.

The breasts or mammary glands are the glands that nourish a baby. They are responsible for the production of milk within the alveolar glands inside the breast. These glands send the milk into milk ducts that come together at the nipple in the area called the *areola*. This process is called *lactation*.

The functions of the reproductive system are:

Male

- To manufacture sperm and the male hormone testosterone

Female

- To manufacture ova (eggs) and the female hormones, estrogen and progesterone
- To provide an environment for the development of a fetus
- To produce milk (lactation) for the nourishment of a baby after birth

Destination: Homeostasis

Homeostasis can be affected by changes in the reproductive system. Stress is one of many factors that can cause males to have a low sperm count. Low sperm count means that the semen a male ejaculates contains fewer sperm than normal. A sperm count can be considered low when there are fewer than 15 million sperm per milliliter of semen. Reducing stress may help increase sperm count, returning the body to homeostasis.

3. Discuss changes in the reproductive system due to aging

Normal age-related changes for the reproductive system include the following:

Male

- The prostate gland enlarges.
- The number and capability of sperm decrease.
- Sexual response slows; it may take longer to achieve an erection and to reach orgasm.

Female

- **Menopause** occurs 12 months after a woman's last menstrual period. It signifies the end of the female's ability to reproduce. Menopause usually occurs between the ages of 45 and 55.

- Decrease in production of estrogen and progesterone leads to a loss of calcium, causing brittle bones and, potentially, osteoporosis. Decrease in estrogen also makes females more prone to urinary tract infections.

- Vaginal walls become drier and thinner; this may cause discomfort during sexual intercourse.

4. Discuss common disorders of the reproductive system

Sexually Transmitted Infections (STIs)

Sexually transmitted infections (STIs), or sexually transmitted diseases (STDs), are caused by sexual contact with an infected person. Sexually transmitted infections do not always have apparent signs and symptoms.

STIs are transmitted through sexual contact, such as sexual intercourse (vaginal and anal), contact of the mouth with the genitals or anus, and contact of the hands with the genital area. The transmission of some STIs can be reduced or stopped by using latex or polyurethane condoms (Fig. 17-3). The human immunodeficiency virus (HIV) can be transmitted sexually as well. HIV and AIDS are discussed in depth in Chapter 24.

Chlamydia infection is caused by bacteria. Symptoms of chlamydia include burning with urination, yellow or white discharge from the penis or vagina, swelling of the testes, painful intercourse, and abdominal and lower back pain. In many cases, no symptoms are apparent. This disorder may cause an eye infection (conjunctivitis, or "pink eye") or pneumonia in babies born to infected mothers. It may also cause infertility and pelvic inflammatory disease (PID) if not

promptly and properly treated. Chlamydia is treated with antibiotics.

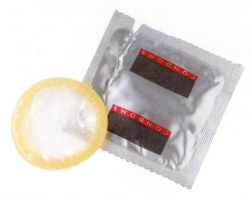

Fig. 17-3. *Using latex or polyurethane condoms reduces a person's risk of being infected with or transmitting some sexually transmitted infections.*

Genital herpes is caused by herpes simplex viruses type 1 (HSV-1) or type 2 (HSV-2). Usually genital herpes is caused by HSV-2. It cannot be treated with antibiotics, nor can it be cured. However, one type of medication makes it less likely that it will be transmitted to others. Once infected with genital herpes, a person may have repeated outbreaks of the disease for the rest of his or her life. Symptoms include itching and painful, red blisters or open sores. Herpes may also cause a burning sensation while urinating or during intercourse, low grade fever, headache, and muscle aches. Herpes sores are infectious and may appear quickly after sexual contact with an infected partner. However, a person can also spread genital herpes when sores are not present. Genital herpes is treated with antiviral medication. The medication does not cure the disease, but it can help lessen the frequency, duration, and intensity of the episodes.

Genital HPV infection is a sexually transmitted infection caused by human papillomavirus (HPV). These viruses are spread primarily through genital contact and can infect the genital area of both men and women. This includes the penis, vulva, lining of the vagina, cervix, rectum, or anus. Many people have no signs or symptoms of HPV. Some HPV infections cause women to have an abnormal pap test. Genital warts may appear. They may also lead to the development of cervical cancer. Treatment to remove warts is done in a doctor's office or through the use of medication. There is no cure for HPV. However, an HPV vaccine, licensed by the Food and Drug Administration (FDA), is available for males and females from age 9 to 26. It may help prevent genital warts and anal, vaginal, and vulvar cancers in women, and genital warts and anal cancer in men.

Gonorrhea is a sexually transmitted infection caused by bacteria. It is easier to detect in men because many women with gonorrhea show no early symptoms. Symptoms in men include painful or burning urination, a white, yellow, or green cloudy pus-like discharge from the penis, and painful or swollen testes. Symptoms in women include cloudy vaginal discharge, along with vaginal bleeding between periods. Rectal symptoms, such as itching, soreness, bleeding, or painful elimination of stool, can occur in both sexes. This disorder can cause blindness, joint infection, or a serious blood infection in babies born to infected mothers. It can also cause sterility and pelvic inflammatory disease (PID) if not treated. Gonorrhea is treated with antibiotics.

Syphilis is caused by bacteria. Syphilis is generally easier to detect in men than in women. The first stage is marked by small, painless sores called *chancres* that form on the penis soon after infection. In women, these sores may form inside the vagina. If left untreated, the infection progresses to the second stage, in which rashes appear on one or more areas of the body. These rashes do not usually cause itching. A headache and a fever may occur, along with sore throat, weight loss, and muscle aches. The third stage usually takes years to develop. During this stage, the symptoms from the second stage disappear. The person will still have the disease, and if not treated with penicillin or other antibiotics, the infection spreads to the heart, brain, and other vital organs. Untreated syphilis will eventually be fatal. The sooner it is treated, the better the chance is of preventing long-term damage and infection to others.

Trichomoniasis is a sexually transmitted infection caused by protozoa (single-celled animals). Men may have no symptoms. However, mild discharge, irritation, or a burning sensation after urination or ejaculation sometimes occurs. Symptoms of infection in women include a green-yellow vaginal discharge with a strong odor, irritation, or itching. The infection may cause discomfort during intercourse or urination. Trichomoniasis is treated with the prescription drug metronidazole.

Trivia

The Scourge of Syphilis

The first epidemic of syphilis affected sailors who returned from Columbus's first voyage to the Americas. At that time, it was called the "Naples Disease" or "French Disease." Paul Ehrlich (1854–1915), a doctor and medical scientist, developed a substance called *Salvarsan* that was effective in treating syphilis. It was used as the primary drug to treat syphilis until antibiotics became the treatment of choice during the 1940s. Ehrlich won the Nobel Prize in Medicine in 1908.

Vaginitis

Vaginitis is an inflammation of the vagina; symptoms include vaginal discharge, itching, and pain. There are many different types of vaginitis. Bacterial vaginosis occurs when there is an overgrowth of normal bacteria inside the vagina. Yeast infections are caused by an overproduction of a fungus called *Candida albicans*. Noninfectious vaginitis is caused by irritation or an allergic reaction to a product, such as bubble bath, soap, or fabric softener. Another cause of noninfectious vaginitis is vaginal atrophy, which is caused by lower estrogen levels that can occur in women after menopause.

Creams, suppositories, antibiotics, and estrogen supplements are used to treat vaginitis.

Noninfectious vaginitis is treated by eliminating the product(s) suspected of causing the vaginitis.

Female Reproductive Cancers

Ovarian cancer begins in the ovaries. It can occur in women at any age. Symptoms are not always apparent, which is why it may not be discovered until it is in a late stage. Some symptoms may occur, including abdominal pressure, indigestion, low back pain, and constipation. There is no definitive screening test for ovarian cancer. Pelvic examinations and ultrasound testing may be performed to help diagnose this type of cancer. Treatment of ovarian cancer includes surgery, radiation, and chemotherapy.

Endometrial cancer begins in the uterus. Symptoms of this type of cancer include vaginal bleeding and pelvic pain. Pelvic examinations and ultrasounds are used to diagnose this type of cancer. If detected early, endometrial cancer is highly curable by removing the uterus.

Cervical cancer begins in the cervix. It can occur at any age. Signs and symptoms are not always apparent, but include vaginal bleeding, change in menstrual cycles, painful intercourse, and blood-tinged vaginal discharge. Pap tests, colposcopies, and biopsies are tests that check for cervical cancer. A vaccine for cervical cancer is available for younger women up to age 26. If detected early, cervical cancer is curable.

Benign Prostatic Hypertrophy

Benign prostatic hypertrophy is a disorder that is common in men over the age of 60. Studies show that one-third to one-half of all men over this age show signs of this disorder. When a man has BPH, the prostate becomes enlarged, which causes pressure on the urethra. When the urethra becomes compressed, urination becomes difficult. Other symptoms are a feeling of incomplete urination, frequent urination, and a weak stream of urine. Dribbling of urine right after urinating, the need to urinate often during the night, and urinary incontinence are symptoms, too. The cause of benign prostatic hypertrophy is unknown. Medications and/or surgery are used to treat this disorder.

Prostate enlargement is not a cancerous condition. However, as men age, they are at increased risk for prostate cancer.

Male Reproductive Cancers

Prostate cancer is a type of cancer that forms in the prostate gland, normally in older men. Certain men have a higher risk of prostate cancer. Risk factors include having a family history of prostate cancer and being 60 years of age or older. Regular prostate checks are often a part of annual exams, and a screening test is available. Symptoms of prostate cancer are urinating during the night, a weak flow of urine, painful urination, blood in urine, and problems with maintaining an erection. This type of cancer tends to be slow-growing and treatable if caught early. Treatment includes radiation therapy, removal of the prostate, and hormone therapy.

Testicular cancer occurs in the testes, the male reproductive glands. It is the most common form of cancer in younger men, from ages 15 to 35, but can also occur in older men. Regular self-examinations and doctor examinations can help diagnose this form of cancer. Symptoms include a noticeable lump in the testes, pain in the testicles, breast tenderness, back pain, an ache in the groin, heaviness in the scrotum, and fluid collection in the scrotum. Testicular cancer is highly curable. Treatment includes surgical removal of the testes, chemotherapy, and radiation therapy.

Additional resources for information relating to reproductive disorders include the following:

- Centers for Disease Control and Prevention, cdc.gov/std

- Office on Women's Health (OWH), U.S. Department of Health & Human Services, womenshealth.gov

Obesity and Disorders of the Reproductive System

Obesity increases the risk for certain reproductive diseases or disorders, including the following:

- Cancers of the reproductive system, such as breast, endometrial, and ovarian cancer
- Frequent yeast infections

5. Describe sexual needs of the elderly

Sexual needs continue throughout a person's life. All people, regardless of age, have sexual needs and desires (Fig. 17-4). The ability to engage in sexual activities, such as intercourse and masturbation, continues unless a disease or injury occurs. Nursing assistants can help by providing privacy whenever necessary for sexual activity and respecting residents' sexual needs.

Some factors that can affect sexual activity in the elderly include the following:

- Illness affecting the ability of men and women to perform sexually
- Medications
- Vaginal atrophy (weakening or wasting away of muscles), pain, and dryness in females
- Erectile dysfunction (ED) in males
- Fear of inadequate sexual performance
- A lack of privacy
- Depression

In the past, erectile dysfunction was often viewed as a normal response to aging. **Erectile dysfunction (ED)** is the inability to have or maintain an erection. However, it is not a normal change of aging. ED may be a sign of a more serious problem; heart disease is one example. Medications can help treat this disorder. The NA should report any resident complaints about erectile dysfunction to the nurse.

For women, special creams and medications can help with vaginal dryness. Complaints about dryness or pain should be reported to the nurse.

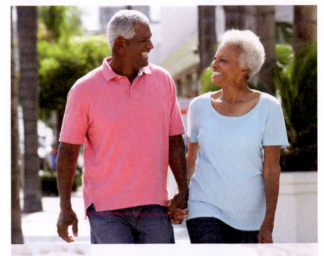
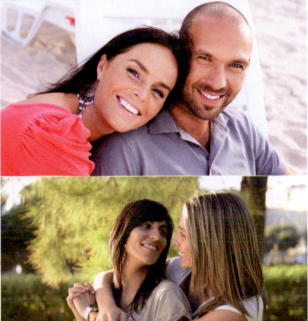
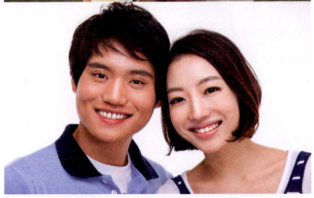

Fig. 17-4. Sexual needs, behavior, and desires are present in all age groups.

Older adults are sexual beings like all humans, and they have the right to choose how they express their sexuality. In all age groups, there is a wide variety of sexual behavior. This is also true of residents who live in long-term care facilities. An attitude that any expression of sexuality by the elderly is cute, funny, or disgusting deprives residents of their right to dignity and respect. All residents have a right to be treated with dignity and to have their privacy respected.

If an NA encounters any sexual situation, such as a resident masturbating or two consenting adult residents engaged in sexual activity, she should provide privacy and leave the area. NAs must not judge any sexual behavior they observe.

Residents' Rights

Gynecological Exams

A gynecological examination may be done in the resident's room or in a special examination room. It can also be performed in an emergency room or an urgent care center. When these exams are done, it is important for the NA to be sensitive to the resident's feelings and concerns. Gynecological examinations may be embarrassing, uncomfortable, and frightening. The NA should listen to residents who want to talk and answer any questions that are within her scope of practice. She should provide privacy throughout the exam. Any questions that the NA cannot answer should be referred to the nurse or doctor.

Chapter Review

1. List the functions of the male and female reproductive systems (LO 2).

2. List all normal age-related changes of the reproductive system for males and females (LO 3).

3. How are sexually transmitted infections (STIs) transmitted (LO 4)?

4. When encountering a sexual situation between consenting adult residents, what should an NA do (LO 5)?

18
The Integumentary System

The Field of Dermatology in Its Infancy

Ferdinand Hebra (1816–1880) was one of the first doctors to specialize in the diseases of the skin. One of the discoveries he made concerned scabies, a disorder that causes intense itching. Hebra noted that when the itch-mite parasite was destroyed, scabies was cured. He also made the important discovery that scabies could be transmitted from one person to another.

"'Tis not a lip or eye we beauty call/But the joint force and full result of all."

Alexander Pope, 1688–1744

"Men should be judged, not by their tint of skin . . . But by the quality of thought they think."

Adela Florence Cory Nicolson, 1865–1904

1. Define important words in this chapter

bony prominences: areas of the body where the bone lies close to the skin.

bruise: a purple, black, or blue discoloration on the skin caused by the leakage of blood from broken blood vessels into the surrounding tissues; also called *contusion*.

cellulitis: a skin infection caused by bacteria moving into the tissues due to a break in the skin.

closed wound: a type of wound in which the skin's surface is not broken.

dermatitis: inflammation of the skin.

dermis: the inner layer of the two main layers of tissue that make up the skin.

epidermis: the outer layer of the two main layers of tissue that make up the skin.

gangrene: death of tissue caused by infection or lack of blood flow.

integument: natural protective covering.

lesion: an area of abnormal tissue or an injury or wound.

melanin: the pigment that gives skin its color.

melanocyte: cell in the skin that produces and contains the pigment called melanin.

necrosis: the death of living cells or tissues caused by disease or injury.

open wound: a type of wound in which the skin's surface is not intact.

pressure injuries: localized damage to the skin (and possibly the underlying soft tissue) that occurs due to shearing or to continued pressure over time; also known as *pressure ulcers, pressure sores, decubitus ulcers,* or *bed sores.*

pressure points: areas of the body that bear the greatest amount of weight.

psoriasis: a chronic skin condition caused by skin cells growing too quickly that results in red, white, or silver patches, itching, and discomfort.

scabies: a contagious skin infection caused by mites burrowing into the skin that results in pimple-like irritations, rashes, intense itching, and sores.

shingles: a viral infection caused by the same virus that causes chickenpox; results in pain, itching, and rashes.

sitz bath: a warm soak of the perineal area to clean perineal wounds and reduce inflammation and pain.

skin cancer: the growth of abnormal skin cells.

tinea: a fungal infection that causes red, scaly patches to appear in a ring shape, generally on the upper body or on the hands and feet.

wart: contagious hard bump caused by a virus.

2. Explain the structure and function of the integumentary system

The integumentary system consists of the following parts: the skin, hair, nails, oil glands, sweat glands, subcutaneous tissue, and nerve endings (Fig. 18-1). The skin is a natural protective covering, or **integument**, and is the largest organ in the human body. It is considered an organ because it has different types of tissues that function together to perform activities of the body. The skin covers and protects the body, provides sensation through nerves, regulates body temperature, and prevents the loss of too much water.

The two basic layers of the skin are the epidermis and the dermis. The **epidermis** is the outer layer of the skin, which is composed of dead cells. These cells are continuously shed as new cells move up from the dermis. The epidermis does not contain blood vessels. Keratin is a protein substance found in the dead skin cells of the epidermis. Keratin has waterproof qualities that protect the inside of the body when the skin gets wet. Beneath the very top of the epidermis lie other types of cells. One type is **melanocyte**, which contains **melanin**, the substance that

gives skin its color. The more melanin skin produces, the darker a person's skin color.

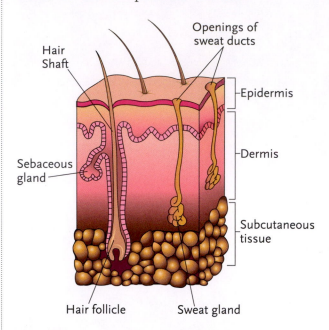

Fig. 18-1. *Cross-section showing the integumentary system.*

The skin is a sense organ. Receptors are found in the skin that give the ability to feel and touch. One type of receptor is found near the surface of the skin and the other is found within the dermis. The **dermis** is the inner layer of the skin. Within the dermis lie the structures responsible for unique fingerprints. These ridges are called *dermal-papillae* and form before birth. Fingerprints and footprints, which grow as a child becomes an adult, will always have the same pattern and can identify people throughout their lives. Hair and nail follicles, sweat and oil glands, blood vessels, and receptors for touch, temperature, pressure, and pain are also located in the dermis.

Hair grows from roots located in the dermis. Every hair consists primarily of dead cells, made up of keratin and the pigment that gives hair its color. Hair protects the body. The hair inside the nose protects against inhaling irritants in the air. Hair on the head, underarms, and genitals protects sensitive areas from injuries. Eyebrows and eyelashes help keep objects from getting into the eyes.

Collagen fibers, which make skin tough, are found within the dermis. Elastic fibers are also found in the dermis. They give the skin its elasticity, or ability to stretch.

The subcutaneous layer is positioned immediately underneath the dermis. This is the area of the body where fat, or adipose tissue, lies. Adipose tissue also serves as a cushion over bone and provides some protection as it insulates the body from cold weather. The fat layer in humans is thinner than the fat layer in some other mammals.

The functions of the integumentary system are to

- Protect internal organs from injury

- Protect the body against bacteria and other pathogens

- Prevent the loss of too much water

- Regulate body temperature

- Respond to heat, cold, pain, pressure, and touch

- Excrete waste products in sweat

- Help with production of vitamin D

Destination: Homeostasis

When cells die or become damaged, homeostasis is disturbed. When the surface of the skin is opened, such as by a cut, the inflammatory response begins. Blood flow increases to the area. Signs of inflammation, such as redness, swelling, heat, and pain, occur. Platelets, along with a substance called *fibrin*, form a clot. White blood cells, called *phagocytes*, travel to the area and start cleaning the wound of bacteria. A scab, which is a hard, protective structure, forms over the area. Normal tissue eventually develops and, over time, the scab is pushed off of the area, leaving new skin. When normal tissue repair is complete, the injured area returns to homeostasis.

Tip

Observing Residents' Skin is a Daily Duty
Every time nursing assistants help residents bathe and/or dress, they should carefully observe their skin. This helps identify any changes in the skin, which need to be reported immediately. Pressure injuries, skin cancer, and contagious skin diseases can pose serious health risks if not caught early and treated. Because NAs see residents most often on a daily basis, their careful observations can help prevent serious illnesses.

3. Discuss changes in the integumentary system due to aging

Normal age-related changes for the integumentary system include the following:

- Amount of fat and collagen decreases, causing skin to sag.

- Elastic fibers lose elasticity, causing wrinkles.

- Hair and nail growth slows.

- Skin becomes drier due to decreased production of perspiration and oil.

- Skin becomes thinner and more fragile, causing more frequent skin injuries, tearing, and infections.

- Protective fatty tissue layer thins, so the person feels colder.

- Hair thins and turns gray, due to a decrease in the melanocyte activity (Fig. 18-2).

- Brown spots on the skin may appear due to an increase in the production of certain melanocytes in areas exposed to the sun.

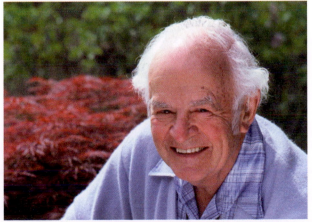

Fig. 18-2. *Hair growth slows, and hair thins and turns gray as a person ages.*

The Integumentary System

Fragile Skin

An elderly person's skin is extremely fragile. Remove dressings, tape, and bandages carefully and gently to help prevent damage and tears to residents' skin.

4. Discuss common disorders of the integumentary system

Pressure injuries, a major complication related to the integumentary system, are discussed in Learning Objective 5 of this chapter.

Burns

Burns and scalds were first discussed in Chapter 8. Burns can be caused by fire, hot liquids, warm water applications (such as warm moist compresses), electrical equipment (such as hair dryers, hair irons, and heaters), hot objects, or certain chemicals.

When a burn occurs, there may be a varying degree of skin damage (Fig. 18-3). Here are the different degrees or classifications of burns:

Degree	Layer of Skin	Damage Involved
First-degree (superficial)	Epidermis (outer layer)	Redness and pain
Second-degree (partial-thickness)	Epidermis and dermis (deeper layer)	Some skin damage; redness, pain, swelling, and blistering
Third-degree (full-thickness)	Epidermis, dermis, and underlying tissue	Serious scarring; muscle and bone may be affected; white or charred skin; pain; swelling; and peeling skin

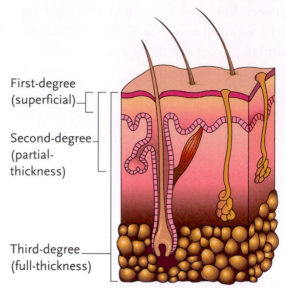

Fig. 18-3. *Different degrees of burns.*

Burns and scalds are very painful and can require surgery. They can cause a resident's condition to deteriorate quickly. When caring for a resident who has burns, the NA should be careful not to cause additional pain. Before giving care, it may be necessary for the nurse to give the resident pain medication. The pain medication can then take effect before the care begins. Being gentle when moving and positioning residents helps reduce pain and the risk of damaging dressings. Special protective devices, such as pads or draw sheets, may need to be used. The NA should encourage fluids, follow diet instructions, and measure intake and output (I&O) carefully (Chapter 14). Pus or other fluids around burned areas, resident complaints of pain, or any decrease in appetite or intake and output should be reported to the nurse.

Scabies

Scabies is a skin infection that causes pimple-like irritations to form on the skin. These irritations are caused by tiny mites that burrow into the skin to lay eggs. A rash, intense itching, and sores can occur, and the sores may become infected. The symptoms may take a month or more to appear.

Scabies is contagious and is usually transmitted by direct person-to-person contact. Using an infected person's towel, washcloth, clothing, or bedding can also spread scabies. The elderly and others with weakened immune systems are at a higher risk of acquiring scabies.

Special lotions are used to treat scabies. NAs do not apply the lotion, but they may assist the nurse with the application. The NA should handle clothing and linens carefully, following instructions. The NA will need to don gloves and additional personal protective equipment when touching areas that have been treated.

Even after treatment, the itching may continue for a while. Anyone who may have been infected with scabies should be treated at the same time, such as residents, their families and friends, and their roommates.

Shingles

Shingles is a viral infection that causes a painful rash. Shingles is also called *herpes zoster* or *zoster*. It is caused by the same virus that causes chickenpox—the varicella-zoster virus (VZV). The disease can occur in anyone who has had chickenpox. The infection begins with pain or itching at the site where the rash will appear. The rash commonly occurs in a single stripe on one side of the body. The person may have fever or chills. Severe pain can occur after the rash is gone; this happens in about 20% of people and is more common in the elderly. The pain may last for many years.

Shingles cannot be transmitted through person-to-person contact. However, the virus that causes shingles can cause chickenpox in someone who has never had chickenpox or has not received the chickenpox vaccine. The virus is spread when the disease is in its blister form (Fig. 18-4). When the blisters have crusts, the disease is no longer contagious. Healthcare workers who have never had chickenpox or who are pregnant should not care for residents who have shingles.

A shingles rash must remain covered at all times. Infected people should wash their hands often and should not touch or scratch the rash. Medication is used to treat shingles. If the medication is started immediately, it can reduce the severity of the disease and shorten the length of the illness. A doctor should be contacted when shingles first appears. Waiting to treat this infection reduces the effectiveness of the medication.

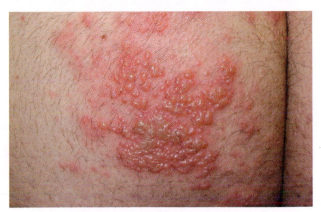

Fig. 18-4. *Shingles in blister form.* (PHOTO COURTESY OF DR. JERE MAMMINO, DO)

There are two recommended vaccines available for preventing shingles—one is for people aged 50 and older, while the other may be used for healthy adults aged 60 and older.

Wounds

Wounds fall into two categories: closed and open. A **closed wound** is a wound where the skin's surface is not broken, such as a bruise or internal bleeding. A *contusion*, also called a **bruise**, is a common type of a closed wound. Trauma to the outside of the body can cause a contusion. The skin's surface generally remains intact, but internal damage and bleeding can occur.

Skin that is not intact is considered an **open wound**. Types of open wounds include the following:

- An *abrasion* is a tearing or wearing away of the surface skin due to friction. Other words for abrasion are *scrape* or *excoriation*. Abrasions usually bleed very little, but the area must be kept clean to help prevent infection.

- An *avulsion* is a tearing away of tissues during a violent act or accident, such as a dog bite, gunshot wound, or an explosion. Bleeding from this type of wound is usually heavy.

- An *incision* is a cut caused by a sharp-edged object, such as glass, a knife, or a razor. Bleeding in this type of wound is generally rapid and heavy; however, when an incision is made during surgery, the bleeding is usually controlled.

- A *laceration* is an irregular or jagged wound that is caused by blunt tearing of soft tissue. For example, it can result from the tearing of skin that occurs during childbirth. A laceration may cause rapid and extensive bleeding.

- A *puncture wound* is a wound from a sharp object that causes a small hole in the tissues. For example, a needle or a nail can cause a puncture wound. Bleeding may be slight or heavy.

Signs and symptoms of wounds are pain, tissue damage, discoloration, drainage, and light or heavy bleeding. Fever, chills, or trouble breathing may occur. If any of these symptoms is observed, the NA must report to the nurse immediately.

There are four types of wound drainage:

- Serous drainage is yellow or transparent.

- Sanguineous drainage is bright red blood from a new cut.

- Serosanguineous drainage is pink drainage that may turn sanguineous.

- Purulent (pus) drainage is yellow, green, brown, or white drainage that may have an odor. It may appear milky or thick. This type of drainage usually contains bacteria and should be treated promptly.

New wounds require immediate medical attention, assessment, and monitoring by a nurse. Treatment includes stopping bleeding and cleaning the wound. A dressing will need to be applied. Stitches or special bandages may be needed. In some cases, a tetanus shot is required. A bite from an animal may require rabies shots.

Skin Lesions

Different types of lesions can occur on the skin. A **lesion** is an area of abnormal tissue or an injury or wound.

Macules are the most simple skin lesion. Macules are flat spots that can be seen but not felt. They are visible because they change the color of the skin. Freckles are an example.

Papules are skin lesions that are raised, little round bumps on the skin. Papules can be felt. They do not contain pus. Contact dermatitis is an example.

Pustules are raised spots filled with pus, such as acne or infected boils.

Vesicles are small blisters that contain fluid. They can occur on the skin or inside the mouth. Chickenpox is an example.

Wheals are large raised, irregular areas that are usually itchy (Fig. 18-5). Hives (urticaria) from an allergic reaction are an example.

Hematoma is a collection of blood in one area. The spot can be visible as a bruise, but may also occur on internal organs. Hematomas can become larger over time. They may also change color.

Purpura are small, purplish spots caused by bleeding under the skin. In elderly people, these spots are called *senile purpura*. Senile purpura occur because blood vessels become more fragile with age.

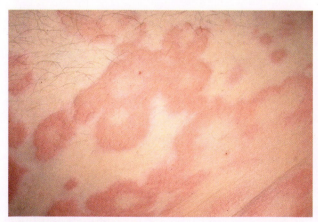

Fig. 18-5. An example of wheals. (PHOTO COURTESY OF DR. JERE MAMMINO, DO)

Gangrene

Gangrene means death of tissue. It is caused by a lack of blood flow due to factors such as burns, diabetes, injuries, circulatory disorders, a weakened immune system, and complications from surgery. Gangrene must be treated immediately.

Symptoms of gangrene include discoloration of the skin (usually black or blue), sores that do not heal, pain, loss of feeling, and foul-smelling discharge. The person may experience chills or have a change in vital signs.

Treatments depend on the extent of the spread of the gangrene and may include antibiotics, surgery, amputation, or hospitalization.

The NA should be familiar with residents' normal vital signs measurements. Elevated temperature, pulse, or respiration rate; a change in blood pressure; or difficulty breathing must be reported to the nurse.

Dermatitis

Dermatitis means inflammation of the skin. There are different types of dermatitis. One form is atopic dermatitis, commonly known as *eczema*, which can be temporary or chronic and has a variety of causes, including stress, allergies, irritating agents, and a family history. Some people who have eczema also have asthma or hay fever (allergic rhinitis). Symptoms of eczema include redness, itching, burning, swelling, cracking, or weeping (oozing fluid) of the skin, and lesions.

Treatment of eczema includes topical steroid creams, soothing or drying lotions prescribed by a dermatologist (a doctor specializing in conditions of the skin), and stronger medications such as immunosuppressants and biologics (drugs that target specific parts of the immune system).

Exposure to sunlight may also be used to treat eczema. Scratching should be avoided; certain types of oral medication can help reduce itching. Avoiding the irritating agent can help prevent the problem.

Contact dermatitis is another type of dermatitis. There are two forms of contact dermatitis: irritant contact dermatitis and allergic contact dermatitis.

Irritant contact dermatitis develops in some people who are exposed to certain chemicals. Soaps and detergents can cause this disorder. Allergic contact dermatitis occurs when the skin comes into contact with a substance that causes an allergic reaction. Such substances include latex, some adhesives, and some types of plants, such as poison ivy, poison oak, and poison sumac.

Symptoms of contact dermatitis include a red or pink rash that may burn, itch, or sting. Treatment includes washing the affected areas immediately to remove traces of the irritating substance, steroids or other creams, oral medications, and special compresses or baths.

Cellulitis

Cellulitis is an infection of the skin that occurs when bacteria move deeper into the tissues. If this infection is not treated promptly, it may worsen and become sepsis, a condition that can be fatal (Chapter 26). Cellulitis is commonly caused by a break in the skin such as from a surgical incision, rash, cut, insect bite, tattoo, or piercing. Diabetes, edema, obesity, and a weakened immune system also put a person at a higher risk for cellulitis. Antibiotics are normally used to treat this condition. The NA should report warm, red, and swollen skin, as well as fever, to the nurse.

Psoriasis

Psoriasis is a chronic skin condition in which skin cells grow too fast, causing red, white, or silver patches to form. The patches can be small or large and usually occur on the arms, elbows, lower back, knees, or feet. Psoriasis can be mild or severe. Larger patches can cause itching and discomfort. People with psoriasis may also have arthritis and pain.

Psoriasis is usually inherited. It may also be caused or aggravated by a dry climate, cold weather, stress, or a weakened immune system.

Treatment includes topical creams, shampoos, lotions, and medications such as immunosuppressants and biologics. Exposure to sunlight or special ultraviolet light, called *phototherapy*, may be prescribed. Dietary changes may be recommended to help treat the disorder.

Fungal Infections

Fungal and yeast (one type of fungus) infections can occur anywhere on the body. However, they most commonly occur in moist areas, such as the toes, under the breasts, and in the groin area. Red, scaly patches appear, accompanied by itching, rawness, and pain. Jock itch, vaginal yeast infections, and athlete's foot are all examples of fungal infections.

Tinea is a contagious fungal infection that causes red scaly patches to appear in a ring shape, generally on the upper body, or on the hands and feet (Fig. 18-6). Tinea is sometimes referred to as *ringworm*. Tinea is spread by direct contact, such as touching an infected person's skin, as well as through indirect contact, such as touching an infected person's brush or clothing. Tinea can also be spread to humans from animals, such as dogs and cats.

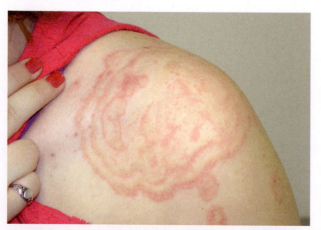

Fig. 18-6. *Tinea is a fungal infection that causes red scaly patches to appear in a ring-like shape.* (PHOTO COURTESY OF DR. JERE MAMMINO, DO)

Fungal infections are caused by an overgrowth of fungus due to overuse of antibiotics, reduced immune system function, and other factors. Perspiration can worsen these infections, as it creates a more favorable environment for fungus to grow. Treatment includes topical antifungal creams and medications. The earlier the treatment begins, the faster the infection heals. Using proper personal hygiene practices, such as handwashing and keeping the body clean and dry, can help prevent the spread of some fungal infections. The NA should report any skin changes, skin abrasions, flaking, redness, sores, or scratching to the nurse.

Warts

A **wart** is a rough, hard bump (Fig. 18-7). Bumps may be spongy-looking with red, yellow, brown, or black spots. Warts are contagious and are caused by a virus that invades the skin, usually through a cut or tear. They may spread to other areas of the body if not treated. People who have a weakened immune system are more prone to developing warts.

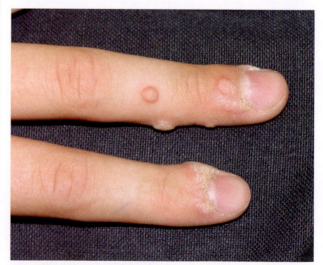

Fig. 18-7. *Warts on the fingers.* (PHOTO COURTESY OF DR. JERE MAMMINO, DO)

Treatment includes medication and/or removal with a laser or special instrument. The NA should wash her hands frequently to help prevent the spread of warts to other parts of the body.

Skin Cancer

Skin cancer is the growth of abnormal skin cells. There are different types of skin cancer. The most serious form is malignant melanoma. If the cancer is caught in its early stages, it is generally treatable. If the skin cancer spreads, it can be fatal. Signs and symptoms of skin cancer include changes in a mole, wart, or spot on the skin, sores that do not heal, itching, pain, and skin that is oozing or bleeding. People with darker skin have a higher risk of skin cancer on the palms of their hands, soles of their feet, and under their nails.

Treatment of skin cancer involves removing the cancerous area and sometimes the surrounding tissue. Advanced melanoma may be treated with interferon, a protein. Reducing sun exposure, wearing sunscreen, and wearing hats and protective clothing can reduce the risk of skin cancer. The skin should be checked regularly by a dermatologist.

The NA should report any changes in residents' skin to the nurse, including the following:

- **A**symmetry: one-half of a mole, spot, or birthmark does not match the other half.
- **B**order: the edges of a mole are irregular or blurred.
- **C**olor: the color of a mole varies with red, pink, black, brown, white, or blue areas.
- **D**iameter: a mole is over six millimeters in size (the size of a pencil eraser). Some melanomas are smaller than this, so any spot observed should be reported.
- **E**volution: any change in size, shape, symptoms, surface (for example, bleeding), or color of a mole.

Additional resources for information relating to integumentary disorders include the following:

- National Pressure Ulcer Advisory Panel (NPUAP, npuap.org)
- The Skin Cancer Foundation, skincancer.org
- National Institutes of Health's MedlinePlus, medlineplus.gov/woundsandinjuries.html

Obesity and Disorders of the Integumentary System

Obesity increases the risk for certain integumentary diseases or disorders, including the following:
- Pressure injuries (next learning objective)
- Skin infections, such as cellulitis
- Excess facial and body hair
- Slow wound healing

5. Discuss pressure injuries and identify prevention guidelines

When a person is confined to bed for long periods of time, the amount of blood that circulates to the skin is reduced. The risk of skin breakdown increases. This breakdown usually occurs at the areas of the body that bear the greatest amount of weight. These points are called **pressure points**, and there are many on the human body. They are mainly located at **bony prominences**, which are areas of the body where the bone lies close to the skin. These areas include the elbows, shoulder blades, sacrum (tailbone), hips and knees (inner and outer parts), ankles, heels, toes, and the back of the neck and the head. Other areas at risk for skin breakdown include the ears, the area under the breasts or scrotum, the area between the folds of the buttocks or abdomen, and skin between the legs (Fig. 18-8).

When skin breaks down due to poor circulation, the amount of oxygen the cells receive is reduced, and necrosis results. **Necrosis** is the death of living cells or tissues. This is due to prolonged pressure on an area or any other cause that interferes with circulation. Moisture and warmth also contribute to skin breakdown. Once skin has broken down and is weakened, sores can occur and may become infected, causing damage to the underlying tissue. The sores or wounds that result from skin deterioration and shearing are called **pressure injuries**. **Shearing** is rubbing or friction resulting from the skin moving one way and the bone underneath it remaining fixed or moving in the opposite direction. Pressure injuries are also called *pressure sores*, *decubitus ulcers*, or *bed sores*.

Lateral Position

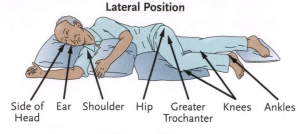

Side of Head | Ear | Shoulder | Hip | Greater Trochanter | Knees | Ankles

Prone Position

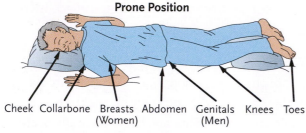

Cheek | Collarbone | Breasts (Women) | Abdomen | Genitals (Men) | Knees | Toes

Supine Position

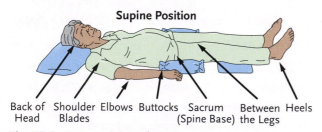

Back of Head | Shoulder Blades | Elbows | Buttocks | Sacrum (Spine Base) | Between the Legs | Heels

Fig. 18-8. Pressure injury danger zones.

Pressure injuries are a common, serious problem in long-term care. If caught early, a break or tear in the skin can heal fairly quickly without other complications. However, if not caught early, a pressure injury can become bigger, deeper, and infected. Pressure injuries are painful and difficult to heal, and can lead to life-threatening infections.

Pressure injuries are much easier to prevent than to cure. Prevention is very important and is the key to skin health. CMS requires that pressure injury prevention be ongoing. Treatment should prevent infection and new injuries from forming. Pressure injuries are categorized by stages, which are as follows:

Stage 1: Skin is intact, but it may look red, and the redness is not relieved after removing pressure. Brown or black skin tones may not look red but may appear to be a different color than the surrounding area. The area may be painful, firm, soft, and warmer or cooler when compared to the area around it.

Stage 2: There is partial-thickness skin loss involving the epidermis and the dermis. The injury is pink or red and moist, and may also look like a blister.

Stage 3: There is full-thickness skin loss in which fat is visible in the injury. Slough and/or eschar may be present. Slough is yellow, tan, gray, green, or brown tissue that is usually moist. Eschar is dead tissue that is hard or soft in texture and black, brown, or tan, and may be similar to a scab. The damage may extend down to, but not through, the tissue that covers muscle.

Stage 4: There is full-thickness skin loss extending through all layers of the skin, tissue, muscle, bone, and other structures, such as joints or tendons. The injury will look like a deep crater and slough and/or eschar may be visible.

Unstageable Pressure Injury: There is full-thickness skin and tissue loss, but the extent of the damage cannot be determined because it is covered with slough or eschar. Once the slough and/or eschar is removed, the injury can then be staged (either Stage 3 or Stage 4).

Deep Tissue Pressure Injury: The skin area is intact or nonintact and is deep red, purple, or maroon. The wound may appear as a blood-filled blister. The area may be painful and may be warmer or cooler than the surrounding tissue. Discoloration may be different in brown or black skin tones.

NAs are in the best position to observe for signs of pressure injuries since they see residents' skin on a daily basis. Each resident's skin should be inspected every time care is given.

Observing and Reporting: Pressure Injuries

- O/R Pale, white, reddened, gray, or purple skin
- O/R Dry, cracked, or flaking skin
- O/R Torn skin
- O/R Blisters, bruises, or wounds on the skin
- O/R Differences in temperature of the skin when compared to the area around it
- O/R Rashes or any skin discoloration
- O/R Tingling, warmth, or burning
- O/R Itching or scratching
- O/R Swelling of the skin
- O/R Wet skin
- O/R Broken skin anywhere on the body, including between the toes or around the toenails
- O/R Changes in existing injuries, including size, depth, drainage, color, or odor

In addition to immobility, there are other risk factors for pressure injuries. Wrinkled linens that do not lie flat under residents, as well as crumbs or other irritating objects in the bed, can increase the risk for pressure injuries. Malnutrition and dehydration increase the risk, too. Urinary and fecal incontinence are also major risk factors for pressure injuries.

Guidelines: Preventing Pressure Injuries

- G Promptly report any changes in a resident's skin.
- G Perform regular skin care, closely inspecting the resident's skin each time it is performed. Check areas that may be irritated by an IV line or an oxygen delivery device. Inspect areas around bandages, dressings, or casts for irritation.
- G Keep skin clean and dry. Pay close attention to folds of skin (for example, the breasts) to make sure they are clean and dry. Give skin care immediately after episodes of incontinence (urine or stool) or when skin is damp or wet from sweat or wound drainage. Do not use hot water when bathing the skin. Do not rub any areas during bathing. Change clothing and bed linens as needed.
- G Use moisturizers as ordered on unbroken skin. Follow the care plan. Do not use creams, lotions, soaps, or other products on nonintact skin.
- G Do not massage any white, red, or purple areas, bony areas, or pressure points.
- G Follow posted turn schedules. Assist immobile residents to change position as ordered, but at least every two hours.
- G Ask or assist every resident in a wheelchair or any other chair to change position at least every hour.
- G Do not pull residents across linen or other surfaces during transfers or repositioning. This causes friction and shearing. Be gentle so that you do not tear fragile skin.
- G Keep linens dry, clean, and wrinkle-free. Keep the bed free from crumbs and other irritating objects.
- G Perform range of motion exercises as ordered.
- G Protect the heels and ankles by using pillows and other positioning devices to keep them from resting on the surface of the bed (Fig. 18-9). Use footrests in chairs and wheelchairs to prevent the feet from touching the floor.
- G Use pillows to separate skin surfaces.
- G Follow diet and fluid orders carefully; encourage fluids and proper nutrition.

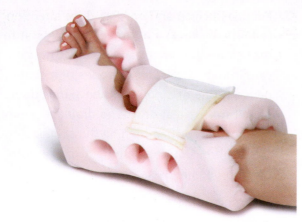

Fig. 18-9. *This foam boot suspends the heel to help reduce pressure.* (© MEDLINE INDUSTRIES, INC. 2019)

6. Explain the benefits of warm and cold applications

Applications of heat or cold can have beneficial effects on injuries, infections, fevers, and other conditions. The body responds to heat and cold in different ways.

Heat helps relieve pain and muscular tension. It elevates the temperature in the tissues, increases waste removal from the area, and increases blood flow due to dilated blood vessels. Increased blood flow brings more oxygen and nutrients to the tissues for healing. However, there are risks associated with warm applications. Heat can cause burns, make bleeding worse, and cause confusion, dizziness, or fainting due to a reduction of blood to the brain. The elderly are at an increased risk for burns and other complications because they have thinner, more fragile skin.

With cold applications, blood flow decreases due to the constriction of the vessels. The movement of oxygen and nutrients into the tissues decreases. Cold applications help stop bleeding, minimize swelling, and reduce pain. Cold helps bring down high temperatures. Risks associated with cold applications include cyanosis or pale skin, chills, and shivering. Lack of blood flow to the application area and the cold temperature may damage tissue.

Warm or cold applications can be either moist or dry. Moisture strengthens the effect of both heat and cold, which means that moist applications are more likely to cause injury. When using these applications, NAs must know how long they should be applied and should use the correct temperature listed in the care plan.

Types of moist applications include the following:

- Compresses (warm or cold)
- Soaks (warm or cold)
- Tub baths (warm)
- Sponge baths (warm or cold)
- Sitz baths (warm)
- Ice packs (cold)

Types of dry applications include the following:

- Aquamatic K-pads (warm or cold)
- Disposable warm packs (warm)
- Ice bags (cold)
- Disposable cold packs (cold)
- Warming blankets (warm)
- Cooling blankets (cold)

Some facilities do not allow NAs to prepare and apply warm and cold applications. NAs should only perform procedures that are assigned and trained to do.

When applying warm and cold applications, the NA should observe and report any of the following signs that may indicate that the application is causing tissue damage:

- Excessive redness
- Pain
- Blisters
- Numbness

Gloves should be donned before applying warm or cold applications if a resident has nonintact skin or open sores. Warm or cold applications should not be applied directly on nonintact skin or open sores. Gloves should always be worn when assisting with a sitz bath. A **sitz bath** is a warm soak of the perineal area to clean perineal wounds and reduce inflammation and pain.

Tip

Heat Opens and Cold Closes

Warm and cold applications have different effects on the body. The following tip serves as a reminder of the body's response to heat and cold:

Heat opens, or dilates, blood vessels.

Cold closes, or constricts, blood vessels.

Tip

The 20-Minute Rule

When warm and cold applications are applied for too long, the opposite effect of what is intended occurs. This means that if an ice bag is left on an affected area for longer than 20 minutes, the blood vessels may start to open again. This can increase bleeding and swelling at the injury site. Warm or cold applications should be limited to 20 minutes at a time.

A washcloth or a commercial warm compress may be used as a warm compress. There are different types of commercial compresses available (Fig. 18-10). If these are provided, the NA should follow the package directions and the nurse's instructions.

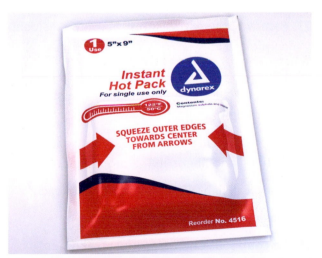

Fig. 18-10. *Disposable heat compresses are used only once and then discarded. The compress shown here must be squeezed and shaken to activate and then applied. It maintains heat for a certain amount of time, usually up to 20 minutes.* (REPRINTED WITH PERMISSION OF DYNAREX CORPORATION, DYNAREX.COM, 845-365-8200)

Applying warm moist compresses

Equipment: washcloth or compress, plastic wrap, towel, basin, water thermometer

1. Identify yourself by name. Identify the resident. Greet the resident by name.

2. Wash your hands.

3. Explain procedure to the resident. Speak clearly, slowly, and directly. Maintain face-to-face contact whenever possible.

4. Provide for the resident's privacy with a curtain, screen, or door.

5. Fill the basin one-half to two-thirds full with warm water. Test the water temperature with the thermometer or against the inside of your wrist to ensure it is safe. Water temperature should be no higher than 105°F. Have the resident check the water temperature. Adjust if necessary.

6. Soak the washcloth in the water and wring it out. Immediately apply it to the area. Note the time. Quickly cover the washcloth with plastic wrap and the towel to keep it warm (Fig. 18-11).

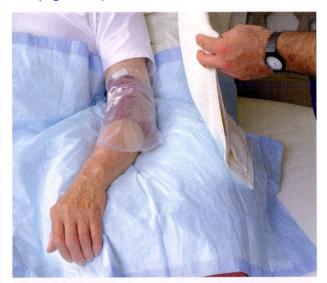

Fig. 18-11. *Cover warm compresses to keep them warm.*

7. Check the area every five minutes. Remove the compress if the area is red or numb or if the resident complains of pain or discomfort.

Change the compress if cooling occurs. Remove the compress after 20 minutes.

8. Remove privacy measures. Make the resident comfortable.

9. Discard the plastic wrap. Empty, rinse, and dry the basin. Place the basin in the area for cleaning or clean and store it according to policy.

10. Place soiled clothing and linens in the proper containers.

11. Leave call light within the resident's reach.

12. Wash your hands.

13. Be courteous and respectful at all times.

14. Report any changes in the resident to the nurse. Document procedure using facility guidelines.

Administering warm soaks

Equipment: towel, basin, water thermometer, bath blanket, disposable absorbent pad

1. Identify yourself by name. Identify the resident. Greet the resident by name.

2. Wash your hands.

3. Explain procedure to the resident. Speak clearly, slowly, and directly. Maintain face-to-face contact whenever possible.

4. Provide for the resident's privacy with a curtain, screen, or door.

5. Fill the basin one-half to two-thirds full with warm water. Test the water temperature with the thermometer or against the inside of your wrist to ensure it is safe. Water temperature should be no higher than 105°F. Have the resident check the water temperature. Adjust if necessary.

6. Place the basin on a disposable absorbent pad (protective barrier) in a comfortable position for the resident.

7. Immerse the body part in the basin. Pad the edge of the basin with a towel (Fig. 18-12). Use a bath blanket to cover the resident if needed for extra warmth.

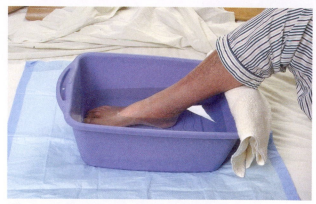

Fig. 18-12. *Pad the edge of the basin to make the resident more comfortable.*

8. Check the water temperature every five minutes. Add warm water as needed to maintain the temperature, but never add water warmer than 105°F. To prevent burns, ask the resident not to add warm water. Observe the area for redness. Discontinue the soak if the resident has pain or discomfort.

9. Soak for 15 to 20 minutes or as ordered.

10. Remove the basin. Use the towel to dry the resident.

11. Remove privacy measures. Make the resident comfortable.

12. Empty, rinse, and dry the basin. Place basin in the area for cleaning or clean and store it according to policy.

13. Discard the disposable pad. Place soiled clothing and linens in the proper containers.

14. Leave call light within the resident's reach.

15. Wash your hands.

16. Be courteous and respectful at all times.

17. Report any changes in the resident to the nurse. Document procedure using facility guidelines.

Applying an Aquamatic K-Pad

Equipment: K-Pad and control unit (Fig. 18-13), covering for pad, distilled water

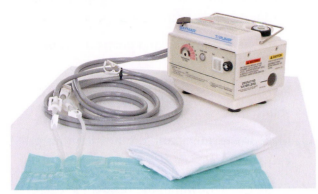

Fig. 18-13. An Aquamatic K-Pad and control unit.

1. Identify yourself by name. Identify the resident. Greet the resident by name.

2. Wash your hands.

3. Explain procedure to the resident. Speak clearly, slowly, and directly. Maintain face-to-face contact whenever possible.

4. Provide for the resident's privacy with a curtain, screen, or door.

5. Make sure the surface of the bedside table is dry. Place the control unit on the bedside table. Make sure the cords are not frayed or damaged. Check that the tubing between the pad and unit is intact.

6. Remove the cover of the control unit to check the water level. If it is low, fill it with distilled water to the fill line.

7. Put the cover of control unit back in place.

8. Plug the unit in and turn pad on. A key is used to set the temperature. If the temperature was not preset, check with the nurse for the proper temperature. If you need to set the temperature, remove the key after doing so. Place the key in the proper place.

9. Place the pad in the cover. Do not pin the pad to the cover.

10. Uncover the area to be treated. Place the covered pad on the area. Note the time. Make sure the tubing is not hanging below the bed. It should be coiled on the bed. Make sure the tubing has no kinks.

11. Return and check the area every five minutes. Remove the pad if the area is red or numb or if the resident reports pain or discomfort.

12. Check the water level and refill with distilled water to the fill line when necessary.

13. Turn off the unit and remove the pad after 20 minutes.

14. Remove privacy measures. Make the resident comfortable.

15. Clean and store supplies.

16. Place soiled linen in the proper container.

17. Leave call light within the resident's reach.

18. Wash your hands.

19. Be courteous and respectful at all times.

20. Report any changes in the resident to the nurse. Document procedure using facility guidelines.

Sitz baths increase circulation to the perineal area. Voiding may be stimulated by a sitz bath. Residents with perineal swelling (such as hemorrhoids) may have orders for sitz baths. Because the sitz bath causes increased blood flow to the pelvic area, blood flow to other parts of the body is decreased. Residents may feel weak, faint, or dizzy after a sitz bath. NAs must always wear gloves when helping with a sitz bath. The NA should stop the bath if the resident complains of feeling dizzy or faint.

A disposable sitz bath fits on the toilet seat and is attached to a rubber bag containing warm water (Fig. 18-14).

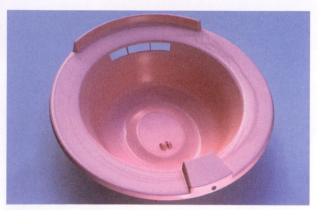

Fig. 18-14. *A disposable sitz bath.* (REPRINTED WITH PERMISSION OF DYNAREX CORPORATION, DYNAREX.COM, 845-365-8200)

Assisting with a sitz bath

Equipment: disposable sitz bath, water thermometer, towels, gloves

1. Identify yourself by name. Identify the resident. Greet the resident by name.

2. Wash your hands.

3. Explain procedure to the resident. Speak clearly, slowly, and directly. Maintain face-to-face contact whenever possible.

4. Provide for the resident's privacy with a curtain, screen, or door.

5. Put on gloves.

6. Fill the sitz bath container two-thirds full with warm water. Place the sitz bath on the toilet seat. Check the water temperature using the water thermometer. Water temperature should be no higher than 105°F.

7. Help the resident undress and sit on the sitz bath. A valve on the tubing connected to the bag allows the resident or you to refill the sitz bath with warm water.

8. You may be required to stay with the resident during the bath for safety reasons. If you leave the room, check on the resident every five minutes to make sure she is not dizzy or weak. Make sure the resident knows how to use the emergency pull cord in the bathroom if it is needed. Stay with a resident who seems unsteady.

9. Help the resident off of the sitz bath after 20 minutes. Provide towels and help with dressing if needed.

10. Empty and rinse the sitz bath container. Discard it properly, according to policy.

11. Place soiled clothing and linens in proper containers.

12. Remove and discard gloves properly. Wash your hands.

13. Make the resident comfortable. Remove privacy measures.

14. Leave call light within the resident's reach.

15. Wash your hands.

16. Be courteous and respectful at all times.

17. Report any changes in the resident to the nurse. Document procedure using facility guidelines.

There are different types of commercial cold packs available, which may be used instead of traditional ice packs (Fig. 18-15). If these are provided, the NA should follow the package directions and the nurse's instructions. Some cold packs are disposable, while others are cleaned and reused.

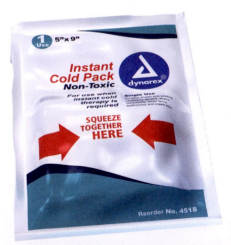

Fig. 18-15. *Disposable cold compresses are used only once and then discarded. The compress shown here must be squeezed to activate before being applied.* (REPRINTED WITH PERMISSION OF DYNAREX CORPORATION, DYNAREX.COM, 845-365-8200)

Applying ice packs

Equipment: cold pack or sealable plastic bag, crushed ice, towel to cover pack or bag

1. Identify yourself by name. Identify the resident. Greet the resident by name.

2. Wash your hands.

3. Explain procedure to the resident. Speak clearly, slowly, and directly. Maintain face-to-face contact whenever possible.

4. Provide for the resident's privacy with a curtain, screen, or door.

5. Fill the plastic bag one-half to two-thirds full with crushed ice. Seal the bag. Remove excess air. Cover the bag or pack with the towel (Fig. 18-16).

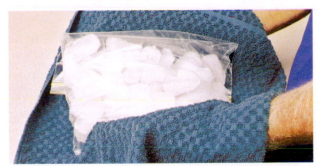

Fig. 18-16. *Seal the bag filled with ice and cover it with a towel.*

6. Apply the bag or pack to the area as ordered. Note the time. Use another towel to cover the bag or pack if it is too cold.

7. Check the area after five minutes for blisters or pale, white, or gray skin. Stop treatment if the resident reports numbness, tingling, burning, or pain.

8. Remove the bag or pack after 20 minutes or as ordered.

9. Remove privacy measures. Make the resident comfortable.

10. Discard supplies or store in the freezer if ordered.

11. Place used linen in the proper container.

12. Leave call light within the resident's reach.

13. Wash your hands.

14. Be courteous and respectful at all times.

15. Report any changes in the resident to the nurse. Document procedure using facility guidelines.

A resident who has a high fever may need to have a cooling or tepid sponge bath. Sponge baths can reduce body temperature. High fevers can have serious side effects, such as seizures and confusion.

Prior to the bath, baseline vital signs, including body temperature, will need to be checked. During the procedure, vital signs will need to be measured at specific intervals. Possible complications of sponge baths are chills, shivering, a sudden change in vital signs, or breathing problems. If any of these occur, the NA should stop the bath, cover the resident completely, and immediately call for the nurse.

7. Discuss nonsterile and sterile dressings

Open wounds increase the risk of infection because breaks in the skin are a way for bacteria and other microorganisms to enter the body. In order to protect wounds from bacteria, dressings are applied. Dressings can be either nonsterile or sterile. Nonsterile dressings are applied to dry wounds that have less chance of infection. Sterile dressings are required when the wound is new, open, or draining. They are also required when there is a higher risk of infection.

NAs may help with nonsterile and sterile dressing changes. The NA should notify the nurse if the resident says that he is allergic to latex.

Assisting the nurse with changing a nonsterile dressing

Equipment: package of square gauze dressings, adhesive tape, scissors, 2 pairs of gloves, plastic bag

1. Identify yourself by name. Identify the resident. Greet the resident by name.

2. Wash your hands.

3. Explain procedure to the resident. Speak clearly, slowly, and directly. Maintain face-to-face contact whenever possible.

4. Provide for the resident's privacy with a curtain, screen, or door.

5. The nurse will prepare a clean, flat, dry surface for the dressing materials. Keep the plastic bag close by for immediate disposal of old dressing materials.

6. You may be asked to open packages for the nurse or cut strips of tape. Cut pieces of tape long enough to secure the dressing. Open the square gauze packages without touching the insides or the gauze.

7. Put on gloves.

8. Only expose the area where the dressing will be changed. The nurse will remove the soiled dressing. Discard used dressing in the proper container.

9. Remove your gloves and discard them in the plastic bag.

10. Wash your hands.

11. Put on new gloves. The nurse will observe the wound and then apply the fresh gauze over the wound and tape it in place (Fig. 18-17). Assist as directed.

12. Remove and discard gloves properly. Wash your hands.

13. Make the resident comfortable. Remove privacy measures.

14. Leave call light within the resident's reach.

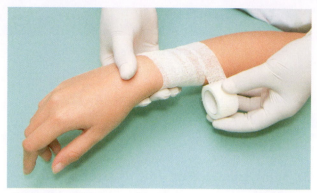

Fig. 18-17. *The nurse will apply and secure the dressing.*

15. Wash your hands.

16. Be courteous and respectful at all times.

17. Report any changes in the resident to the nurse. Document procedure using facility guidelines.

Sterile gloves will be used for sterile dressing care. A sterile field—the area that is kept sterile—is created when performing sterile dressing care. The NA may need to assist the nurse with sterile dressing care. Examples of supplies that are considered sterile are sterile dressings, drapes, and pads. Packages are generally marked in some way to indicate whether the supply is sterile or nonsterile. The NA should check expiration dates on packaging to make sure gloves and other supplies can be used.

Care must be taken so that neither the sterile field nor the sterile gloves become contaminated. If any part of the sterile field becomes contaminated, the entire process must be restarted.

Applying sterile gloves

Equipment: 2 pairs of sterile gloves in correct size

1. Wash your hands.

2. Using a clean, flat, dry surface, remove the outer wrapper from the gloves. Place the inner wrapper on the clean surface. The word *Left* should be on your left side, and the word *Right* should be on your right side.

3. Slowly open the inner wrapper, only touching the small flaps of the wrapper.

4. The gloves will have been placed palm-side up with cuffs in place. Pick up the first glove by the bottom end of the cuff. Slip your fingers into the glove without touching the outside of the glove (Fig. 18-18). If you touch the outside of the glove, it will be contaminated. You will have to start over with a new pair of gloves. Wait to adjust the glove until the second glove is on your other hand.

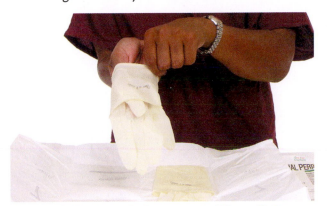

Fig. 18-18. *Touching the bottom end of the cuff, slip your fingers into the glove without touching the outside of the glove.*

5. Slip your gloved hand into the second glove in the area under the cuff.

6. Slowly slip the fingers of your ungloved hand into the second glove, and pull it completely over your hand and wrist (Fig. 18-19).

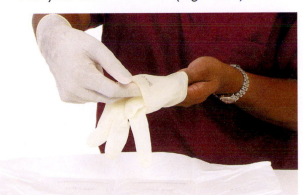

Fig. 18-19. *Touching the area under the cuff of the second glove, slip the fingers of your ungloved hand inside.*

7. With your gloved second hand, finish pulling the first glove up and over the wrist.

Adjust the fingers now if any adjustment is necessary.

8. If either glove has a tear in it, stop and start again with the second set of sterile gloves.

9. Keep your gloved hands in front of you and above the level of your waist at all times during the procedure.

10. Assist the nurse with the sterile procedure.

Trivia

The History of the Rubber Glove

In the early 20th century, William Halsted developed rubber gloves to protect his nurse's (and future wife's) hands. A student suggested that surgeons adopt them. The gloves were very thick, though, and many surgeons would not wear them. Some surgeons wore cloth gloves over the rubber ones. Over the years, rubber gloves became thinner and easier to wear. Today's gloves are made of different materials, such as latex, vinyl, or nitrile.

Chapter Review

1. List four functions of the integumentary system (LO 2).

2. List eight normal age-related changes of the integumentary system (LO 3).

3. Briefly describe the damage and/or symptoms caused by first-, second-, and third-degree burns (LO 4).

4. How is scabies usually transmitted (LO 4)?

5. Under what circumstances are nonsterile dressings usually used? When are sterile dressings used (LO 7)?

Multiple Choice

6. Where does skin breakdown often occur (LO 5)?
   (A) At pressure points.
   (B) On the tops of the hands.
   (C) On all exposed skin.
   (D) At the fingertips.

7. How often should a resident in a wheelchair change positions in order to help prevent pressure injuries (LO 5)?
   (A) Every hour
   (B) Every 90 minutes
   (C) Every three hours
   (D) Every 30 minutes

8. Generally speaking, for how long should warm or cold applications be applied (LO 6)?
   (A) 5 minutes
   (B) 10 minutes
   (C) 15 minutes
   (D) 20 minutes

19
The Circulatory or Cardiovascular System

Discovering the Pathways of the Blood

An English physician named William Harvey (1578–1657) wrote *On the Movement of the Heart and Blood in Animals*, which was published in 1628. He noted that blood moves throughout the body in a closed system. He came to the conclusion that the blood recycles itself and moves inside the body in a single direction, not back and forth.

Harvey also identified that the heart is a pump and that it works by using the force of muscle. He found the heart has two phases: systole, when the heart contracts and empties itself of blood, and diastole, when the chambers of the heart are filled with blood.

"It ennobled our hearts and enriched our blood."

Richard Leveridge, 1670–1758

"So in my veins red life might stream again."

John Keats, 1795–1821

1. Define important words in this chapter

anemia: a condition in which the amount of red blood cells or hemoglobin in the body is less than normal.

angina pectoris: chest pain, pressure, or discomfort.

arrhythmia: irregular heartbeat.

artery: vessel that carries blood away from the heart.

atria: the upper two chambers of the heart.

capillaries: tiny blood vessels in which the exchange of gases, nutrients, and waste products occurs between blood and cells.

cardiomyopathy: a weakening of the heart muscle due to enlargement or thickening, which reduces the heart's ability to pump blood effectively.

congestive heart failure (CHF): a condition in which the heart muscle is damaged and fails to pump effectively.

coronary artery disease (CAD): a condition in which the coronary arteries become damaged and narrow over time, causing chest pain and other symptoms.

deep vein thrombosis (DVT): a condition in which a blood clot forms in a large vein in the body, most often in the leg.

diastole: phase when the heart muscle relaxes.

elastic stockings: stockings that are used to prevent swelling and blood clots and to promote circulation; also called *compression* or *antiembolic stockings*.

embolism: the blockage of a blood vessel by a blood clot or a foreign substance.

heart: four-chambered pump that is responsible for the flow of blood in the body.

hypoxia: a condition in which the body does not receive enough oxygen.

ischemia: a lack of blood supply to an area.

myocardial ischemia: a condition in which the heart muscle does not receive enough blood and lacks oxygen; can cause angina pectoris.

nitroglycerin: medication that relaxes the walls of the coronary arteries.

occlusion: a complete obstruction of a blood vessel.

orthopnea: shortness of breath when lying down that is relieved by sitting up.

peripheral vascular disease (PVD): a condition in which the legs, feet, arms, or hands do not have enough blood circulation.

phlebitis: inflammation of the veins, usually in the lower extremities.

pulmonary edema: a condition in which there is an accumulation of fluid in the lungs; usually due to heart failure.

pulmonary embolism (PE): a blockage in the pulmonary artery, usually by a blood clot.

sequential compression device (SCD): a plastic, air-filled sleeve that is placed around the leg and inflates and deflates regularly to help improve circulation, reduce fluid buildup, and prevent blood clots.

stable angina: chest pain that occurs when a person is active or under severe stress.

sudden cardiac arrest: a serious, often fatal condition in which there is a loss of heart function, breathing, and consciousness.

systole: phase where the heart is at work, contracting and pushing blood out of the left ventricle.

thrombus: a blood clot in a blood vessel.

unstable angina: chest pain that occurs while a person is at rest and not exerting himself.

vein: vessel that carries blood to the heart.

ventricles: the lower two chambers of the heart.

2. Explain the structure and function of the circulatory system

The circulatory, or cardiovascular, system is made up of the heart, blood vessels, and blood (Fig. 19-1). The **heart** is the pump of the circulatory system. It is positioned between the lungs, slightly to the left of the middle of the chest. The heart muscle is made up of three layers: the pericardium, the myocardium, and the endocardium.

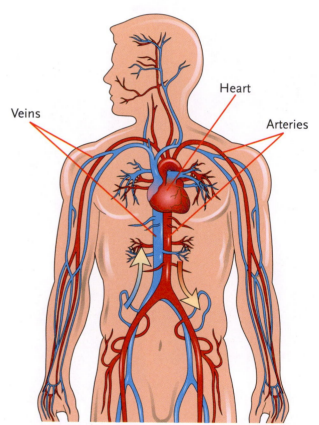

Fig. 19-1. *The heart, blood vessels, and blood are the main parts of the circulatory system.*

The heart is composed of four main chambers: the **atria** (the upper left and right chambers) and the **ventricles** (the lower left and right chambers). The right atrium receives deoxygenated blood from the body. It is delivered via the superior vena cava from the head and upper extremities and via the inferior vena cava from the rest of the body (Fig. 19-2).

The heart functions in two phases: systole and diastole. During **systole**, the lower chambers of the heart, the ventricles, contract. This contraction causes blood to move out of the ventricles of the heart and into the arteries. The ventricles relax after contraction and fill up with blood again. This part of heart function is known as **diastole**. This is the relaxation phase of the heart, or when the heart rests.

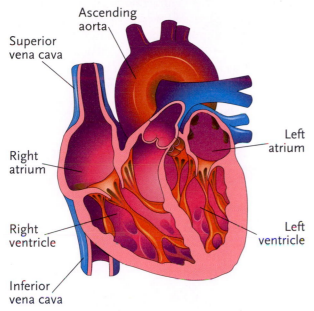

Fig. 19-2. *The four chambers of the heart connect to the body's largest blood vessels.*

Blood is pumped from the right atrium to the right ventricle. The right ventricle pumps the deoxygenated blood into the lungs via the pulmonary arteries. These are the only arteries in the body that carry deoxygenated blood; the other arteries carry oxygen-rich blood. The exchange of carbon dioxide for oxygen is made during this process. The blood then travels back into the heart through the pulmonary veins. These are the only veins in the body that carry oxygen-rich blood.

While in the lungs, carbon dioxide is removed when a person exhales, or breathes out, and oxygen is added when a person inhales, or takes a breath. This exchange of gases returns oxygen-rich blood to the left ventricle. The left ventricle then pumps the oxygen-rich blood out of the heart via the largest **artery** in the body, the aorta. The blood is delivered to all of the arteries in the body through the arterial system (Fig. 19-3).

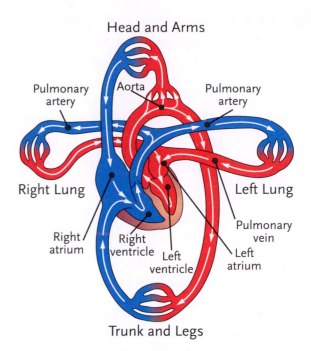

Fig. 19-3. *The flow of blood through the heart.*

With the exception of the pulmonary arteries, the arteries carry oxygen-rich blood away from the heart to deliver the oxygen to the cells. When blood arrives at the cell level, it moves into arterioles, the tiniest of the arterial vessels. The arterioles deliver the blood to the tiny blood vessels called **capillaries**. Gas, nutrient, and waste exchanges happen within capillaries. Capillaries have very thin walls, allowing blood to move in and out of the tiny vessels. During capillary exchange, oxygen and nutrients move from the blood into the tissues, and fluid and waste products move from the tissues into the blood.

Capillaries connect to small veins called *venules.* The venules collect the deoxygenated blood from the capillaries and then drain this blood into the veins. The **veins** carry the deoxygenated blood back to the heart, and the whole process begins again.

Blood is made up of solids and liquids: cells and plasma. Blood cells make up about 45% of blood; plasma makes up the remaining 55%. Blood is composed of three different types of blood cells: red blood cells, or erythrocytes; white blood cells, or leukocytes; and platelets, or thrombocytes.

Red blood cells (erythrocytes) contain hemoglobin, which carries oxygen through the blood vessels. Red blood cells also transport carbon dioxide from the cells through the heart to the lungs. The lungs are responsible for the elimination of carbon dioxide from the body via exhaling. Red blood cells are produced by bone marrow, a substance found inside hollow bones. Iron, found in bone marrow and red blood cells, is essential to blood. It gives blood its red color. Iron in the diet allows the body to produce new red blood cells. Red blood cells function for a short time, and then they die. They are filtered out of the blood by the liver and spleen.

White blood cells (leukocytes) protect the body from bacteria and viruses and other foreign substances. When the body becomes aware of these invaders, white blood cells rush to the site of infection and multiply rapidly. The bone marrow, spleen, and thymus gland produce white blood cells.

Platelets (thrombocytes) cause the blood to clot, which prevents excess bleeding. Platelets are also produced by the bone marrow.

Plasma, the liquid portion of the blood, is made up mostly of water. The plasma carries oxygen, nutrients, waste products, hormones, salts, antibodies, and the substance necessary for the blood to clot.

The functions of the circulatory system are

The heart

- Pumps blood through blood vessels to every cell in the human body

The blood

- Transports oxygen, nutrients, hormones, salts, and antibodies to cells

- Removes carbon dioxide and other waste products from the cells

- Controls pH level and body temperature

- Clots and fights pathogens and poisons

Destination: Homeostasis

A sudden decrease in blood pressure, as in the case of shock (decrease in amount of blood to organs and tissues) or a severe hemorrhage (loss of blood), causes an imbalance in homeostasis. The body responds to this change by triggering the sympathetic nervous system to increase the heart rate, along with the force of the contraction of the heart. This increases the output of blood from the heart. The change in the output of blood increases blood pressure. The heart tries to restore an adequate volume of blood to all body tissues. When blood volume is back to normal levels, the body has returned to homeostasis.

3. Discuss changes in the circulatory system due to aging

Normal age-related changes for the circulatory system include the following:

- Heart pumps less efficiently.

- Blood vessels narrow.

- Blood vessels become less elastic.

- Blood flow decreases.

4. Discuss common disorders of the circulatory system

Hypertension (HTN) or High Blood Pressure

When systolic blood pressure consistently measures 130 mm Hg or higher or diastolic pressure regularly measures 80 mm Hg or higher, a person is diagnosed as having *hypertension*, or high blood pressure. (Systolic and diastolic readings do not both need to be high for a reading to be considered high.) The major cause of hypertension is the hardening and narrowing of the blood vessels. It can also result from kidney disease, tumors of the adrenal glands, pregnancy, extreme stress or pain, and certain medications. Arteries may become hardened, or narrower, because of a buildup of plaque on the walls of the blood vessels, and this can also cause hypertension (Fig. 19-4).

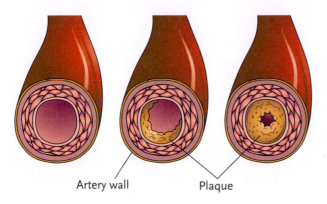

Artery wall   Plaque

Fig. 19-4. Arteries may harden or narrow because of a buildup of plaque. Hardened arteries cause high blood pressure.

Hypertension can develop in people of any age. Signs and symptoms of hypertension are not always obvious, especially in the early stages of the disease. Often the illness is only discovered when a blood pressure measurement is taken by a healthcare provider. Persons with the disease may complain of headache, blurred vision, and dizziness.

Hypertension can lead to a myocardial infarction (heart attack). This is often caused by fatty deposits completely blocking off a coronary artery. This is called an *occlusion* or a *coronary occlusion*. An **occlusion** is an obstruction of a blood vessel. Occlusions cause damage to a part of the heart muscle from the lack of blood supply. **Ischemia** is a lack of blood supply to an area. If hypertension is not treated promptly, it can also result in a cerebrovascular accident (CVA), or stroke (Chapter 22). Hypertension can also lead to kidney disease or blindness.

Medication is usually ordered to treat hypertension. This helps lower blood pressure and can prevent the complications listed above. Extra fluid can increase blood volume and weight, which increases the workload on the heart. Diuretic medications help reduce fluid in the body. Residents may have prescribed exercise programs and special diets, such as low-fat or low-sodium diets. Reducing the intake of sodium

(salt) in the diet can help reduce extra fluid in the body. Stopping smoking can increase the size of the blood vessels, increasing the flow of blood. Nicotine constricts (closes) blood vessels. Lowering stress levels can also help people with hypertension.

NAs may be asked to measure blood pressure often. They can also assist by encouraging residents to follow their prescribed diets and exercise programs.

> **Tip**
>
> **The Silent Killer**
>
> Signs of hypertension include nosebleeds, eye hemorrhages (blood showing up in the white of an eye), dizziness, trembling, shortness of breath, and headaches. Hypertension puts a person at high risk for a heart attack or stroke. Any of these signs and symptoms should be reported to the nurse.

Coronary Artery Disease (CAD)

The coronary arteries supply blood to the heart. **Coronary artery disease (CAD)** occurs when the coronary arteries become damaged. Over time, a buildup of arterial plaque forms and the arteries narrow. This plaque can partially or completely block the arteries.

When the blood supply to the heart is reduced, myocardial ischemia occurs. **Myocardial ischemia** is a condition in which the heart muscle does not get enough blood, and therefore lacks enough oxygen. When the heart is deprived of oxygen, chest pain can occur. However, myocardial ischemia can occur without causing pain or discomfort. Chest pain, pressure, or discomfort due to coronary artery disease is known as **angina pectoris** (Fig. 19-5). Angina pectoris is a symptom of myocardial ischemia.

Angina pectoris is classified as stable or unstable. **Stable angina** is chest pain that occurs when a person is active or under severe stress. **Unstable angina** is chest pain that occurs while a person is at rest and not exerting himself.

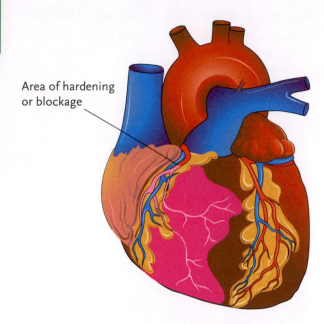

Fig. 19-5. Angina pectoris is chest pain that results from the heart not getting enough oxygen.

Area of hardening or blockage

The pain of angina can be mild or severe. Angina is usually described as intense pressure in the chest, a tightness in the chest, or pain in the back, neck, jaw, or shoulder. Some people have pain that radiates down the inside of the left arm. Other signs and symptoms are sweating, trouble breathing, dizziness, and cyanosis of the lips, nailbeds, and mucous membranes.

Guidelines: Angina

G Reduce stress as much as possible. Stress can cause or worsen angina.

G Notify the nurse immediately if the resident needs help taking medication prescribed for angina. **Nitroglycerin** is usually prescribed for this condition, and is a medication that relaxes the walls of the coronary arteries. This medication comes in various forms, such as pills, sprays, or patches. If pills are used, the resident places a pill under his tongue as soon as chest pain occurs. Nitroglycerin pills must be kept within reach at all times, even when residents leave the facility. Nitroglycerin spray is sprayed onto or under the tongue.

A nitroglycerin patch is placed on the upper body or upper arm; it is normally worn up to 14 hours a day. Remember that NAs are not allowed to give medication, which includes nitroglycerin. Your responsibilities are to report any side effects from the nitroglycerin, such as headache, dizziness, blurred vision, fainting, slow or rapid pulse rate, and a drop in blood pressure. Report if a nitroglycerin patch loosens or falls off.

G Make sure residents get enough rest. Rest is very important for people suffering from angina pectoris. It reduces the heart's need for extra oxygen. However, rest may not help unstable angina.

G Residents will need to avoid overeating, especially right before bedtime.

G Encourage residents to follow their exercise plans as ordered by the doctor. During exercise, observe for chest pain. Report to the nurse if a resident has pain or difficulty during exercising.

G Climate can affect symptoms of coronary artery disease. Humid weather can cause breathing problems. Residents may need to avoid hot and humid weather.

G Be encouraging if residents have quit or are trying to quit smoking.

Cardiomyopathy

Coronary artery disease can cause **cardiomyopathy**, or a heart muscle that no longer pumps effectively due to the heart thickening or becoming enlarged. Cardiomyopathy can also be caused by a virus, diabetes, thyroid problems, drug and alcohol use, or a birth defect. The cause may also be unknown. The prognosis for cardiomyopathy is not good. This condition is the most common reason for heart transplants.

Myocardial Infarction (MI) or Heart Attack

When all or part of the blood flow to the heart muscle is blocked, oxygen and nutrients fail to reach the cells in that area. Waste products are not removed and muscle cells die. This is called a *myocardial infarction (MI)* or a heart attack (Fig. 19-6). When a clot (thrombus) causes an MI by blocking the blood supply to an area of the heart, it is called *coronary thrombosis*.

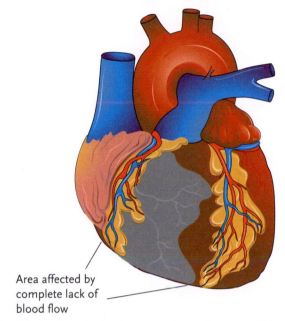

Area affected by complete lack of blood flow

Fig. 19-6. *A heart attack occurs when all or part of the blood flow to the heart is blocked.*

After a myocardial infarction, the area of the heart that has been damaged can no longer function and usually turns into scar tissue. The undamaged part of the heart muscle must then compensate (take over) for the part of the heart that has died. This can increase the workload on the part of the heart that is still able to function.

Sudden Cardiac Arrest

Sudden cardiac arrest is a serious, often fatal condition in which the heart suddenly stops beating, breathing stops, and consciousness is lost. Blood flow to the brain and other organs ceases, and death can occur within minutes.

SCA is often caused by an **arrhythmia** (irregular heartbeat), which is a result of a problem with the electrical signals within the heart.

Risk factors for SCA include heredity, aging, hypertension, and diabetes, which can lead to heart disease. Signs and symptoms include dizziness, shortness of breath, and fainting.

Because an SCA is a medical emergency, it must be treated with a defibrillator right away. If a person survives an SCA, ongoing treatment includes medication and possibly surgery.

A myocardial infarction (MI) is different from an SCA. MIs occur when the circulation to a part of the heart is compromised due to a blockage in one or more blood vessels. The blood flow to the heart may be reduced or stopped. MIs can cause SCA.

Cardiac Rehabilitation

After a myocardial infarction, cardiac rehabilitation is usually ordered. Cardiac rehabilitation is ongoing. This comprehensive program consists of a variety of components, including the following:

- A low-fat, low-sodium diet
- A regular exercise program
- Medications to regulate the heart rate and blood pressure, to lower cholesterol, and to lower triglycerides
- Regular blood testing
- Stopping smoking
- Avoiding cold temperatures
- A stress management program
- Mental health care to help deal with depression and anxiety

Peripheral Vascular Disease (PVD)

Peripheral vascular disease (PVD) is a condition in which the blood supply to the legs, feet, arms, or hands is decreased due to poor circulation. This is primarily due to a buildup of arterial plaque over time. Peripheral vascular disease refers to disease of the blood vessels; it does not include the vessels of the heart and brain. Other causes of peripheral vascular disease are a reduction in cardiac output (amount of blood being pumped out of the heart with each contraction), trauma, and inflammation of the veins, called **phlebitis**. When the blood supply is reduced, the oxygen supply is reduced, causing damage to tissues.

The most common type of peripheral vascular disease is peripheral arterial disease (PAD). It is similar to coronary artery disease. A blockage is created by arterial plaques that build up in the artery walls. Blood circulation decreases, mostly in the arteries leading to the kidneys, stomach, arms, legs, and feet. Pain occurs because there is not enough blood supply to the muscles during exercise. Pain or cramping in the legs due to decreased blood flow is the most common symptom of peripheral arterial disease.

Signs and symptoms of peripheral vascular disease include the following:

- Painful cramping in the hips, thighs, or calves when walking, climbing stairs, or doing other exercise

- Painful cramping in the legs that does not go away when exercise stops

- Cyanotic (blue or gray-tinged) hands or feet

- Bluish nailbeds

- Arms and/or legs that feel warm or cold to the touch

- Edema (swelling) in the hands or feet

- Ulcers on the legs or feet, especially sores that do not heal

- Gangrene (Chapter 18)

Identifying and managing the cause of peripheral vascular disease can improve circulation to the peripheral blood vessels. For example, if the cause is arterial plaque, a low-fat diet may be ordered to try to prevent further plaque from forming.

NAs can help by carefully observing residents for signs and symptoms or changes that might signal poor circulation. Following orders for weighing residents daily and measuring intake and output (I&O) is important. Residents must be encouraged to follow any ordered fluid restrictions and/or special diets. The NA should be encouraging and should offer support if the resident has quit smoking.

Observing and Reporting: Peripheral Vascular Disease (PVD)

- °/ʀ Resident complaints of pain or discomfort or any change in the hands, legs, or feet

- °/ʀ Change in any vital sign, especially in pulse or blood pressure

- °/ʀ Change in edema

- °/ʀ Weight gain

- °/ʀ Intake or output change

- °/ʀ Any pain or discomfort in the head, neck, jaw, shoulder, chest, or back

- °/ʀ Complaints about the inability to see clearly

- °/ʀ Disorientation, dizziness, or confusion

Being bedbound or sitting for long periods of time can increase a person's risk of developing a blood clot, called a **thrombus**. **Deep vein thrombosis (DVT)** is a condition in which a blood clot forms in a large vein in the body, most often in the leg. When a blood clot or thrombus breaks loose from a vein, it becomes an **embolism**. An embolism can travel from where it was formed to another part of the body, blocking blood flow. It can cause serious damage and even death. When a clot travels to the lungs, it becomes a **pulmonary embolism (PE)**, which can be fatal if not treated immediately. Venous thromboembolism (VTE) is a term that refers both to deep vein thrombosis (DVT) and pulmonary embolism (PE).

To help prevent blood clots and swelling, special stockings are ordered for people who have poor circulation or who have reduced mobility. These stockings increase blood circulation and help reduce fluid retention. They are called **elastic**

stockings (or *compression* or *antiembolic stockings*). These stockings help prevent embolisms. Because some people should not use these stockings, they should only be used with a doctor's order.

Antiembolic stockings increase blood circulation by causing smooth, even compression of the legs so that the blood moves better through the vessels. Measurements are taken so that the person is given the correct size of stocking. There are two styles: thigh-high and knee-high.

Each stocking has a seamed hole in the fabric around the toe or underneath the foot. This allows the skin color of the feet and toes to be observed without taking the stockings all the way off. For residents who wear elastic stockings, NAs should check their toes and feet for cyanosis regularly.

Using these stockings poses some risks. If the stocking is turned over at the top, the compression can double, causing the blood flow in the leg to be blocked. These stockings should be applied in the morning when legs are at their smallest size. It is more difficult to apply them later in the day. They should be put on while feet are still elevated, before the resident gets out of bed. The stockings are usually removed in the evening.

Applying knee-high elastic stockings ▶

Equipment: elastic stockings

1. Identify yourself by name. Identify the resident. Greet the resident by name.

2. Wash your hands.

3. Explain procedure to the resident. Speak clearly, slowly, and directly. Maintain face-to-face contact whenever possible.

4. Provide for the resident's privacy with a curtain, screen, or door.

5. Adjust the bed to a safe level, usually waist high. Lock bed wheels.

6. The resident should be in the supine position (on her back) in bed. With the resident lying down, remove her socks, shoes, or slippers, and expose one leg. Expose no more than one leg at a time.

7. Take one stocking and turn it inside out at least to the heel area (Fig. 19-7).

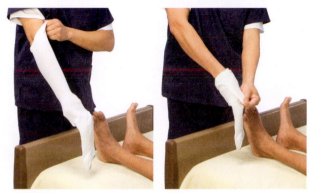

Fig. 19-7. *Turning the stocking inside out allows the stocking to roll on gently.*

8. Gently place the foot of the stocking over the toes, foot, and heel (Fig. 19-8). Make sure the heel is in the right place. The heel of the foot should be in the heel of the stocking.

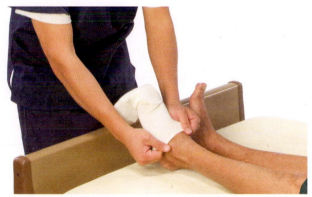

Fig. 19-8. *Place the foot of the stocking over the toes, foot, and heel. Promote the resident's comfort and safety.*

9. Gently pull the top of the stocking over the foot, heel, and leg. Move the foot and leg gently and naturally to avoid force and overextension of the limb and joints.

10. Make sure there are no twists or wrinkles in stocking after it is on the leg. It must fit smoothly and be comfortable (Fig. 19-9). Make sure the heel of stocking is over the

heel of the foot. If the stocking has an opening in the toe area, make sure the opening is either over or under the toe area. This depends on the manufacturer's instructions. Check toes for pressure from the stocking and adjust if needed.

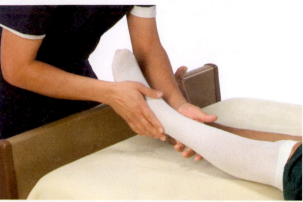

Fig. 19-9. *Make the stocking smooth. Wrinkles cause the stocking to be too tight, which reduces circulation.*

11. Repeat steps 7 through 10 for the other leg.

12. Make the resident comfortable.

13. Return bed to its lowest position. Remove privacy measures.

14. Leave call light within resident's reach.

15. Wash your hands.

16. Be courteous and respectful at all times.

17. Report any changes in the resident to the nurse. Document procedure using facility guidelines.

A **sequential compression device (SCD)** is a plastic, air-filled sleeve that is applied to the leg to improve circulation, reduce fluid buildup, and prevent blood clots. The sleeve is hooked up to a machine with an on/off switch. The machine inflates and deflates the sleeves regularly, causing alternating compression of the legs. It acts in the same way that the muscles do during normal activity (Fig. 19-10).

This device is sometimes used along with elastic stockings. A measurement is needed to order

the correct size of sequential compression stockings. As with any electrical equipment, the NA should report damage or problems with the device to the nurse.

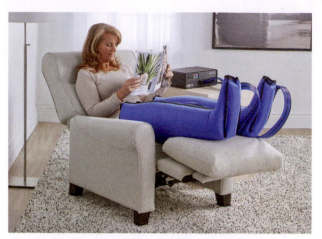

Fig. 19-10. *A sequential compression device.* (PHOTO COURTESY BIO COMPRESSION SYSTEMS, INC., BIOCOMPRESSION.COM, 800-888-0908)

Congestive Heart Failure (CHF)

Coronary artery disease, myocardial infarction, hypertension, heart valve problems, or other disorders may damage the heart. When the heart muscle has been damaged, it fails to pump effectively. When the left side of the heart is affected, blood backs up into the lungs. When the right side of the heart is affected, blood backs up into the legs, feet, or abdomen. When one or both sides of the heart stop pumping blood effectively, it is called **congestive heart failure (CHF)**. Congestive heart failure occurs when the normal cardiac output cannot meet the body's needs for activities of daily living (ADLs). Signs and symptoms of CHF include the following:

- Fatigue

- Reduction in the ability to exercise or be active

- Difficulty breathing, or dyspnea

- Shortness of breath, or **orthopnea** (shortness of breath when lying down that is relieved by sitting up)

- Increased pulse

- Irregular heartbeat

- Chest pain
- Dizziness
- Lack of appetite
- Edema, especially in the feet or ankles
- Swollen abdomen (ascites)
- Abdominal pain
- Increased urination, especially at night
- Confusion
- Weight gain

Other symptoms may occur, depending on the side of the heart that is affected. In right-sided failure, the blood buildup causes swelling of the feet and ankles and can cause the liver and the abdomen to retain fluid. In left-sided heart failure, the buildup of fluid in the lungs causes shortness of breath. These are the symptoms of congestive heart failure associated with each side of the heart:

- Left-sided failure: fatigue, orthopnea, coughing, rapid pulse, and weight gain
- Right-sided failure: fatigue, weakness, edema of the extremities (especially the ankles), bulging neck veins, irregular heartbeat, and fainting

Congestive heart failure may be treated and controlled through medication. Diuretic medications help reduce excess fluid buildup inside the body, thereby reducing edema. Other medications may also help the heart contract more effectively, which increases the movement of blood through the body. Certain medications improve the flow of blood, which helps reduce the workload of the heart.

Guidelines: Congestive Heart Failure

G Follow orders for activity and exercise. Low-intensity exercises may be ordered to help residents improve strength and quality of life.

Have the resident sit or lie down if dizziness or fainting (syncope) occur.

G Measure daily weight and intake and output accurately.

G Encourage residents to follow orders for fluid restrictions, reduced caffeine intake, and low-sodium diets.

G Be encouraging if residents have quit or are trying to quit smoking.

G Use special stockings as ordered.

G Provide extra pillows for residents who have trouble breathing while lying flat in bed.

G Assist with personal care and activities of daily living (ADLs) as needed.

G Assist with range of motion exercises to improve muscle tone when activity is limited.

G Report any of the following signs and symptoms to the nurse:

- Changes in activity level
- Fatigue
- Dizziness, confusion, or fainting
- Increased respiratory rate, pulse, or blood pressure
- Irregular heartbeat
- Palpitations
- Chest tightness or chest pain
- Dyspnea
- Coughing
- Wheezing
- Lack of appetite
- Abdominal swelling or pain
- Edema
- Bulging neck veins
- Weight gain from fluid retention
- Change in urinary output

Arrhythmias

An arrhythmia is an irregular heartbeat. It occurs when the electrical impulses that control the heartbeat do not work properly. The heart then beats irregularly, too slowly, or too rapidly. Some arrhythmias can be life-threatening. Signs and symptoms include chest pain, dizziness, or shortness of breath. Factors increasing the risk for developing an arrhythmia include hypertension, diabetes, and smoking.

A pacemaker (a small device that is implanted near the heart), an implantable cardioverter defibrillator (ICD), medications, cardioversion (a procedure that provides a shock to the heart in an attempt to regain a normal heart rhythm), or ablation (tubes or catheters used to direct bursts of energy in order to change the tissues within the heart) are used to treat arrhythmias. Some devices contain both a pacemaker and an ICD.

Pulmonary Edema

With left-sided heart failure, fluid builds up in the lungs, which presses on the air sacs, causing shortness of breath. This can cause **pulmonary edema**. Pulmonary edema is a life-threatening condition that can be caused by an infection or can be a complication of congestive heart failure or myocardial infarction.

Symptoms of pulmonary edema include shortness of breath, wheezing, coughing, gurgling when breathing, anxiety, and restlessness. A person may feel like he is drowning. Emergency treatment is necessary with acute pulmonary edema. Oxygen will be ordered, and a ventilator may be necessary to help the person breathe. Other follow-up treatments include medication and cardiac rehabilitation.

Blood Disorders

Anemia is a condition in which the amount of red blood cells or hemoglobin in the body is less than normal. This prevents adequate oxygen from reaching the organs and tissues, a condition called **hypoxia**. Anemia is the most common blood disorder. It is diagnosed by a blood test.

Symptoms of anemia include fatigue, weakness, pale skin, a sore or swollen tongue, brittle nails, and difficulty concentrating. A deficiency of iron (iron deficiency anemia) is the most common form of anemia. Treatment includes a high-iron diet and iron supplements. In some cases, an iron transfusion may need to be done. Constipation may occur with an increased intake of dietary iron. A high-fiber diet, additional fluids, and exercise may be ordered to prevent or treat constipation. If excessive bleeding is the suspected cause of the anemia, additional tests may be performed.

Pernicious anemia is a form of anemia caused by a lack of a substance that absorbs vitamin B12 from the digestive tract. This type of anemia is common in people over the age of 60. Symptoms include bleeding gums; a bright red, smooth tongue; rapid pulse; unsteadiness; shortness of breath; pale skin; diarrhea; and numbness and tingling in the hands and feet. Treatment includes monthly vitamin B12 injections. For less severe cases, large doses of B12 pills may be recommended. B12 is also available as a nose gel and spray.

Here are a few additional resources for information relating to circulatory disorders:

- American Heart Association, heart.org

- Centers for Disease Control and Prevention, cdc.gov/ncbddd/dvt

- Centers for Disease Control and Prevention, cdc.gov/bloodpressure

Obesity and Disorders of the Circulatory System

Obesity increases the risk for certain circulatory diseases or disorders, including the following:

- Coronary artery disease (CAD)
- Congestive heart failure (CHF)
- Hypertension (HTN)
- Deep vein thrombosis (DVT)
- Pulmonary embolism (PE)

Chapter Review

1. List four functions of blood (LO 2).

2. List three normal age-related changes of the circulatory system (LO 3).

3. List three ways that hypertension is treated (LO 4).

4. How is the pain of angina pectoris commonly described (LO 4)?

5. List three common symptoms of anemia (LO 4).

Multiple Choice

6. When should elastic stockings be applied (LO 4)?
   (A) During the night
   (B) In the morning
   (C) In the early afternoon
   (D) Before going to bed at night

20
The Respiratory System

Respiration and the "Vapours" of the Heart

Galen, an early physician and author of many medical works, studied the process of respiration. He formed a belief that respiration actually cooled a person's heart. Galen also thought that chest movement added air that helped get rid of certain "vapours" of the heart. Much later, William Harvey, a doctor and researcher, developed the theory that the lungs change venous blood to arterial blood.

"Full of sweet dreams, and health, and quiet breathing."

John Keats, 1795–1821

"Nothing to breathe but air. Quick as a flash 'tis gone."

Benjamin Franklin King, Jr., 1857–1894

1. Define important words in this chapter

alveoli: tiny, grape-like sacs in the lungs where the exchange of oxygen and carbon dioxide occurs.

asthma: a chronic and episodic inflammatory disease that makes it difficult to breathe and causes coughing and wheezing.

bronchi: branches of the passages of the respiratory system that lead from the trachea into the lungs.

bronchiectasis: a condition in which the bronchi become permanently dilated (widened) and damaged.

bronchitis: an irritation and inflammation of the lining of the bronchi.

chest percussion: clapping the chest to help lungs drain with the force of gravity.

chronic obstructive pulmonary disease (COPD): a chronic, progressive, and incurable lung disease that causes difficulty breathing.

emphysema: a chronic, incurable lung disease in which the alveoli in lungs become filled with trapped air; usually results from smoking and chronic bronchitis.

expiration: the process of exhaling air out of the lungs.

hemoptysis: the coughing up of blood from the respiratory tract.

inspiration: the process of breathing air into the lungs.

lungs: main organs of respiration responsible for the exchange of oxygen and carbon dioxide.

multidrug-resistant TB (MDR-TB): a form of tuberculosis caused by an organism that is resistant to medication that is used to treat TB.

oxygen therapy: the administration of oxygen to increase the supply of oxygen to the lungs.

pneumonia: acute inflammation in the lung tissue caused by a bacterial, viral, or fungal infection or chemical irritants.

respiration: the process of inhaling air into the lungs and exhaling air out of the lungs.

sputum: mucus coughed up from the lungs.

trachea: an air passage that goes from the throat (pharynx) to the bronchi; also called *windpipe.*

tuberculosis (TB): a contagious disease caused by a bacterium called *Mycobacterium tuberculosis* that is transmitted through the air; usually affects the lungs, but other body parts can also be affected, such as the spine, brain, and kidneys.

2. Explain the structure and function of the respiratory system

The respiratory system is composed of the nose, nasal cavity, pharynx, larynx, trachea, bronchi, lungs, and alveoli (Fig. 20-1). The nose serves as the front line of the body's air filtration. Air enters the nose and moves through the nasal cavity. Nasal hairs are located in the nasal cavity, which has a mucous membrane lining. The hairs and mucus work to filter particles, such as bacteria and other microbes, dust, smoke, and pollen, from the air as it moves through the cavity. These particles are then moved by the cilia, fine, threadlike projections that work to sweep away particles and fluid, to the pharynx, or throat, to be eliminated from the body.

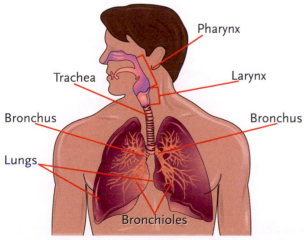

Fig. 20-1. An overview of the respiratory system.

The nasal cavity also warms and humidifies the cooler inhaled air before it continues along toward the pharynx. The pharynx allows for the passage of air and food. The air then moves through the pharynx down to the larynx, or voice box. The larynx is made up of nine pieces of cartilage, including the thyroid cartilage (often called the *Adam's apple*) and the epiglottis. The epiglottis acts like a lid, shutting off the larynx during the swallowing process. This blocks food from entering the **trachea**, or windpipe, which can cause choking.

The larynx enables speech. Exhaled air passes over the vocal cords and causes them to vibrate. Males have lower voices because they have thicker and longer vocal cords than females. This causes their vocal cords to vibrate more slowly, which lowers the overall pitch of their voices.

The trachea transfers air to the lungs. The trachea is lined with a mucous membrane. During the movement through the trachea, more foreign particles attach to the mucus, and the cilia there move the particles up toward the pharynx for elimination from the body.

From the trachea, the air travels into the **bronchi**, the branches of the respiratory system that enter into the lungs. The bronchi turn into the tiniest branches, called *bronchioles*. These tiny branches end in the grape-like clusters called **alveoli**. These are known as the air sacs of the lungs. The exchange of oxygen and carbon dioxide occurs in the alveoli.

The **lungs** are large organs in the chest cavity. They are covered by a membrane called the *pleura*, which covers and protects the lungs. The pleura is made up of two layers that have a small amount of fluid in between them. This fluid allows the pleura to move easily without rubbing together as the lungs expand and contract.

The lungs expand and contract the chest cavity when a person breathes in, or inhales **(inspiration)**. Inspiration is an active process. Expiration is a passive process. The lungs relax and the chest cavity gets smaller when a person exhales **(expiration)**. The process of inspiration uses more energy than the process of expiration. **Respiration**, the body taking in oxygen and removing carbon dioxide, involves inspiration (inhaling) and expiration (exhaling).

Oxygen is a colorless, odorless, and tasteless gas that makes up about 21% of the atmosphere. Oxygen nourishes cells, aids in respiration, and provides energy for cell metabolism. Carbon dioxide is a colorless, odorless, and tasteless gas that makes up about 1% of the atmosphere. Carbon dioxide is a waste product produced by the cells.

Two oxygen and carbon dioxide gas exchanges occur in the lungs and in the cells. The exchange in the lungs is called *external respiration*. During external respiration, oxygen moves into the blood, and carbon dioxide moves into the alveoli. The carbon dioxide is transported from the alveoli when a person exhales through the nose and the mouth.

The second exchange of gases inside the cells is called internal respiration. During internal respiration, oxygen moves into the cells and carbon dioxide moves into the blood. The second exchange is now complete. The cells have oxygen, and carbon dioxide is headed to the lungs to be exhaled. This process of breathing air in and out is continuous; it never stops. Cells must constantly be filled with a fresh supply of oxygen.

The functions of the respiratory system are to

- Serve as an air filter, cleaning the inhaled air
- Supply oxygen to body cells
- Remove carbon dioxide from the cells
- Produce the sounds associated with speech

Destination: Homeostasis

When a stressor increases the blood carbon dioxide level in the blood, the area in the brain responsible for respiratory control, the medulla, sends out nerve impulses. These impulses cause the diaphragm and the other respiratory muscles to contract more forcefully and more often. This is known as *hyperventilation*, or rapid and deep breathing. This increase in breathing removes the excess carbon dioxide, thereby increasing the oxygen to meet cellular needs. When the carbon dioxide level returns to normal, homeostasis is restored.

3. Discuss changes in the respiratory system due to aging

Normal age-related changes for the respiratory system include the following:

- Lung strength decreases.
- Air sacs (the alveoli) become less elastic and decrease in number.
- Airways become stiff and less elastic.
- Lung capacity decreases.
- Chest muscles become weaker.
- Cough reflex becomes less effective and cough becomes weaker.
- Oxygen in the blood decreases.
- Decreased lung capacity causes voice to weaken.

4. Discuss common disorders of the respiratory system

Chronic Obstructive Pulmonary Disease (COPD)

Chronic obstructive pulmonary disease (COPD) is a chronic, progressive disease. Progressive means that the disease gets worse. COPD leads to difficulty breathing due to the obstruction of the airways, especially during exhalation. Many people live with this disease for years. It is irreversible and cannot be cured, but treatment may slow its progression. Two chronic lung diseases are grouped under COPD: chronic bronchitis and emphysema.

Bronchitis is an inflammation of the lining of the bronchi. There are two types of bronchitis:

acute and chronic. Acute bronchitis is caused by an infection. It is often associated with severe colds and usually lasts a brief period of time. Symptoms include coughing, yellow or green **sputum** (mucus coughed up from the lungs), and trouble breathing. Acute bronchitis is generally treated with antibiotics and/or anti-inflammatory medications.

Chronic bronchitis is a condition that occurs when the lining of the bronchial tubes becomes inflamed. This later causes scarring. The irritation of these tubes continues for a long period of time, which then causes excessive mucus production. A long-lasting, mucus-producing cough occurs. Air flow may be restricted and the lungs become scarred. Lung infections can occur more easily when this happens. Chronic bronchitis is caused by cigarette smoking, second-hand smoke, and air pollution or other irritants in the air.

Treatment usually consists of reducing the triggers that cause irritation. Quitting smoking is encouraged. Medications may be ordered.

Emphysema is a chronic condition in which the walls between the alveoli (air sacs) in the lungs become overstretched. The air sacs weaken and break. Air is trapped in the air sacs and normal breathing is impaired. Emphysema usually results from cigarette smoking and chronic bronchitis. Symptoms of emphysema include shortness of breath, coughing, and difficulty breathing.

There is no cure for emphysema. Treatment focuses on providing comfort and relieving symptoms. Quitting smoking is very important. Oxygen may be ordered to help with breathing. Medication and regular respiratory therapy, including breathing exercises, may reduce discomfort.

General symptoms of COPD include the following:

- Coughing or wheezing

- Dyspnea (difficulty breathing)

- Shortness of breath, especially during activity

- Chest pain or tightness

- Cyanosis

- Weakness

- Weight loss or loss of appetite

- Fear and anxiety

- Confusion

Guidelines: COPD

G COPD causes difficulty with breathing. Residents may be constantly anxious or fearful about not being able to breathe. They may fear suffocation. Be supportive and calm. Be empathetic. Not being able to breathe properly is very frightening.

G Use pillows to help residents sit upright or lean forward. This may help them breathe more comfortably.

G Be supportive of residents who are quitting smoking.

G Offer plenty of fluids, and encourage a healthy diet.

G Encourage periods of rest. Try to get residents to save their energy for important tasks.

G Use proper infection prevention practices. Wash your hands often and help residents do the same if help is needed. Discard used tissues immediately in the nearest no-touch waste container.

G Colds can make COPD worse. Report signs and symptoms of colds or the flu immediately to the nurse.

G Medications that relax the air passages may be prescribed. These may be taken orally or inhaled directly into the lungs using sprays or inhalers. It is important for residents to take medications as ordered.

G Oxygen must be supplied to the resident exactly as ordered. Follow safety guidelines for oxygen therapy (Chapter 7).

G Report any of the following signs and symptoms to the nurse:

- Change in breathing patterns, especially shortness of breath

- Change in color or consistency of mucus or sputum

- Chest pain

- Fever

- Refusal to take ordered medications

- Inability to sleep due to anxiety or fear

- Confusion or changes in mental state

Asthma

Asthma is a chronic, episodic disorder in which irritants, allergens such as pollen or dust, infection, and cold air cause inflammation and swelling within the air passages in the lungs (Fig. 20-2). Exercise and stress can also cause or worsen asthma. When the bronchi become irritated due to any one of these conditions, they constrict, making it difficult to breathe. Thick mucus is produced by the mucous membranes, which further inhibits breathing. Air is trapped in the lungs, which causes heavy wheezing, coughing, and a tight feeling in the chest.

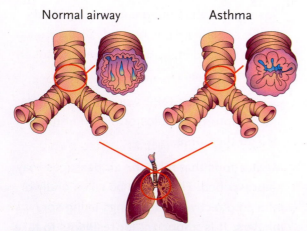

Fig. 20-2. *When a person has asthma, air passages in the lungs become inflamed and swollen.*

The cause of asthma is unknown. Medications are usually ordered to treat asthma. Residents should carry a rescue inhaler with them at all times (Fig. 20-3). They should also avoid the triggers that cause asthma attacks. A resident with asthma should not be exposed to strong-smelling cleaning agents, perfume, cologne, aftershave, or scented soaps and lotions. Smoking and secondhand smoke should be avoided as much as possible. Because stress is a trigger for asthma attacks, reducing stress levels can help. Nursing assistants can help by talking with and listening to residents.

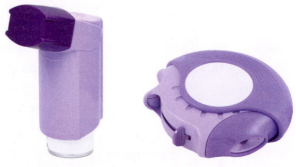

Fig. 20-3. *Two different types of asthma inhalers. Residents with asthma should be encouraged to carry their inhalers at all times.*

Observing and Reporting: Asthma

O/R Changes in vital signs, especially respiratory rate or pulse

O/R Wheezing, shortness of breath, or dyspnea

O/R Cyanosis

O/R Chest pain or tightness

O/R Refusal to use inhaler when needed

Bronchiectasis

Bronchiectasis is a condition in which the bronchi become permanently dilated (widened) and damaged. A person may be born with this disorder, or may develop it later. Bronchiectasis is caused by an infection of the airways. Cystic fibrosis, tumors, or inhaling foreign material are causes of bronchiectasis.

Bronchiectasis is a serious illness that can result in chronic coughing, shortness of breath, wheezing, weight loss, cyanosis, and coughing up blood. Respiratory infections may occur. Over time, foul-smelling sputum may cause halitosis, or bad breath.

Treatment includes proper positioning for drainage (postural drainage) and **chest percussion** (clapping the chest to help the lungs drain with the force of gravity). Recognizing infections early can reduce the severity of the condition. The NA should report fever, chest pain, and a change in mucus or phlegm production to the nurse right away. Prompt treatment of infections will reduce the risk of complications.

Pneumonia

Pneumonia is an inflammation of the lungs caused by a viral, bacterial, or fungal infection or chemical irritants. The air sacs in the lungs fill with pus and other liquid.

There are different types of pneumonia. *Community-acquired pneumonia* occurs when a person develops pneumonia in the community (not in a healthcare facility). Pneumonia developed when a person is in or was in a healthcare facility, such as a long-term care facility, a hospital, an outpatient center, etc., is called *healthcare-associated pneumonia*. If pneumonia is caused by a ventilator, which is a device that performs the process of breathing for someone who cannot breathe on his own, it is considered a *ventilator-associated event (VAE)*. Chapter 26 has more information.

With pneumonia, a person experiences signs and symptoms such as a high fever, chest pain (especially when inhaling), coughing, difficulty breathing, shortness of breath, chills, and a rapid pulse. Thick secretions may be coughed up from the lungs. The NA should report these symptoms to the nurse.

People with weaker immune systems, such as young children and the elderly, are at a higher risk of developing pneumonia. Pneumonia can be a serious and potentially fatal disease, especially for the elderly, who may take longer to recover.

The CDC recommends two vaccines to protect against pneumonia. The pneumococcal conjugate vaccine is recommended for children younger than 2 years old, adults 65 years or older, and for people who are 2–64 years old with certain medical conditions. The pneumococcal polysaccharide vaccine is recommended for adults 65 years or older, people who are 2–64 years old with certain medical conditions, and adults 19–64 years old who smoke cigarettes.

Treatment of pneumonia includes antibiotics and other medications, along with an inhaler. Fluid intake and a proper diet should be encouraged.

Tuberculosis (TB)

Tuberculosis, or TB, is a highly contagious disease caused by a bacterium, *Mycobacterium tuberculosis*, that is carried on mucous droplets suspended in the air. The bacteria usually affect the lungs, known as *pulmonary tuberculosis*. However, the bacteria can also affect other parts of the body such as the spine, brain, and kidney, which is known as *extrapulmonary tuberculosis*. TB is an airborne disease. People can be exposed to TB when they spend time with a person who is infected with TB. The infected person can spread the disease by coughing, breathing, singing, sneezing, or even laughing.

Pulmonary TB causes coughing, difficulty breathing, fever, weight loss, and fatigue. TB can be cured by taking all prescribed medication. However, if left untreated, TB may cause death.

There are two types of TB: latent TB infection (LTBI) and TB disease. Someone with latent TB infection carries the disease but does not show symptoms and cannot infect others. A person with TB disease shows symptoms of the disease and can spread TB to others. Latent TB infection can progress to TB disease. Signs and symptoms of TB include the following:

- Prolonged coughing
- Coughing up blood **(hemoptysis)**
- Shortness of breath
- Dyspnea
- Chest pain
- Slight fever and chills
- Night sweats
- Loss of appetite
- Weight loss
- Fatigue

Tuberculosis is more likely to be spread in areas with poor ventilation or small, confined spaces. People are more likely to get active TB (TB disease) if their immune systems are weakened by illness, malnutrition, cancer, HIV/AIDS, alcoholism, or drug abuse.

Multidrug-resistant TB (MDR-TB) is a form of tuberculosis caused by an organism that is resistant to medication used to treat TB. It may develop when a person infected with TB does not take all of his prescribed medication. Drug resistance can also develop if the TB medication is used incorrectly or the medication is ineffective due to poor quality or poor storage conditions.

Guidelines: Tuberculosis

G Follow Standard Precautions and Airborne Precautions.

G Wear personal protective equipment (PPE) as instructed during care. Use an N95 or HEPA respirator to provide care (Chapter 6).

G Residents will be placed in an *airborne infection isolation room (AIIR)*. These rooms have a controlled flow of air. All of the air inside the room will be exhausted directly to the outside, or all air will first be recirculated through a special HEPA filter before returning to circulation. Keep doors to these rooms closed except when entering or exiting the room. When entering the room, do not open or close the door rapidly. This pulls contaminated room air into the hallway.

G Be careful when handling sputum.

G Residents must take all of the medication prescribed. Failure to take all medication is a major factor in the spread of TB.

Additional resources for information relating to respiratory disorders include the following:

- American Lung Association, lung.org
- National Heart, Lung, and Blood Institute, nhlbi.nih.gov
- COPD Foundation, copdfoundation.org
- Centers for Disease Control and Prevention, cdc.gov/asthma/links.htm

Obesity and Disorders of the Respiratory System

Obesity increases the risk for certain respiratory diseases or disorders, including the following:

- Asthma
- Sleep apnea (OSA)
- Repeated occurrences of pneumonia or bronchitis
- Pulmonary hypertension

Trivia

The History of the Mask
Masks were first regularly used in medical practice during the 1940s and 1950s. It is hard to believe, but many surgeons left their noses uncovered and wore masks only over their mouths. If only they had known how risky this practice really was.

5. Describe oxygen delivery

Every living cell in the human body needs oxygen to survive. The oxygen level in the air is adequate for most people. However, when a person has low oxygen levels, supplemental oxygen is required.

Oxygen therapy is the administration of oxygen to increase the supply of oxygen to the lungs. Because oxygen is considered a drug, in most states oxygen delivery can only be administered by certain licensed healthcare professionals such as nurses and respiratory therapists.

There are different ways to deliver additional oxygen to a person. Oxygen may be piped into a room at a healthcare facility from a wall outlet. Compressed oxygen comes in large cylinders or smaller, portable cylinders, which do not require electricity. Liquid oxygen in special reservoirs can be used in facilities and is also supplied in special containers for use in the home and the community. The liquid oxygen warms and becomes a gas that the person can then breathe. Oxygen concentrators are machines that run on electricity, removing oxygen from the air and storing it for use.

The doctor determines which oxygen delivery device best suits a resident who needs additional oxygen. Residents who require oxygen therapy will need it either continuously or periodically. Continuous oxygen means the oxygen must be on at all times. It is important that NAs understand that oxygen is considered a drug and NAs cannot adjust oxygen levels. Common types of oxygen delivery devices include the following:

Nasal cannula: This device has a set of two prongs which are placed into the nostrils and a plastic tube that fits behind the ears (Fig. 20-4).

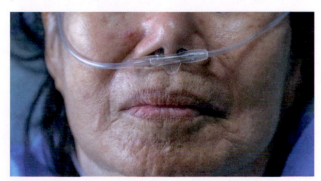

Fig. 20-4. *A nasal cannula.*

The tubing is attached to the oxygen delivery source, which is generally a wall outlet. A small plastic slide moves up and down on the tubing below the chin and adjusts it for comfort and stability. A nasal cannula is the simplest oxygen delivery device. It is a low-flow oxygen delivery system. It is the device seen most often in long-term care facilities.

Simple face mask: This plastic device is shaped to fit over the nose and mouth. It is held in place with an elastic band that slides over the head and above the ears (Fig. 20-5). The band can be adjusted for comfort and stability. The person breathes in through the nose and mouth, and oxygen is delivered. Plastic tubing connects the mask to the oxygen source. Simple face masks deliver low-flow oxygen. These masks can irritate the skin and may feel hot and cause claustrophobia. Masks make it difficult for a person to talk and must be removed before eating or drinking.

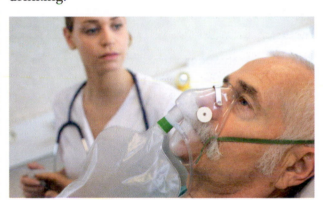

Fig. 20-5. *One type of face mask for oxygen delivery.*

Oxygen concentrator: An oxygen concentrator filters oxygen from normal room air. It delivers low-flow oxygen. It is generally used in conjunction with a nasal cannula. The cannula is placed on the person and is then attached to the oxygen concentrator. Oxygen concentrators are quiet and efficient. They can either be large units that remain in a room, or small, portable ones that can be used when leaving the facility or the home (Fig. 20-6). Oxygen concentrators plug into electrical outlets and may not be usable during power outages. It may take a while for the oxygen concentrator to reach full power after it is turned on.

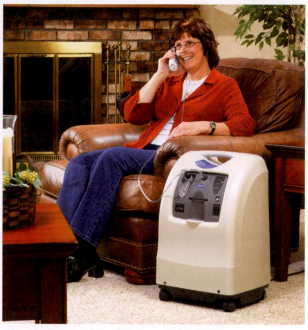

Fig. 20-6. *One type of oxygen concentrator.* (© INVACARE CORPORATION. USED WITH PERMISSION. WWW.INVACARE.COM)

Guidelines: Care of the Resident Using Oxygen

G Perform frequent skin care on areas of the face where the oxygen device rests, such as by the nose, behind the ears, and around the mouth. Special cushions may be used to pad areas that the cannula may irritate.

G Observe for redness, sores, bruising, or discomfort in the ear, nose, mouth, or chin area.

G Lubricate sensitive areas on the nose and mouth using water-based lubricants. Do not use any oil, petroleum-based products, alcohol, or acetone on the tubing; these can be a fire hazard.

G Check the oxygen delivery device often for proper fit and comfort.

G Do not remove an oxygen delivery system or adjust oxygen levels. That is the nurse's responsibility.

G Check vital signs as ordered. A pulse oximeter measures a person's blood oxygen level and pulse rate. Chapter 26 contains more information about pulse oximetry.

G Notify the nurse if the oxygen equipment does not seem to be working. Tell the nurse if the tubing is clogged or dirty and/or if the tank level drops to the point where replacement is needed.

G Make sure that portable oxygen tanks are always in an upright position and in a proper oxygen cylinder holder when in use or when stored.

G Post *No Smoking* and *Oxygen in Use* signs. These should be posted on each door and over the resident's bed. Do not allow smoking or open flames anywhere around oxygen equipment. Remove fire hazards from the room. Chapter 7 has more information.

G Avoid using synthetic or wool fabrics that can cause static electricity discharges. Cotton bedding, clothing, and towels should be used.

G Know the location of the fire alarms and fire extinguishers.

G Add pillows as needed to improve breathing.

G Encourage fluids as directed.

G Encourage activity as permitted so resident does not withdraw or feel isolated.

G Provide emotional support; some oxygen delivery devices are difficult to use and can cause feelings of claustrophobia.

G If you notice any of the following, notify the nurse:

- Sores or crusts on nasal area
- Dry and/or reddened areas on the skin by the ears, nose, mouth, or chin
- Complaints of discomfort or pain
- Shortness of breath or dypsnea
- Changes in vital signs, especially respiratory rate or pulse
- Cyanosis or any change in skin, nail, or mucous membrane color
- Chest pain or tightness

CPAP

Obstructive sleep apnea (OSA) is a sleep disorder that can put a person at higher risk for certain diseases or disorders, such as type 2 diabetes, cardiovascular disease, obesity, and depression. Continuous positive airway pressure (CPAP) is a device used to treat obstructive sleep apnea by promoting breathing during sleep. A small machine supplies steady air pressure and is hooked to a hose and mask or nose piece that the person wears while sleeping. Complications such as dry mouth or nose, sore throat, congestion, and eye or skin irritation can result from using this device.

6. Describe how to collect a sputum specimen

It is sometimes necessary to collect a specimen of mucus that comes from inside the respiratory system for testing. Sputum is not the same as saliva, which comes from the salivary glands inside the mouth. Sputum may show evidence of cancer or bacteria. The lab will study the sputum, looking for abnormal cells, microorganisms, or blood.

Some facilities allow NAs to collect sputum specimens. Early morning is the best time to collect sputum. When people are flat on their backs for an entire night, mucus tends to collect inside the respiratory passages. This makes it easier to collect the sputum specimen.

The resident should rinse her mouth with water before the NA obtains the sputum specimen. This removes any leftover food and any excess saliva. The resident should not rinse with mouthwash before a sputum specimen collection. Mouthwash kills certain kinds of bacteria and other organisms that need to remain within the sputum for analysis.

Collecting a sputum specimen

Equipment: specimen container and lid, completed label (labeled with resident's name, date of birth, doctor's name, room number, date, and time), biohazard specimen bag, tissues, gloves, N95 or other ordered mask, emesis basin, lab slip

1. Identify yourself by name. Identify the resident. Greet the resident by name.

2. Wash your hands.

3. Explain procedure to the resident. Speak clearly, slowly, and directly. Maintain face-to-face contact whenever possible.

4. Provide for the resident's privacy with a curtain, screen, or door.

5. Put on the required mask and gloves.

6. Ask the resident to rinse her mouth with water. Assist as necessary. Have her spit the rinse water in the emesis basin if she does not use the sink.

7. Stand behind the resident if the resident can hold the specimen container by herself. Ask the resident to cough deeply, so that sputum comes up from the lungs. To prevent the spread of infectious material, give the resident tissues to cover her mouth while coughing. Ask the resident to spit the sputum into the specimen container.

8. When you have obtained a good sample (about two tablespoons of sputum), cover the container tightly. Wipe any sputum off the outside of the container with tissues. Discard the tissues. Apply the label and place the specimen in a clean biohazard specimen bag.

9. Remove and discard gloves and mask properly.

10. Wash your hands.

11. Leave call light within the resident's reach.

12. Wash your hands.

13. Be courteous and respectful at all times.

14. Report any changes in the resident to the nurse. Document procedure using facility guidelines. Take specimen and lab slip to designated place promptly.

7. Describe the benefits of deep breathing exercises

Deep breathing exercises help expand the lungs, clearing them of mucus and preventing infections such as pneumonia. Residents who have had surgery, such as hip replacement or abdominal surgery, are instructed to do deep breathing exercises to regularly expand the lungs. The care plan may include using a deep breathing device called an *incentive spirometer* (Fig. 20-7). Incentive spirometry encourages the resident to take long, slow, deep breaths. Regular use can help open the airway, help clear the lungs of fluid and mucus, and strengthen the breathing muscles.

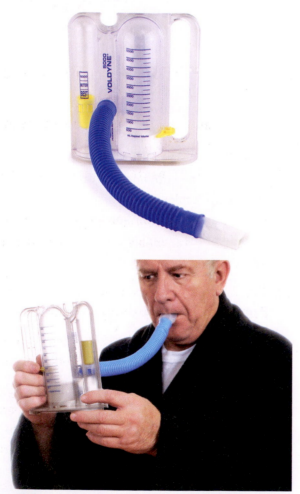

Fig. 20-7. Incentive spirometers are used for deep breathing exercises.

Incentive spirometers should not be shared among residents; each spirometer should be labeled with the resident's name. The NA must make sure that both she and the resident wash their hands prior to using the spirometer. Assisting with this procedure requires that the NA don gloves, and additional personal protective equipment may be necessary. Incentive spirometry should not be done directly after eating.

The resident may need encouragement to use this device. The NA should encourage the resident to use the device as ordered, but should not insist that he do so. If the resident refuses to do the procedure, the NA should report to the nurse.

The incentive spirometer should remain upright during use. If the resident becomes dizzy or lightheaded while he is using it, he should remove the mouthpiece and take normal breaths.

The device should be cleaned and stored after each use, following the care plan and the nurse's instructions. The NA should not assist with these exercises if she has not been trained.

Assisting with deep breathing and coughing exercises

Equipment: gloves, pillow, tissues, emesis basin

1. Identify yourself by name. Identify the resident. Greet the resident by name.

2. Wash your hands.

3. Explain procedure to the resident. Speak clearly, slowly, and directly. Maintain face-to-face contact whenever possible.

4. Provide for the resident's privacy with a curtain, screen, or door.

5. Put on gloves.

6. Position the resident in the Fowler's position with a pillow over the abdomen if needed. You may be instructed to position the resident in a dangling position instead.

7. Ask the resident to wrap his arms around the pillow and hold the pillow tightly against his abdomen.

8. Tell the resident to take a deep breath and hold the breath for a few seconds.

9. Ask the resident to exhale for as long as possible through lips that are pursed.

10. Tell the resident to then repeat the deep breathing exercise a few more times. Ideally the deep breathing exercise should be repeated five times in a row.

11. Make sure the tissues are nearby. Ask the resident to hold the pillow tightly, breathe in once deeply, and then cough as forcefully as possible. Collect any secretions with the tissues and place tissues temporarily in the emesis basin.

12. Repeat the sequence above the designated number of times or the number of times the resident is able to perform the exercises.

13. Discard tissues in the nearest no-touch receptacle.

14. Empty, rinse, and dry emesis basin. Place the basin in the designated dirty supply area or return to storage, depending on facility policy.

15. Remove and discard gloves properly. Wash your hands.

16. Make the resident comfortable. Remove privacy measures.

17. Leave call light within the resident's reach.

18. Wash your hands.

19. Be courteous and respectful at all times.

20. Report any changes in the resident to the nurse. Document procedure using facility guidelines.

Assisting with an incentive spirometer

Equipment: clean incentive spirometer, gloves

1. Identify yourself by name. Identify the resident. Greet the resident by name.

2. Wash your hands.

3. Explain procedure to the resident. Speak clearly, slowly, and directly. Maintain face-to-face contact whenever possible.

4. Provide for the resident's privacy with a curtain, screen, or door.

5. Adjust the bed to a safe level, usually waist high. Lock bed wheels.

6. Position the resident sitting upright in bed or upright in a chair.

7. Put on gloves.

8. Clean the mouthpiece as directed prior to the procedure.

9. Slide the indicator to the correct level, as indicated in the care plan.

10. Ask the resident to grasp the spirometer and to fully exhale.

11. Ask the resident to wrap his lips around the mouthpiece and inhale very slowly, as deeply as possible.

12. Ask the resident to keep the indicator at the designated level for as long as possible.

13. Let the resident know he should then exhale slowly once he cannot keep the indicator at the correct level any longer.

14. Repeat the steps as ordered in the care plan. Spirometry may need to be done every 1 to 2 hours, repeating these steps anywhere from 3 to 15 times during the treatment.

15. If the resident needs to cough during the procedure, give him time to do so. Following surgery, the resident may need to hold a

pillow against his chest or abdomen during spirometry in order to cough successfully.

16. If the resident becomes dizzy during the procedure, stop the procedure and notify the nurse.

17. Place the spirometer in the area for cleaning or clean and store according to policy.

18. Remove and discard gloves properly.

19. Make the resident comfortable.

20. Return bed to its lowest position. Remove privacy measures.

21. Leave call light within the resident's reach.

22. Wash your hands.

23. Be courteous and respectful at all times.

24. Report any changes in the resident to the nurse. Document procedure using facility guidelines.

Chapter Review

1. List three functions of the respiratory system (LO 2).

2. List six normal age-related changes of the respiratory system (LO 3).

3. Why might a person with COPD be fearful or anxious (LO 4)?

4. What is the difference between latent TB infection and TB disease (LO 4)?

5. Why is it important for a resident to take all prescribed medication if he has TB (LO 4)?

6. What conditions can be helped by deep breathing exercises (LO 7)?

Multiple Choice

7. The process of inhaling and exhaling is referred to as (LO 2)
   (A) Inspiration
   (B) Respiration
   (C) Expiration
   (D) Resuscitation

8. Which of the following is one of the duties of an NA with regard to oxygen therapy (LO 5)?
   (A) The nursing assistant orders the type of oxygen delivery device needed for the resident.
   (B) The nursing assistant orders the amount of oxygen the resident needs.
   (C) The nursing assistant performs skin care on the areas of the face where the oxygen device rests.
   (D) The nursing assistant refills oxygen cylinders once they are empty.

9. What time of day is best to collect a sputum specimen (LO 6)?
   (A) Middle of the night
   (B) Late afternoon
   (C) After lunch
   (D) Early morning

21 The Musculoskeletal System

Roentgen and the Discovery of the X-ray

On November 8, 1895, Wilhelm Konrad Roentgen (1845–1923) passed electric current through a tube and noted afterward that a specially coated cardboard material nearby was glowing. He discovered that the glow came from the radiation coming out of the tube. He named the radiation *X-rays*. One of his early X-rays was of his wife's hand. The tremendous impact of this discovery was felt throughout the world. Fractures and diseases of the bones could now be made visible.

"And the muscular strength . . . has lasted the rest of my life."
Lewis Carroll, 1832–1898
from *Alice's Adventures in Wonderland*

"His bones ache with the day's work that earned it."
Ralph Waldo Emerson, 1803–1882

1. Define important words in this chapter

abduction: moving a body part away from the midline of the body.

adduction: moving a body part toward the midline of the body.

amputation: the surgical removal of part or all of a body part.

arthritis: a general term that refers to inflammation of the joints.

atrophy: weakening or wasting away of muscles.

bones: rigid connective tissues that make up the skeleton, lend support to body structures, allow the body to move, and protect the organs.

bursae: tiny sacs of fluid that are located near joints and help reduce friction.

bursitis: a condition in which the bursae become inflamed and painful.

cartilage: the protective substance that covers the ends of bones and makes up the discs that are found between vertebrae.

flexion: bending a body part.

fracture: a broken bone.

full weight-bearing (FWB): a doctor's order stating that a person has the ability to support full body weight on both legs and has no weight-bearing limitations.

joints: the points where two bones meet; provide movement and flexibility.

ligaments: strong bands of fibrous connective tissue that connect bones or cartilage and support the joints and joint movement.

muscles: groups of tissues that contract and relax, allowing motion, supporting the body, protecting organs, and creating heat.

muscular dystrophy: an inherited, progressive disease that causes a gradual wasting away of muscle, resulting in weakness and deformity.

non-weight-bearing (NWB): a doctor's order stating that a person is unable to touch the floor or support any body weight on one or both legs.

osteoarthritis: a type of arthritis that usually affects weight-bearing joints, especially the hips and knees; also called *degenerative joint disease*.

osteopenia: a condition in which the bones have reduced density, but not enough to be classified as osteoporosis.

osteoporosis: a condition in which the bones become brittle and weak, causing them to break easily.

partial weight-bearing (PWB): a doctor's order stating that a person is able to support some body weight on one or both legs.

phantom limb pain: pain in a limb (or extremity) that has been amputated.

phantom sensation: warmth, itching, or tingling from a body part that has been amputated.

prosthesis: an artificial device that replaces a body part, such as an eye, hip, arm, leg, tooth, or heart valve; used to help improve function and/or appearance.

rheumatoid arthritis: a type of arthritis in which joints become red, swollen, and very painful; movement is restricted and deformities of the hands are common.

sling: a bandage or piece of material that is suspended from the neck for the purpose of holding and supporting a forearm.

tendons: tough fibrous bands that connect muscle to bone.

total hip replacement (THR): a surgical replacement of the head of the femur (long bone of the leg) and the socket it fits into where it joins the hip with artificial materials.

total knee replacement (TKR): a surgical replacement of a damaged or painful knee with artificial materials.

2. Explain the structure and function of the musculoskeletal system

The musculoskeletal system is composed of muscles, bones, joints, tendons, and ligaments. The musculoskeletal system gives the body shape and structure. It allows the body to move and support itself. It also provides protection for the body and creates heat.

Muscles are made up of groups of tissues that help the body move by contracting and relaxing. They support the body, protect organs, and create heat. There are over 600 muscles in the human body. There are three types of muscles:

1. Skeletal muscles, also called *voluntary muscles*, control body movements by contracting and relaxing. A voluntary muscle is a muscle that can be controlled voluntarily, or at will. Skeletal muscles work together—one muscle moves the bone in one direction, and another moves it back. For example, the biceps are skeletal muscles that flex or contract when a person bends at the elbow.

2. Smooth muscles, also called *involuntary muscles*, make up the walls of organs, such as the bladder and uterus. Involuntary muscles are controlled automatically and are not under a person's conscious control. This type of muscle has the ability to stretch without putting a lot of stress on the muscle.

3. Cardiac muscles are involuntary muscles that are found only in the heart. The cardiac muscles contract and relax anywhere from 60 to 100 times each minute.

Bones are the rigid connective tissues that make up the skeleton, which is the framework of the human body (Fig. 21-1). Bones lend support to body structures, allow the body to move, and protect the organs. The outer layer of bone is hard or compact, while the inner layer at the end of a long bone is soft and spongy. Bone marrow lies within the spongy area of long bones. Bone marrow is responsible for the production of red and white blood cells and platelets. There are 206 bones in the human adult skeleton. There are four types of bones:

1. Long bones: the humerus (upper arm bone), the femur (upper leg or thigh bone)

2. Short bones: carpals (wrist bones), tarsals (ankle bones)

3. Flat bones: the sternum (breastbone) and the scapula (shoulder blade)

4. Irregular bones: bones of the vertebrae (spine)

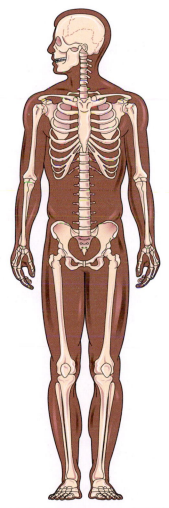

Fig. 21-1. The skeleton is composed of 206 bones that help movement and protect organs.

Joints are found at the places where two bones come together (articulate). The joints or articulations provide movement and flexibility. Joint movements depend on the way in which the joint is formed. There are three types of joints: immovable, slightly movable, and movable.

Examples of immovable joints are the bones of the cranium (skull). The joints of the skull bones are called *sutures*. An example of a slightly movable joint is the joint between the pubic bones. The joint between the scapula and the humerus is an example of a freely movable joint. Other types of movable joints are the hip and shoulder joints, which are ball-and-socket joints, and the elbow and knee joints, which are hinge joints (Fig. 21-2).

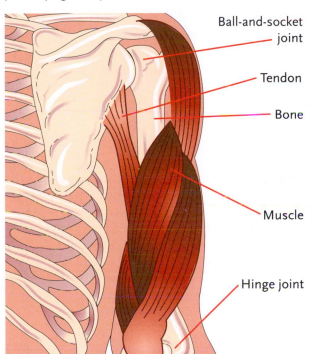

Ball-and-socket joint

Tendon

Bone

Muscle

Hinge joint

Fig. 21-2. Muscles are connected to bones by tendons. Bones meet at different types of joints. Examples of the ball-and-socket joint and the hinge joint are shown here.

Joints are found within a cavity or "capsule" that is lined with a synovial membrane. This membrane produces a fluid called *synovial fluid* that aids in joint lubrication. The ends of movable bones are covered with a flexible, protective substance called **cartilage** that allows free joint movement. Cartilage is also found in other parts of the body, such as the nose. **Bursae** are tiny sacs of fluid located near joints. They reduce friction during body movement.

Tendons are tough bands of connective tissue that anchor or connect muscles to bones. **Ligaments** are strong, fibrous bands that connect bones or cartilage and help support the joints and joint movement. Ligaments can become injured during sports or other strenuous activity. Torn ligaments can take a long time to heal following an injury.

The functions of the musculoskeletal system are to

- Give shape and form to the body
- Maintain posture
- Permit movement
- Protect internal organs
- Store calcium and phosphorus
- Produce heat
- Produce some blood cells

Destination: Homeostasis

The musculoskeletal system helps to regulate the calcium levels in the blood. Bones serve as a calcium storage area. When blood calcium decreases to abnormally low levels, bones are alerted to release some of the stored calcium back into the blood. The calcium level then returns to normal range, and homeostasis is restored.

Tip

Shoulder Joints are Delicate

Pulling too hard on a person's arm can easily dislocate a shoulder joint. Because of this, nursing assistants should never jerk a resident's arm or attempt to lift or reposition a resident by pulling on his arm. Dislocations can cause extreme pain, as well as permanent damage.

3. Discuss changes in the musculoskeletal system due to aging

Normal age-related changes for the musculoskeletal system include the following:

- Muscles weaken and lose tone.

- Bones lose calcium, causing them to become porous and brittle (easily broken).

- Height is gradually lost due to shrinkage of the space between the vertebrae in the spine.

- Loss of muscle mass in the body causes weight loss.

- Joints are less flexible and are stiffer, which slows normal body movements and decreases range of motion.

4. Discuss common disorders of the musculoskeletal system

Muscular Dystrophy (MD)

Muscular dystrophy is a hereditary, progressive disease that causes various disabilities. With this disease, muscle tissue is destroyed, and the muscles atrophy. Muscle **atrophy** means the muscle wastes away, decreases in size, and weakens. MD causes muscle weakness, stiffness, and twitching of the hands and arms. People with this disorder may be confined to a wheelchair.

Muscular dystrophy is a genetic disorder caused by a specific gene. It generally appears at birth or during childhood. Duchenne's muscular dystrophy is a type of MD that is more common in males. Currently there is no cure for muscular dystrophy.

Guidelines: Muscular Dystrophy

G   Allow enough time for the person to move about with braces or in wheelchair.

G   Give frequent skin care to prevent pressure injuries.

G   Reposition resident often as ordered to help prevent pressure injuries or contractures, which are the permanent and painful stiffening of a muscle, tendon, or ligament.

G   Perform range of motion as directed. A physical therapist may perform special stretching exercises as well.

G Assist with activities of daily living (ADLs) as needed. Encourage independence with ADLs so functioning muscles will not atrophy.

G If any of the following occurs, notify the nurse:

- Red or discolored skin, or other signs of the beginning of a pressure injury (Chapter 18)

- Stiffening of muscles

- Pain, swelling, or burning (especially back pain, pain in the lower leg or calf)

- Swallowing problems

- Symptoms of a urinary tract infection

- Constipation

- Signs of pneumonia, such as fever, chills, cough, and chest pains

- Shortness of breath

- Changes in blood pressure or pulse rate

Osteoporosis

Osteoporosis is a condition in which the bones lose density, which causes them to be brittle and easily broken. Osteoporosis is caused by any one or a combination of the following: a lack of calcium in the diet, the loss of estrogen, a lack of regular exercise, reduced mobility, or age. Osteoporosis is more common in women, especially after menopause. Signs and symptoms of osteoporosis are low back pain, loss of height, fractures, and stooped posture (Fig. 21-3). A person may develop osteopenia before developing osteoporosis. **Osteopenia** is a condition in which bones lose density, but not enough to be classified as osteoporosis.

Osteoporosis is treated with medication, exercise, and supplements. Some osteoporosis medication helps maintain bone density and reduce the risk of fractures. Medication will need to be taken weekly, monthly, biannually, or yearly, and comes in pill or injectable form. Oral medication may

require that the person remains upright for at least 30 to 60 minutes after taking it.

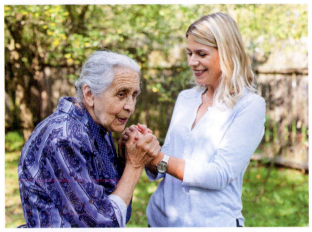

Fig. 21-3. *Stooped posture is a common sign of osteoporosis.*

The NA should be patient and allow residents enough time to move. Residents with osteoporosis must be repositioned and moved very carefully. The NA should encourage ambulatory residents to walk and keep canes or walkers close by. Any decline in activity or movement should be reported to the nurse.

> **Tip**
>
> **Fragile Bones**
>
> When a person has osteoporosis, bones are weak and fragile and can break easily. Movements that a person may take for granted, such as turning in bed, sitting down, or standing, can cause osteoporotic bones to break. NAs must be very careful when moving residents.

Arthritis

Arthritis is a general term for the inflammation of the joints that can cause pain, stiffness, and swelling. Decreased mobility may also result. Two common types of arthritis are osteoarthritis and rheumatoid arthritis.

Osteoarthritis, also called *degenerative arthritis* or *degenerative joint disease (DJD)*, is a condition in which the cushiony cartilage that rests between the bones and pads the ends of the bones begins to slowly erode. The cartilage also loses its elasticity. Without the padding of the cartilage, the bones begin to rub together causing pain, redness, swelling, stiffness, and limited motion. If the condition worsens, the area may eventually become deformed. Osteoarthritis generally occurs with aging and may also be due to a joint injury. It usually affects weight-bearing joints, especially the hips and knees. Joints in the fingers, thumbs, and spine can also be affected. Cold, damp weather can increase pain and stiffness caused by osteoarthritis.

Rheumatoid arthritis is a form of arthritis that may become crippling. It affects the synovial membrane, which is a membrane that lines the joint capsule, causing stiffness, swelling, intense pain, and deformities that can be severe and disabling. Fever, fatigue, and weight loss are also symptoms of rheumatoid arthritis. The synovial membrane may eventually be completely destroyed. When this occurs, the joint becomes fixed and unable to move. It usually affects smaller joints first before progressing on to larger ones. Often rheumatoid arthritis develops early in middle age, but it can affect people of any age.

Rheumatoid arthritis is considered an autoimmune, inflammatory disease. An autoimmune illness occurs when the body's immune system attacks normal tissue in the body. A type of virus or bacteria acts as a trigger, which causes the body to turn on itself.

Treatment for arthritis includes rest and controlled exercise. Range of motion exercises may be ordered. Anti-inflammatory medications, such as ibuprofen, as well as other medications, are used to relieve pain. Weight loss can help reduce stress on the joints. Heat applications are often useful to lessen inflammation and pain. With a serious deformity, joint replacement can help.

Guidelines: Arthritis

G   Assist with the exercise program as needed. Encourage gentle activity and ambulation as

ordered. Keep canes or walkers close by if needed.

G   Perform range of motion exercises as directed.

G   Let the nurse know about 30 minutes prior to exercise if pain medication is supposed to be given beforehand.

G   Assist with ADLs as needed. Using assistive devices for bathing, dressing, and eating can promote independence (Fig. 21-4).

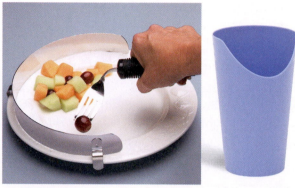

Fig. 21-4. *Special equipment, such as this plate, fork, and cup, can help a person with arthritis remain independent.* (PHOTO COURTESY OF NORTH COAST MEDICAL, INC., WWW.NCMEDICAL.COM, 800-821-9319)

G   Encourage the use of handrails and safety bars in the bathroom.

G   Be positive and supportive.

G   If any of the following occurs, notify the nurse:

   •   Pain

   •   Stiffness

   •   Swelling

   •   Reduced ability to perform range of motion exercises

   •   Decline in activity

Fibromyalgia

Fibromyalgia syndrome (FMS) is a disorder with no clear cause. It can occur in some people following surgery, infection, or extreme stress. Symptoms include widespread pain, fatigue, sleep disturbances, problems with thinking and memory (sometimes referred to as *fibro fog*), and depression. Women are more prone to have fibromyalgia syndrome. There is no cure for this disorder. There are various treatments, including medications, exercises, and some complementary and alternative therapies, such as massage or acupuncture.

Bursitis

Bursitis is a condition in which the bursae (tiny sacs of fluid found near joints) become inflamed. The tissues around the joint may become painful, swollen, and tender. The shoulder, elbow, hip, and knee are joint areas that are commonly affected. Bursitis may also occur in the foot. Treatment for bursitis includes application of ice, immobilization to rest the joint, and the use of anti-inflammatory and pain medications. Removing fluid from the joint with a needle may be necessary. Cortisone injections may be administered. If the area becomes infected, antibiotics will be ordered.

Amputations

An **amputation** is the surgical removal of some or all of a body part, such as an arm, hand, finger, leg, foot, or toes. Amputations are necessary due to disease, such as diabetes, which can cause severe circulatory problems. They are also performed due to cancer or injuries. Traumatic amputations are due to car accidents or an accident involving some type of machinery or equipment.

Limb amputations are performed either above or below the knee or elbow joint. The surgeon determines the extent of the removal of tissue. Some skin will be left in place to cover the residual stump. Postoperatively, the surgical site may be closed immediately or left open for a few days. A temporary prosthesis may be used until the permanent prosthesis is ready. A **prosthesis** is an artificial device that replaces a body part, such as an eye, tooth, arm, leg, hip, or heart valve (Fig. 21-5). It is used to improve function and/or appearance.

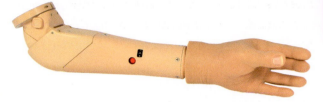

Fig. 21-5. A type of prosthetic arm. (MOTION CONTROL UTAH ARM. PHOTO BY KEVIN TWOMEY.)

A prosthesis is created specifically for each amputee. The prosthesis may take weeks to make and can cost tens of thousands of dollars. People who have stumps may require special, costly wheelchairs.

Prostheses for limbs are very lifelike and give greater movement and flexibility. People can walk, exercise, and do other activities, such as dancing or writing, with an artificial limb. Artificial eyes (ocular prosthetics), dentures, and hearing aids are other types of prostheses.

Transplants of certain body parts are done on some amputees. One serious complication of transplants is rejection of the surgically attached part. The person may need medication for the rest of his life to prevent rejection of the transplanted body part.

After an amputation, a person may feel that the amputated limb is still a part of his body. Three conditions that can occur following an amputation are phantom limb pain, phantom sensation, and stump pain. With **phantom sensation**, the person may have the feeling that the body part is still there. This involves sensations such as warmth, tingling, or itching in the area where the limb existed. **Phantom limb pain** occurs when the person feels pain in a limb (or extremity) that has been amputated. There is a variety of possible causes for phantom sensation and phantom limb pain. Causes include remaining damaged nerve endings, the level of pain the person had prior to the amputation, cold weather, surgery that was not performed correctly, scar tissue from surgery, stress, fatigue, lack of blood flow, infections, viruses, excessive pressure on the body part, swelling in the area, and inactivity. Phantom sensation and limb pain are real and should not be ignored or ridiculed. Medication or physical therapy may be used to treat these conditions.

Stump pain is pain felt in the area of the part of the limb that is still there. With stump pain, the prosthesis may need to be altered for a better fit.

Guidelines: Amputation and Prosthesis Care

G   Be careful when handling prostheses and special wheelchairs. This equipment is very expensive.

G   The nurse will demonstrate how to apply a prosthesis. Follow instructions to apply and remove the prosthesis. Do not apply a prosthesis unless you have been trained and instructed to do so. Assist the resident as needed.

G   Apply special compression bandages and/ or stump shrinkers as ordered to help with swelling. A stump shrinker is an elastic, compression-like bandage that fits snugly, but not too tightly, around the stump. Bandages should not be applied too tightly and should not cause pain. Stump bandages may be changed many times a day. When they are removed, inspect the skin carefully.

G   Socks of different layers (for example, one-ply, two-ply, etc.), are used to cover and protect the stump before the prosthesis is applied. Change socks often and place seams on the sock to the outside to prevent abrasions, which increase the risk of infection. Make sure there are no foreign objects inside the socks before applying. Place used socks in a bag or hamper for laundering.

G   Regular skin care is vital to avoid complications with the stump and the prosthesis. The residual limb can suffer complications, including trauma, allergic reactions to the materials used, and infections. Give careful skin care to the area under a prosthesis.

Make sure the skin is always clean and dry. Ask resident not to use a sharp object to scratch the stump or the nonamputated limb. Report signs of skin problems to the nurse immediately.

G   The prosthesis must be removed prior to going to bed. Bathe the stump gently. Use mild, scent-free soap and warm water (not hot). Avoid other products, such as iodine-based cleansers, because they can injure the stump. If an abrasion, rash, or other problem occurs, do not use soap, and report to the nurse. Clean the stump thoroughly and rinse completely. Use a soft, nonabrasive towel to dry the area. Apply creams to the stump area as ordered.

G   Clean the socket of the prosthesis when it is removed. Use warm water and mild soap for cleaning, following instructions. Use a soft cotton cloth to wipe and dry the prosthesis. Avoid using other products on the socket. Dry the prosthesis, especially the socket, completely. Leaving moisture in any area can increase the risk of infection.

G   Before applying a prosthesis, make sure the area is completely dry. If you observe any complications in the stump area, report to the nurse immediately.

G   Do not react negatively to the stump or the prosthesis during care.

G   Special positioning to prevent pressure injuries is usually necessary. The doctor may order stump elevation postoperatively, which can help reduce swelling of the residual limb. The prone position may be ordered for limited time periods. Carefully follow orders for bed elevation and positioning.

G   Follow orders for positioning of the leg. Flexion, elevation of the knee, and crossing of the legs may be restricted. **Flexion** is bending a body part. Pillows cannot be used under or between the limbs.

G Assist the resident as needed with ADLs. Occupational therapists may work with the resident to help with ADLs.

G Encourage activity as ordered. Check with the nurse 30 minutes prior to exercising to see if pain medication is needed.

G To prevent contractures and other complications, follow the exercise program exactly as ordered. Perform range of motion exercises as directed.

G Physical therapists will teach the resident how to bear weight on the prosthesis. Follow any weight-bearing orders.

G Provide support for phantom pain, phantom sensation, or stump pain. The pain or sensation is real and should be treated that way.

G A resident may have difficulty adjusting physically and emotionally to a new prosthesis. Residents may be depressed, sad, angry, or frustrated. Be supportive during the continuing process of adjustment.

G If any of these occur, notify the nurse:

- Redness or swelling of the stump or extremity

- Drainage, bleeding, or sores of any kind on the stump or extremity

- Stump pain, burning, phantom pain, or phantom sensation

- Reduced ability to move extremity

- Cyanosis of any portion of the extremity

- Problems with the prosthesis

Trivia

An Early Method of Amputation

Amputation was a very difficult procedure prior to the discovery of anesthesia. People requiring amputations experienced excruciating pain during surgery. Patients were often given alcohol to drink prior to the procedure to help them manage the pain. The surgical staff would hold the patient down while the amputation was being performed. The discovery of anesthesia allowed these surgeries to be performed without the unbearable pain.

Fractures

A **fracture** is a broken bone. Fractures are usually caused by some sort of trauma or accident. Fractures can also occur spontaneously due to diseases such as osteoporosis. Elderly people are more prone to falling, which is a common cause of fractures. Falling also contributes to other serious physical problems, including head injuries and soft tissue injuries. A fractured hip is a very serious problem that can occur with a fall.

Common signs and symptoms of fractures are pain, swelling, and bruising. The pain can be severe, and the area may be painful to touch. Pain may increase if treatment is not obtained soon after the injury. Movement may be limited. Bleeding can occur with some fractures. Different types of fractures include the following:

- **Closed or simple fracture**: The skin is closed. Bone is in the proper position and has not dislocated.

- **Hairline fracture**: The skin is closed. Bone has fine-line crack noted on X-ray or magnetic resonance imaging (MRI) scan, and has not dislocated.

- **Open or compound fracture**: The skin is open. Bone may come through the skin. The person has an increased risk of infection.

- **Greenstick fracture**: The skin is usually closed. The fracture is incomplete. Only one side of the bone is broken; the other side is bent. Greenstick fractures are more common in children.

- **Comminuted fracture**: The skin is open or closed. Bone has fractured in two or more places.

- **Compression fracture**: The fracture occurs in the spine. The skin is usually closed. Bone may break with trauma or without significant trauma. This fracture can be due to osteoporosis, tumors, or other conditions. It is commonly seen in the elderly.

- **Pathologic fracture**: A fracture that occurs in a bone that is weakened by disease. Causes include tumors, metastatic cancers, and infection.

Preventing Falls

In addition to causing fractures, falls can contribute to other problems related to physical injuries, such as immobility, dehydration, and pressure injuries. Falls can have psychological consequences as well, such as triggering fear, anxiety, and depression. If a resident is less confident, he may be unwilling to perform routine activities. Problems related to falls are often long-lasting and costly. Elderly residents take longer to heal from injuries. Preventing falls is very important. As the people who often spend the most time with residents, NAs play an important role in preventing falls. Chapter 7 contains a comprehensive list of fall prevention guidelines.

Fractures are generally diagnosed with an X-ray. During the healing process, X-rays are often used to check the progress. Fractures are treated by specialists. The bones must be set and allowed to heal in normal alignment. The joints above and below the fracture are immobilized. New bone develops to heal a fractured bone. The ends of the broken bones need to be snugly set in order for them to heal properly. Bone healing can take four to eight weeks or longer. However, fractures can take even longer to heal in the elderly. When bones heal properly, there is a greater chance the area of the fracture will return to normal function.

Some fractures require a cast. Casts keep the fractured bones in place so that they can heal. Casts are generally made of fiberglass. Fiberglass casts dry very rapidly. The edges of the cast may need to be padded to reduce sharp edges. Special material may be used for this padding. The stocking under the cast can also be used to help pad the rough edges. Padding the cast helps avoid skin injury from the cast. Sharp objects should never be placed inside a cast because they can pierce the skin. This increases the chance of infection in the area under the cast.

Guidelines: Cast Care

G Pad the cast edges as needed; ask the nurse for help with this.

G Do not get the cast wet. Wet casts can lose their shape. If showers are allowed, tape a plastic bag securely around the cast before showering.

G Keep the cast clean. Protect the cast from soiling during elimination.

G Follow orders exactly on moving and repositioning. Tell the nurse prior to moving if pain medication is needed.

G The extremity in a cast may need to be elevated to reduce swelling. Use pillows to assist with elevation (Fig. 21-6).

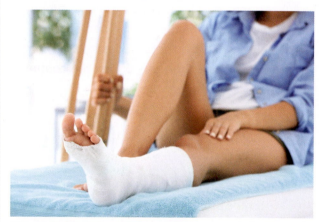

Fig. 21-6. Elevating the extremity in a cast helps to reduce swelling.

G Help with range of motion exercises as ordered.

G Allow enough time for the person to move.

G Assist with the use of cane, walker, or crutches as needed.

G Use bed cradles to reduce pressure from the bed linens.

G If any of the following occurs, notify the nurse:

- Numbness, tingling or increased swelling
- Resident complains cast feels too tight

- Pain, burning, or pressure
- Redness, drainage, bleeding, or sores of any kind
- Wetness in or around a cast
- Odor around the cast
- Changes in temperature of the skin (hot or cold skin)
- Cyanosis or pale skin
- Resident places sharp object inside the cast

A person may need physical therapy while the fracture heals and after the cast is removed because muscle atrophy and weakness can occur. Physical therapy helps return the limb to normal strength and function.

A sling is sometimes used to support an injured or broken arm in a cast. A **sling** is a bandage or piece of material that is suspended from the neck for the purpose of holding and supporting a forearm (Fig. 21-7). A sling also helps reduce swelling by keeping the arm elevated. When a resident has a sling, the NA should make sure the arm is positioned comfortably and elevated properly.

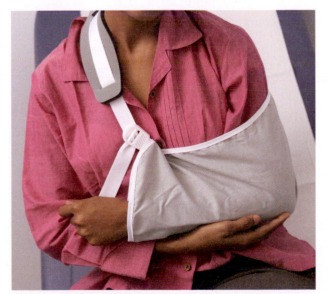

Fig. 21-7. A sling can support an injured or broken arm, as well as reduce swelling.

Fractured Hip

Older people, especially those who have osteoporosis or arthritis, are at risk for hip fractures. Hip fractures can result from falls or even from simple movements. If the bones are already weak, they can fracture easily.

Surgery is often performed on fractured hips. **Total hip replacement (THR)** is a surgical replacement of the head of the femur (long bone of the leg) and the socket it fits into where it joins the hip. THR may be performed due to a fractured hip that does not heal properly, a hip weakened by age and decreased bone strength, or a hip that is painful, stiff, and no longer able to bear weight. After surgery is complete, the doctor will write an order to restrict weight-bearing on the operative leg while the hip heals. The order will be either partial weight-bearing or non-weight-bearing. **Partial weight-bearing (PWB)** means the resident is able to support some body weight on one or both legs. **Non-weight-bearing (NWB)** means the resident is unable to touch the floor or support any body weight on one or both legs. Once the resident can bear full weight again on both legs, the order will be for **full weight-bearing (FWB)**.

One of the goals of care for a postoperative hip replacement is to avoid dislocating the operative hip. To accomplish this, an abduction pillow will normally be used after hip replacement surgery. **Abduction** means moving a body part away from the midline of the body. The abduction pillow immobilizes and positions the hips and lower extremities. The pillow is placed in between the legs. The legs are secured to the sides of the pillow using straps (Fig. 21-8). The NA should follow instructions for application and positioning.

Adduction of the operative hip must be prevented. This means the hip cannot be bent or flexed more than 90 degrees. It cannot be turned inward or outward. If the hip is adducted, it can dislocate, which can cause serious complications. A second surgery may be required, and each surgery an elderly person has to undergo can further weaken him.

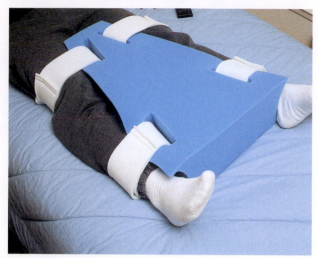

Fig. 21-8. An abduction pillow is placed in between the legs to immobilize and position the hips and lower extremities. (PHOTO COURTESY OF NORTH COAST MEDICAL, INC., WWW.NCMEDICAL.COM, 800-821-9319)

Guidelines: Total Hip Replacement (THR)

G Follow the care plan exactly. If the resident wants to do more than is ordered, inform the nurse. Follow orders for weight-bearing.

G Physical therapy is usually ordered after a hip replacement. Encourage residents to attend their physical therapy appointments. Assist with physical therapy exercises as instructed.

G Follow the care plan regarding positioning and elevation of the head of the bed. Use abduction pillows as directed.

G Do not perform range of motion exercises on a leg on the side of a hip replacement.

G Caution the resident not to cross legs in bed or in a chair or turn toes inward or outward. The hip cannot be bent or flexed more than 90 degrees even when sitting in a chair or on the toilet. It cannot be turned inward or outward. Pivoting or twisting must be avoided on the operative leg.

G Assist with dressing the resident, starting with the weaker, or affected, side first.

G Deep vein thrombosis (DVT) and pulmonary embolism (PE) are complications that can occur postoperatively. Apply elastic stockings as ordered to aid circulation.

G Assistive devices, such as a reaching aid (a tool that helps a person grab an item out of reach), may be ordered to help the resident remain independent. A raised toilet seat may be helpful for elimination.

G Ask resident to use available handrails when moving into or out of a shower.

G Ask the nurse to give pain medication prior to moving and positioning if needed.

G Assist with coughing and deep breathing exercises and incentive spirometry as ordered (see Chapter 20 for more information on these exercises).

G Encourage fluids to prevent complications of immobility, such as urinary tract infections and constipation. Using a fracture pan rather than a regular sized bedpan may be easier for elimination.

G Never rush the resident. Use praise and encouragement often.

G Keep often-used items, such as the call light, telephone, tissues, and water, within easy reach.

G If any of the following occurs, notify the nurse:

   • Incisions that are red, draining, bleeding, or warm to the touch

   • An increase in pain or a burning sensation, especially on the operated side or in the calves

   • Fever or other change in vital signs

   • Numbness or tingling

   • Edema (swelling) of the legs

- Cyanosis or pale skin

- Problems with appetite

- Constipation

- Resident is not following the doctor's orders for exercise and activity

Total Knee Replacement

Total knee replacement (TKR) is a surgical replacement of a knee with artificial materials. This may be necessary due to damage from injuries or arthritis or to help stabilize a knee that buckles repeatedly. The person may also need a knee replacement due to severe knee pain.

Care of a resident recovering from TKR is similar to that for a total hip replacement, but the recovery time is usually longer and may be more painful. Self-care should be promoted as much as possible.

Guidelines: Total Knee Replacement

G   To prevent blood clots, apply special stockings or sleeves, such as elastic stockings or sequential compression devices (SCD) as ordered (see Chapter 19).

G   Physical therapy exercises may be ordered. Assist with physical therapy exercises as instructed. Do not perform range of motion exercises unless told to do so.

G   Assist with coughing and deep breathing exercises as ordered.

G   Encourage fluids to prevent complications of immobility, such as urinary tract infections and constipation.

G   Ask the nurse to give pain medication prior to moving and positioning if needed.

G   If any of the following occurs, notify the nurse:

- Incisions that are red, draining, bleeding, or warm to the touch

- An increase in pain or a burning sensation, especially on the operated side or in the calves

- Fever or other change in vital signs

- Numbness or tingling

- Edema (swelling) of the legs

- Cyanosis or pale skin

- Problems with appetite

- Constipation

- Resident is not following the doctor's orders for exercise and activity

- Reduced mobility in the extremity

A device called a continuous passive motion (CPM) machine may be used for people who have had a total knee replacement (Fig. 21-9). A CPM machine passively moves a specific joint repetitively through its normal range of motion. It helps to prevent stiffness and swelling that can occur postoperatively. It aids in increasing circulation. By continuously cycling through the knee's normal range of motion, it also helps prevent scar tissue and contractures from developing.

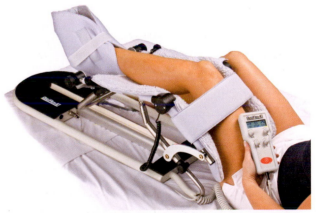

Fig. 21-9. One type of CPM machine. (PHOTO COURTESY OF THE MEDCOM GROUP, LTD., 800-231-4276, WWW.MEDCOMGROUP.COM)

A nurse or physical therapist will position the leg, set the machine rate, and turn on the machine. The NA may be asked to stay with the resident until the resident is comfortable with the movement of the machine. If the resident complains of pain or discomfort or if the extremity moves out of proper position in the machine, the NA should notify the nurse. The nurse or therapist will turn off the machine and remove the leg when the therapy has been completed.

Traction

Traction is a method of treating fractures by keeping bones in the proper position. Traction is also used to reduce pain and pressure or to relieve muscle spasms. Traction is used to treat a fracture by using weights and pulleys to keep the broken bones in proper position in order for the injury to heal. Careful observation of the resident is required to prevent complications.

The NA should not disconnect the traction assembly. The resident must be kept in proper body alignment at all times. The weights should not be touching the floor, the bed, or the bed frame. The NA should not adjust the weights on a traction unit.

Observing and Reporting: Traction

If any of the following occurs, notify the nurse:

- %R Numbness or tingling
- %R Pain, burning, pressure, or swelling
- %R Redness, drainage, bleeding, or sores
- %R Wetness on sling
- %R Odor around sling or boot
- %R Changes in skin temperature
- %R Cyanosis or pale skin
- %R Resident moves to the side or slides down in bed
- %R Sling or boot loosens or comes off or weights come off, touch the floor, or move

Tip

The Trapeze
The trapeze is a triangular piece of equipment that attaches to the bed frame of a person in traction or a person who requires help with movement in bed. Residents grasp the trapeze with their hands and are able to lift themselves more easily. This helps caregivers change bed linens, pads, and gowns and perform other tasks. The resident must be shown how to use the trapeze. The NA should check that the trapeze is secure before the resident uses it.

Additional resources for information relating to musculoskeletal disorders include the following:

- National Institute of Arthritis and Musculoskeletal and Skin Diseases, niams.nih.gov
- medlineplus.gov/hipreplacement

Obesity and Disorders of the Musculoskeletal System

Obesity increases the risk for certain musculoskeletal diseases or disorders, including the following:

- Osteoarthritis (degenerative joint disease)
- Chronic back pain
- Gout (a form of inflammatory arthritis that affects the joints, causing severe pain, swelling, redness, and tenderness)

5. Describe elastic bandages

Elastic bandages, also called *nonsterile* or *self-adhering bandages*, are stretchy bandages that are wrapped around an injured body part. They are also referred to as *ACE bandages* or *ACE wraps*, which is a common brand name for these bandages. Elastic bandages are used to keep dressings in place, hold splints in place, and provide protection, compression, and support for body parts (Fig. 21-10). These bandages are also used to decrease swelling from injuries.

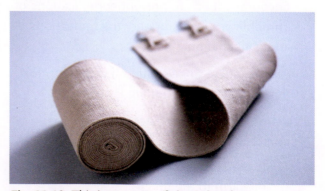

Fig. 21-10. *This is one type of elastic bandage.*

Elastic bandages must be wrapped in a distal to proximal (far to near) direction. They should be wrapped snugly enough so that the proper amount of compression and support is provided. However, if they are applied too snugly, they can interfere with circulation. The bandages must be smooth and wrinkle-free to prevent too much compression to the area.

Observing and Reporting: Elastic Bandages

Check on a resident 10 to 15 minutes after the bandage has been applied to make sure it is not interfering with circulation. After that, check on the resident periodically. If any of the following signs and symptoms of poor circulation occur, notify the nurse:

O/R Numbness or tingling

O/R Resident complains of the bandage feeling too tight

O/R Swelling

O/R Indentation marks on the skin

O/R Pain or discomfort

O/R Skin that is cold to the touch

O/R Pale, gray, cyanotic, or white skin

Chapter Review

1. List the three types of muscles that are found in the human body (LO 2).

2. What are three functions of bones (LO 2)?

3. List five normal age-related changes of the musculoskeletal system (LO 3).

4. What happens when a muscle atrophies (LO 4)?

5. What can happen to bones when they become brittle (LO 4)?

6. Why is preventing falls so important for elderly residents (LO 4)?

7. List six signs and symptoms of poor circulation due to elastic bandages that need to be reported to the nurse (LO 5).

Multiple Choice

8. After an amputation, a resident may experience phantom sensation. Phantom sensation is (LO 4)
   (A) Not real
   (B) Tingling from a body part that has been amputated
   (C) An artificial body part
   (D) The removal of a body part

9. When helping a resident who has had a hip replacement get dressed, how should the NA begin (LO 4)?
   (A) Start with the stronger side
   (B) Start with the left side
   (C) Start with the weaker side
   (D) Start with the feet and move upward

10. A person recovering from a total hip replacement should not bend or flex the hip more than _____ degrees (LO 4).
    (A) 30
    (B) 45
    (C) 90
    (D) 120

11. Which of the following means that the resident can bear some weight on one or both legs postoperatively (LO 4)?
    (A) Non-weight-bearing (NWB)
    (B) Full weight-bearing (FWB)
    (C) 100% weight-bearing (1WB)
    (D) Partial weight-bearing (PWB)

22
The Nervous System

Galen and the Persian Patient

Galen was a physician who lived and worked in ancient Rome. He treated a man from Persia who had a loss of sensation only in certain parts of his hand. Galen determined the patient had fallen on his back and that caused the injury. He believed nerve damage caused the loss of sensation. Galen was amazed that the man could still move his hand. To him, this meant that different nerves controlled different parts of the body. In addition, Galen thought that an injury could affect feeling, but perhaps not always movement. This was a new and exciting idea at the time.

"The harvest of old age is the recollection and abundance of blessings previously secured."
Marcus Tullius Cicero, 106–43 B.C.

"He that wrestles with us strengthens our nerves and sharpens our skill."
Edmund Burke, 1729–1797

1. Define important words in this chapter

age-related macular degeneration (AMD): a condition in which the macula degenerates, gradually causing central vision loss.

agitated: the state of being excited, restless, or troubled.

Alzheimer's disease (AD): a progressive, degenerative, and incurable disease that causes proteins to build up in and around nerve cells, which results in memory loss, cognitive impairment, and behavioral changes.

bipolar disorder: a type of mental health disorder that causes a person to have mood swings and changes in energy levels and the ability to function.

brain: the part of the nervous system housed in the skull that is responsible for motor activity, memory, thought, speech, and intelligence, along with regulation of vital functions, such as heart rate, blood pressure, and breathing.

burnout: mental or physical exhaustion due to a prolonged period of stress and frustration.

cataract: a condition in which the lens of the eye becomes cloudy, causing vision loss.

catastrophic reaction: reacting to something in an unreasonable, exaggerated way.

central nervous system: part of the nervous system made up of the brain and spinal cord.

cerebrovascular accident (CVA): a condition caused when the blood supply to the brain is cut off suddenly by a clot or a ruptured blood vessel; also called *stroke*.

cognition: the ability to think clearly and logically.

cognitive behavioral therapy (CBT): a type of psychotherapy that is usually short-term and focuses on skills and solutions that a person can use to modify negative thinking and behavior patterns; often used to treat anxiety disorders.

concussion: a head injury that occurs from a banging movement of the brain against the skull.

delusion: a belief in something that is not true or is out of touch with reality.

dementia: a serious, progressive loss of mental abilities such as thinking, remembering, reasoning, and communicating.

disruptive behavior: any behavior that disturbs others.

elope: in medicine, when a person with Alzheimer's disease wanders away from a protected area and does not return on his own.

epilepsy: a disorder that causes recurring seizures.

farsightedness: the ability to see distant objects more clearly than objects that are near; also called *hyperopia.*

glaucoma: a condition in which the pressure in the eye increases, damaging the optic nerve and causing blindness.

hallucinations: seeing, hearing, smelling, tasting, or feeling things that are not there.

hearing aid: a small device placed in the ear that amplifies sound.

hemianopsia: loss of vision in one-half of the visual field, due to CVA, tumor, or trauma.

hoarding: collecting and putting things away in a guarded way.

intervention: a way to improve or change an action or development.

irreversible: unable to be reversed or returned to the original state.

Meniere's disease: a disorder of the inner ear caused by a buildup of fluid, which causes vertigo, hearing loss, tinnitus (ringing in the ear), and pain or pressure.

mental health: the normal functioning of emotional and intellectual abilities.

mental health disorder: a disorder that disrupts a person's ability to function in the family, home, or community and often causes inappropriate behavior.

multiple sclerosis (MS): a progressive disease in which the protective covering of the nerves, spinal cord, and white matter of the brain breaks down over time; causes problems with balance, walking, and many other symptoms.

nearsightedness: the ability to see objects that are near more clearly than distant objects; also called *myopia.*

neuron: the basic nerve cell of the nervous system.

obsessive-compulsive disorder (OCD): a type of mental health disorder characterized by intrusive, repetitive thoughts or behaviors that cause anxiety or stress.

otitis media: an infection in the middle ear that causes pain, pressure, fever, and reduced ability to hear.

pacing: walking back and forth in the same area.

panic disorder: a type of mental health disorder characterized by panic attacks, which are repeated episodes of intense fear, along with physical symptoms such as rapid heartbeat, dizziness, chest pain, shortness of breath, and an upset stomach.

paraplegia: the loss of function of the lower body and legs.

Parkinson's disease: a progressive disease that causes a portion of the brain to degenerate; causes rigid muscles, shuffling gait, pill-rolling, mask-like face, and tremors.

peripheral nervous system: part of the nervous system made up of the nerves that extend throughout the body and connect to the spinal cord.

perseveration: the repetition of words, phrases, questions, or actions.

phobia: an intense, irrational fear of or anxiety about an object, place, or situation.

posttraumatic stress disorder (PTSD): a type of mental health disorder caused by witnessing or experiencing a traumatic event.

progressive: something that continually gets worse or deteriorates.

psychotherapy: a method of treating mental health disorders that involves talking about one's problems with mental health professionals.

quadriplegia: the loss of function of the legs, trunk, and arms.

reminiscence therapy: type of therapy that encourages people with Alzheimer's disease to remember and talk about the past.

remotivation therapy: type of group therapy that promotes self-esteem, self-awareness, and socialization for people with Alzheimer's disease.

rummaging: going through items that belong to other people.

schizophrenia: a type of mental health disorder that may involve acute episodes; affects a person's ability to think, communicate, make decisions, and understand reality.

social anxiety disorder: a type of mental health disorder characterized by excessive anxiety about social situations; also called *social phobia*.

spinal cord: the part of the nervous system inside the vertebral canal that conducts messages between the brain and the body and controls spinal reflexes.

substance abuse: the repeated use of legal or illegal substances in a way that is harmful to oneself or others.

sundowning: a condition in which a person becomes restless and agitated in the late afternoon, evening, or night.

trigger: a situation that leads to agitation.

validating: giving value to or approving.

validation therapy: a type of therapy that lets people with Alzheimer's disease believe they are living in the past or in imaginary circumstances.

violence: forceful actions that include attacking, hitting, or threatening someone.

wandering: walking aimlessly around the facility or facility grounds.

2. Explain the structure and function of the nervous system

The nervous system controls and coordinates all body functions. It sends messages throughout the body and senses and interprets information from outside the body.

The **neuron**, or nerve cell, is the basic working unit of the nervous system. Neurons send and receive nerve impulses from the receptors through the spinal cord to the brain. Neurons are also involved in thought processes, directing the functioning of glands and the movement of muscles. The neuroglia hold together, support, and protect the neurons.

The nervous system is divided into two main parts: the central nervous system (CNS) and the peripheral nervous system (PNS). The brain and the spinal cord make up the **central nervous system**. The nerves connected to the spinal cord that extend throughout the body are classified as the **peripheral nervous system** (Fig. 22-1).

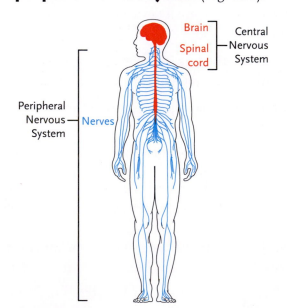

Fig. 22-1. The brain, spinal cord, and nerves throughout the body make up the nervous system.

The Central Nervous System (CNS)

The **brain** is housed within the cranium. It weighs approximately three pounds, which makes it one of the largest organs in the human body. The brain controls speech, motor and sensory activity, intelligence, reasoning, coordination, reflexes, breathing, emotions, and heart rate. It is responsible for memory and regulation of certain glands, such as the adrenal gland. The brain is divided into three main parts: the cerebrum, the cerebellum, and the brainstem (Fig. 22-2).

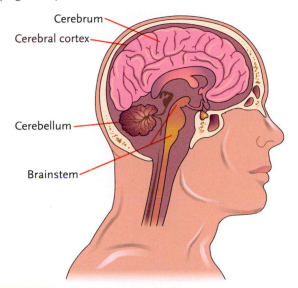

Fig. 22-2. *The three main sections of the brain are the cerebrum, the brainstem, and the cerebellum.*

The cerebrum is the largest section of the brain; it is the center of the brain where thought and intelligence exist. There are two sides, or cerebral hemispheres, in the brain. The right side of the brain, or right hemisphere, controls the motor activity on the left side of the body. The left side, or left cerebral hemisphere, controls the motor activity on the right side of the body (Fig. 22-3). The cerebellum is the center of coordination. It regulates the movements of the body and controls balance.

The cerebrum and cerebellum are connected to the spinal cord by the brainstem. The midbrain, pons, and the medulla oblongata rest within the brainstem. The medulla controls several major functions of the body, including breathing, opening and closing of blood vessels, and heart rate. The medulla controls swallowing, gagging, coughing, and vomiting.

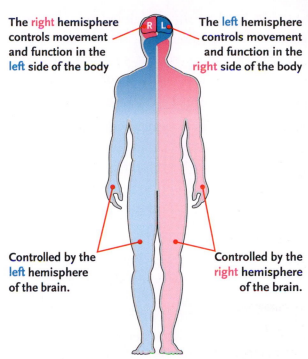

Fig. 22-3. *The right hemisphere controls movement and function in the left side of the body. The left hemisphere controls movement and function in the right side of the body.*

The **spinal cord** is located inside the vertebral canal in the spinal cavity of the body. It is about 18 inches long and is connected to the brain. The spinal cord conducts messages between the brain and the body within its pathways. The spinal cord is also the center that controls the body's reflex activities. An example of a reflex activity is when a person blinks because dirt has come into contact with his eye.

The brain and the spinal cord are protected by bone. They are also surrounded by and suspended in cerebrospinal fluid (CSF). This fluid helps cushion the brain and the spinal cord from shocks, serves as a delivery system for certain types of nutrients, and eliminates waste products and toxins. Protective membranes called the *meninges* cover the brain and the spinal cord.

The Peripheral Nervous System (PNS)

The peripheral nervous system (PNS) consists of the cranial and spinal nerves. Nerves carry the messages to and from the brain from the rest of the body. There are 12 pairs of cranial nerves, and they have different functions. Cranial nerves direct aspects of the senses, such as taste, smell, and vision, deal with hearing and balance, and control certain muscles in the body.

There are 31 pairs of spinal nerves that emerge from the spinal cord. Spinal nerves carry messages back and forth from the brain to the spinal cord. They also transmit messages to and from areas of the body to the spinal cord.

The peripheral nervous system is divided into the somatic nervous system (SNS) and the autonomic nervous system (ANS). The SNS helps with conscious movement of the skeletal muscles. The ANS has two parts: the parasympathetic and sympathetic nervous systems. The parasympathetic nervous system works to conserve the body's energy and provide for relaxation of the body. The parasympathetic nervous system is responsible for slowing body functions, such as heart rate and blood pressure.

The sympathetic nervous system activates the *fight-or-flight* response. This response occurs when a person faces excessive stress and must act quickly. The body prepares for fight or flight, or fighting or running away, by increasing blood pressure and heart rate. This creates a surge in adrenaline (epinephrine) and increases the blood glucose (sugar) to be used for the needed energy.

Tip

The 3 Rs vs. Art
The left hemisphere of the brain is usually involved in a person's ability to do the "3 Rs," reading, writing and 'rithmetic, or mathematics. The right hemisphere of the brain is more involved in artistic and creative abilities.

The Sense Organs

The skin, tongue, nose, eyes, and ears are the body's sense organs. They receive impulses from the environment and relay these impulses to the brain.

Nerve endings within the dermis sense touch, temperature, pain, and pressure. Taste buds are found on papillae on the tongue. These papillae make the tongue bumpy. The nasal cavity is the receptacle of smell. Within the upper part of the nasal cavity, there is an area called the *olfactory area*. That area begins the process of sensing odors. It then sends messages to the brain where the odors are identified. The nose and tongue work together in order for a person to taste the foods she eats. Smell influences the ability to taste.

The eye is about an inch in diameter and is located in a bony socket in the skull (Fig. 22-4). The socket protects the eye and is surrounded by muscles that control eye movements. Within the eye are the receptors that enable the ability to see. The thickest layer and outer part of the eyeball is called the *sclera*, which is the white of the eye. The front part of the sclera is called the *cornea*, and it is transparent. It appears colored because it is positioned over the iris. The iris is the part of the eye that is genetically colored and gives the eyes their unique appearance. The pupil is the circular opening in the center of the iris, which dilates (opens) and constricts (closes) to adjust the amount of light coming into the eye. Inside the back of the eye is the retina. It contains cells that respond to light and send messages to the brain, where the picture is interpreted so a person can see.

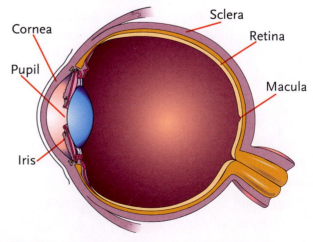

Fig. 22-4. *The parts of the eye.*

The ear is the sense organ that provides balance and hearing. It is divided into three sections: the outer, middle, and the inner ear (Fig. 22-5). The outer ear collects sound waves and directs them inward through the external auditory canal toward the middle ear. Hairs and earwax (cerumen) in the outer ear help protect the ear from foreign particles. The eardrum, or tympanic membrane, separates the outer ear from the middle ear. The middle ear amplifies and transfers sound waves to the inner ear. Tiny hair cells (stereocilia) within the inner ear send nerve impulses to the brain.

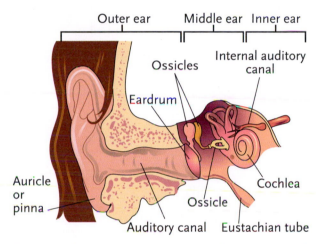

Fig. 22-5. *The outer ear, middle ear, and inner ear are the three main divisions of the ear.*

Hearing occurs when the sounds enter the ear canal. The structures of the middle ear transfer vibrations into the inner ear. This happens when the eardrum vibrates. The three tiny bones within the middle ear, known as the *ossicles*, pick up these vibrations and send impulses to the brain.

The functions of the nervous system are to

- Control and coordinate mental processes and voluntary movements
- Provide reflex centers for heartbeat and respiration
- Sense and respond to changes occurring both inside and outside of the body

Destination: Homeostasis

To maintain homeostasis, the human body has to respond quickly to sudden changes in the environment. A reflex is a rapid, automatic response to a specific change in a person's environment. The body does not formally initiate its response; it is simply automatic. A reflex arc is the path that different types of neurons (nerve cells) travel in order to make the body respond to a sudden change or a stimulus. For example, if a finger touches a hot stove, the finger immediately withdraws from the intense heat. This is called a *withdrawal reflex*. Neurons send the message to the spinal cord that the surface is hot. Following the reflex, neurons return to their normal state until they are needed again. Homeostasis is restored.

3. Discuss changes in the nervous system due to aging

Normal age-related changes for the nervous system include the following:

- Responses and reflexes slow.
- Some memory loss occurs, especially short-term memory loss.
- Sensitivity of nerve endings in skin decreases, resulting in diminished sense of touch.
- Some hearing loss occurs.
- Senses of vision, smell, and taste weaken.

4. Discuss common disorders of the nervous system

Cerebrovascular Accident (CVA)

A **cerebrovascular accident (CVA)**, or stroke (sometimes called *brain attack*), occurs when blood supply to a part of the brain is blocked, or a blood vessel leaks or ruptures within the brain. An ischemic stroke is the most common type of stroke (Fig. 22-6). With this type of stroke, the blood supply is blocked. Without blood, part of the brain does not receive oxygen. Brain cells will begin to die, and additional damage can occur due to leaking blood, clots, and swelling of the tissues. Swelling can also cause pressure on other areas of the brain.

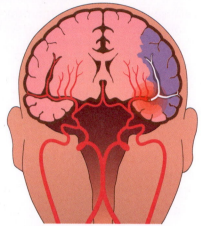

Fig. 22-6. An ischemic stroke is caused by an obstruction of a blood vessel, which cuts off the blood supply to a part of the brain.

Another type of stroke called a *hemorrhagic stroke* occurs when there is leaking or a rupture of a blood vessel inside the brain.

A transient ischemic attack (TIA) is a warning sign of a CVA. It occurs when the brain loses a portion of its blood supply. The attack is usually quite sudden, and symptoms may last only a few minutes or up to 24 hours. Signs and symptoms that a TIA or CVA is occurring are listed in Chapter 8.

CVAs occur on either the right or left side of the brain. Blood flow is affected during a CVA and can cause brain damage and a variety of symptoms. Symptoms differ, depending on which side of the brain is affected. Strokes that occur on the right side of the brain affect functioning on the left side of the body. Strokes that occur on the left side of the brain affect functioning on the right side of the body. The following problems can result from right-sided or left-sided brain damage from a CVA:

- Hemiparesis (weakness on one side of the body)

- Hemiplegia (paralysis on one side of the body)

- One-sided neglect (tendency to ignore a weak or paralyzed side of the body)

- Loss of ability to tell where affected body parts are

- Expressive aphasia (difficulty communicating through speech or writing)

- Receptive aphasia (difficulty understanding spoken or written words)

- Emotional lability (inappropriate or unprovoked emotional responses, including crying, laughing, and anger)

- Loss of sensations, such as temperature or touch

- Loss of bowel or bladder control

- Cognitive impairments, such as poor judgment, memory loss, loss of problem-solving abilities, and confusion

- Changes in personality

- Loss of thinking and learning abilities

- Dysphagia (difficulty swallowing) or the total inability to swallow

- Vision impairments or blurred vision

- **Hemianopsia** (loss of vision in one-half of the visual field due to CVA, tumor, or trauma)

Tip

Left- and Right-Sided CVAs

When referring to a stroke, a nurse may say that a resident has had a "right-sided CVA," which means the person has a left-sided deficit (experiences symptoms on the left side of the body). A left-sided CVA results in a deficit on the right side of the body. Nursing assistants should know how strokes are documented and referred to in their facility. If unsure which side of the body is affected, the NA should ask the nurse.

Guidelines: Residents Recovering from CVA

G   Encourage independence and self-esteem. Use assistive devices when needed to promote self-care.

G   Be patient with self-care. Tasks may take longer. Never rush residents.

G   Encourage resting in between self-care tasks so as not to tire, confuse, or agitate residents.

G   Assist with range of motion exercises as ordered to prevent contractures and to strengthen muscles.

G   Reposition often to help prevent pressure injuries and contractures. Position in proper alignment. Use positioning devices when necessary.

G   Residents who have hemiplegia or hemiparesis will have a weaker side of the body. Do not refer to the weaker side as "bad," such as the "bad leg" or "bad arm." Use the terms *weaker*, *affected*, or *involved* instead.

G   Assist with ambulation to prevent falls. When transferring, stand on and support the weaker side of the body. Lead with the stronger side (Fig. 22-7). Use a transfer belt as needed.

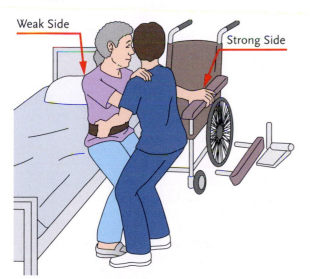

Fig. 22-7. *When helping a resident transfer, support the weaker side while leading with the stronger side.*

G   For one-sided neglect, remind residents often about the weaker side of the body.

G   When assisting with eating, always place food in the unaffected, or stronger, side of the mouth.

G   Observe for and report any signs of swallowing problems. Thickening agents may be ordered to help with swallowing problems.

G   Encourage fluids and proper nutrition to prevent unintended weight loss, constipation, and dehydration.

G   Carefully assist with shaving, grooming, and bathing. Diminished sensation or one-sided paralysis causes a lack of awareness about such things as water temperature and sharpness of razors. Be careful so that injury does not occur.

G   Make sure a clock and calendar are visible to help remind residents regularly of the day and time.

G   For a resident who has emotional lability, redirect her attention when she has an emotional outburst. Try asking a question or pointing out something in the room. Be patient and supportive.

G   Use praise often, even for small successes. Encourage the resident's progress.

G   Prevent withdrawal and feelings of isolation. Listen to the resident if she wants to talk.

Many people have trouble with communication after having a stroke. The level of difficulty a person has depends on the severity of the stroke, as well as the resulting effects on speech and cognition. Use these guidelines to help communicate with a resident who has had a CVA:

G   Speak clearly and face the resident when communicating.

G   Be patient. Problems with speech and thinking may make communication difficult. Do not rush the resident.

G   Use signals such as nodding the head and pointing to assist with communication.

G   Use questions that can be answered with a "yes" or "no," such as "Would you like to eat your vegetables first?"

G   Keep questions and directions simple. Break instructions down into short sentences. Use communication boards or cards as directed to make communication easier (Fig. 22-8).

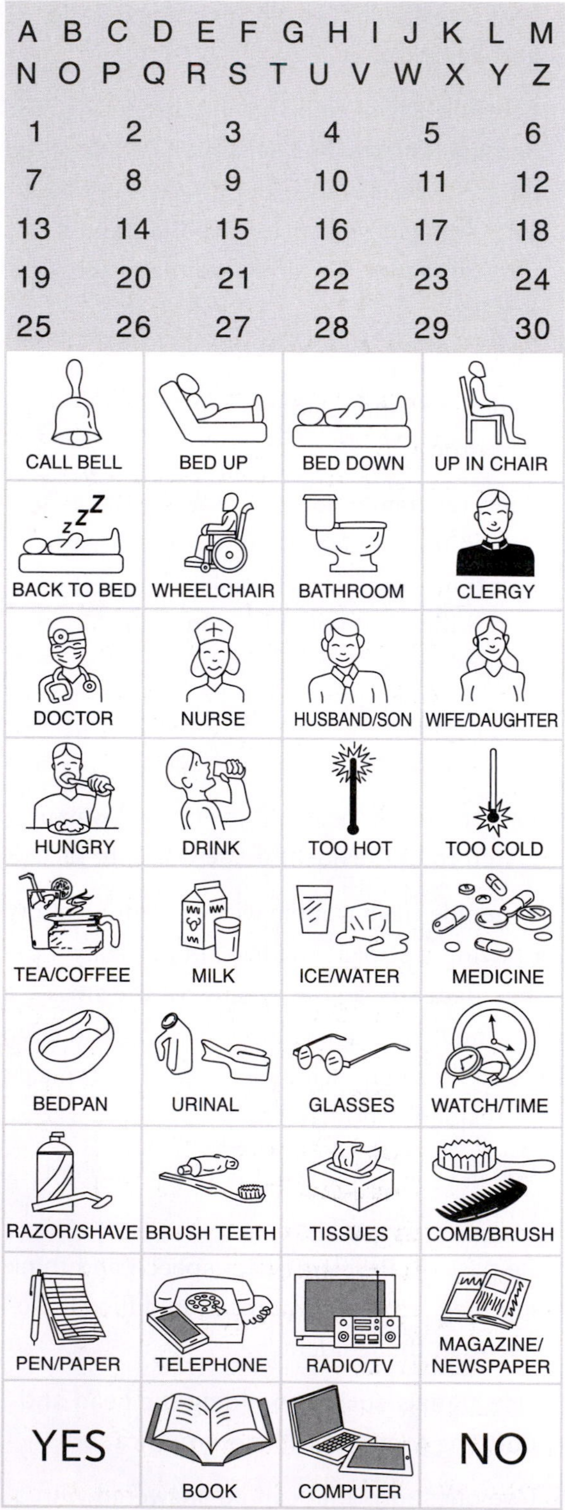

A	B	C	D	E	F	G	H	I	J	K	L	M
N	O	P	Q	R	S	T	U	V	W	X	Y	Z

1	2	3	4	5	6
7	8	9	10	11	12
13	14	15	16	17	18
19	20	21	22	23	24
25	26	27	28	29	30

CALL BELL	BED UP	BED DOWN	UP IN CHAIR
BACK TO BED	WHEELCHAIR	BATHROOM	CLERGY
DOCTOR	NURSE	HUSBAND/SON	WIFE/DAUGHTER
HUNGRY	DRINK	TOO HOT	TOO COLD
TEA/COFFEE	MILK	ICE/WATER	MEDICINE
BEDPAN	URINAL	GLASSES	WATCH/TIME
RAZOR/SHAVE	BRUSH TEETH	TISSUES	COMB/BRUSH
PEN/PAPER	TELEPHONE	RADIO/TV	MAGAZINE/NEWSPAPER

YES   BOOK   COMPUTER   NO

Fig. 22-8. A sample communication board.

Parkinson's Disease

Parkinson's disease is a progressive disorder that causes a part of the brain to degenerate. **Progressive** means that the disease gets worse with time. Neurons in the brain that produce the substance called dopamine, a neurotransmitter, begin to break down and die. This causes symptoms, such as tremors or shaking, that are uncontrollable. Tremors can make it difficult for a person to write, eat, and perform other ADLs. This disease also causes a mask-like face, pill-rolling (moving the thumb and first finger together like rolling a pill), rigid muscles, and a shuffling gait, or walk. Movement may slow, called *bradykinesia*. Postural and balance changes may occur. In addition, movements such as eye blinking or smiling may diminish. Speech may be affected, causing words to be slurred. The voice may become monotone and softer or breathy. Other symptoms are mood swings and gradual behavior changes. Parkinson's disease may also cause cognitive problems such as memory loss and dementia.

The average age for a person to be diagnosed with Parkinson's disease is 60, although some people are diagnosed at a younger age. Drug therapy is one way to treat Parkinson's disease. Some people are candidates for surgery that can help reduce the need for medications.

Guidelines: Parkinson's Disease

G   Encourage self-care. Be patient with self-care and communication. Allow the resident time to do and say things.

G   Assist with activities of daily living (ADLs) as necessary.

G   Assist with range of motion exercises as ordered to prevent contractures and to strengthen muscles (Fig. 22-9).

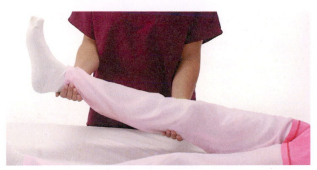
Fig. 22-9. *Range of motion exercises help prevent contractures, strengthen muscles, and increase circulation.*

G Residents are at a high risk for falls. Assist with ambulation to prevent falls due to shuffling walk or gait.

G Encourage resident to stand as straight as possible when ambulating.

G Encourage fluids and proper nutrition to prevent weight loss, constipation, and dehydration.

G People who have Parkinson's disease may have depression and anxiety. Listen to the resident if she wants to talk. Try relaxation techniques such as massage. Report any signs and symptoms of depression to the nurse, such as fatigue and apathy.

G If any of the following occurs, notify the nurse:

- Severe trembling
- Severe muscle rigidity/contractures
- Mood swings
- Sudden incontinence
- Constipation
- Dehydration
- Weight loss
- Signs of depression

Multiple Sclerosis (MS)

Multiple sclerosis (MS) is a progressive nervous system disorder that affects the way impulses are transmitted to and from the brain. When a person has MS, there is a loss of myelin, the protective covering over the nerves and spinal cord. Without this covering, nerves cannot send clear messages to and from the brain in a normal way.

This diseases progresses unpredictably. A person with MS will have varying abilities (Fig. 22-10). Symptoms will vary as well, and may include the following:

- Numbness and tingling
- Muscle weakness
- Extreme fatigue
- Tremors
- Vertigo (a spinning feeling)
- Reduced sensation
- Blurred or double vision, along with jerky eye movements
- Poor balance
- Difficulty walking
- Incontinence of bladder and bowel
- Paralysis in advanced cases

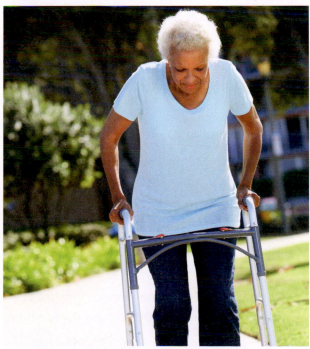
Fig. 22-10. *Multiple sclerosis is an unpredictable disease that causes varying symptoms and abilities. MS can cause a range of problems, including fatigue, poor balance, and trouble walking.*

Multiple sclerosis is often diagnosed in young adulthood. The exact cause of multiple sclerosis is not known. It may be an autoimmune disease triggered by a type of virus. There is no cure for the disease.

Multiple sclerosis is treated with medication. Some people who have MS use complementary medicine or treatments (Chapter 1).

Guidelines: Multiple Sclerosis

G   Be patient with self-care and movement. Allow the resident time to do things independently. Assist with activities of daily living as needed.

G   Offer rest periods as necessary.

G   Assist with range of motion exercises as ordered to prevent contractures and to strengthen muscles.

G   Encourage residents to follow their prescribed exercise programs.

G   Assist with ambulation to prevent falls due to lack of coordination, fatigue, and vision impairments.

G   Give frequent skin care to help prevent pressure injuries. Reposition residents at least every two hours.

G   Encourage proper nutrition and fluid intake.

G   People with MS may have difficulty communicating their thoughts. Do not rush or interrupt residents.

G   Stress can worsen the effects of MS. Be calm. Listen to residents, and try to provide a stress-free environment as much as possible.

G   Symptoms of MS sometimes change from day to day; offer support and encouragement.

G   If any of the following occurs, tell the nurse:

   •   Red skin, pale skin, or the beginning of a pressure injury

   •   The start of a contracture

   •   Urinary tract infection symptoms, such as frequency or burning during urination, increased incontinence, or cloudy urine

   •   Signs of depression

Head and Spinal Cord Injuries

Accidents, such as motor vehicle accidents, sporting injuries, gunshot wounds, stab wounds, or falls may cause head or spinal injuries. Head injuries are injuries that occur to the scalp, skull, or brain. They can be open or closed injuries. A head injury that occurs from a banging movement of the brain against the skull is a **concussion**. A head injury that is a bruise on the brain is a contusion. A traumatic brain injury (TBI) occurs when there is a violent blow, jolt, or other injury to the head that causes damage to the brain.

A person can have a head injury and show few or no symptoms initially. Head injuries can cause confusion or disorientation, along with serious complications like coma or death. Other symptoms include headaches, drowsiness, loss of consciousness, seizures, fractures, drainage from the ears, nose, or mouth, irritability, poor coordination, slurred speech, blurred vision, unequal pupil size, vomiting, a stiff neck, and a decreased sense of smell. A traumatic brain injury can cause permanent disability from brain damage.

When a person sustains a spinal cord injury, it means that the spinal cord is cut or damaged in some way. Symptoms include paralysis and loss of function, depending on where the spine is injured. The higher the injury, the greater the loss of function. **Paraplegia** is the loss of function of the lower body and legs. It is caused by injuries in the thoracic or lumbar area of the spinal cord. **Quadriplegia** is the loss of function of the arms, trunk, and legs. It is caused by injuries in the cervical area of the spine (Fig. 22-11).

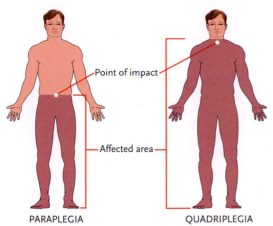

Fig. 22-11. *Loss of function depends on where the spine is injured.*

PARAPLEGIA

QUADRIPLEGIA

Point of impact

Affected area

Spinal cord injuries can be treated with some success if the cord is not completely cut or severed. The results of these injuries range from spasms, weakness, and difficulty coordinating movements to complete paralysis. Sometimes rehabilitation helps a person regain some of his former abilities. In other cases, movement or sensation cannot be recovered. Research relating to the regeneration of spinal cord tissue is ongoing.

Guidelines: Head or Spinal Cord Injuries

G   Allow as much independence as possible with activities of daily living (ADLs).

G   Offer rest periods as necessary.

G   Perform range of motion exercises to prevent contractures and to strengthen muscles.

G   Give frequent skin care to prevent pressure injuries. A lack of sensation will prevent awareness that a pressure injury is developing. Change position at least every two hours.

G   Be gentle when turning and repositioning. Logrolling may be required when turning in bed.

G   Protect residents from harm due to lack of sensation. Residents with paralysis are at a higher risk of injury from heat, cold, and sharp objects. Keep residents away from

heaters, radiators, hot plates, or any other source of heat. Check for sharp edges or objects when repositioning residents.

G   Check water temperature carefully to prevent burns due to lack of sensation. Make sure hot drinks have cooled enough before offering them.

G   Lack of activity can lead to poor circulation and fatigue. Use special stockings to help increase circulation as ordered.

G   Immobility can lead to constipation. Encourage fluids and a proper diet that is high in fiber.

G   Problems with bladder function can lead to the need for a urinary catheter. Urinary tract infections are common. Give careful catheter care and encourage a high intake of fluids.

G   If vomiting occurs, logroll the resident on her side to try to prevent aspiration.

G   Help resident with bladder and bowel retraining as directed.

G   Difficulty coughing and shallow breathing can lead to pneumonia. Encourage deep breathing exercises as ordered.

G   Male residents may have involuntary erections. Provide for privacy and be sensitive if this happens. Behave professionally to put residents at ease.

G   Listen to residents. They will need emotional support, as well as physical assistance. Anger, irritation, and frustration are some emotions they may experience while dealing with these injuries. Try not to take it personally, and be supportive.

G   If any of the following occurs, notify the nurse:

•   Red skin, pale skin, or the beginning of a pressure injury

•   Start of a contracture

•   Urinary tract infection symptoms

- Shortness of breath
- Constipation
- Dehydration
- Weight loss
- Any change in level of consciousness or confusion or disorientation
- Depression

Seizures (Convulsions)

Seizures are involuntary muscular contractions. They can involve a small area of the body or the entire body. Some causes of seizures are tumors, head injuries, medications, injuries to the brain during birth, high fevers, stroke, dementia, genetic factors, and alcohol and drug abuse.

Epilepsy is a disorder that causes recurring seizures. With epilepsy, electrical signals within the brain are generated that cause these seizures.

Treatment for seizures includes medication. Surgery may be performed. For seizures caused by drug and alcohol abuse, rehabilitation can help. Chapter 8 contains more information on types of seizures and how to care for a resident who is having a seizure.

Vision Impairment

Vision changes can affect people of all ages. **Nearsightedness** (myopia) is the ability to see objects that are near more clearly than distant objects. **Farsightedness** (hyperopia) is the ability to see distant objects more clearly than objects that are near. Eyeglasses, contact lenses, or surgery can be used to correct these eye problems (Fig. 22-12).

Other vision problems include cataracts and glaucoma. A **cataract** develops when the lens of the eye, which is normally clear, becomes cloudy. Light is prevented from entering the eye, which causes decreased vision. The first symptom is blurred vision. Other symptoms are glare

when driving at night or a yellowing of vision. A cataract can eventually cause blindness in one or both eyes.

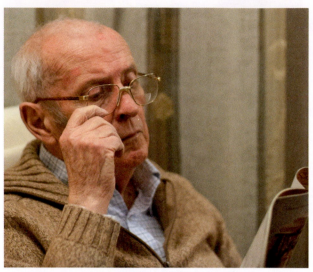

Fig. 22-12. *Nearsightedness and farsightedness are often corrected with the use of eyeglasses.*

Cataracts may be inherited. They can be caused by diabetes or an eye injury, or they may just be a result of normal aging.

Treatment depends upon the level of maturity of the cataract. Surgery is often performed to remove the cataract. The lens that has turned cloudy is removed, and an artificial lens, or lens implant, called an *intraocular lens (IOL)*, is placed and remains there. The implanted lens is made of plastic or silicone. The eye must be carefully measured for the lens implant prior to the surgery. This implant is permanent; it rarely has to be removed. It is only removed if inflammation occurs or the implant moves out of place.

Glaucoma is the leading cause of blindness in the United States. The pressure inside the eye, called *intraocular pressure*, increases, causing damage to the optic nerve. This increase in the intraocular pressure can ultimately cause a loss of vision and blindness if left untreated.

There are many forms of glaucoma. The majority of people have open-angle, or primary, glaucoma. Risk factors for open-angle glaucoma include elevated intraocular pressure, being over

45, family history of the disease, certain diseases and eye conditions, some medications, and ethnic background. All people with a family history of glaucoma should have their intraocular pressure checked regularly.

Symptoms of open-angle glaucoma may not be apparent. Over time, a person experiences a decrease in vision, especially in the peripheral vision.

Angle-closure glaucoma is a less common form of glaucoma. Angle-closure glaucoma can be chronic or acute. With acute angle-closure glaucoma, symptoms include pain, nausea, vomiting, seeing a halo around lights, reddening of the eye, and blurred vision. If not treated immediately, it can cause blindness very quickly.

Treatment of glaucoma includes eye drops and other medications. The NA should report if the resident has any difficulty using the eye dropper. Regular or laser surgery may also be used to treat glaucoma. The surgery does not work on every patient.

Age-related macular degeneration (AMD) is a condition in which the part of the retina that allows people to see detail, the *macula*, degenerates. Central vision is gradually destroyed, which can affect a person's ability to drive, read, write, and do other tasks. Peripheral vision (side vision) is not affected. AMD is the most common cause of vision loss in those 60 and older. There is no pain associated with this disorder, and it may evolve slowly. Vision problems may be different for each eye.

The two forms of this condition are wet and dry age-related macular degeneration; the dry form is more common. The exact cause of AMD is unknown. Risk factors include aging, smoking, sun exposure, heredity, gender, and race. Treatments for wet AMD include laser surgery and injections. Dry AMD may be treated with zinc and antioxidants to slow its progression. When dry AMD reaches the advanced stage, it cannot be treated, and vision loss results.

Guidelines: Vision Impairment

G Encourage the use of eyeglasses or contact lenses (contacts) if worn.

G Keep eyeglasses clean and in a safe place. If eyeglasses are damaged or do not fit well, notify the nurse.

G Cases for contact lens storage should be changed regularly to avoid the build up of bacteria. Follow any policies concerning replacement of contact lens cases (Fig. 22-13).

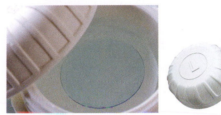

Fig. 22-13. *Contact lenses are made of different types of plastic. Some can be worn and discarded daily. Others are worn for longer periods and need to be cleaned and disinfected regularly. When not in the eye, they should be stored in a case filled with contact lens solution.*

G Always identify yourself as you enter the room. Do not touch the resident until you have done so. When leaving the room, let the resident know you are going.

G Keep doors completely open or closed, not partially open or closed.

G Leave furniture in place; never move furniture without the nurse's or the resident's permission.

G Use the face of an imaginary clock as a guide to explain the position of objects in a room.

G Make sure there is enough light in every room. Lighting should allow the resident to read in comfort without eye strain. However, harsh, bright lighting should not be used because it can put a strain on the eyes.

G Walk a little ahead of the resident while he touches your arm. This allows you to guide the person and warn him of steps, curbs, etc.

G   Walk at the resident's pace, not yours.

G   Assist residents who need help completing menus. Set up meal trays, cut meat and vegetables, and open containers as needed. Use the face of an imaginary clock to explain the position of food and drink on the tray.

G   Use special large-print books, audiobooks, and digital books if available.

G   Read to residents as often as time permits if they desire it. Volunteers and visitors can also help with this.

G   Assist with vision screenings as needed.

Tip

Using Braille

Braille is a system of touch reading for blind people that uses tiny raised dots (Fig. 22-14). Braille was developed in the 1800s by Louis Braille when he was a teenager. It was based on a code used to help soldiers communicate in the dark. Braille is composed of an alphabet of "cells" that consists of dots. Learning to read Braille takes a long time and requires special training.

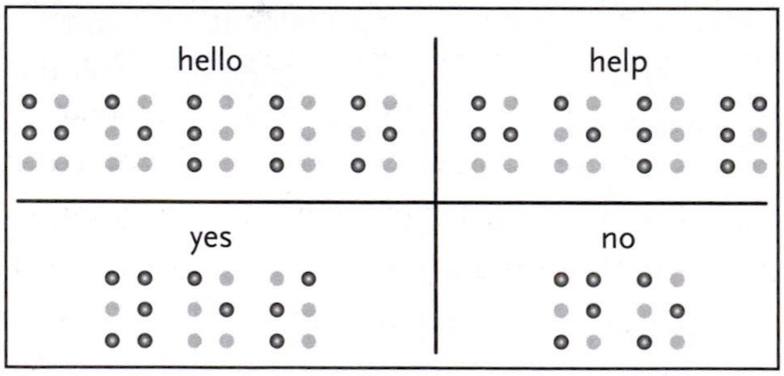

Fig. 22-14. *Examples of words in Braille.*

Tip

Resources for Visual Impairments

Residents who have print disabilities may require digital books or audiobooks. Many websites and smartphone apps sell, rent, or share these books:

*   Bookshare.org
*   Audible.com
*   Amazon.com

Microsoft offers an app, Seeing AI, to help people who are blind or who have low vision by narrating the world around them.

Chapter 4 contains more information about visual impairment.

Caring for eyeglasses

Equipment: emesis basin, special cleaning fluid, 2 lens cloths, towel

1. Identify yourself by name. Identify the resident. Greet the resident by name.

2. Wash your hands.

3. Explain procedure to the resident. Speak clearly, slowly, and directly. Maintain face-to-face contact whenever possible.

4. Provide for the resident's privacy with a curtain, screen, or door.

5. Gently remove the eyeglasses and place them in the emesis basin.

6. Line the sink with the towel.

7. Clean the eyeglasses over a lined sink with the proper solution and a cloth. While cleaning, observe for loose screws or loose or broken lenses.

8. Dry the eyeglasses with a soft, 100% cotton cloth or lens cloth. Do not use tissues to dry, as they can scratch eyeglasses.

9. Gently assist the resident to replace her eyeglasses on her face. Place over the ears and position comfortably. Observe for proper fit.

10. Make the resident comfortable. Remove privacy measures.

11. Leave call light within the resident's reach.

12. Wash your hands.

13. Be courteous and respectful at all times.

14. Report any changes in the resident to the nurse. Document procedure using facility guidelines.

The artificial eye is a type of prosthesis, sometimes referred to as an *ocular prosthetic*. An artificial eye does not provide vision. It can, however, improve appearance. It may be used when a person has lost an eye due to disease or injury, such as cancer or a gunshot wound. Artificial eyes can be made of plastic or glass; however, most artificial eyes are made from a special kind of plastic. Plastic eyes can adapt to changes in the eye socket as a person ages, while a glass eye cannot be changed once it is made. Plastic eyes do not require replacement very often, and they can be cleaned and polished repeatedly.

An artificial eye is held in place by suction. Some artificial eyes do not require frequent removal unless the eye becomes uncomfortable. Others need daily removal and cleaning. Each eye specialist will give individual instructions to their patients. NAs must carefully follow the instructions for residents regarding care for their artificial eyes.

Guidelines: Artificial Eye

G   If the artificial eye has been removed, clean or rinse the resident's eye socket carefully using a clean gauze square and warm water or saline solution.

G   Clean the empty socket from the inner canthus (inner part of the eye) toward the outer canthus (outer part of the eye).

G   Clean the eyelid last with a clean gauze square.

G   If the artificial eye is in place in the eye socket, clean the area, moving in the opposite direction. Clean from the outer part of the eye toward the inner part of the eye. Cleaning in this direction helps prevent accidental movement and dislodging of the eye.

G   Use an eyecup or a small clean basin when removing and transporting an artificial eye.

G   Follow manufacturer's instructions regarding cleaning. Do not use products that contain alcohol, antibacterial soaps, or abrasives such as cleansers or toothpaste. The artificial eye can be permanently damaged by improper cleaning. It needs to be stored in water or saline solution. Always cover the eye completely with the proper solution; the eye must never be allowed to dry out.

Hearing Impairment

There are many different kinds of hearing loss. A person may be born with a hearing impairment or it may happen gradually. Deafness is a partial or total hearing loss that occurs most often in people over the age of 65 but can occur in younger people.

Some disorders affect a person's ability to hear. **Otitis media** is an infection in the middle ear. Bacteria grow inside the middle ear, which cause symptoms such as pain, pressure, fever, and reduced ability to hear. Otitis media is treated with antibiotics, and the full course of antibiotics must be taken. Vital signs, especially body temperature, may need to be monitored. Because ear drainage can occur, the resident's pillowcase may need to be changed regularly.

Meniere's disease is a disorder of the inner ear caused by a buildup of fluid. It usually only affects one ear. The exact cause is unknown, but Meniere's disease may be caused by infections, allergies, or a genetic link. This disorder usually affects people between the ages of 40 and 60. Symptoms include vertigo, hearing loss, tinnitus (ringing in the ear), and pain or pressure. Vertigo can lead to nausea and vomiting. Some people who have sudden attacks of vertigo fall down; these are sometimes called *drop attacks*.

Treatment includes medications, salt restriction and other dietary changes (including no alcohol, caffeine, and chocolate), cognitive therapy (a type of talk therapy), antibiotic or corticosteroid injections, and, in extreme cases, surgery. The person may be advised to stop smoking. Immediate treatment for a drop attack or severe vertigo is to have the person lie down and lower the lighting in the area. The FDA has approved a device for treatment of Meniere's disease. This device is inserted into the outer ear and sends pressure pulses to the middle ear, which can help decrease vertigo.

A person who has a hearing impairment may read lips, use sign language to communicate, or use a hearing aid. A **hearing aid** is a small device placed in the ear to amplify sound. There are many different kinds of hearing aids (Fig. 22-15).

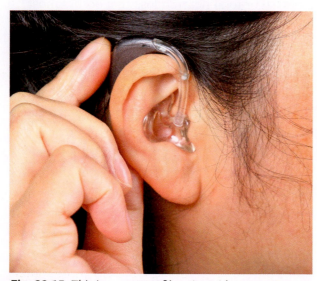

Fig. 22-15. This is one type of hearing aid.

Guidelines: Hearing Aids

G   Handle hearing aids carefully; they are very expensive.

G   Before inserting a hearing aid, turn the volume down. Be gentle when inserting the device. Make sure it sits snugly in place before turning it on. The hearing aid should feel comfortable when in place. If the hearing aid does not fit properly, notify the nurse.

G   Turn off the hearing aid when not in use. Always store it inside its case when it is not being worn. The case should be labeled with the resident's name and room number. It should be stored in a cool, dry area. Heat can damage the device.

G   Some hearing aids have rechargeable batteries. Some need to be recharged nightly. Follow the care plan's instructions. Replace batteries as needed. The correct battery size must be used, and batteries need to be firmly in place.

G   If the hearing aid does not work, check the batteries. If this does not solve the problem, notify the nurse.

G   Follow instructions for cleaning hearing aids. In general, they need to be cleaned daily using a soft cloth and mild cleanser and water. Do not submerge a hearing aid in water or allow the section that houses the battery to get wet.

G   Remove hearing aids before bathing, showering, or shampooing hair.

G   Do not spray hair care products near hearing aids.

G   Check for hearing aids before removing bed linens and meal trays.

G   Report any signs of sores or abrasions in the ear, as well as wax buildup, to the nurse.

Chapter 4 contains more information about properly communicating with someone who has a hearing impairment.

Here are a few additional resources for information relating to nervous system disorders:

*   National Stroke Association, stroke.org

*   Alzheimer's Association, alz.org

*   National Institute of Mental Health, nimh.nih.gov

5. Discuss dementia and related terms

Cognition is the ability to think clearly and logically. A person with a cognitive impairment has a reduced ability to perform these mental tasks. Focus and memory, as well as self-awareness and judgment, may be impaired. Some loss of cognitive ability is a result of normal changes of aging in the brain.

Dementia is a general term that refers to a more serious loss of mental abilities, such as thinking, remembering, reasoning, and communicating. It interferes with normal functioning, and a person may lose the ability to perform activities of daily living (ADLs), such as eating, bathing, and toileting. Social skills may be affected. Dementia is not a normal part of aging (Fig. 22-16).

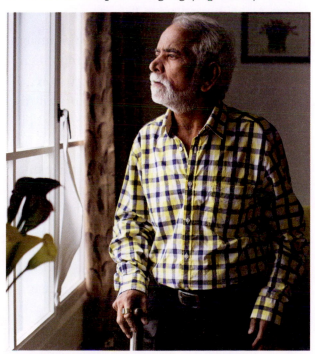

Fig. 22-16. Some loss of cognitive ability is normal; however, dementia is not a normal part of aging.

Alzheimer's disease is the most common form of dementia. Dementia may also be caused by these disorders:

- Vascular or multi-infarct dementia (a series of strokes causing damage to the brain)

- Lewy body dementia (abnormal structures, called *Lewy bodies*, develop in areas of the brain, causing a variety of symptoms)

- Parkinson's disease

- Acquired immunodeficiency syndrome (AIDS) (Chapter 24)

- Huntington's disease (an inherited disease that causes certain nerve cells in the brain to waste away)

- Excessive alcohol or drug use

- Head injuries

- Thyroid disorders

- Nutritional deficiencies, especially of the B vitamins

Some forms of dementia can be treated. Dementia caused by thyroid disorders or vitamin deficiencies can often be reversed with proper treatment. However, many forms of dementia are **irreversible**, meaning the disease cannot be cured. With those types of dementia, symptoms are managed with specific care techniques and different medications.

Diagnosing dementia is difficult, involving many physical and mental tests to rule out other causes. Testing is sometimes begun after a person develops two or more problems with brain functioning, such as a loss of speech or language abilities, math skills, or memory skills.

6. Discuss Alzheimer's disease and identify its stages

Alzheimer's disease (AD) is a progressive, degenerative, and incurable disease that causes proteins (plaques and tangles) to build up in and around nerve cells in the brain. They eventually cause dementia. As the disease progresses, it causes a greater loss of health and abilities. People with Alzheimer's disease have significant physical and mental changes. Most are eventually completely unable to care for themselves. There is no known cause of Alzheimer's disease, and there is no cure.

The Alzheimer's Association estimates that there are 5.8 million people living in the United States with Alzheimer's disease. Most of these people are age 65 or older, and almost two-thirds are women. The disease affects people from all races, backgrounds, socioeconomic statuses, and cultures. The Alzheimer's Association estimates that by 2050, the number of people with Alzheimer's disease will reach 14 million.

Alzheimer's disease generally progresses in stages. In each stage, the symptoms become progressively worse. The majority of people with Alzheimer's disease are eventually completely dependent on others for care.

Each person with AD may show different symptoms at different times. For example, one resident may continue to read, but not be able to recognize a family member. Another may be able to play a musical instrument, but does not know how to use the phone. Skills a person has used over a lifetime are usually retained longer (Fig. 22-17).

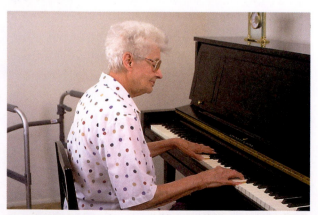

Fig. 22-17. *A person with AD may continue to have skills she has used her whole life.*

The Alzheimer's Association identifies three general stages of Alzheimer's disease:

Mild Alzheimer's disease (early stage)

At this stage, the person may show some problems, such as memory loss and forgetting some words and the location of familiar objects. The person's medical examination may show problems with memory and concentration. However, the person may still be independent and able to work, drive, and do other activities.

Moderate Alzheimer's disease (middle stage)

Generally speaking, this stage has the longest duration. At this stage, the person may show signs and symptoms such as forgetting recent events, forgetting some of one's own past experiences and background, changes in personality and behavior, and being moody or withdrawn. Other changes include needing help with some activities of daily living, such as elimination needs and choosing clothing appropriately. There may be changes in sleep patterns, increased wandering, suspiciousness or delusions, and confusion about time and place.

Severe Alzheimer's disease (late stage)

During this final stage, a person may be unable to communicate with others, control movement, or respond to his surroundings. The person needs significant help with activities of daily living, including eating and eliminating. The ability to walk, sit, and swallow may be affected.

It is important for NAs to encourage independence, regardless of what signs and symptoms a resident with Alzheimer's disease shows. The resident should be encouraged to do whatever he is able to do. This helps keep the resident's mind and body as active as possible. Working, socializing, reading, problem-solving, and exercising should all be encouraged (Fig. 22-18).

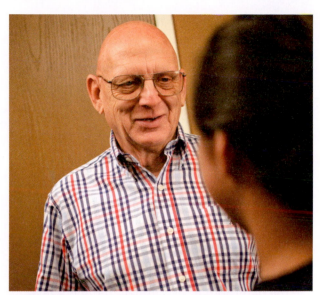

Fig. 22-18. NAs should encourage residents with AD to socialize, read, work, problem-solve, and exercise to keep their minds and bodies active.

7. List strategies for better communication with residents with Alzheimer's disease

Many things can be done to improve communication with residents who have Alzheimer's disease. Some communication guidelines follow:

Guidelines: Communicating with Residents Who Have Alzheimer's Disease

G   Always approach from the front, and do not startle the resident.

G   Smile and look happy to see the resident. Be friendly.

G   Determine how close the resident wants you to be.

G   Communicate in a calm area with little background noise and distraction.

G   Always identify yourself and use the resident's name when greeting him. (Never touch first; this may upset the person.) Continue to use the resident's name during the conversation.

G   Look at the resident the entire time you are speaking with him.

G   Speak slowly, using a lower tone of voice than normal. This is calming and easier to understand.

G   Repeat yourself, using the same words and phrases, as often as needed.

G   Only talk about one subject at a time. Be patient. Use simple, short sentences.

G   Use signs, pictures, gestures, or written words to help communicate.

G   Break complex tasks into smaller, simpler ones. Give simple, step-by-step instructions as necessary.

Communication with residents with AD can also be helped by following these specific techniques:

If the resident is frightened or anxious:

G   Speak slowly in a low, calm voice. Speak in a quiet area with few distractions (Fig. 22-19).

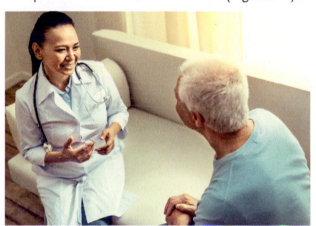

Fig. 22-19. Find a room with little background noise and distraction when communicating with residents with AD.

G   Try to see and hear yourself as the resident might. Always describe what you are going to do.

G   Use simple words and short sentences. If helping with care, list steps one at a time.

G   Check your body language; make sure you are not tense or hurried.

If the resident forgets or shows memory loss:

G   Repeat yourself, using the same words if you need to repeat an instruction or question.

However, you may be using a word the resident doesn't understand, such as *tired*. Try other words like *nap*, *lie down*, or *rest*. Repetition can be soothing for a resident with AD. Many people with AD will repeat words, phrases, questions, or actions. This is called **perseveration**. Do not try to stop a resident who is perseverating. Answer the questions, using the same words each time, until he stops. Even though responding over and over may frustrate you, it communicates comfort and security.

G   Keep messages simple. Break complex tasks into smaller, simpler steps.

If the resident has trouble finding words or names:

G   Suggest a word that sounds correct. If this upsets the resident, learn from it and try not to correct a resident who uses an incorrect word. As words (written and spoken) become more difficult, smiling, touching, and hugging can help show care and concern (Fig. 22-20). Remember, however, that some people find touch frightening or unwelcome.

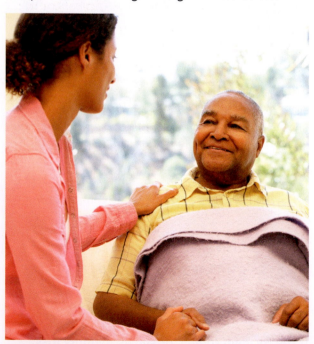

Fig. 22-20. Touch, smiles, and laughter will be understood longer, even after a resident's speaking abilities decline.

If the resident seems to not understand basic instructions or questions:

G   Ask the resident to repeat your words. Use short words and sentences, allowing time to answer.

G   Note the communication methods that are effective and use them.

G   Watch for nonverbal cues as the ability to talk lessens. Observe body language—eyes, hands, and face.

G   Use signs, pictures, gestures, or written words. For example, a picture of a toilet on the bathroom door can help remind a resident where the bathroom is. Combining verbal and nonverbal communication is helpful. For example, you can say "Let's get dressed now" while holding up clothes.

If the resident wants to say something but cannot:

G   Encourage the resident to point, gesture, or act it out.

G   If the resident is obviously upset but cannot explain why, offer comfort with a smile, or try to distract him. Verbal communication may be frustrating.

If the resident does not remember how to perform basic tasks:

G   Break each activity into simple steps. For instance, "Let's go for a walk. Stand up. Put on your sweater. First the right arm..." Always encourage residents to do what they can.

If the resident insists on doing something that is unsafe or not allowed:

G   Redirect activities toward something else. Try to limit the times you say "Don't."

If the resident hallucinates (sees or hears things that are not really happening), or is paranoid or accusing:

G   Try not to take it personally.

G   Try to redirect behavior or ignore it. People with AD often have a limited attention span. This behavior usually passes quickly.

If the resident is depressed or lonely:

G   Take time, one-on-one, to ask how he is feeling and really listen to the response.

G   Try to involve the resident in activities. Always report signs of depression to the nurse.

If the resident repeatedly asks to go home:

G   Ask the resident to tell you what his home was like and how he felt being there.

G   Redirect or guide the conversation and/or the resident's activities to something he enjoys.

G   Expect that the resident may continue to ask to go home and be patient and gentle in your response.

If the resident is verbally abusive or uses bad language:

G   Remember it is the dementia speaking, not the person. Try to ignore the language, and redirect attention to something else.

If the resident has lost most verbal skills:

G   Use nonverbal skills. As speaking abilities decline, people with AD will still understand touch, smiles, and laughter for much longer. However, remember that some people do not like to be touched. Approach touching slowly and be gentle. Softly touching the hand or smiling can express affection and say you want to help (Fig. 22-21).

G   Remember that even after verbal abilities are lost, signs, labels, and gestures can reach people with dementia.

G   Assume that residents with AD can understand more than they can express. Do not talk about them as though they were not there or treat them like children.

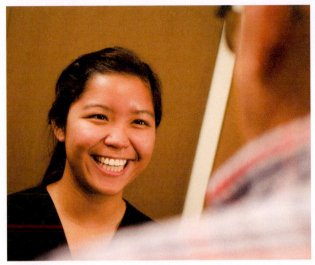

Fig. 22-21. *Smiling can communicate positivity and a willingness to help.*

8. Identify personal attitudes helpful in caring for residents with Alzheimer's disease

These attitudes will help NAs give the best possible care for residents with Alzheimer's disease:

Do not take things personally. Alzheimer's disease is a devastating mental and physical disorder that affects everyone who cares for the person with AD. People with AD do not always have control over their words or actions. They may often be unaware of what they say or do. A resident with AD may not recognize a caregiver or do what he is supposed to do. He may ignore, accuse, or insult staff members. When this happens, it is important to remember that the behavior is due to the disease.

Be empathetic. It is helpful if the NA thinks about what it would be like to have Alzheimer's disease. She can imagine being unable to do activities of daily living and being dependent on others for care. It would be very frustrating for anyone to have no memory of recent events or to be unable to find words for what one wants to say. NAs should assume that people with AD have insight and are aware of the changes in their abilities. They should treat residents with AD with dignity and respect.

Work with the symptoms and behaviors noted. Each person with Alzheimer's disease is an individual. Residents with AD will not all show the same symptoms at the same times. Each resident will do some things that others will never do. The best plan is to work with the behaviors that are seen on any particular day. For example, a resident who has AD may want to go for a walk one day, when the day before he did not want to go to the bathroom without help. If it is allowed, the NA should try to go for a walk with him. NAs should notice and report changes in behavior, mood, and independence.

Work as a team. Symptoms and behaviors change daily. When NAs observe and report carefully, as well as listen to others' reports, the care team may be better able to develop solutions. Being with residents often allows NAs to have insights that others may not have. They should make the most of this opportunity. Residents with AD may not be able to recognize or distinguish between aides, nurses, or administrators. All staff members should be prepared to help when needed.

Be aware of difficulties associated with caregiving. Caring for someone with dementia can be physically and emotionally exhausting, as well as incredibly stressful. NAs should take care of themselves so they can continue to provide the best care (Fig. 22-22). Being aware of the body's signals to slow down, rest, or eat better is important. Each NA's feelings are real; they have a right to them. Mistakes should be viewed as learning experiences.

Work with family members. Family members can be a wonderful resource. They can help an NA learn more about a resident. They also give stability and comfort to the resident with AD. NAs should build relationships with family members and keep the lines of communication open.

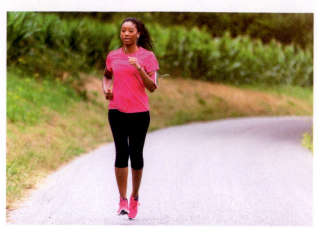

Fig. 22-22. Regular exercise is an important part of taking care of oneself.

In addition, NAs should be reassuring to family members. It is very difficult for families to see a loved one's health and abilities decline. When residents with AD exhibit problem behaviors, it can be stressful for the family. NAs can help by reassuring family members that they understand that this behavior is part of the disease.

Remember the goals of the care plan. Along with the practical tasks that NAs perform, the care plan will also call for maintaining residents' dignity and self-esteem. NAs should help residents be as independent as possible.

Tip

Burnout

Caregivers of residents with Alzheimer's disease tend to experience burnout. **Burnout** is mental or physical exhaustion due to a prolonged period of stress and frustration. Burnout can include feelings of failure about the work a person does. Unmanaged stress can cause physical and emotional problems. NAs can talk to their supervisors if they need help addressing stress or would like to find support groups in their areas. Chapter 28 contains more information about stress management.

9. Describe guidelines for problems with common activities of daily living (ADLs)

As Alzheimer's disease worsens, residents will have trouble with their activities of daily living. Below are interventions to help make caring for a resident with AD easier. An **intervention** is a way to improve or change an action or development.

Guidelines: Assisting with ADLs for Residents Who Have Alzheimer's Disease

If a resident has problems with bathing:

G   Schedule bathing when the resident is least agitated. Be organized so the bath can be quick. Give sponge baths if the resident resists a shower or tub bath.

G   Prepare the resident before bathing. Hand her the supplies (washcloth, soap, shampoo, towels). This serves as a visual aid.

G   Take a walk with the resident down the hall, stopping at the tub or shower room, rather than talking directly about the bath.

G   Make sure the bathroom is well lit and at a comfortable temperature.

G   Provide privacy during the bath.

G   Be calm and quiet when bathing a resident and keep the process simple.

G   Give the resident a washcloth to hold, which can help distract her while you finish the bath.

G   Always follow safety precautions. Ensure safety by using nonslip mats, tub seats, and handholds.

G   Be flexible about when to bathe a resident. A resident may not always be in the mood. Also, be aware that not everyone bathes with the same frequency. Understand if a resident does not want to bathe.

G   Be relaxed and allow the resident to enjoy the bath. Offer encouragement and praise.

G   Let the resident do as much as possible during the bath.

G   Observe the skin for any signs of breakdown or irritation during the bath.

If a resident has problems with grooming and dressing:

G   Assist with grooming to help the resident feel attractive and dignified (Fig. 22-23).

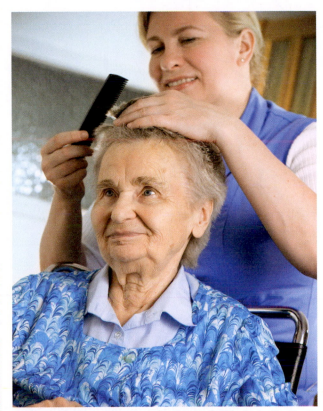

Fig. 22-23. NAs should assist residents with grooming to promote dignity and self-esteem.

G   Avoid delays or interruptions while dressing.

G   Show the resident some of her clothing. This brings up the idea of dressing. Tell her you are going to help her get dressed.

G   Provide privacy by closing doors and curtains. Dress the resident in her room.

G   Encourage the resident to pick clothes to wear. Simplify this task by giving just a few choices. Make sure the clothing is clean and appropriate, and lay out clothes in the order in which they are put on (Fig. 22-24). Choose clothes that are simple to put on, such as slip-on instead of lace-up shoes and pants or skirts instead of dresses. Some people with Alzheimer's disease make a habit of layering clothing regardless of the weather.

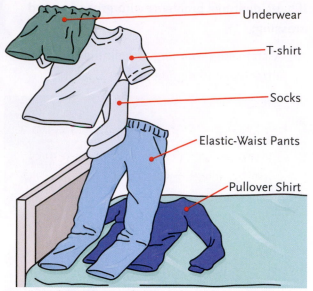

Underwear

T-shirt

Socks

Elastic-Waist Pants

Pullover Shirt

Fig. 22-24. Clothes should be laid out in the order in which they should be put on.

G   Break the task down into simple steps. Introduce one step at a time and do not rush the resident.

G   Use a friendly, calm voice when speaking. Praise and encourage the resident at each step.

If a resident has problems with elimination:

G   Encourage fluids. Never withhold or discourage fluids because a resident has urinary incontinence. Report to the nurse if the resident is not drinking fluids. Follow the schedule in the care plan for drinking fluids.

G   Mark the bathroom with a sign or a picture as a reminder of where it is and to use the toilet.

G   Make sure the path to the bathroom and the bathroom are well lit.

G   Note when the resident is incontinent over two to three days. Check her every 30 minutes. This can help determine "bathroom times." Take the resident to the bathroom just before her bathroom time.

G   Observe incontinence patterns for two to three nights to try to determine nighttime bathroom times.

G   Take the resident to the bathroom before and after meals and before bed. Make sure the resident actually urinates before getting off the toilet.

G   Put lids on trash cans, wastebaskets, or other containers if the resident urinates or defecates in them.

G   Follow the toileting schedule carefully and document urination and bowel elimination as required.

G   Family or friends may be upset by their loved one's incontinence. Be professional when cleaning after episodes of incontinence. Do not show disgust or irritation.

If a resident has problems with nutrition:

G   Encourage nutritious foods. Food may not interest a resident with AD, or she may forget to eat. It may be of great interest, but she may only want to eat a few types of food. A resident with AD is at risk for malnutrition.

G   Have meals at regular times each day. You may need to remind the resident that it is mealtime. Familiar, appetizing foods should be served.

G   Make sure there is adequate lighting.

G   Keep noise and distractions to a minimum during meals. The dining area should be as pleasant and calm as possible.

G   Keep the task of eating simple. If the resident is restless during meals, the NA can try smaller, more frequent meals. Finger foods (foods that are easy to pick up with the fingers) work best. Bite-sized pieces of food may also work well. They allow residents to choose the food they want to eat.

G   Do not serve steaming or very hot foods or drinks.

G   Use a simple place setting with a single eating utensil and remove other items from the table. Plain plates without patterns or colors work best (Fig. 22-25).

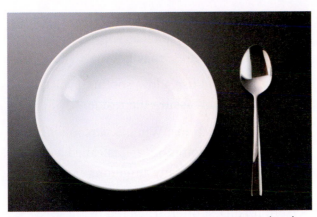

Fig. 22-25. Plain white plates on a contrasting-colored surface may help avoid confusion and distraction.

G   Put only one item of food on the plate at a time. Multiple kinds of food on a plate or a tray may be overwhelming.

G   Give simple, clear instructions. Residents with AD may not understand how to eat or use utensils. Help the resident taste a sample of the meal first. Place a spoon to the lips. This will encourage the resident to open her mouth. Ask the resident to open her mouth.

G   Guide the resident through the meal, providing simple instructions. Offer regular drinks of water, juice, and other fluids to prevent dehydration.

G   Use assistive devices for eating, such as special spoons and bowls, as needed.

G   If the resident needs to be fed, do so slowly. Offer small pieces of food.

G   Make mealtimes simple and relaxed, not rushed. Give the resident time to swallow before each bite or drink.

G   Seat the resident with others at small tables. This encourages socializing. If helping a resident eat, sit directly in front of the resident and make simple conversation during the meal.

G   Observe and report eating or swallowing problems, as well as changes in eating habits.

G   Report changes in intake or output. Monitor weight accurately and frequently.

Chapter 14 contains more information about nutrition.

To promote the resident's physical health:

G   Prevent infections and follow Standard Precautions.

G   Help residents wash their hands frequently.

G   Observe the resident's physical health and report any potential problems. People with dementia may not notice their own health problems.

G   Reduce the risk of falls; fractures can cause severe pain and a lengthy recovery.

G   Provide careful skin care to prevent pressure injuries.

G   Watch for signs of pain. A person who has AD may not be able to express that she is in pain. Nonverbal signs that a resident may be in pain include grimacing or clenching fists (Fig. 22-26). A resident may be agitated or have an angry outburst. Report possible signs of pain to the nurse. Chapter 13 contains more information about pain and pain management. Special pain management techniques for residents who are close to death may be found in Chapter 27.

G   Maintain a daily exercise routine.

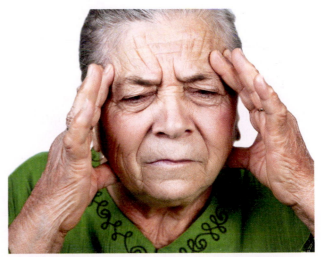

Fig. 22-26. Be aware of nonverbal signs of pain, such as holding or rubbing a body part. The NA should report these signs to the nurse immediately.

To promote the resident's mental and emotional health:

G   Maintain self-esteem by encouraging independence in activities of daily living.

G   Share in enjoyable activities, such as looking at pictures, talking, and reminiscing.

G   Reward positive and independent behavior with smiles and warm touches.

Residents' Rights

Residents' Rights and Alzheimer's Disease

Because people with Alzheimer's disease may not be aware of what they are doing, it is especially important to protect their dignity. For example, if a resident lifts up her skirt often, she should wear pants. If a resident is a messy eater, he should have privacy when he is eating. NAs should actively protect residents' privacy and promote their dignity, even if the residents seem unaware of these concerns.

10. Describe interventions for common difficult behaviors related to Alzheimer's disease

Below are some common difficult behaviors that NAs may face when working with residents who have Alzheimer's disease. Interventions for each behavior are also included. Each resident is different, and NAs should work with each person as an individual. Details of behavior should be reported to the nurse.

Agitation: A resident who is excited, restless, or troubled is said to be **agitated**. Feeling insecure or frustrated, encountering new people or places, and changing a routine can all trigger this behavior. A **trigger** is a situation that leads to agitation. Even watching television can cause agitation, as a person with AD may lose his ability to distinguish fiction from reality. If a resident is agitated, the NA should

*   Try to eliminate triggers, keep a routine, and avoid frustration. Redirecting the resident's attention may help.

*   Reduce noise and distractions. Focusing on a familiar activity, such as sorting things or looking at pictures, may help.

*   Stay calm and use a low, soothing voice to speak to and reassure the resident.

Catastrophic Reactions: When a person with AD overreacts to something, it is called a **catastrophic reaction**. Many situations can cause this reaction, and they differ from person to person. It is most often triggered by these conditions:

*   Fatigue

*   Change of routine, environment, or caregiver

*   Overstimulation (too much noise or activity)

*   Difficult choices or tasks

*   Physical pain or discomfort, including hunger or a need to use the toilet

An NA can respond to catastrophic reactions as she would to agitation. For example, she can try to eliminate triggers and help the resident focus on a soothing activity.

Violent Behavior: A resident who attacks, hits, or threatens someone is using **violence**. Violent behavior also includes being violent to oneself. For example, a resident may bang his head repeatedly against a wall. Violence may be triggered by many situations. These include frustration, overstimulation, or a change in routine, environment, or caregiver. If a resident is violent, the NA should

*   Notify the nurse immediately.

*   Block blows but never hit back.

*   Not try to restrain the resident.

*   Step out of reach and stay calm.

*   Avoid leaving the resident alone.

*   Try to remove triggers and remove other residents or visitors from the area.

*   Use the same calming techniques as for agitation.

A care conference may be needed to discuss the behavior, especially if it is new behavior. Chapter 4 contains more information about aggressiveness, anger, and combativeness.

Hallucinations or Delusions: A resident who sees, hears, smells, tastes, or feels things that are not there is having **hallucinations**. A resident who believes things that are not true is having **delusions**. If a resident is experiencing hallucinations or delusions, the NA should

- Ignore harmless hallucinations and delusions.

- Reassure a resident who seems agitated or worried.

- Not argue with a resident who is imagining things. Challenging the resident serves no purpose and can make matters worse. The feelings are real to the resident. The NA should not tell the resident that she sees or hears his hallucinations. She should redirect the resident to other activities or thoughts.

- Be calm and reassure the resident that she is there to help.

Depression: People who become withdrawn, isolated, lack energy, and stop eating or doing things they used to enjoy may be depressed. Losing independence and facing the reality of an incurable disease can cause depression. Feelings of failure and fear are other causes. Chemical imbalances can cause depression. A person who has depression is at risk of suicide. Suicide is the act of taking one's own life intentionally and purposefully. Suicide is more common in people who have been recently diagnosed with Alzheimer's disease. Learning Objective 13 in this chapter has more information on depression and its symptoms. If a resident is depressed, the NA should

- Report signs of depression to the nurse immediately. It is an illness that can be treated with medication and psychotherapy.

- Observe for triggers that cause changes in mood.

- Encourage independence, self-care, and activity.

- Find ways to help foster social interaction and relationships, such as group activities.

- Listen to residents if they want to share their feelings or talk about their moods. Offering comfort and concern, as well as being as pleasant as possible, may help.

- Report any comments about suicide immediately. Report any possible signs that a resident may be considering suicide such as saying or writing goodbyes, abusing alcohol, or making changes to wills or trusts.

Disruptiveness: **Disruptive behavior** is anything that disturbs others, such as yelling, banging on furniture, and slamming doors. Often this behavior is triggered by pain, constipation, frustration, or a wish for attention. To prevent or respond to disruptive behavior, the NA should

- Be calm and friendly, and try to find out why the behavior is occurring. There may be a physical reason, such as pain or discomfort.

- Gently try to direct the resident to a private area.

- Notice and praise improvements in the resident's behavior, being sensitive to avoid treating the resident like a child.

- Tell the resident about any changes in schedules, routines, or the environment in advance. Involving the resident in developing routine activities and schedules may help.

- Encourage the resident to join in independent activities that are safe (for example, folding towels). This helps the resident feel in charge and can prevent feelings of powerlessness. Independence is power.

- Help the resident find ways to cope. Focusing on activities the resident may still be able to do, such as knitting or crafts, can provide a diversion.

Inappropriate Sexual Behavior: Inappropriate sexual behavior, such as removing clothing, touching one's own genitals in public, or trying to touch others can disturb or embarrass those who see it. It is helpful to stay calm and be professional when this behavior occurs. The NA should not overreact or be judgmental. Trying to determine the cause of the problem may help. Is the behavior actually intentional? Is it consistent? If distracting the resident does not work, the NA can gently direct him to a private area and inform the nurse. A resident may be reacting to a need for physical stimulation or affection. Ways to provide physical stimulation include giving back rubs, offering a soft doll or stuffed animal to cuddle, providing comforting blankets, or giving physical touch that is appropriate. More information about inappropriate sexual behavior may be found in Chapter 4.

Inappropriate Social Behavior: Inappropriate social behavior may include cursing, name-calling, or yelling. As with violent or disruptive behavior, there may be many reasons why a resident is behaving in this way. The NA should try not to take this behavior personally. The resident may only be reacting to frustration or other stress. The NA should remain calm and be reassuring. She can try to find out what caused the behavior. Possible causes include too much noise, too many people, and too much stress, pain, or discomfort. If the resident is disturbing others, the NA should gently direct him to a private area if possible. Any physical abuse or verbal abuse should be reported to the nurse.

Perseveration or Repetitive Phrasing: Residents who have dementia may repeat words, phrases, or questions over and over again. This is called *perseveration* or *repetitive phrasing*. They may also repeat an action or task, such as tapping fingers and folding or cleaning things. Such behavior may be caused by several factors, including disorientation or confusion. The NA should be patient with this behavior and not try to silence or stop the resident. She should answer questions each time they are asked, using the same words each time.

Hoarding and Rummaging: **Hoarding** is collecting and putting items away in a guarded way. **Rummaging** is going through drawers, closets, or personal items that belong to oneself or to other people. These behaviors are not within the control of a person who has Alzheimer's disease. Hoarding and rummaging should not be considered stealing. Stealing is planned and requires a conscious effort. In most cases, the resident is only collecting something that catches his attention. It is common for those with AD to wander and collect things. They may carry these objects around for a while and leave them in other places. This is not intentional. Residents with AD will often take their own things and leave them in another room, not knowing what they are doing. If a resident hoards or rummages, the NA should

- Label all personal belongings with the resident's name and room number. This way there is no confusion about what belongs to whom.

- Place a label, symbol, or object on the resident's door. This helps the resident find his own room.

- Not tell the family that their loved one is "stealing" from others.

- Prepare the family so they are not upset when they find items that do not belong to their family member.

- Ask the family to tell staff if they notice unfamiliar items in the room.

- Regularly check areas where residents store items. They may store uneaten food in these places. Providing a rummage drawer—a drawer with items that are safe for the resident to take with him—can help.

Sundowning: When a resident with AD becomes restless and agitated in the late afternoon, evening, or night, it is called **sundowning**.

Sundowning may be caused by hunger, fatigue, a change in routine or caregiver, or any new or frustrating situation. If a resident experiences sundowning, the NA should

- Provide adequate lighting before it gets dark.

- Avoid stressful situations during this time. Activities, appointments, trips, and visits should be limited.

- Play soft music.

- Try to discourage residents from taking naps during the day.

- Set a bedtime routine and keep it.

- Recognize when sundowning occurs and plan a calming activity just before.

- Serve the evening meal long before bedtime.

- Remove caffeine from the diet.

- Provide snacks.

- Give a soothing back massage.

- Distract the resident with a simple, calm activity like looking at a magazine.

- Maintain a daily exercise routine.

Suspicion: A person with Alzheimer's disease often becomes suspicious as the disease progresses. Residents may accuse staff or family members of lying to them or stealing from them. Suspicion may escalate to paranoia (having intense feelings of distrust and believing others are "out to get" them). When a resident is acting suspicious, the NA should not argue with him. Arguing just increases defensiveness. Instead, the NA should offer reassurance and be understanding and supportive.

Pacing and Wandering: A resident who walks back and forth in the same area is **pacing**. A resident who walks aimlessly around the facility or the facility grounds is **wandering**. Pacing and wandering may have some of the following causes:

- Restlessness

- Hunger

- Disorientation

- Incontinence or the need to use the bathroom

- Constipation

- Pain

- Forgetting how or where to sit down

- Too much daytime napping

- Need for exercise

If a resident paces and wanders, the NA should

- Remove causes when possible. For example, give nutritious snacks, encourage an exercise routine, and maintain an elimination schedule.

- Discourage daytime napping.

- Let the resident pace or wander in a safe, locked area where staff can keep an eye on him. The resident should not be restrained.

- Redirect attention to something the resident enjoys, such as taking a walk together.

- Mark rooms with signs or pictures, such as stop signs or "closed" signs, may prevent residents from wandering into areas where they should not go.

- Report to the nurse immediately if a resident wanders away from a protected area and does not return, or **elopes**. In order to guard against elopement, facilities often have secured areas so that residents with AD will not wander away. There may be a coded entry system. This system requires a code to be entered to open a door. The code is available to oriented residents, visitors, and staff. It is very important for all staff members to keep doors locked when leaving an Alzheimer's unit or area.

11. Discuss ways to provide activities for residents with Alzheimer's disease

Activities are very important for residents with Alzheimer's disease. Activities that residents enjoy help them stay focused and prevent frustration and boredom.

When a person is first diagnosed with Alzheimer's disease or is admitted to the facility, staff should request a detailed biography from family or friends. Information that would be helpful includes likes, dislikes, cultural needs, work history, hobbies and interests, and a description of the person's personality. These can all be used to plan the most beneficial types of activities for residents with AD.

Meaningful activities help people with Alzheimer's disease maintain or improve their ability to function in daily life. They draw on past skills the resident has used throughout his life to help provide a focus. For example, if a resident once filed medical records for work, giving her papers or folders to file can help her stay focused on a task.

Other activities—sometimes referred to as *doing activities*—keep residents busy (Fig. 22-27). Folding towels can help the resident stay focused. Separating cards into groups can help with motor coordination and keep the resident engaged.

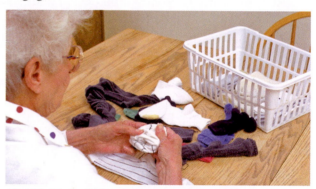

Fig. 22-27. Activities that are not frustrating can help keep residents busy and engaged.

Residents may only be able to focus on specific activities for 20 to 30 minutes at a time. NAs should not try to push them to continue the activity. If an activity is not engaging a resident, another one can be offered.

Some of the things staff can do to provide meaningful activities include the following:

- Encourage family participation in activities.

- Limit some activities to small groups.

- Use quiet places for activities and maintain a comfortable temperature in activity areas.

- Set short time frames for activities to allow for limited attention spans.

- Help plan events that are of interest to residents, based on their interests and past experiences.

- Plan activities at times of the day when residents are feeling their best and are most engaged.
- Encourage residents to exercise in specially designated areas.
- Plan activities that allow residents to make things that can be utilized by others.
- Encourage each resident's specific skills, such as playing a musical instrument.
- Provide opportunities for residents who are immobile as well. Reading to them or playing music in their rooms are ways to provide activity for residents who are bedbound.

In addition to encouraging participation in activities, the NA must make sure residents are dressed and ready to go to activities at the designated time. Residents should be well-groomed, have had a meal or snack, and have been taken to the bathroom. The NA may need to take a resident to the activity site.

12. Describe therapies for residents with Alzheimer's disease

There are different types of therapies that can improve the quality of life for people with Alzheimer's disease. These include the following:

Validation therapy means letting residents believe they live in the past or in imaginary circumstances (Fig. 22-28). **Validating** means giving value to or approving and making no attempt to reorient the resident to actual circumstances. It is used for residents with advanced dementia. For example, Mrs. Montego tells the NA she is late for prom. Instead of telling her that prom happened many years ago, the NA asks her to describe her prom dress. The NA can also ask who her date is and how late she can stay out. This allows the resident to work through the memory without forcing her back to reality.

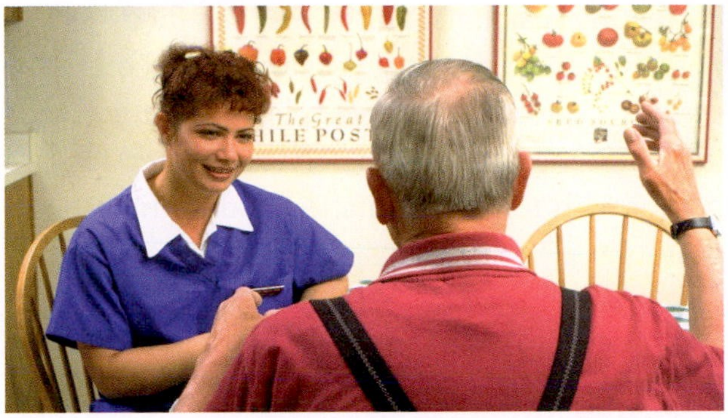

Fig. 22-28. *Validation therapy accepts a resident's statements without attempting to reorient him to reality.*

Reminiscence therapy involves encouraging residents to remember and talk about past experiences (Fig. 22-29). The NA can explore memories by asking about details. If a painful past memory is triggered, the NA should not hurry the resident through the memory, but should not dwell on it either. He should be ready to move on when the resident signals he is done discussing the memory. Reminiscence therapy can help elderly people remember pleasant times in their past and allow caregivers to increase their understanding of residents. This therapy encourages more interaction between residents with Alzheimer's disease and the care team.

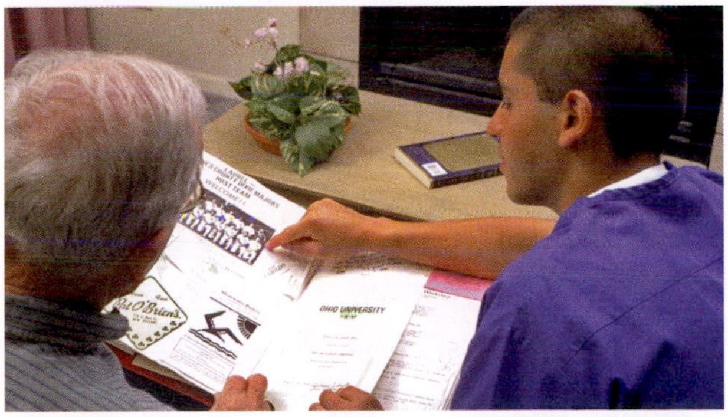

Fig. 22-29. *Reminiscence therapy encourages a resident to remember and talk about his past.*

Remotivation therapy promotes self-esteem, self-awareness, and socialization by having residents gather in small groups. Discussion focuses on facts rather than emotion. For example, participants may discuss their former professions in detail. This type of therapy discourages correcting residents, and it does not focus on personal problems. Discussion is based on the cognitive abilities of the people within the small group. Remotivation therapy can be used together with reality orientation and reminiscence therapy.

13. Discuss mental health and mental health disorders

Mental health is the ability of a person to use cognition and emotion appropriately throughout each day. A mentally healthy person will have successful relationships with family, friends, neighbors, and coworkers (Fig. 22-30). He will perform well in professional and home settings and will meet his responsibilities. He can control his desires and impulses properly. He will develop ways to deal with difficulties that occur throughout life.

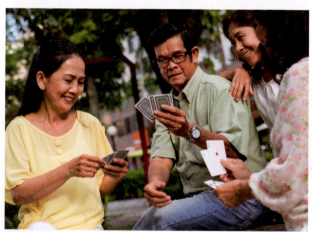

Fig. 22-30. Interacting well with others is a trait of mental health.

A **mental health disorder** is a disorder that affects a person's ability to function within family, home, work, or community settings. It often causes inappropriate behavior. It produces signs and symptoms and affects the body's ability to function. Certain factors cause or make mental health disorders worse, such as certain illnesses, substance abuse, physical abuse, unstable or traumatic relationships, genetic tendencies toward mental health disorders, and extreme

stress. Some types of mental health disorders are discussed below.

Anxiety Disorders: Anxiety was first discussed in Chapter 4. Anxiety is characterized by excessive worrying, tension, and unease, even when there is no apparent cause of these feelings. Symptoms include headaches, muscle aches, sweating, shaking, difficulty swallowing, and irritability. Anxiety disorders are often treated with psychotherapy and medication. **Psychotherapy** is a method of treating mental health disorders that involves talking about one's problems with mental health professionals. **Cognitive behavioral therapy (CBT)** is a type of psychotherapy often used to treat anxiety disorders and depression. This type of therapy is usually short-term and focuses on skills and solutions that a person can use to modify negative thinking and behavior patterns.

Panic disorder is characterized by panic attacks, which are repeated episodes of intense fear, along with physical symptoms such as rapid heartbeat, dizziness, chest pain, shortness of breath, and an upset stomach. During a panic attack, the person may think she is having a heart attack or is dying. A person who has panic disorder has regular panic attacks or lives with chronic anxiety about having another attack. Psychotherapy and medication are used to treat panic disorder.

Social anxiety disorder, also called *social phobia*, is a disorder in which a person has excessive anxiety about social situations. A **phobia** is an intense, irrational fear of or anxiety about an object, place, or situation, such as a fear of dogs or a fear of flying. It causes extreme self-consciousness in common situations. The person may feel as if he is being judged or criticized by others, and may avoid being around other people. A person with social anxiety disorder is unable to manage his fears, which interferes with the ability to attend school, work, social functions, and family events. Symptoms include sweating, shaking, and upset stomach. Psychotherapy and medication are used to treat this disorder.

Obsessive-Compulsive and Related Disorders: Obsessive-compulsive disorder (OCD) is a disorder characterized by intrusive repetitive thoughts or behaviors that cause anxiety or stress. For example, a person with OCD may wash his hands over and over again, or check repeatedly to make sure the door is locked. A person with OCD cannot control this behavior. Obsessive-compulsive disorder is treated with psychotherapy and medication.

Trauma and Stressor-Related Disorders: Post-traumatic stress disorder (PTSD) is a disorder caused by witnessing or experiencing a traumatic event, such as being in combat while in the military. PTSD can also develop after a crime, tornado or other natural disaster, domestic violence, or a severe accident. Symptoms include flashbacks, nightmares and sleep disturbances, avoiding reminders of the event (people, places, objects, or situations), negative thoughts, and irritability and anger. Flashbacks are episodes in which the person experiences the event again and again. PTSD is treated with psychotherapy and medication.

Depressive Disorders: Major depressive disorder, also called *clinical depression*, is a type of mental health disorder that causes withdrawal, apathy (lack of interest), and lack of energy. Other symptoms are pain, fatigue, weight loss or gain, insomnia, irritability, feelings of worthlessness, and sadness. It is important to note that sadness is only one symptom of this disorder. Not all people who have major depressive disorder complain of sadness or appear sad.

This disorder makes it difficult for a person to function normally. A person who is depressed may not be able to perform normal tasks or participate in daily activities (Fig. 22-31).

Major depressive disorder is an illness and must be treated as such. A person cannot simply overcome depression through sheer will. Depression is more common in the elderly population. It can occur due to the death of loved ones, or along with other illnesses, such as cancer, Alzheimer's disease, HIV or AIDS, and after a heart attack.

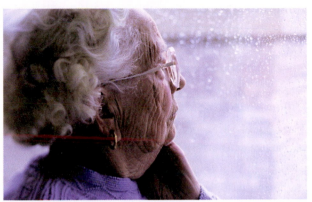

Fig. 22-31. *Signs of major depressive disorder, such as apathy, withdrawal, insomnia, irritability, and being unable to perform normal tasks, are important to report.*

Major depressive disorder may be caused by abnormal levels of chemicals in the brain. It may lead to thoughts of death and suicide. The CDC reports that suicide is the 10th leading cause of death in the US and that 45,000 people died from suicide in 2016. If an NA ever hears a resident make comments, even jokes, about hurting himself or others, she must report them immediately to the nurse. Depression is treated with medication and psychotherapy.

Bipolar and Related Disorders: Bipolar disorder causes a person to have mood swings and changes in energy levels and the ability to function. The mood swings can go from extreme happiness to extreme sadness. The state of extreme excitement or joy is a *manic episode* and the state of extreme hopelessness or sadness is called a *depressive episode*. High energy, little sleep, high self-esteem, and poor judgment are other symptoms of this disorder. Suicide or thoughts of suicide can occur. Bipolar disorder requires long-term treatment with medication. It is important to note that a person with this disorder often has difficulty taking medication as prescribed. During manic episodes, the person may believe he no longer needs his medication and will stop taking it.

Schizophrenia and Other Psychotic Disorders: **Schizophrenia** is a mental health disorder that may involve acute episodes. It is a brain disorder that affects a person's ability to think and communicate clearly. Problems with emotions, decision-making, and understanding reality may occur. A person may think she is hearing voices that tell her what to do or that someone is controlling her thoughts. Symptoms include hallucinations, delusions, disorganized thinking and speech, and a lack of interest in life and in planning activities. The person may have poor hygiene. Problems with memory may develop.

Guidelines: Mental Health Disorders

G Encourage self-care.

G Encourage independence with ADLs and activities. Watch for any change in a resident's ability to perform ADLs.

G Know your residents. Observe and watch for changes in behavior, such as manic episodes in people with bipolar disorder.

G Watch your body language when caring for the resident. He may be sensitive to this.

G Do not treat residents like children. Always treat residents like adults.

G Do not yell or use a harsh tone of voice. Never argue with the resident.

G Use eye contact when communicating.

G Provide support for the resident and family and friends. Do not judge the behavior of the resident, friends, or family. Notify the nurse if you become concerned about any specific behavior.

G If you observe any of the following, notify the nurse:

- Change in ability to perform ADLs

- Changes in mood, such as sadness, irritability, or crying

- Change in behavior, such as the inability to make decisions, the inability to concentrate, or low self-esteem

- Behavior that seems extreme, dangerous, or frightening to others

- Excessive fatigue or insomnia

- Headaches

- Constipation

- Weight loss or weight gain, appetite changes

- Social withdrawal, or lack of participation in activities

- Hallucinations or delusions

- Concerns that the resident is not properly taking a medication or is hiding medication

- Any person(s), activity, program, telephone call, specific date, object, article of clothing, or place that makes the person's behavior change in some way

- Any comments about suicide, even jokes

14. Discuss substance abuse and list signs of substance abuse to report

Substance abuse is the repeated use of legal or illegal substances in a way that is harmful to oneself or others. Many different substances can be abused, including alcohol, tobacco, legal and illegal drugs, glue, paint, and permanent markers (Fig. 22-32). These substances are considered *mood-altering substances* because they create a change in the person's perception or the control of his body. For example, alcohol is a depressant. It can cause slurred speech, slower reflex response, unsteadiness, irritability, and poor decision-making. Because of these effects, it is unsafe to drive under the influence of alcohol.

Opioids are drugs used to relieve severe pain (such as from surgery or from diseases like cancer). Opioid medications work to block pain signals to the brain and boost feelings of relaxation, happiness, and pleasure. Some opioids, such as codeine, fentanyl, morphine, and oxycodone, are available legally by prescription. Illegal opioids include heroin and illegally made fentanyl. Opioid abuse has become a pervasive problem in the US. The positive feelings they create can make a person feel dependent on the drugs, which can lead to addiction.

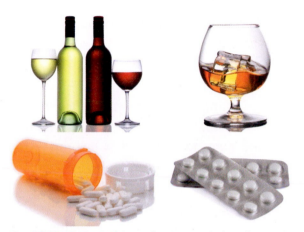

Fig. 22-32. *Prescription and nonprescription drugs, cigarettes, and alcohol are examples of legal substances that may be abused.*

In a 2016 CDC survey, more than 11.5 million people in the US reported abusing prescription opioids. Some people seek illegal drugs to alleviate pain when they are no longer able to obtain the prescribed drugs from physicians.

In addition, when taking prescribed opioids, a person's tolerance for the medication can increase, requiring higher doses. At higher doses, a person's breathing slows and may even stop, which can be fatal. The CDC estimates that 130 people die every day from opioid overdoses. Someone experiencing an opioid overdose can be given an antidote called naloxone, but it must be given within a certain time frame in order to successfully reverse the potentially deadly effects of the drug.

Risk factors for substance abuse include a family history of addiction, the presence of a mental health disorder, an unstable home environment, poor coping skills or a lack of social support,

and taking a highly addictive drug (such as opioid painkillers or certain illegal drugs). Elderly people are at a greater risk for substance abuse when they have poor or absent relationships with family or friends. Substance abuse can cause even more problems for elderly people because of possible interactions with prescribed medications they may be taking.

Observing and Reporting: Substance Abuse

If you observe any of the following signs, report them to the nurse. Simply report what you see, not what you think the cause may be.

- °/R Changes in physical appearance (torn clothing, red eyes, weight loss)
- °/R Changes in personality (moodiness, mood swings, strange behavior, lying)
- °/R Smell of alcohol, cigarettes, or other substances in resident's room or on clothing
- °/R Strong smell of room fresheners
- °/R Increased use of breath fresheners
- °/R Constricted or dilated pupils
- °/R Slurred speech
- °/R Loss of appetite
- °/R Forgetfulness
- °/R Confusion
- °/R Blackouts or memory loss
- °/R Hiding substances or alcohol
- °/R Stealing money or valuables
- °/R Problems with other residents, staff, friends, or family
- °/R Comments about thoughts of suicide

Without treatment, substance abuse can cause injury or even death. When a person stops using an addictive substance, physical and mental symptoms can occur. It is usually necessary for people to receive treatment to help them through the process of quitting. Substance abuse is treated with medication and cognitive behavioral therapy (or other types of psychotherapy). Residential treatment centers are facilities where people can live while completing a structured course of treatment. This can also be an effective way to treat substance abuse.

Chapter Review

1. What is the basic working unit of the nervous system (LO 2)?

2. What makes up the central nervous system? What makes up the peripheral nervous system (LO 2)?

3. List three functions of the nervous system (LO 2).

4. List four normal age-related changes of the nervous system (LO 3).

5. Why is it important not to use rubbing alcohol to clean artificial eyes (LO 4)?

6. What is the most common cause of dementia (LO 5)?

7. Why is it important for NAs to encourage independence for as long as possible for residents who have AD (LO 6)?

8. If a resident with Alzheimer's disease loses interest in an activity, what should the NA do (LO 11)?

9. Does a person usually overcome major depressive disorder through sheer will (LO 13)?

10. What should an NA do if a resident makes comments or jokes about suicide (LO 13)?

Multiple Choice

11. When a cerebrovascular accident (CVA) occurs on the left side of the brain, which side of the body will be affected (LO 4)?
    (A) The left side
    (B) The right side
    (C) The underside
    (D) The front side

12. When assisting a resident who has had a CVA with eating, in which side of the resident's mouth should food be placed (LO 4)?
    (A) Stronger side
    (B) Affected side
    (C) Weaker side
    (D) Right side

13. When a resident with Alzheimer's disease repeats an action over and over, he is (LO 7)
    (A) Babbling
    (B) Intervening
    (C) Strategizing
    (D) Perseverating

14. One morning a resident with Alzheimer's disease says he does not like eating with others and wants to eat breakfast by himself in his room. The next morning he tells his NA that he does not like to eat alone and wants help going to the dining room. What would be the best response by the NA to this shift in the resident's preferences (LO 8)?
    (A) The NA should remind him that he prefers eating alone in his room.
    (B) The NA should explain that it is difficult for him to eat in the dining room because he requires additional help.
    (C) The NA should take the resident to the dining room.
    (D) The NA should tell the resident that he must eat in his room because it is the facility's policy.

15. Which of the following is a way for an NA to help a resident who has Alzheimer's disease with his nutritional needs (LO 9)?
    (A) The NA should use a plain plate without a pattern and a single eating utensil for meals.
    (B) The NA should put multiple kinds of food, in different colors and textures, on the resident's plate.
    (C) The NA should serve steaming hot foods.
    (D) The NA should avoid talking to the resident while he is eating.

16. When a resident with Alzheimer's disease continues to ask the same question, the NA should (LO 10)
    (A) Ask the resident to stop asking that question
    (B) Answer the question, using the same words each time
    (C) Remind the resident that he has asked that question several times before
    (D) Ignore the behavior until it stops

17. A resident with Alzheimer's disease tells his NA that he is not going to eat dinner today because he is meeting his wife for dinner at their favorite restaurant. The NA knows his wife has been dead for many years. What would be the best response by the NA (LO 12)?
    (A) The NA should tell the resident that he cannot eat in restaurants due to his disease.
    (B) The NA should remind the resident that his wife is no longer alive.
    (C) The NA should ask him what restaurant he is going to and what he will have.
    (D) The NA should let him know that if he does not go to the dining room soon, he will miss dinner.

18. Which of the following puts a person at a higher risk for substance abuse (LO 14)?
    (A) Having many friends
    (B) Exercising often
    (C) Having a mental health disorder
    (D) Not having tried illegal drugs

23
The Endocrine System

1. Define important words in this chapter

diabetes: a condition in which the pancreas does not produce insulin or does not produce enough insulin; causes problems with circulation and can damage vital organs.

glands: organs that produce and secrete chemicals called hormones.

hormones: chemical substances produced by the body that control numerous body functions.

hyperglycemia: high blood glucose (blood sugar).

hyperthyroidism: a condition in which the thyroid gland produces too much thyroid hormone, which causes body processes to speed up and metabolism to increase.

hypoglycemia: low blood glucose (blood sugar); also known as *insulin reaction* or *insulin shock*.

hypothyroidism: a condition in which the body lacks thyroid hormone, which causes body processes to slow down.

prediabetes: a condition in which a person's blood glucose levels are above normal but not high enough for a diagnosis of type 2 diabetes.

thyroid: a butterfly-shaped gland in the neck that is responsible for regulating metabolism and growth.

2. Explain the structure and function of the endocrine system

The endocrine system regulates many important body functions. The endocrine system is made up of glands in different areas of the body (Fig. 23-1). The **glands** are organs that produce and secrete chemicals called hormones. **Hormones** are chemical substances created by the body that control numerous body functions. They are vital to survival. Hormones are carried in the blood for delivery to target tissues or organs.

The pituitary gland, also referred to as the *master gland,* is located at the base of the brain and is attached to the hypothalamus. It is called the master gland due to its ability to control the hormone production of other glands. There are two parts, or lobes, of the pituitary gland: the anterior (front) and the posterior (back). The anterior lobe releases the hormones, while the posterior lobe stores hormones for release when needed.

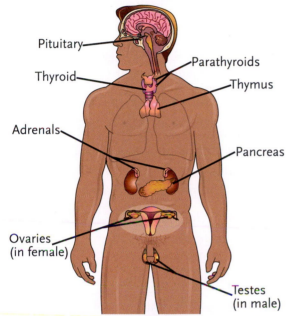

Pituitary
Thyroid
Parathyroids
Thymus
Adrenals
Pancreas
Ovaries
(in female)
Testes
(in male)

Fig. 23-1. The endocrine system includes glands that produce hormones that regulate body processes.

The **thyroid** gland is located in the neck below the larynx, or voice box. Thyroid hormones primarily regulate metabolism and growth. Metabolism is the process of breaking down and transforming all nutrients that enter the body to provide energy, growth, and maintenance. Thyroid hormones also stimulate the growth of nervous tissue.

Four tiny parathyroid glands are embedded in the thyroid gland. They are responsible for the production of parathyroid hormone. This hormone regulates the levels of vitamin D, calcium, and phosphate in the bloodstream.

Two adrenal glands are located on top of the kidneys. They secrete adrenaline (epinephrine) and noradrenaline (norepinephrine), aldosterone, and cortisol. During stressful situations, adrenaline, and the less potent noradrenaline, increase

the efficiency of muscle contractions, increase heart rate and blood pressure, and also increase blood glucose levels to provide extra energy. This is called the *fight-or-flight response.* It enhances body performance during stressful or threatening situations. Aldosterone regulates the balance of sodium, potassium, and water. Cortisol (hydrocortisone) maintains metabolism by regulating the amount of glucose (natural sugar) in the blood.

The pancreas is a gland located in the back of the abdomen and behind the stomach. The pancreas produces the hormone insulin. Insulin regulates the amount of glucose available to the cells for metabolism. Cells cannot absorb sugar without insulin.

Male and female sex glands, called the *gonads,* are endocrine glands. The ovaries in the female secrete estrogen and progesterone. The testes in the male secrete testosterone.

The functions of the endocrine system are to

- Maintain homeostasis through hormone secretion

- Influence growth and development

- Regulate levels of vitamin D, calcium, and phosphate in the body

- Maintain blood sugar levels

- Regulate the body's ability to reproduce

- Determine how quickly cells burn food for energy

Destination: Homeostasis

The parathyroid glands work to maintain calcium levels in the body. If the blood calcium gets too low—for example, due to surgery or cancer—the parathyroid glands increase production of parathyroid hormone (PTH). PTH controls vitamin D, calcium, and phosphate levels in the blood. When the blood calcium reaches the proper level, the parathyroid glands stop the production of PTH. This quick response by the parathyroid glands helps the body return to homeostasis.

3. Discuss changes in the endocrine system due to aging

Normal age-related changes for the endocrine system include the following:

- Levels of estrogen and progesterone decrease, which signals the onset of menopause in women.

- Testosterone levels in males usually decrease, but production does not stop.

- Insulin production decreases.

- The body is less able to handle stress.

4. Discuss common disorders of the endocrine system

Diabetes

Diabetes mellitus, commonly called *diabetes*, is a disease that can affect people of any age. **Diabetes** is a condition in which the pancreas does not produce insulin or does not produce enough insulin. Without insulin to process glucose, or natural sugar, glucose builds up in the blood. This causes **hyperglycemia**, or high blood sugar. Because the body is unable to get energy from the sugar in the blood, it has to find energy another way. Usually the energy is obtained by burning fat. Diabetes is common in people with a family history of the illness, in the elderly, and in people who are obese.

Diabetes can cause many complications, including the following:

- **Hypoglycemia** (insulin reaction) and diabetic ketoacidosis are complications of diabetes that can be life-threatening (Chapter 8).

- Decreased blood flow can cause problems with circulation, such as coronary artery disease or peripheral vascular disease (Chapter 19). These problems increase the risk of heart attack, stroke, or impaired circulation in the legs. Poor circulation in the legs can increase the risk of infection and the loss of toes, feet, or legs to gangrene.

- Diabetic retinopathy, or damage to blood vessels in the retina, can cause blindness.

- Damage to vital organs, such as the kidneys being unable to properly filter the blood, is another complication of diabetes.

- Diabetic peripheral neuropathy can result from diabetes. It causes numbness, pain, or tingling of the legs and/or feet and causes nerve damage over time.

There are a few different types of diabetes:

Prediabetes is a condition in which glucose levels are elevated, but not high enough to establish a diagnosis of diabetes. The CDC estimates 84 million people in the US have prediabetes, and approximately 90% are unaware they have it. Some damage to vital organs may have occurred already with prediabetes.

In order to be diagnosed with prediabetes, a fasting blood sugar level must be between 100 mg/dL (milligrams per deciliter) to 125 mg/dL. Prediabetes can be delayed or prevented with certain lifestyle changes. A change in the diet, along with daily exercise, can reduce weight and lower the risk of prediabetes or diabetes.

Type 1 diabetes is a condition that is usually diagnosed in children and young adults. It was formerly known as *juvenile diabetes*. In type 1 diabetes, the pancreas does not produce any insulin. This condition will continue throughout a person's life. Daily injections of insulin are needed, but these injections do not always prevent complications of diabetes. Special diets help treat this disorder and must be followed carefully. Blood glucose testing must also be done to monitor diabetes.

Type 2 diabetes is the most common form of diabetes; it can occur at any age. It was formerly known as *adult-onset diabetes*. In type 2 diabetes, either the body does not produce enough insulin or the body fails to properly use insulin. This is known as *insulin resistance*.

Type 2 diabetes is the milder form of diabetes. It usually develops after age 35. However, the number of children with type 2 diabetes is growing rapidly. This form of diabetes often occurs in obese people or those with a family history of the disease.

Treatment for type 2 diabetes includes careful monitoring of blood glucose levels. It can often be controlled with diet, weight loss, and medication. Oral medications or injections of insulin will be used to control blood glucose. Smoking will be discouraged. Exercise may be ordered by a doctor to help with weight loss.

People with diabetes may have many different signs and symptoms, including the following:

- Excessive thirst
- Excessive hunger
- Excessive urination
- High blood sugar levels
- Glucose in the urine
- Very dry skin
- Fatigue
- Blurred vision or visual changes
- Slow-healing sores, cuts, or bruises
- Tingling or numbness in hands or feet
- Unexplained weight loss
- Increased number of infections

Hypothyroidism (Underactive Thyroid Gland)

Hypothyroidism is a condition in which the body lacks thyroid hormone, which causes body processes to slow down. It is an autoimmune disorder in which the body produces antibodies that attack the thyroid, interfering with the production of thyroid hormone.

Hypothyroidism is often caused by Hashimoto's thyroiditis (formerly known as *Hashimoto's disease*). Other causes include surgical removal of the thyroid gland, radioactive iodine therapy, and thyroiditis (inflammation of the thyroid). Symptoms of hypothyroidism include the following:

- Fatigue and weakness
- Weight gain
- Constipation
- Intolerance to cold
- Dry skin
- Thinning hair or hair loss
- Brittle hair or fingernails
- Slow heart rate
- Low blood pressure
- Abnormally low body temperature
- Enlarged thyroid (goiter)
- Hoarseness
- Heavier than normal menstrual periods or absent menstrual periods
- Depression

Blood tests, neck examinations, and ultrasounds of the thyroid diagnose this condition. Treatment is thyroid hormone replacement therapy.

Hyperthyroidism (Overactive Thyroid Gland)

Hyperthyroidism is a condition in which the thyroid gland produces too much thyroid hormone. Body processes speed up, and metabolism increases, causing weight loss, a rapid heartbeat, and sweating. Nervousness and irritability may result.

Hyperthyroidism is primarily caused by Graves' disease, an autoimmune disorder in which antibodies cause the thyroid gland to produce excessive thyroid hormone. Nodules (lumps in the gland), thyroiditis, or taking too much thyroid medication can also cause hyperthyroidism. Symptoms of hyperthyroidism include the following:

- Nervousness
- Trembling, especially of the hands
- Restlessness
- Fatigue
- Visual problems or eye irritation
- Bulging or protruding eyes (exophthalmos)
- Intolerance to heat
- Excessive perspiration
- Rapid heartbeat
- High blood pressure
- Increased appetite
- Weight loss
- Changes in bowel movements
- Irregular or absent menstrual periods
- Enlarged thyroid (goiter)

Blood tests and physical examinations help diagnose this condition. Treatment includes antithyroid drugs, other medications called beta blockers, or radioactive iodine to destroy the thyroid gland. If a goiter is large, surgery may be done. If the thyroid is removed, the person will need to take medication for the rest of her life.

Here are a few additional resources for information relating to endocrine system disorders:

- American Diabetes Association, diabetes.org
- American Thyroid Association, thyroid.org

Obesity and Disorders of the Endocrine System

Obesity increases the risk for certain endocrine system diseases or disorders, including the following:

- Type 2 diabetes
- Insulin resistance

5. Describe care guidelines for diabetes

Care of the person with diabetes includes a plan of care associated with every system in the body. Diabetes must be carefully controlled to prevent complications and serious illness. The care plan must be followed closely.

Guidelines: Diabetes

G   Give frequent skin care. Keep the skin clean and dry.

G   Observe the skin carefully for sores, blisters, cuts, or any other breaks in the skin. Report any of these signs immediately to the nurse (Fig. 23-2). Wounds, skin breaks, and pressure injuries must be prevented. A small sore can grow into a large wound that may not heal, which can require amputation.

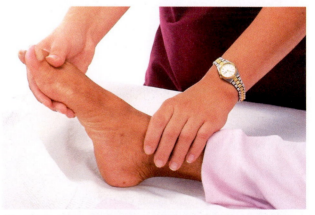

Fig. 23-2. Observe the legs and feet carefully when giving care. Poor circulation can increase the risk of infection and the loss of toes, feet, or legs to gangrene.

G   Encourage residents to follow their exercise plans (Fig. 23-3). Exercise will be ordered to help with circulation and maintaining a healthy weight. Walking, range of motion exercises, frequent position changes, or other activity may be ordered. Report muscle weakness, change in gait, and any change in the ability to ambulate.

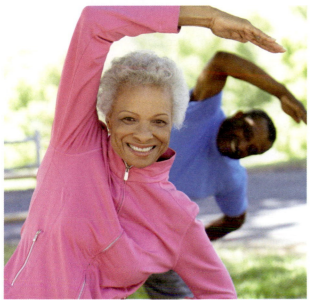

Fig. 23-3. Exercise programs are very important for residents with diabetes. They help to increase circulation and maintain a healthy weight.

G Report complaints of pain, numbness, or tingling in the arms or legs immediately.

G Perform foot care carefully and as directed. Report any changes in the feet. Do not clip or trim the resident's toenails. A doctor will do this.

G Encourage residents to wear supportive, comfortable shoes. Shoes should fit well and not hurt the feet. Shoes made of material that breathes, such as leather, cotton, or canvas, help prevent moisture buildup. Socks made of natural fibers such as cotton or wool are best because they absorb sweat. Residents with diabetes should not go barefoot or wear tight clothing on the legs and feet.

G Carefully following dietary instructions is very important to help manage diabetes. Meals must be served at the same time every day. Meals and snacks, including protein shakes and other supplements, must be completely consumed in order to keep blood sugar stable. Document intake accurately. Always report to the nurse if meals and snacks are not being eaten. Report if visitors bring snacks or treats to residents.

G The American Diabetes Association (ADA) recommends that people with diabetes work with a registered dietitian nutritionist (RDN) or a certified diabetes educator (CDE) to help develop individualized meal plans. The ADA's website, diabetes.org, contains many ideas for planning meals.

G Keep track of any special tests the resident may have. Tests can affect diet and insulin dosage. If a resident is fasting for a blood test, for example, food and insulin may need to be withheld until after the test is completed. Notify the nurse immediately when the test has been completed.

G Perform blood glucose tests only as directed and if trained. Not all states allow NAs to perform this testing. Follow facility policy.

G Insulin dosage is based upon a variety of factors. Balancing factors like caloric intake, metabolism, exercise levels, stress levels, and the relative condition of the resident is important. Report if the resident is not following the care plan exactly.

G If any of the following occurs, notify the nurse:

• Any sign of skin breakdown anywhere on the body, especially on the feet and toes

• Visual changes, especially blurred vision

• Changes in appetite or increased thirst

• Fruity or sweet-smelling breath

• Weight change

• Nausea or vomiting

• Change in urine output, any signs of urinary tract infection, fruity or sweet-smelling urine

- Changes in mobility
- Numbness or tingling in the arms or legs
- Nervousness or anxiety
- Dizziness or loss of coordination
- Irritability or confusion

Blood Glucose Monitoring

Depending on state requirements, NAs may assist the nurse with blood glucose monitoring or may receive special training on how to do this themselves. The blood glucose meter measures the level of glucose in a person's blood at any given time. Normal fasting blood glucose for a person who does not have diabetes is from 70 to 100 mg/dL (milligrams per deciliter). Fasting blood glucose for a person who has diabetes is 126 mg/dL or higher. Strips are used, along with a blood glucose meter, a special glucose monitoring machine (Fig. 23-4). The strips must not have expired. The NA should always wear gloves when assisting with this procedure. Sharps must be handled and discarded properly (Chapter 6).

The A1C (also known as *HbA1c* or *glycated hemoglobin*) and estimated average glucose (eAG) tests are used to help track and regulate glucose levels. The A1C level provides information on blood glucose over two to three months and may be tested twice a year or more. Normal A1C is considered below 5.7%. A1C ranges between 5.7 and 6.4% when a person has prediabetes and is 6.5 % or higher when diabetes is present. The eAG number is calculated using the A1C result. However, the eAG is shown in milligrams per deciliter (mg/dL).

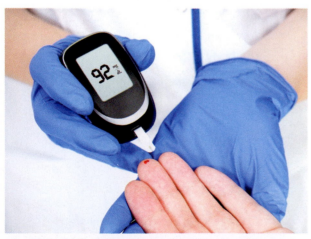

Fig. 23-4. A blood glucose meter is one type of equipment used to measure glucose levels in the blood.

6. Discuss foot care guidelines for diabetes

Quality foot care is vital for people with diabetes. Diabetes weakens the immune system, which reduces resistance to infections. Poor circulation due to the narrowing of the blood vessels also increases the risk of infection. Infections of the feet, when noted in the early stages, can be treated successfully. However, when foot infections are not caught early, they can take months to heal. If wounds do not heal, amputation of a toe, an entire foot, or a leg may be necessary.

Foot care to prevent infection should be a part of daily care of residents and is required by CMS. Keeping the feet clean and dry is a way to help prevent complications. It is important that NAs observe the feet carefully during care.

Guidelines: Safe Diabetic Foot Care

G Inspect and clean resident's feet every day during bathing. Make sure to check the entire foot and between the toes. See the list at the end of these guidelines for items to observe and report to the nurse.

G Avoid harsh soaps and hot water when bathing feet. Use only warm water and mild soaps.

G Always dry feet thoroughly, especially between toes. Do not rub the skin; pat it dry.

G Never cut toenails, corns, or calluses for any reason.

G Do not use any object, such as a nail stick, to try to remove dirt from a toenail.

G Use a doctor-recommended cream or lotion on the feet, but do not apply anything between the toes. Do not use powders. Make sure the feet are completely dry after applying lotion or cream.

G Check shoes for rocks or other objects before putting them on residents.

G Remind residents not to walk around barefoot. Always use clean cotton socks with comfortable shoes or nonskid slippers. Do not turn socks down at the top, as this can decrease circulation. Make sure shoes fit properly.

G If any of the following occurs, notify the nurse:

- Painful, tender, soft, or fragile areas, or burning in the feet

- Rashes or bruises

- Change in color of the skin or nails, especially reddening or blackening

- Change in the temperature of the skin

- Excessive dryness of the skin of the feet

- Breaks or tears in the skin

- Drainage or bleeding on the feet or toes

- Corns, blisters, calluses, or warts

- Ingrown toenails

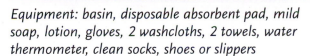

Providing foot care for a resident with diabetes

Equipment: basin, disposable absorbent pad, mild soap, lotion, gloves, 2 washcloths, 2 towels, water thermometer, clean socks, shoes or slippers

1. Identify yourself by name. Identify the resident. Greet the resident by name.

2. Wash your hands.

3. Explain procedure to the resident. Speak clearly, slowly, and directly. Maintain face-to-face contact whenever possible.

4. Provide for the resident's privacy with a curtain, screen, or door.

5. If the resident is in bed, adjust the bed to its lowest position. Lock bed wheels.

6. Fill the basin halfway with warm water. Test the water temperature with a thermometer or against the inside of your wrist. Water

temperature should be no higher than 105°F. Have the resident check water temperature to see if it is comfortable. Adjust if necessary.

7. Place the basin on a disposable absorbent pad (protective barrier) on the floor, at a comfortable position for the resident. If the resident cannot sit up on the side of the bed to do this, place the basin on the pad at the foot of the bed. Support the foot and ankle throughout the procedure.

8. Put on gloves.

9. Remove the resident's socks. Completely submerge the resident's feet in water. Soak the feet for 15 to 20 minutes.

10. Put soap on a wet washcloth. Remove one foot from the water. Wash the entire foot gently, including between the toes and around nail beds (Fig. 23-5).

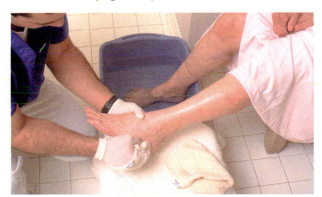

Fig. 23-5. While supporting the foot and ankle, wash the entire foot with a soapy washcloth.

11. Rinse the entire foot, including between the toes.

12. With a clean, dry towel or washcloth, pat the foot dry gently, including between the toes.

13. Repeat steps 10 through 12 for the other foot.

14. Put lotion in one hand. Warm the lotion by rubbing your hands together.

15. Starting at the toes and working up to the ankles, gently rub lotion into the feet with circular strokes. Do not put lotion between

the toes. Remove excess lotion (if any) with a towel or washcloth. Make sure lotion has been absorbed and the feet are completely dry.

16. Observe the feet, ankles, and legs carefully, checking for things like dry skin, skin tears, red areas, corns, blisters, calluses, warts, rashes, or bruises.

17. Help the resident put on clean socks and shoes or slippers.

18. Empty, rinse, and dry basin. Place basin in the designated dirty supply area or return to storage, depending on facility policy.

19. Place soiled linen in the proper container.

20. Remove and discard gloves properly. Wash your hands.

21. Make the resident comfortable.

22. Remove privacy measures.

23. Leave call light within the resident's reach.

24. Wash your hands.

25. Be courteous and respectful at all times.

26. Report any changes in the resident to the nurse. Document procedure using facility guidelines.

Chapter Review

1. List four functions of the endocrine system (LO 2).

2. List three normal age-related changes of the endocrine system (LO 3).

3. What are three conditions that make it more likely for a person to develop diabetes (LO 4)?

Multiple Choice

4. Which form of diabetes is the most common (LO 4)?
   (A) Prediabetes
   (B) Type 1 diabetes
   (C) Type 2 diabetes
   (D) Diabetes mellitus

5. What is a common symptom of hypothyroidism (LO 4)?
   (A) Rapid heartbeat
   (B) Weight gain
   (C) High blood pressure
   (D) Bulging eyes

6. Which of the following is an appropriate guideline for a resident who has diabetes (LO 5)?
   (A) The resident will need to eat meals at the same time every day.
   (B) The resident will need to avoid exercising.
   (C) The NA will need to trim and clean the resident's toenails.
   (D) The resident should go barefoot to avoid having material against his feet.

7. Which of the following should an NA do when giving foot care to a resident with diabetes (LO 6)?
   (A) The NA should use hot water to kill bacteria on the feet.
   (B) The NA should massage lotion in between the resident's toes to keep the area soft.
   (C) The NA should use clippers to remove corns or calluses.
   (D) The NA should pat the feet completely dry after washing them.

24
The Immune and Lymphatic Systems and Cancer

The Amazing Phagocytes

Elie Metchnikoff (1845–1916), a Russian zoologist and microbiologist, discovered that bacteria could be destroyed by certain cells that seemed to consume or "eat" them. He called these cells *phagocytes* (from the Greek meaning "devouring cells") and named the process *phagocytosis*. This process is an important part of the immune system's response to harmful bacteria. He won the Nobel Prize in 1908 for this discovery.

"Healing is a matter of time, but it is sometimes also a matter of opportunity."

Hippocrates, 460–377 B.C.

"There are some remedies worse than the disease."

Publilius Syrus, circa 42 B.C.

1. Define important words in this chapter

acquired immunodeficiency syndrome (AIDS): the final stage of HIV infection, in which infections, tumors, and central nervous system symptoms appear due to a weakened immune system that is unable to fight infection.

autoimmune disease: a disease in which the body is unable to recognize its own tissues and begins to attack these tissues.

benign: noncancerous.

biopsy: the removal of a sample of tissue for examination and diagnosis.

breakthrough pain: a type of severe pain that happens unexpectedly in people who have cancer.

cancer: a general term used to describe a disease in which abnormal cells grow in an uncontrolled way.

homophobia: a fear of homosexuality.

human immunodeficiency virus (HIV): a virus that attacks the body's immune system and gradually disables it; eventually can cause AIDS.

lymph: a clear yellowish fluid that carries disease-fighting cells called lymphocytes.

malignant: cancerous.

metastasize: to spread from one part of the body to another.

opportunistic infection: an illness caused by microorganisms that do not affect people with healthy immune systems but cause disease in people with weakened immune systems.

remission: the disappearance of signs and symptoms of cancer or other diseases; can be temporary or permanent.

tumor: a group of abnormally growing cells.

2. Explain the structure and function of the immune and lymphatic systems

The Immune System

The immune system protects the body from harmful substances, such as disease-causing bacteria, viruses, and microorganisms. There are two types of immunity: nonspecific immunity and specific immunity.

Nonspecific immunity is present at birth. It protects the body from disease in general. Nonspecific immunity is the first line of defense against invading bacteria or organisms. When foreign materials try to enter the body, it produces a response in which additional white blood cells begin fighting against the disease-causing organisms. Examples of things within the body that help nonspecific immunity are intact (unbroken) skin, saliva, mucous membranes, and tears. The inflammatory response, including redness, swelling, heat, and pain, is another defense. This response removes foreign toxins and other materials and begins tissue repair. Fever can also help fight infection.

Specific immunity is a type of immunity that is acquired by the body. Specific immunity is either active or passive. In active immunity, the body manufactures antibodies as a response to an antigen, or foreign substance, in the body. For example, when a person gets chickenpox (varicella-zoster virus), antibodies are created. The body will then "remember" the pathogen each time it is exposed to it in the future. The second time the virus tries to invade the body, the antibodies that formed during the first illness work to prevent a second infection.

Active immunity is also acquired by a vaccine. Vaccines cause the body to produce antibodies to protect against a particular disease. These antibodies will usually protect the person from getting the disease in the future. Vaccines help people develop immunity to diseases without first having the disease. Vaccines can be made with live organisms or with organisms killed by heat or chemicals.

With passive immunity, a person is given the antibodies needed to defend against the antigen. The antibodies can be passed from mother to baby or via an injection. Passive immunity is temporary because the antibodies have a limited life span.

The Lymphatic System

The lymphatic system is composed of the lymph, lymph vessels, lymph nodes, spleen, and thymus gland. The lymphatic system produces and moves lymph fluid from the body's tissues to the circulatory system. The lymphatic system works to remove excess fluids and waste products from the tissues. It transports fat and vitamins from the gastrointestinal tract to the circulatory system. The lymphatic system also helps the immune system fight infection.

Lymph is a clear yellowish fluid that moves into the lymph system from the tiny capillaries in the circulatory system. Lymph carries disease-fighting cells called lymphocytes. The lymph fluid flows in only one direction.

Lymphatic vessels, or capillaries, are tiny vessels found all over the body. They carry the lymph from the tissues into larger lymphatic vessels. While in the vessels, the lymph travels through and is filtered by the lymph nodes. The larger lymphatic vessels transport lymph into the lymph ducts, from which the lymph drains back into the blood.

The lymph nodes are clumps of lymphatic tissue found in groups along the lymph vessels. These nodes work as filters to clean the lymph fluid of microorganisms, such as bacteria, along with other foreign substances. Lymph nodes are strategically located in places where pathogens can be trapped and prevented from harming the body (Fig. 24-1). Tonsils are large clumps of lymphatic tissue at the back of the oral cavity at the entrance to the throat (pharynx). Tonsils work to prevent microorganisms from entering the body, especially through the mouth or nose.

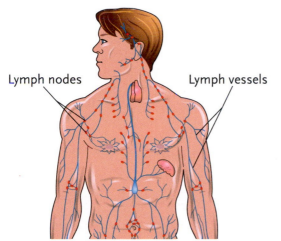

Fig. 24-1. *Lymph nodes work as filters and are located throughout the body.*

The spleen is an organ that contains the biggest cluster of lymph tissue in the human body. One of its main functions is as a type of storage shed for blood. The spleen works as a filter to clean old red blood cells and bacteria from the blood.

The thymus gland is located in the upper chest, just behind the sternum. Its duty is to make T-cells, or CD4+ lymphocytes, which attack and destroy specific types of pathogens. The thymus reaches its greatest size at puberty and shrinks as a person becomes an adult. Once its work is completed, the gland turns into fat and other tissue.

The functions of the immune and lymphatic systems are to

- Protect against the invasion of foreign substances and pathogens

- Return extra fluid to the circulatory system

- Store blood for future needs

- Remove excess fluids and waste products from the tissues

Destination: Homeostasis

A hemorrhage is an excessive, sudden loss of blood that occurs either externally or internally. When a hemorrhage occurs, the spleen readies for action.

The blood that the spleen has held for the body in its reservoir (as much as a full pint or more), is released into the bloodstream. This release of blood helps the body's blood supply and blood pressure return to normal. When bleeding has stopped and the body's blood supply and blood pressure have returned to normal levels, homeostasis is restored.

Tip

Allergies and Anaphylaxis

Allergies occur in people who are hypersensitive to a foreign substance called an allergen. Examples of allergens include pollen, dust, molds, colognes, animals, latex, and certain foods. The immune system responds to the allergen by releasing histamine and other substances that cause the characteristic runny nose and watery eyes. Allergens can sometimes trigger a life-threatening response, called *anaphylaxis*, *anaphylactic reaction*, or *anaphylactic shock*. The bronchi narrow, causing wheezing and difficulty breathing. Loss of consciousness and death may result if not treated immediately with an injection of a medication called epinephrine (often into the thigh). Some people who have allergies carry epinephrine auto-injectors with them. Other treatments may be administered as well, such as oxygen and CPR.

3. Discuss changes in the immune and lymphatic systems due to aging

Normal age-related changes for the immune and lymphatic systems include the following:

- Immune system weakens, causing increased risk of all types of infections.

- Antibody response slows.

- T-cells decrease in number.

- Response to vaccines decreases.

4. Describe a common disorder of the immune system

Acquired Immunodeficiency Syndrome (AIDS)

Acquired immunodeficiency syndrome (AIDS) is a disease caused by the **human immunodeficiency virus (HIV)**. HIV attacks the body's immune system and damages or destroys its cells. HIV gradually weakens and disables the immune system. AIDS is caused by acquiring HIV through blood or body fluids from an infected person. AIDS is the final stage of HIV infection in which infections, tumors, and central nervous system symptoms appear, due to a weakened immune system that is unable to fight infection. It can take years for HIV to develop into AIDS.

Specific behaviors put people at high risk for acquiring HIV. HIV is most commonly transmitted by the following:

- Having unprotected or poorly protected anal sex with an infected person
- Having unprotected or poorly protected vaginal sex with an infected person
- Having sexual contact with many partners
- Sharing drug needles or syringes

In the healthcare setting, infections can be spread through accidental contact with contaminated blood or body fluids, needles or other sharp objects, or contaminated supplies or equipment. The Occupational Safety and Health Administration (OSHA) requires that healthcare facilities provide safety equipment for staff members to prevent exposure to bloodborne pathogens.

Common Misconceptions about HIV Transmission

HIV cannot survive outside the body for very long. According to the Centers for Disease Control and Prevention (CDC), HIV is not spread in any of these ways:

- Through air or water
- By pets or insects, including mosquitoes
- In saliva, tears, or sweat
- Through casual contact, such as hugging, shaking hands, sharing dishes, or touching doorknobs or toilet seats
- Through closed-mouth or casual kissing, such as kissing someone's cheek

Ways to prevent HIV infection and protect against the spread of HIV and AIDS include the following:

- Following Standard Precautions at work
- Handling and disposing of any type of sharps properly
- Covering cuts, sores, tears, breaks, or rashes before caring for residents
- Never sharing needles or syringes
- Not having unprotected sex (always using condoms during sexual contact)
- Staying in a monogamous relationship (being monogamous means having only one sexual partner)
- Practicing abstinence (abstinence means not having sexual contact with anyone)
- Getting tested for HIV and retested if necessary. (HIV is able to be detected in most people within three to eight weeks after exposure. However, it can take up to three months for HIV to be able to be detected and up to six months in rare cases.)
- Following the pre-exposure prophylaxis (PrEP) approach, which involves taking a specific medication every day to lower an uninfected person's risk of getting HIV

The beginning stages of HIV involve flu-like symptoms along with swollen glands. Symptoms like headache, fever, fatigue, and swollen lymph glands can appear, last for a few months, and then disappear. Additional symptoms may appear soon after, or they can take many years to develop.

Over time, HIV destroys the type of white blood cells called T-cells. Specifically, the virus reduces the number of T-cells that work to fight infections in the body. This weakens the immune system and makes the person more susceptible to illness. The diagnosis of AIDS is made when a person's T-cell count falls to 200 or below. At this point, the infected person will normally show symptoms, conditions, and diseases that are consistent with a diagnosis of AIDS.

Signs and symptoms of HIV infection and AIDS include the following:

- Flu-like symptoms, including fever, cough, and severe or constant fatigue
- Headaches
- Blurred vision
- Loss of appetite
- Nausea and vomiting
- Weight loss
- Night sweats
- Shaking, chills
- Dry cough
- Shortness of breath
- Swollen lymph nodes
- Sore throat
- Cold sores or fever blisters on the lips
- Mouth sores
- White patches in the mouth or on the tongue
- Cauliflower-like warts on the skin and in the mouth
- Bleeding, inflamed gums
- Yeast infections
- Skin rashes or sores
- Bruising that does not go away
- Dry skin
- Memory loss

Other diseases can develop in people who have AIDS. Due to the weakened immune system, opportunistic infections can occur and may be fatal. An **opportunistic infection** is an illness caused by microorganisms that do not affect people with healthy immune systems but cause disease in people with weakened immune systems.

Other diseases that can develop in people with AIDS are *Pneumocystis jiroveci* pneumonia (PJP), a lung infection, and cryptococcal meningitis, a nervous system disorder. Tuberculosis, herpes, bacterial infections, and hepatitis can also result.

People with AIDS can also develop certain types of cancers. Cervical cancer and a form of cancer called *Kaposi's sarcoma* are examples. Kaposi's sarcoma is a form of skin cancer that appears as purple, red, or brown skin lesions. The lesions may be painful.

In the late stages of AIDS, a form of dementia called *AIDS dementia complex* (*ADC*) can develop due to damage to the central nervous system. Symptoms of ADC include memory loss, limited attention span, irritability, poor coordination, lack of judgment, withdrawal from social situations, and depression.

There is no cure for this disease, and there is no vaccine to prevent the disease. People who are infected with HIV are treated with drugs that slow the progress of the disease. Without medication, the HIV-infected person's weakened resistance to infections may lead to AIDS and eventually to death.

Many people are living longer with HIV by taking combinations of medications every day. HAART, or highly active antiretroviral therapy, has been shown to control HIV. Three or more medications are used for this therapy.

Treatments used for HIV must be taken at specific times throughout the day. They have many unpleasant side effects. Gastrointestinal symptoms like nausea, vomiting, and diarrhea, as well as fever and skin rashes, are some of the side effects. Certain medications can be effective, but the length of time they will continue to work for each infected person varies.

Here are a few additional resources for information relating to immune system disorders:

- AIDSinfo, a service of the U.S. Department of Health and Human Services, aidsinfo.nih.gov

- Centers for Disease Control and Prevention, cdc.gov/hiv
- American Cancer Society, cancer.org

Obesity and Disorders of the Immune System

Obesity increases the risk for certain immune system diseases or disorders, including the following:

- Kidney, prostate, breast, endometrial, and ovarian cancers

Autoimmune Diseases

The immune system protects the body from microorganisms and toxic substances. With an **autoimmune disease**, the body is unable to recognize its own tissue. The immune mechanism sees the normal body tissues as foreign and begins to attack these tissues.

Types of organs and tissues that may be affected by this disease are blood cells, the pancreas, the joints, and the skin. Examples of autoimmune diseases are systemic lupus erythematosis (SLE) and rheumatoid arthritis (RA) (Chapter 21).

Some causes of autoimmune diseases are genetics, specific microorganisms, and medications. Treatment depends upon the disorder but include medications, hormone supplements, blood transfusions, and insulin.

5. Discuss infection prevention guidelines for a resident with HIV/AIDS

Overall care of a resident who has HIV/AIDS involves protecting him from infections, managing his symptoms, providing a safe environment, and offering him emotional support.

Guidelines: Infection Prevention for HIV/AIDS

G Follow Standard Precautions. You cannot tell by looking at someone whether or not he has a bloodborne disease. Follow Transmission-Based Precautions in addition to Standard Precautions if ordered (Chapter 6).

G Cover all open sores, cuts, abrasions, rashes, or skin breaks or tears with appropriate bandages or dressings before performing care.

Notify the nurse if you have cuts, sores, or breaks in the skin before beginning care.

G Wear gloves and other personal protective equipment (PPE), such as goggles, if you anticipate having contact with blood or other body fluids that might contain blood, like urine and feces. Wear goggles, masks, and/or face shields if splashes or spills may occur.

G Wash hands and any other areas of the body immediately after contact with blood or other body fluids.

G Handle sharps carefully. Dispose of all sharps properly and safely. Never attempt to recap sharps.

G Remind residents and visitors to wash their hands frequently to avoid infection.

G Do not share residents' personal items, such as toothbrushes, hairbrushes, razors, etc., with other residents. Clean and store equipment, following facility policy, after it has been used.

G Properly disinfect surfaces soiled with blood or body fluids according to facility policy.

Residents' Rights

HIV Testing and Confidentiality

The right to confidentiality is especially important to people with HIV/AIDS because others may pass judgment on people with this disease. A person cannot be fired from a job because of the disease; however, a healthcare worker with HIV/AIDS may be reassigned to job duties with a lower risk of transmitting the disease and a reduced risk of acquiring certain infections from patients.

HIV testing requires consent. That means no one can force a person to be tested for HIV unless he agrees. HIV test results are confidential and should not be shared with a person's family, friends, or employer without consent. If a nursing assistant is HIV-positive, he should consider confiding in his supervisor so his assignments can be adjusted to avoid increased risk for exposure to infections. Everyone has a right to privacy regarding their health status. An NA should not discuss a resident's status with anyone except care team members who are directly involved with the resident's care.

6. Discuss care guidelines for a resident with HIV/AIDS

Helping residents with HIV or AIDS avoid infection and live safely and comfortably is important. An NA's careful care and attention may positively impact residents who have this disease.

Guidelines: HIV/AIDS

G Wash your hands often and help residents to wash their hands.

G Disinfect surfaces in the resident's room and bathroom often.

G Protect the resident from people who have known contagious diseases, including the common cold virus.

G Change linen whenever it is soiled. Linen should be clean and dry and should lie flat, without wrinkles.

G Observe the skin closely for skin changes. Keeping skin clean and dry will help prevent skin breakdown. Follow the care plan on the use of soaps and other cleansers.

G Change position at least every two hours or as directed. Be careful when moving and positioning residents to prevent bruising.

G Give back rubs for comfort.

G Monitor vital signs often, especially temperature. Fever can occur with infections.

G Residents with HIV/AIDS may have fatigue and severe weakness. Allow enough rest and recognize limitations.

G Encourage residents to be as independent as possible.

G Ambulate carefully. Provide assistance as needed.

G Allow plenty of time to perform activities of daily living (ADLs), and help as needed.

G Perform range of motion exercises as ordered (Chapter 25).

G Give mouth care frequently. Special mouth rinses may be ordered for mouth sores.

G Use special soft toothbrushes or swabs when cleaning the mouth and performing oral care.

G Carefully measure weight and intake and output.

G Because weight loss is a problem for people with HIV/AIDS, special diets may be ordered to assist with maintaining or gaining weight. For example, a high-calorie diet can help maintain weight. Report to the nurse if a resident does not seem to be eating or enjoying his food.

G Special diets may also be ordered to help prevent complications. For example, a high-fiber diet may aggravate diarrhea, so fiber will be reduced or eliminated in the diet. Soft or pureed foods may be easier to swallow for residents who have mouth infections. Cool or warm (not hot) food may be easier to eat. Eliminating spices and foods high in acids may be ordered. Encourage residents to follow their special diets.

G Encourage fluids. Purified water may be ordered by the doctor. If so, make sure the resident does not drink regular water or fluids made with regular water, such as tea. Do not use ice made from regular water.

G Small meals given throughout the day can help nausea, vomiting, and diarrhea. Extra fluids may be ordered to help replace fluid lost. A BRAT (bananas, rice, applesauce, and toast) diet can also help diarrhea.

G People with AIDS are prone to having diarrhea. Offer a trip to the bathroom or bedpan as often as needed.

G Give emotional support, as well as physical care. A resident who has AIDS may have been abandoned by family or friends due to the fear of the disease itself. Some people avoid a person with AIDS due to **homophobia**, or a fear of homosexuality. They may also have lost friends who have died from AIDS.

Emotions the resident may be experiencing include anxiety, stress, fear, guilt, sadness, depression, and loneliness. It is important to treat residents with respect and help provide the emotional support they need. Listen if the resident wants to talk.

G   Other support systems include family, friends, and the person's clergyperson, along with various HIV/AIDS support groups. Special religious or community groups may be of assistance. Depending on your community, many resources and services may be available. These include counseling, meal services, access to experimental drugs, and other services. Look online for resources available in your area (AIDS.gov is one resource), or speak to your supervisor if you feel a resident needs additional help. Report any comments about suicide immediately to the nurse.

G   Notify the nurse if any of the following occurs:

- Changes in vital signs, especially fever

- Loss of appetite; nausea, vomiting, or diarrhea

- Reduced intake of fluids

- Weight loss

- Dysphagia (difficulty swallowing)

- Mouth sores or discomfort

- Bruising of the skin

- Cracks, breaks, rashes, lumps, or sores anywhere on the skin

- Pressure injuries

- Bleeding from anywhere on the body

- Blood in the stool

- Nervousness, withdrawal, severe mood swings, or depression

- Any behavior that puts the resident or others at risk; suicidal comments

Residents' Rights

HIV/AIDS

NAs should not avoid residents who have HIV or AIDS. HIV/AIDS cannot be transmitted by breathing the same air as someone who is infected. These residents need the same attentive and thoughtful care that NAs give to all residents. Residents may want someone to read to them or to sit and talk with them. NAs can also help by encouraging participation in activities.

More information about HIV/AIDS may be found in Chapter 6.

7. Describe cancer

Cancer is a general term used to describe a disease in which abnormal cells grow in an uncontrolled way. These cancerous cells do not die like normal cells; they live longer and can continue to increase in number.

Cancer usually occurs in the form of a tumor that grows on or within the human body. A **tumor** is a group of abnormally growing cells. Tumors are either **benign** (noncancerous) or **malignant** (cancerous). Benign tumors grow slowly and do not spread to other parts of the body. Malignant tumors grow rapidly and invade surrounding tissue. Cancer can **metastasize** or spread from the site where it first appeared to other areas of the body.

Known causes of cancer include the following:

- Genetic factors

- Certain lifestyle choices, such as tobacco use

- Alcohol use

- Poor diet/obesity

- Lack of physical activity

- Certain infections

- Environmental exposure, such as radiation

- Sun exposure (Fig. 24-2)

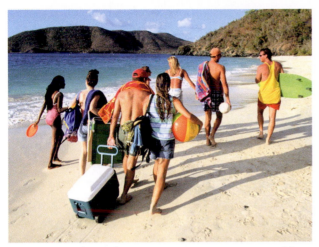

Fig. 24-2. *Prolonged sun exposure puts a person at risk for skin cancer.*

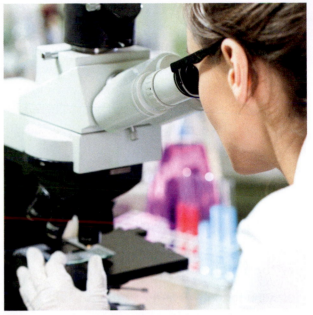

Fig. 24-3. *Tissue that is collected during a biopsy is checked for malignant cells.*

Early identification and treatment of cancer are critical factors in how the disease can progress. The American Cancer Society (ACS) has identified these signs and symptoms of cancer:

- Unexplained weight loss
- Fever
- Fatigue
- Pain
- Skin changes, such as change in skin color (e.g., reddened skin, jaundice)
- Change in bowel/bladder function
- Sores that do not heal
- White patches inside the mouth or white spots on the tongue
- Unusual bleeding or discharge
- Thickening or lump in the breast, testicle, or other part of the body
- Indigestion or difficulty swallowing
- New mole or a change in the appearance of an existing mole, wart, or spot
- Nagging cough or hoarseness

A diagnosis of cancer is made after various tests, such as a biopsy, have been performed. A **biopsy** is the removal of a sample of tissue for examination and diagnosis (Fig. 24-3).

After the diagnosis of cancer is made, the treatment plan is developed by an oncologist. Oncology is the branch of medicine that deals with the study of and treatment of cancer. Treatment is based on whether or not the cancer has spread to other parts of the body. The choice of therapy is determined by the person's prognosis, or outlook. Common treatments for cancer, which may be used in combination, are as follows:

Surgery to remove malignant tumors is performed for some types of cancer, such as breast, skin, and colon. The goal of the operation(s) is to try to remove as much of the cancer as possible.

Radiation therapy (radiotherapy) uses high-energy rays to attempt to destroy cancer cells in a specific area. It can also be used to control cancerous growths. Radiation treatments do not cause pain. However, side effects of radiation therapy include fatigue and skin irritation and burns, which may cause pain. Other side effects depend on the area being treated. Post treatment, special instructions may be given, such as short-term isolation. Radiation therapy may also cause an increased risk of infection. People undergoing this therapy might be asked to avoid others who are sick or to avoid public places.

Chemotherapy involves chemical agents or medications being administered, usually intravenously, to kill malignant cells and tissues. Chemotherapy is used to cure cancer, slow the growth of cancer, or prevent the cancer from spreading to another part of the body. There are many side effects from this treatment, including bone or joint pain, temporary hair loss, nausea and vomiting, diarrhea, fatigue, weakness, mouth sores, peripheral neuropathy (Chapter 23), anxiety, depression, and a higher risk of infections. Chemotherapeutic agents are generally given into a vein through an IV, but some are given by mouth or by injection.

Hormone therapy uses medications to alter the hormones in the body. This can be effective when the tumors rely on specific hormones to survive and grow. Hormone therapy reduces certain hormones in the body. It also changes the ability of the tumors to use the hormones. Side effects include hot flashes, weight gain, and fluid retention.

Immunotherapy (also called *biological therapy*) is another form of cancer treatment. This therapy uses the body's immune system to fight the malignant tumors. Cancer vaccines are a form of immunotherapy. Currently the only FDA-approved vaccine in the US is Provenge (sipuleucel-T). This vaccine treats advanced prostate cancer and might extend a person's life. Other vaccines, such as the HPV vaccine, may reduce the risk of certain cancers. Another form of immunotherapy is the administration of antibodies.

Immunotherapy works in different ways. One way is to interfere with the growth of cancer cells. Side effects depend upon the specific treatment used and include fatigue, muscle aches, fever, weakness, nausea, vomiting, diarrhea, and allergic reactions. This form of therapy is often combined with chemotherapy or other cancer therapies.

The goal of treating cancer is to cure the cancer, have it go into remission, or provide palliative care if it is incurable. **Remission** is the disappearance of signs and symptoms of cancer or other diseases. It can be partial or complete. A remission can be temporary or permanent.

Palliative care will be provided for someone with advanced cancer. This type of care helps to relieve symptoms and reduce pain and suffering caused by the disease. Complications are treated early, which helps reduce discomfort. Care conferences include family and friends, along with a palliative care team. This team is devoted to providing the resident with the best quality of life possible. Chapter 27 contains more information on palliative care.

8. Discuss care guidelines for a resident with cancer

A resident who has cancer will require attentive, person-centered care.

Guidelines: Cancer

G **Preventing infection**. Due to weakened immune systems, preventing infection is important. Follow Standard Precautions and keep everything clean. A resident undergoing chemotherapy may require additional precautions. Wear personal protective equipment (PPE) as required, and follow facility policies for discarding PPE and soiled linens in a biohazard container.

G **Skin care**. Observe the skin carefully to help prevent pressure injuries. Change position at least every two hours or as directed. Be careful when moving and positioning residents to reduce bruising. Follow any special skin care orders exactly (for example: no hot or cold packs; no soap, lotion, or other cosmetics; no garters or tight stockings). Special mattresses or pads used in beds and chairs can help reduce the risk of pressure injuries. Keep the skin clean and dry. Apply lotion to dry skin if ordered. Do not use lotion on areas having radiation therapy and do not remove any markings that are used with radiation therapy. Notify the nurse if you observe any signs of infection, such as swelling, warmth, redness, or draining wounds.

G **Mouth care**. Give mouth care often. Be gentle when brushing the teeth; soft brushes or special swabs can help with mouth pain or sores or lip sores. Mild mouth rinses (avoid mouthwashes) can reduce a bad taste in the mouth due to medication or vomiting.

G **Nutrition**. Proper nutrition is important for people with cancer. They need to eat and drink enough to maintain their energy levels. Unintended weight loss can occur with cancer or with cancer treatment. Provide small, frequent meals or snacks to reduce nausea and help prevent weight loss. Serving favorite foods is best; however, dairy products, spicy foods, fried foods, and high-fiber foods may need to be restricted due to nausea. Fortified liquid nutrition supplements may be used in addition to, not in place of, meals. Try cool or cold foods if hot foods increase nausea. Cut food into small pieces if necessary. Use plastic utensils if silver utensils cause a bitter taste in the mouth.

Certain foods may need to be eliminated while a person is undergoing chemotherapy due to a lowered resistance to infection. These foods may include raw or undercooked meat, eggs, seafood, or sprouts.

Weigh residents as ordered, and report weight loss or gain. Carefully monitor intake and output and report changes.

G **Bladder and bowel changes**. Urinary output may decrease, and blood may appear in the urine. Urine can become more concentrated and have an odor. Diarrhea can occur, along with blood in the stool. Assist residents to the bathroom or offer the bedpan often. Measure output as directed. Give catheter care as needed. Assist with careful perineal care as needed. Test stool as ordered for hidden (occult) blood.

G **Mobility**. People with cancer may have fatigue and weakness, which can make movement difficult. Allow plenty of time for rest and recognize limitations. Gently assist with ambulation if needed.

G **Pain**. Cancer can cause severe pain that happens unexpectedly, called **breakthrough pain**. This type of pain can occur in between doses of pain medication. It can affect the ability to sleep, eat, and move. Fast-acting medications and other measures are used to treat pain. Be alert for signs of pain and notify the nurse as soon as pain occurs. Provide comfort measures to reduce pain. Give back rubs and help residents change positions in bed or in a chair. Other techniques include playing soft music, reading, or talking quietly with residents.

Pain medications can cause side effects, including constipation, nausea, and fatigue. Notify the nurse if these side effects occur. If a resident has a transdermal patch on the skin to help with pain, report redness, swelling, irritation, or hives. A resident who has a transdermal patch will need to avoid direct exposure to heating sources like heating pads, electric blankets, and hot baths. The nurse is responsible for applying and removing these patches. Notify the nurse if you see more than one patch on a resident's body.

The resident may be using a patient-controlled analgesia (PCA) pump for pain relief. A PCA pump allows the person to press a button that releases pain medication. Observe and report redness, swelling, or warmth around the insertion site.

G **Vital signs**. Changes in vital signs can occur with cancer and with cancer therapy. Monitor all vital signs, especially temperature, and report changes to the nurse. Fever can occur with some forms of cancer therapy. Do not apply a blood pressure cuff on a swollen extremity due to lymphedema (a collection of lymph in the tissues). Do not measure blood pressure on the side of the body that has had surgery.

G **Self-image**. Hair loss, weakness, changed appearance, and dependency on caregivers can change a person's self-image. Help residents stay clean and well-groomed. Offer wigs, scarves, or hats for hair loss. Assist with application of makeup as requested.

G **Mental status and emotional needs**. Some people with cancer want to talk about their diagnosis and treatment; others withdraw and avoid discussing their disease. Be sensitive to this and follow residents' wishes. Listen and allow them to express their feelings. Spend as much time with residents as possible. Encourage involvement in activities if possible. There are many support groups available for people with cancer. The nurse can ask the social worker to help the resident contact a support group. When talking with residents, do not use clichés (phrases used over and over again that do not really mean anything) such as, "You will be just fine." Provide support during painful episodes and difficult times. Remind residents that there can still be good days and special times ahead (Fig. 24-4). Observe and report signs of depression, including comments about suicide.

G Notify the nurse if any of the following occurs:

- Pain or increased pain
- Changes in vital signs, especially fever
- Signs of any new bumps or lumps or any other changes in the skin
- Rashes, cracks, sores, breaks, or reddened areas on the skin
- Burns or skin irritation

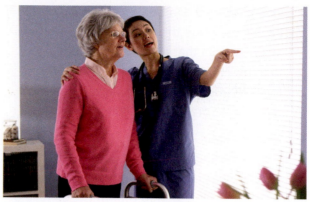

Fig. 24-4. *Have a positive attitude when spending time with a resident who has cancer. For example, comment if the sun is shining brightly outside or if a resident seems stronger that day.*

- Bruising of the skin
- Dry, sore mouth and mouth or lip sores
- Inflammation or irritation of the mucous membranes in the mouth
- Bleeding from the gums or anywhere inside the mouth
- Nausea or vomiting
- Flatus, diarrhea, or constipation
- Blood in the stool
- Appetite changes or weight loss
- Difficulty chewing or swallowing
- Change in output
- Any change in urine or blood in the urine
- Signs of urinary tract infection
- Odors
- Difficulty with ambulation
- Increased fatigue or weakness
- Fainting
- Chest pain or tightness
- Shortness of breath
- Anxiety, fear, or anger
- Change in mental status or confusion
- Signs of depression
- Suicidal comments

Residents' Rights

Cancer

The term *cancer* is frightening to some people. Understanding the facts may help lessen fears. Cancer is not a contagious disease. It cannot be transmitted through touch or hugs or by being close to a person who has the disease. NAs should not avoid residents who have cancer. Being available when residents want to talk is one way NAs can provide person-centered care.

Tip

Pets and Weakened Immune Systems

Some facilities have one or more cats and/or dogs living on the premises. Due to their weakened immune systems, people who have HIV, AIDS, cancer, or another disorders that compromise the immune system may not be able to be around pets due to the risk of different types of infection. NAs should always wash their hands with soap and water after touching a pet and before touching any resident. Visitors should do the same.

Chapter Review

1. Briefly describe nonspecific immunity and specific immunity (LO 2).

2. List four normal age-related changes of the immune and lymphatic systems (LO 3).

3. What is the difference between benign and malignant tumors (LO 7)?

Multiple Choice

4. What is one way that the human immunodeficiency virus (HIV) is transmitted (LO 4)?
   (A) By insects such as mosquitoes
   (B) By hugging an infected person
   (C) By touching a contaminated doorknob
   (D) By contact with contaminated needles

5. What is one of the NA's responsibilities when caring for a resident who has acquired immunodeficiency syndrome (AIDS) (LO 5)?
   (A) The NA should help determine when the resident should change medication.
   (B) The NA should inform others of the resident's diagnosis.
   (C) The NA should help protect the resident from infections.
   (D) The NA should help keep the resident as isolated as possible.

6. A diet that is low in _____ may help residents who have diarrhea (LO 6).
   (A) Fiber
   (B) Fluids
   (C) Bananas
   (D) Applesauce

7. Which type of treatment for cancer involves using high-energy rays to attempt to destroy cancer cells in a specific area (LO 7)?
   (A) Immunotherapy
   (B) Radiation therapy
   (C) Chemotherapy
   (D) Surgery

8. If a resident with cancer expresses fear about her condition, which of the following would be the best response by the NA (LO 8)?
   (A) "Every cloud has a silver lining."
   (B) "Good things come to those who wait."
   (C) "It will be over before you know it."
   (D) "I understand you're scared. How can I help?"

25 Rehabilitation and Restorative Care

A View from the Past: Rehabilitation

In 1918 there were many injured veterans returning to the US from World War I (WWI). Doctors developed a type of care that would enable an injured person to be able to return to work. Following WWI, ideas about rehabilitation grew. Facilities and programs were created, and when the thousands of victims of the war returned to the US (many without arms or legs), they were able to begin their rehabilitation.

"You cannot run away from a weakness. You must some time fight it out or perish."

Robert Louis Stevenson, 1850–1894

"The best of healers is good cheer."

Pindar, 522–438 B.C.

1. Define important words in this chapter

abduction: moving a body part away from the midline of the body.

active assisted range of motion (AAROM): exercises to put a joint through its full arc of motion that are done by a resident with some assistance from a staff member.

active range of motion (AROM): exercises to put a joint through its full arc of motion that are done by a resident himself, without help.

adduction: moving a body part toward the midline of the body.

assistive devices: special equipment that helps a person who is ill or disabled perform activities of daily living.

dorsiflexion: bending backward.

extension: straightening a body part.

flexion: bending a body part.

foot drop: weakness of muscles in the feet and ankles that interferes with the ability to flex the ankles and walk normally.

hyperextension: extending a joint beyond its normal range of motion.

opposition: touching the thumb to any other finger.

orthotic devices: devices applied externally to limbs to support, protect, improve function, and prevent complications.

passive range of motion (PROM): exercises to put a joint through its full arc of motion that are done by a staff member, without the resident's help.

physiatrists: doctors who specialize in rehabilitation.

pronation: turning downward.

range of motion (ROM): exercises that put a joint through its full arc of motion.

rehabilitation: care that is managed by professionals to restore a person to the highest possible level of functioning after an illness or injury.

restorative care: care given after rehabilitation to maintain a person's function and increase independence.

rotation: turning the joint.

supination: turning upward.

2. Discuss rehabilitation and restorative care

A disability results from physical, personal, and environmental factors that, when combined, limit a person's ability to function properly. When a person develops a change in her ability to function, rehabilitation may be necessary. **Rehabilitation** is care used to restore a person to her highest level of functioning possible after an accident, illness, or injury. Rehabilitation revolves around person-centered, holistic (treating the whole person) care. All of the resident's individual needs, preferences, and capabilities are assessed, and a plan is formulated. The amount of progress made with rehabilitive and restorative programs depends upon many factors, including the following:

- How soon rehabilitation began

- Any preexisting diseases or injuries that the resident may have

- The resident's overall motivation

- Type of facility where the resident is living

- Combined efforts of the staff and the resident's family and friends

- Attitude of the rehabilitation team

- Consistency in following the care plan

For rehabilitation to succeed, all staff members must work together to return the resident to her highest level of functioning. The rehabilitation team consists of highly skilled and trained professionals, including the following (Fig. 25-1):

- **Physiatrists** (doctors who specialize in rehabilitation) and other doctors

- Speech-language pathologists and physical and occupational therapists

- Nurses

- Social workers

- Discharge planners

- Nursing assistants

- Resident

- Resident's family and friends

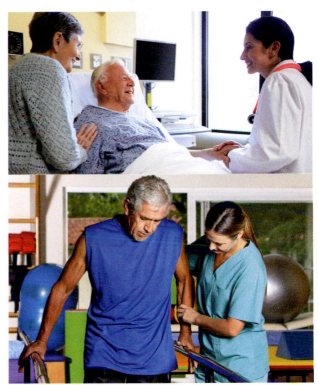

Fig. 25-1. *A team of specialists, including doctors, nurses, physical therapists, and other kinds of therapists, helps assist residents with rehabilitation.*

The nursing staff will develop a care plan based on goals for restoring and maintaining the resident's function as well as for providing person-centered care. Each body system will be considered when creating the care plan. For example, the team will work to prevent contractures, a musculoskeletal condition and a serious complication of immobility. In addition, the resident's individuality, choices, and abilities will be taken into account.

Goal-setting is done with the participation of all departments. For each task requiring improvement, the team will develop specific steps to meet the goals. The rehabilitation team will carefully follow the goals listed in each resident's care plan. The goals of rehabilitative care include the following:

- Assist the resident in maintaining and/or regaining the ability to perform activities of daily living (ADLs)

- Promote resident's independence and help resident adapt to the new disability

- Prevent complications of immobility

Nursing assistants are vital members of the rehabilitation team. The Omnibus Budget Reconciliation Act (OBRA) states that NAs must be properly trained to work with residents who are in a rehabilitative setting. Not only will they provide quality physical care, but they will also help with the resident's emotional needs. NAs should work to make the environment as safe and secure for the resident as possible.

When the goals of rehabilitation have been met, restorative care may be ordered. **Restorative care** may also be ordered when rehabilitation is not an option for a resident and/or when restorative needs arise during a resident's length of stay. Restorative care works to maintain a person's functioning, to improve his quality of life, and to increase independence. Restorative care programs include help with the following:

- Elimination
- Range of motion exercises
- Positioning
- Mobility and ambulation
- Transferring
- ...ooming
- ...d drinking
- ...aces
- ...ication

The care and services residents receive are planned to improve their quality of life. The attitude of staff members has a great impact on the success of the program. During rehabilitation and restorative care, the team should work together to prevent complications. Residents must retain their independence to the extent possible.

Guidelines: Rehabilitation and Restorative Care

G   Understand the diagnosis and the disability. Know any limitations the resident may have. Be familiar with the resident's ability to perform activities of daily living (ADLs). OBRA requires that residents must receive all of the therapy listed in the care plan each day.

G   Be patient with the resident and his family and friends. Offer praise frequently, even if the improvement is small. For example, a resident can hold a spoon on Monday. On Tuesday, he is able to lift the spoon. Praise each success.

G   Maintain a positive attitude at all times. Be empathetic. An optimistic and positive attitude is a key to success (Fig. 25-2). Never become frustrated or angry with the resident or his family or friends. The nursing staff should serve as positive role models.

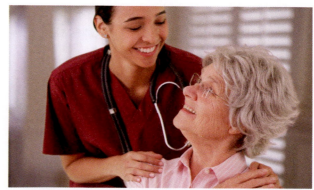

Fig. 25-2. *Being optimistic and encouraging can have a positive effect on residents.*

G   Spend as much time as possible listening to the resident's thoughts and feelings about the process. Sitting quietly and listening can be very helpful.

G Provide plenty of privacy while working with residents. Privacy helps to avoid distractions and promotes dignity.

G Encourage residents' independence, along with personal choice. They must do as much for themselves as possible. Ask family and friends to encourage residents' independence, too. Residents' personal choices and preferences should be honored whenever possible. This is part of providing person-centered care. See Learning Objective 3 of this chapter for more on independence.

G Encourage activity and exercise daily, as ordered. Inactivity causes complications and can cause setbacks in rehabilitation, along with other problems. Some residents will be following exercise programs. They may include things like walking, stretching, lifting light weights, or playing active video games.

G Accept that the resident may have setbacks. Each person is different. Focus on the things that the resident can do, and not on what he cannot do.

G NAs are often the first staff members who observe a potential problem or complication with the rehabilitative process. Report any of the following signs and symptoms to the nurse:

- Any change in ability, positive or negative
- Decreased strength
- Lack of motivation
- Signs of withdrawal or depression

Residents' Rights

The Restorative Environment

A resident's surroundings are very important to the success of rehabilitation. The environment should be set up to encourage a positive outcome. The rehabilitation team should

- Create a secure, quiet, and pleasant rehabilitative environment.
- Encourage residents to make choices and decisions.

- Ensure that residents are bathed, dressed, and well groomed every day.
- Maintain privacy and allow for private visits from family and friends.
- Encourage friendly relationships between residents.
- Spend time with residents as often as possible.
- Encourage participation in appropriate activities.

3. Describe the importance of promoting independence

An injury or illness that results in a loss of function can cause dependence on others for help with daily activities. Residents may never have needed help before with bathing, dressing, eating, or other tasks during their entire adult lives. Being required to accept help with activities of daily living can cause anger, frustration, depression, and embarrassment, along with a decline in independence.

Promoting each resident's independence is an important duty of the care team and is a vital part of making rehabilitation successful. Encouraging independence has positive effects on self-image, attitude, and abilities. Sometimes it will appear easier for the NA to do things for residents, rather than allowing them to accomplish tasks independently. However, residents should do as much as they can for themselves, regardless of how long it takes or how well they do it. Even if an NA thinks she could do a task better or faster, she should be patient. Independence helps self-esteem, along with speeding recovery. Self-care also helps the body stay active and prevents complications of immobility.

Cues

A common approach to promoting independence with rehabilitative care involves using verbal or physical cues. A verbal cue is a short sequence of words that directs the person to complete a specific step. For example, the NA can say, "Take a sip of water." A physical cue is showing the person how to do the activity. For example, the NA places her hand over the resident's hand around the cup, helping him bring it to his mouth for a drink. Cues may be used with residents during rehabilitation and also for residents with other conditions, such as Alzheimer's disease. Chapters 14 and 22 contain more information on cues.

Residents' Rights

The Right to Make Choices

Residents should make as many choices as possible. They have the right to choose their food, clothing, doctors, visitors, and how to spend their time. This is not just their legal right; it also encourages independence and promotes person-centered care.

4. Explain the complications of immobility and describe how exercise helps maintain health

Activity is an essential part of a person's life. When a person becomes immobile and inactive, the body does not respond well. Complications that result from a lack of exercise and activity, organized by body system, include the following:

- Gastrointestinal: constipation

- Urinary: urinary tract infection (UTI)

- Integumentary: pressure injuries and slow-healing wounds

- Circulatory: blood clots, especially in the legs

- Respiratory: pneumonia

- Musculoskeletal: muscle atrophy and contractures

- Nervous: depression or insomnia

- Endocrine: weight gain

Just as inactivity and immobility have negative effects, regular activity and exercise have many benefits for the body:

- Gastrointestinal: promotes appetite and aids in regular elimination

- Urinary: improves elimination, helping to decrease infection

- Integumentary: improves the quality and health of the skin

- Circulatory: improves circulation

- Respiratory: reduces the chance of infections, such as pneumonia, and improves oxygen level

- Musculoskeletal: increases blood flow to the muscles and improves strength

- Nervous: improves relaxation and sleep

- Endocrine: increases metabolism, helping to maintain healthy weight

5. Describe canes, walkers, and crutches

Residents may require temporary or permanent walking aids. Canes, walkers, and crutches are assistive devices that help a person with ambulation. Chapter 11 contains information about how to assist with ambulation.

A cane is used to help with balance. It is not meant to completely support a person's weight. Residents who use a cane should be able to bear some weight on both legs, even if one leg is weaker. If one leg is weaker, the cane should be held on the stronger side. The proper height of the cane will be determined by a physical therapist. Types of canes include the C cane, the functional grip cane, and the quad cane. The C cane is a common style of cane; it is straight with a curved handle at the top (shaped like a candy cane). It has a rubber-tipped bottom to prevent slipping. A functional grip cane is like a C cane, except that it has a straight grip handle, rather than a curved one. This helps the person grip the handle better. A quad cane has four rubber-tipped feet and a rectangular base. It is able to bear more weight than the other canes (Fig. 25-3).

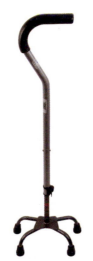

Fig. 25-3. A quad cane has four rubber-tipped feet and can bear more weight than other canes.

A walker is a type of walking aid that offers additional support and provides stability when a person is unsteady or has some weakness. Residents who use a walker should be able to bear some weight on both legs. The frame of the walker may have rubber-tipped feet and/or wheels (Fig. 25-4). Other types of walkers are designed with a seat in the back to allow a person to rest during ambulation. When using a walker, the walker is moved first, then the weak leg, then the strong leg.

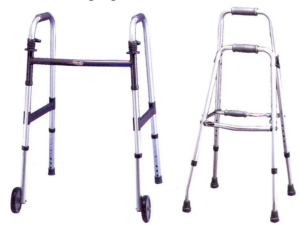

Fig. 25-4. The photo on the left shows a standard walker and the photo on the right shows a Hemi Walker, which is a walker that is designed for people who have difficulty using one arm or hand. (© INVACARE CORPORATION. USED WITH PERMISSION. WWW.INVACARE.COM)

Crutches are used when a person can only bear limited weight or cannot bear any weight at all on one leg. Crutches have rubber-tipped feet to prevent sliding. One or two crutches may be used. When a resident uses crutches, the NA should stay on the resident's weaker side.

Canes, walkers, and crutches are specially fitted to each resident. A physical therapist takes measurements for walking aids and will give instructions to residents about how to use this equipment. When helping residents, NAs should know how to assist with each device. Any questions should be directed to the nurse.

Guidelines: Canes, Walkers, and Crutches

G Carefully check the cane, walker, or crutches for any damage before using these devices. Make sure there are no cracks and that the device is not bent. Make sure any rubber pieces are snugly in place and are in good condition.

G Watch for and avoid unsafe environmental situations, such as wet floors or clutter in the hallways. Wipe up spills and keep walkways clear.

G Make sure the resident is wearing nonskid shoes with the laces tied or straps fastened. Clothing should not be so loose or long that it catches in the equipment when moving.

G Have the resident hold the cane on his stronger side.

G Do not hang heavy items on a walker.

G Encourage residents to use proper posture when walking.

G While the resident is ambulating, stay near on the weaker side.

G Do not rush the resident during ambulation.

G If the resident has pain while ambulating, move him to a chair or back to the bed, if near, then notify the nurse.

G Return the resident safely back to the bed or chair after activity is completed.

Assisting with ambulation for a resident using a cane, walker, or crutches

Equipment: transfer belt; nonskid shoes; cane, walker, or crutches

1. Identify yourself by name. Identify the resident. Greet the resident by name.

2. Wash your hands.

3. Explain procedure to the resident. Speak clearly, slowly, and directly. Maintain face-to-face contact whenever possible.

4. Provide for the resident's privacy with a curtain, screen, or door.

5. Adjust the bed to its lowest position. Lock bed wheels. Assist the resident into a sitting position with his feet flat on the floor. Adjust the bed height if needed.

6. Before ambulating, put nonskid footwear on the resident and securely fasten.

7. Stand in front of and face the resident. Stand with your feet about shoulder-width apart.

8. Place the transfer belt around the resident's waist over his clothing (not on bare skin). Check to make sure that skin or skin folds (for example, breasts) are not caught under the belt. Grasp the belt securely on both sides, with hands in an upward position.

9. If the resident is unable to stand without help, brace (support) the resident's lower extremities. This can be done by placing one or both of your knees against the resident's knees. Or you can stand toe to toe with the resident. Bend your knees and keep your back straight.

10. On the count of three, with your hands still grasping the transfer belt on both sides and moving upward, help the resident to stand.

11. Help as needed with ambulation.

a. **Cane**. Resident places the cane about six inches, or a comfortable distance, in front of his stronger leg (Fig. 25-5). He brings his weaker leg even with the cane. He then brings his stronger leg forward slightly ahead of the cane. Repeat.

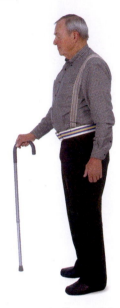

Fig. 25-5. *The cane moves in front of the stronger leg first.*

b. **Walker**. Resident picks up or rolls the walker. He places it about six inches, or a comfortable distance, in front of him. All four feet or wheels of the walker should be on the ground before the resident steps forward to the walker. The walker should not be moved again until the resident has moved both feet forward and is steady. The resident should never put his feet ahead of the walker.

c. **Crutches**. Resident should be fitted for crutches and taught to use them correctly by a physical therapist. The resident may use the crutches several different ways. It depends on his weakness. No matter how they are used, weight should be on his hands and arms. Weight should not be on the underarm area.

12. Walk slightly behind and to one side of resident for the full ordered distance, while holding onto the transfer belt. Stand on the weaker side if the resident has one.

13. Watch for obstacles in the resident's path. Ask the resident to look forward, not down at the floor, during ambulation.

14. Encourage the resident to rest if he is tired. When a person is tired, it increases the chance of a fall. Let the resident set the pace. Discuss how far he plans to go based on the care plan.

15. After ambulation, remove the transfer belt. Help the resident to the bed. Make the resident comfortable. Remove footwear. Check that the resident is in proper alignment.

16. Leave bed in its lowest position. Remove privacy measures.

17. Leave call light within resident's reach.

18. Wash your hands.

19. Be courteous and respectful at all times.

20. Report any changes in the resident to the nurse. Document procedure using facility guidelines.

Tip

Robotic Exoskeleton

The US Food and Drug Administration approved a robotic exoskeleton to allow people with spinal cord injuries to sit, stand, and walk independently. The device is worn over the legs and part of the upper body, and it requires help from someone who has been trained in its use. The device is in use at rehabilitation centers and homes around the US. The company that developed the exoskeleton system, ReWalk, has more information on its website: rewalk.com.

6. Discuss other assistive devices and orthotics

People in rehabilitation may struggle to perform their activities of daily living (ADLs), such as dressing, eating, bathing, oral care, hair care, moving, nail care, elimination, and eating and drinking. The rehabilitation team works to help restore a resident's ability to do these activities. **Assistive devices** can help people who are recovering from an illness or adapting to a physical disability. They also help promote a person's independence. Examples are special combs, plate guards, and prostheses (Chapter 21). There are many types of assistive devices. Some examples are shown in Figure 25-6.

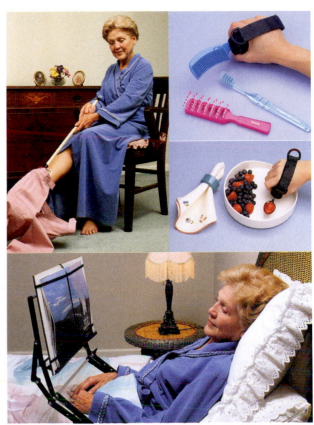

Fig. 25-6. *Many assistive devices are available to help residents adapt to physical changes.* (PHOTOS COURTESY OF NORTH COAST MEDICAL, INC., WWW.NCMEDICAL.COM, 800-821-9319)

Positioning devices are used to help prevent complications from inactivity and immobility. These devices aid in proper body alignment and positioning. They include the following:

- Backrests can be regular pillows or special wedge-shaped foam pillows. They provide support and comfort and maintain proper body alignment.

- Footboards are padded boards or pillow-like devices placed against the resident's feet to keep them properly aligned. They help prevent foot drop. **Foot drop** is a weakness of muscles in the feet and ankles that interferes with the ability to flex the ankles and walk normally. Footboards are also used to keep bed linens off the feet.

- Bed cradles or foot cradles are used to keep bed covers from resting on the resident's legs and feet.

- Abduction pillows/wedges/splints/pads (hip wedges) keep hips in proper position after hip surgery.

- Trochanter rolls are rolled bath blankets or towels that prevent the hip and leg from turning outward.

- Handrolls are cloth-covered or rubber grips that keep the hand and/or fingers in a normal, natural position. Handrolls help prevent finger, hand, or wrist contractures.

- Finger cushions are stuffed devices made of terry cloth or a similar material that keep the fingers separated. They help prevent contractures of the thumb or fingers.

- Elbow protectors are padded protectors wrapped around elbows to help prevent rubbing, irritation, and pressure injuries.

- **Orthotic devices**, or *orthoses*, are devices applied externally to a limb for support and protection (Fig. 25-7). They keep the joints in the correct position and are used to improve function and prevent complications, such as contractures. Splints are a type of orthotic device.

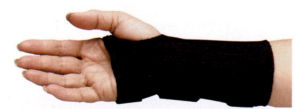

Fig. 25-7. *This is one type of orthotic splint.* (PHOTO COURTESY OF NORTH COAST MEDICAL, INC., WWW.NCMEDICAL.COM, 800-821-9319)

7. Discuss range of motion exercises

Because being immobile causes a wide range of complications, range of motion exercises are often ordered to prevent complications from inactivity and immobility. **Range of motion (ROM)** exercises put a joint through its full arc of motion. The goals of range of motion exercises are to decrease or prevent contractures and atrophy, increase circulation, and improve strength and movement.

Range of motion exercises may need to be performed at various times during the day. There will be guidelines for how many times an exercise for a particular joint should be done during each session. The procedure below states that these exercises should be performed at least three times for each joint per session. However, the NA should follow the care plan, which may require more exercises to be completed.

Three types of range of motion exercises are

Active range of motion (AROM) exercises put a joint through its full arc of motion and are done by a resident alone, without help.

Active assisted range of motion (AAROM) exercises put a joint through its full arc of motion and are done by a resident with some help from a staff member.

Passive range of motion (PROM) exercises put a joint through its full arc of motion and are done by a staff member, without the resident's help. These are ordered when a resident cannot move on his own.

Range of motion exercises are specific for each area of the body. They include these movements (Fig. 25-8):

- **Abduction**: moving a body part away from the midline of the body

- **Adduction**: moving a body part toward the midline of the body

- **Extension**: straightening a body part

- **Flexion**: bending a body part

- **Dorsiflexion**: bending backward

- **Rotation**: turning the joint

- **Pronation**: turning downward

- **Supination**: turning upward

- **Opposition**: touching the thumb to any other finger

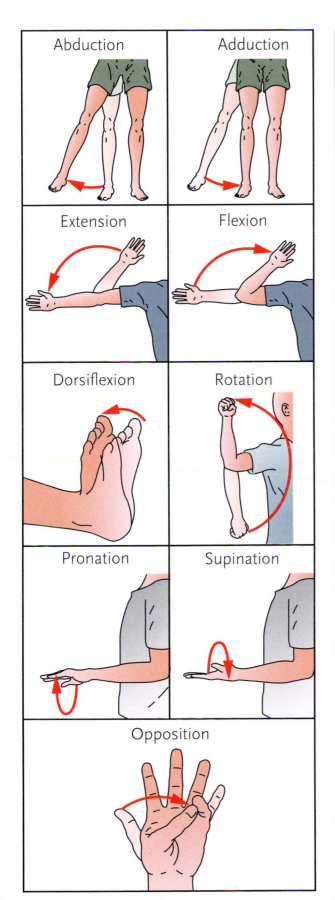

Fig. 25-8. *The different range of motion body movements.*

Guidelines: Range of Motion (ROM) Exercises

G   Follow the care plan carefully. A doctor will give the order for ROM exercises to be performed. NAs do not usually exercise the head and neck without specific instructions from a nurse or doctor.

G   Maintain privacy at all times when doing ROM exercises. Expose only the area being exercised at one time.

G   Use proper body mechanics when performing ROM exercises.

G   Support the joint, both above and below, while doing these exercises.

G   Keep the resident's body in proper alignment. Use pillows as needed (see Chapter 11).

G   You will work on both sides of the body, unless instructed otherwise. Begin at the shoulders and work down the body. The upper extremities (arms) should be exercised before the lower extremities (legs).

G   Follow instructions for limiting ROM exercises. Do not exercise a joint that is bandaged or has a dressing, cast, or special tubing. Never exercise a joint that has reddened areas, rashes, bruises, or sores, or one that is draining fluid.

G   Never push the resident to move further than what is comfortable. **Hyperextension**, extending a joint beyond its normal range of motion, can cause injury. If a resident reports pain or any other problem, such as difficulty breathing, stop the exercises and report to the nurse.

G   Use these exercises as an opportunity to provide holistic care to residents. For example, listen to and talk with the resident while performing these exercises. Let the resident voice any problems or concerns he may have. Give praise often.

Exercise Should Not Hurt

Range of motion exercises are important to help keep muscles strong and healthy, and must be done properly. If these exercises are performed in an aggressive or rough way, they can cause pain and injury. Causing unnecessary pain during these exercises is considered abusive behavior. If a resident reports pain during ROM exercises, stop immediately and inform the nurse.

Assisting with passive range of motion exercises

1. Identify yourself by name. Identify the resident. Greet the resident by name.

2. Wash your hands.

3. Explain procedure to resident. Speak clearly, slowly, and directly. Maintain face-to-face contact whenever possible.

4. Provide for the resident's privacy with a curtain, screen, or door.

5. Adjust the bed to a safe level, usually waist high. Lock bed wheels.

6. Position the resident lying supine—flat on her back—on the bed. Use proper alignment. Ask the resident to let you know if she has any pain during the procedure.

7. While supporting the limbs, move all joints gently, slowly, and smoothly through the range of motion to the point of resistance. Repeat each exercise at least three times. Ask the resident if an exercise is causing pain. Watch for signs of pain. Stop if the resident appears to be in pain or reports pain.

8. **Shoulder**. Support the resident's arm at the elbow and wrist while performing ROM for the shoulder. Place one hand under the elbow and the other hand under the wrist. Raise the straightened arm from the side position upward toward the head to ear level and return the arm down to side of the body (extension/flexion) (Fig. 25-9).

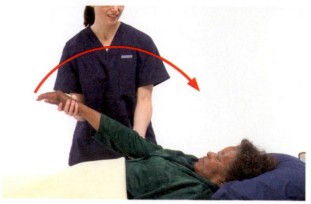

Fig. 25-9. Raise the straightened arm upward toward the head to ear level and return it to the side of the body.

Keep one hand under the elbow and one hand under the wrist. Move the straightened arm away from the side of the body to shoulder level. Return the arm to the side of the body (abduction/adduction) (Fig. 25-10).

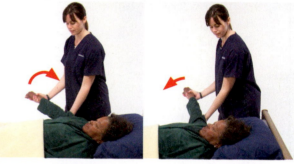

Fig. 25-10. Move the straightened arm away from the side of the body to shoulder level and return the arm to the side.

9. **Elbow**. Hold the resident's wrist with one hand and the elbow with the other hand. Bend the elbow so that the hand touches the shoulder on that same side (flexion). Straighten the arm (extension) (Fig. 25-11).

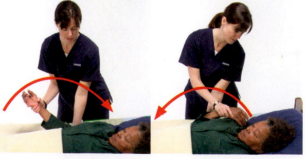

Fig. 25-11. Bend the elbow so that the hand touches the shoulder on the same side. Then straighten the arm.

Rehabilitation and Restorative Care

Exercise the forearm by moving it so the palm is facing downward (pronation) and then the palm is facing upward (supination) (Fig. 25-12).

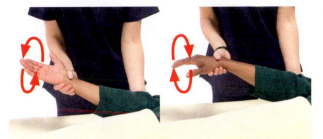

Fig. 25-12. Exercise the forearm so that the palm is facing downward and then upward.

10. **Wrist**. Hold the wrist with one hand. Use the fingers of your other hand to help move the joint through the motions. Bend the hand down (flexion). Bend the hand backward (dorsiflexion) (Fig. 25-13).

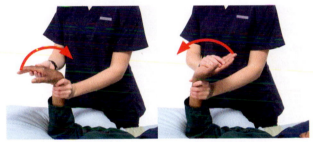

Fig. 25-13. While supporting the wrist, gently bend the hand down and then backward.

Turn the hand in the direction of the thumb (radial flexion). Then turn the hand in the direction of the little finger (ulnar flexion) (Fig. 25-14).

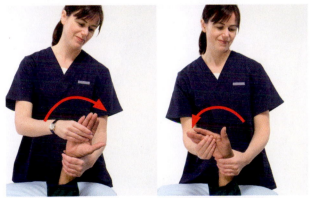

Fig. 25-14. Turn the hand in the direction of the thumb, then turn it in the direction of the little finger.

11. **Thumb**. Move the thumb away from the index finger (abduction). Move the thumb back next to the index finger (adduction) (Fig. 25-15).

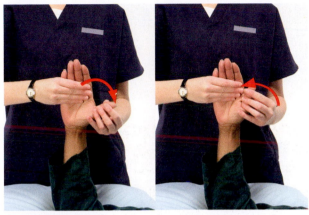

Fig. 25-15. Move the thumb away from the index finger and then back next to the index finger.

Touch each fingertip with the thumb (opposition) (Fig. 25-16).

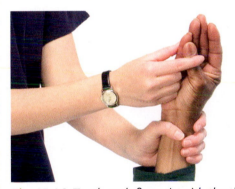

Fig. 25-16. Touch each fingertip with the thumb.

Bend the thumb into the palm (flexion) and out to the side (extension) (Fig. 25-17).

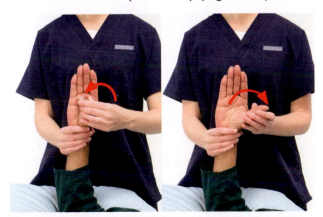

Fig. 25-17. Bend the thumb into the palm and then out to the side.

12. **Fingers**. Make the hand into a fist (flexion). Gently straighten out the fist (extension) (Fig. 25-18).

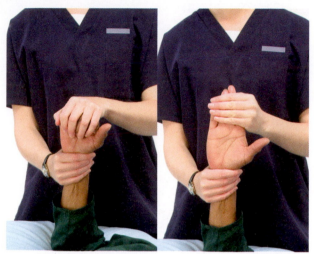

Fig. 25-18. *Make the fingers into a fist and then gently straighten out the fist.*

Spread the fingers and the thumb far apart from each other (abduction). Bring the fingers back next to each other (adduction) (Fig. 25-19).

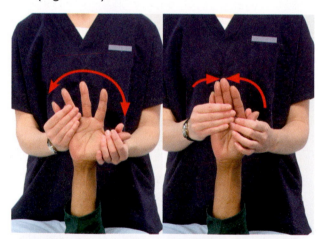

Fig. 25-19. *Spread the fingers and thumb far apart from each other and then bring them back next to each other.*

13. **Hip**. Support the leg by placing one hand under the knee and one under the ankle. Straighten the leg and gently raise it upward. Move the leg away from the other leg (abduction). Move the leg toward the other leg (adduction) (Fig. 25-20).

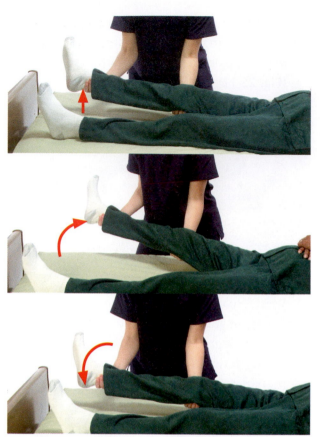

Fig. 25-20. *Straighten the leg and gently raise it. Move the leg away from the other leg and then back toward the other leg.*

Gently turn the leg inward (internal rotation), then turn the leg outward (external rotation) (Fig. 25-21).

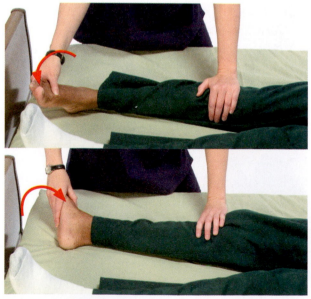

Fig. 25-21. *Gently turn the leg inward and then outward.*

14. **Knee**. Support resident's leg under the knee and ankle while performing ROM for the knee. Bend the knee to the point of resistance (flexion). Return the leg to the resident's normal position (extension) (Fig. 25-22).

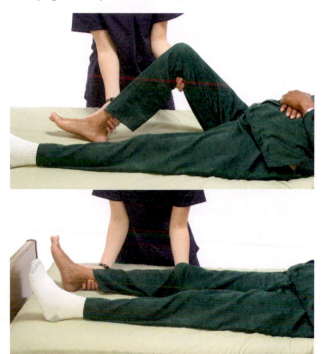

Fig. 25-22. Gently bend the knee to the point of resistance and return the leg to its normal position.

15. **Ankle**. Support the foot and under the ankle close to the bed while performing ROM for the ankle. Push/pull the foot up toward the head (dorsiflexion). Push/pull the foot down, with the toes pointed down (plantar flexion) (Fig. 25-23).

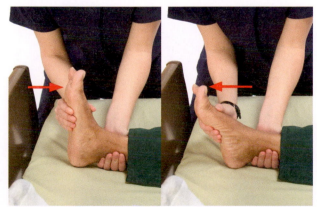

Fig. 25-23. Push the foot up toward the head and then push it back down.

Turn the inside of the foot inward toward the body (supination). Bend the sole of the foot so that it faces away from the body (pronation) (Fig. 25-24).

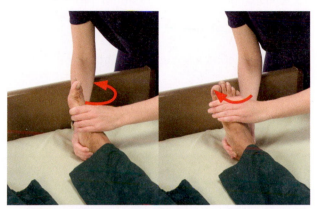

Fig. 25-24. Turn the inside of the foot inward, toward the body, and then bend it to face away from the body.

16. **Toes**. Curl and straighten the toes (flexion and extension) (Fig. 25-25).

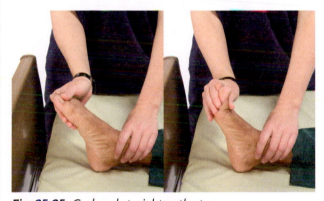

Fig. 25-25. Curl and straighten the toes.

Gently spread the toes apart (abduction) (Fig. 25-26).

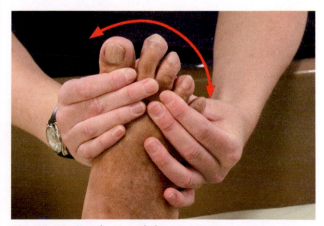

Fig. 25-26. Gently spread the toes apart.

17. Make the resident comfortable. Return the bed to its lowest position. Remove privacy measures.

18. Leave call light within resident's reach.

19. Wash your hands.

20. Be courteous and respectful at all times.

21. Report any changes in the resident to the nurse. Document procedure using facility guidelines.

Tip

Osteoporosis

Range of motion exercises may not be recommended for residents who have osteoporosis or other conditions that cause brittle bones or weak joints. NAs should never perform ROM exercises without a doctor's order.

Chapter Review

1. List three goals of rehabilitation (LO 2).

2. List three positive effects that encouraging independence and self-care can have on a resident (LO 3).

3. List one complication for each body system that results from a lack of exercise and activity (LO 4).

4. List one benefit for each body system that results from regular activity and exercise (LO 4).

Multiple Choice

5. Which type of cane has four rubber-tipped feet (LO 5)?
   (A) C cane
   (B) Quad cane
   (C) Functional grip cane
   (D) Crutch cane

6. When a resident uses a cane, walker, or crutches, on which side should the NA stay (LO 5)?
   (A) Right
   (B) Left
   (C) Stronger
   (D) Weaker

7. A type of device that is applied externally to a limb for support and protection is called a(n) (LO 6)
   (A) Prosthetic device
   (B) Musculoskeletal device
   (C) Chiropractic device
   (D) Orthotic device

8. When performing ROM exercises, where on the body should the NA begin (LO 7)?
   (A) Shoulder
   (B) Wrist
   (C) Hip
   (D) Ankle

26
Subacute Care

1. Define important words in this chapter

central venous line: a type of intravenous line (IV) that is inserted into a large vein in the body.

chest tubes: hollow drainage tubes that are inserted into the chest to drain air, blood, pus, or fluid that has collected inside the pleural space/cavity.

delirium: a sudden state of severe confusion due to a change in the body; also called *acute confusional state* or *acute brain syndrome.*

gastrostomy: a surgically created opening in the abdomen and stomach.

intubation: the insertion of a plastic tube through the mouth or nose and into the trachea or windpipe in order to place an artificial airway.

mechanical ventilator: a machine used to inflate and deflate the lungs when a person cannot breathe on his own.

nasogastric tube: a feeding tube that is inserted through the nose and into the stomach.

percutaneous endoscopic gastrostomy (PEG) tube: a tube placed through the abdominal wall into the stomach to deliver liquid nutrients and medications.

pulse oximeter: device that measures a person's blood oxygen level and pulse rate.

sedation: the use of medication to calm a person.

sepsis: a serious illness caused by an infection, usually bacterial, that requires immediate care.

telemetry: the application of a cardiac monitoring device that transmits information about the heart rhythm and heart rate to a monitoring station for assessment.

total parenteral nutrition (TPN): the intravenous infusion of nutrients in a basic form that is absorbed directly by the cells, bypassing the digestive tract.

2. Discuss the types of residents who are in a subacute setting

A subacute setting is a special unit or facility for people who need more care than most long-term care facilities can provide. Hospitals and long-term care facilities may offer subacute care. Residents in subacute care settings need a higher level of care than other residents. They require more care, treatment, and monitoring by staff members. The cost for subacute care is usually less than care received in a hospital, but more expensive than the cost of long-term care.

Recent surgery or acute conditions, such as total joint replacements, cardiac surgery, or recent stroke, or chronic illnesses, such as AIDS or cancer, may require subacute care. Other conditions that warrant subacute care are serious burns, the need for special administration of nutrients or medicine, or dialysis. Dialysis cleans the body of wastes that the kidneys cannot remove due to renal failure. Residents in subacute care units may also be on a **mechanical ventilator**, a machine used to inflate and deflate the lungs when a person cannot breathe on his own.

3. Describe preoperative and postoperative care

Residents who have outpatient or inpatient surgery require special care. Care given before surgery is known as *preoperative care*. Care given after surgery is called *postoperative care*. Preoperative and postoperative care varies, depending on the facility, the surgery, and the resident's condition. A resident who undergoes surgery requiring general anesthesia will recover in an area called a *postanesthesia care unit (PACU)*. When he has stabilized, he will either be transferred directly to a unit within the acute care facility where the surgery took place or back to his long-term care facility. The following are general care guidelines:

Guidelines: Preoperative and Postoperative Care

G Follow orders for fluid restrictions. The resident may have a nothing by mouth (NPO) medical order for up to eight hours before surgery, although the amount of time can vary. This helps prevent vomiting and aspiration.

G Before surgery the resident may be nervous, frightened, or anxious. Be calm and compassionate, and listen to the resident. Answer questions that are within your scope of practice. Notify the nurse if anxiety is getting worse or if the resident has questions that are outside your scope of practice.

G The resident will usually need to remove contact lenses, eyeglasses, dentures, hearing aids, and jewelry before surgery. Follow facility policy on storage of these items. Be ready to return these items or ask the nurse for the items directly after surgery as requested. This is part of respecting Residents' Rights and providing person-centered care. It allows the resident to see or hear properly again, and to be free of concern about the whereabouts of personal property.

G An indwelling catheter may be inserted temporarily. Provide catheter care as needed. Report to the nurse when the resident voids for the first time following surgery.

G Vital signs are monitored frequently after surgery. A pulse oximeter is used to check pulse rate and blood oxygen levels (as described in the next learning objective). Measure vital signs and monitor the pulse oximeter as ordered. Report changes in vital signs immediately.

G To improve lung functioning, assist with the use of an incentive spirometer as needed.

G A sequential compression device may be ordered to help prevent postoperative blood clots. Apply this device as ordered.

G   Encourage the resident to follow any special postoperative diet orders.

4. List care guidelines for pulse oximetry

When residents are on oxygen, require surgery, or have bleeding or breathing problems, a pulse oximeter may be used. A **pulse oximeter** measures a person's blood oxygen level and pulse rate. Oxygen is carried by the arteries. Hemoglobin carries the oxygen. Blood oxygen is the oxygen level inside the arteries and is also called *oxygen saturation (SpO2)*, sometimes referred to as *O_2 sat*.

A sensor is clipped on a finger, earlobe, or toe (Fig. 26-1). Adhesive probes may be used on fingers, the forehead, or the nose. The sensor warns of a low blood oxygen level before any observable signs or symptoms develop. It works by moving infrared and red light through the skin. The sensor measures the amount of each type of light absorbed by the hemoglobin in the blood. Blood with oxygen absorbs more of the infrared light, while blood without oxygen absorbs more red light.

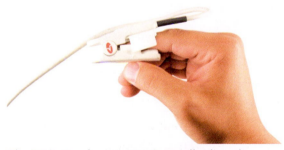

Fig. 26-1. A pulse oximeter is usually clipped on a person's finger.

Normal blood oxygen levels measure between 95% and 100%. However, normal ranges may differ from person to person. Diseases such as chronic obstructive pulmonary disease (COPD) (Chapter 20) can lower a person's blood oxygen levels. Other factors that affect pulse oximetry readings include the following:

- Reduced circulation to the extremities

- Smoking
- Recent exposure to various dyes for health-care testing
- Oxygen therapy
- Exposure to a fire or carbon monoxide
- Nail polish or artificial nails
- Skin tones (people with brown or black skin tones may have inaccurate readings due to increased pigmentation of their skin)
- Exposure of the probe to bright light

Guidelines: Pulse Oximeter

G   The nurse will set the alarm so it will alert staff to a resident's low oxygen saturation. The alarm must be placed in the 'on' position. If the alarm on the pulse oximeter sounds, report it to the nurse immediately.

G   Do not place the sensor on an artificial nail. Remove nail polish from the index finger or other finger to be used for the sensor.

G   Be careful when moving and positioning residents to make sure the oximeter does not dislodge or come off. Make sure the device does not get wet.

G   Report dyspnea (difficulty breathing) or shortness of breath.

G   Report cyanotic, pale, grayish, or darkening skin or mucous membranes.

G   Check the skin around and under the oximeter. Observe and report any signs of skin breakdown, such as irritation, rash, breaks, cracking, sores, bleeding, or drainage. Sometimes the adhesive on the sensor does not adhere to the skin and needs to be changed. Obtain a new sensor if needed.

G   Carefully monitor all vital signs and report changes to the nurse. Do not measure blood pressure on the side where the pulse oximeter is placed. Pulse oximetry readings between 95% and 100% are generally considered normal. Promptly report readings that are considered abnormal for the resident.

Applying a pulse oximetry device

Equipment: pulse oximetry clip-on sensor, cleansing wipe (facility approved)

Measure blood pressure and count pulse rate before placing the device if needed.

1. Identify yourself by name. Identify the resident. Greet the resident by name.

2. Wash your hands.

3. Explain procedure to the resident. Speak clearly, slowly, and directly. Maintain face-to-face contact whenever possible.

4. Provide for the resident's privacy with a curtain, screen, or door.

5. Using the cleansing wipe, clean the finger or other body area on which the sensor will be placed, following facility policy.

6. Remove the sensor from the package and place on the index finger, toe, or earlobe. The sensor must be placed fully onto the finger or toe; it should not be placed on the tip of the finger or toe.

7. Turn on the device. The pulse oximetry reading should appear on the screen quickly. If the device does not seem to be working, make sure the wires on the pulse oximeter are in place and that device is plugged in.

8. Ask the resident not to remove or adjust the pulse oximetry device. Let him know that he should press the call light if the device dislodges or comes off.

9. Make the resident comfortable.

10. Remove privacy measures.

11. Leave call light within the resident's reach.

12. Wash your hands.

13. Be courteous and respectful at all times.

14. Report any changes in the resident to the nurse. Document procedure (both the pulse and the oxygen saturation) using facility guidelines. Leave the sensor in place, turned on, following the care plan and the nurse's instructions.

5. Describe telemetry and list care guidelines

Telemetry is the application of a cardiac monitoring device that transmits information about the heart's rhythm and rate to computer screens at a monitoring station (Fig. 26-2). This data is monitored and assessed constantly by specially trained staff members.

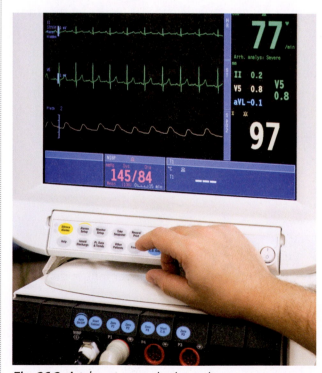

Fig. 26-2. *A telemetry monitoring unit.*

The device is connected to different parts of a person's chest using wires with sponge-like adhesive pads or patches called *electrodes* (Fig. 26-3). Portable units may be used that are attached to the chest and are carried in a pack that allows for movement (Fig. 26-4).

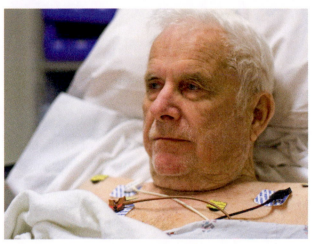

Fig. 26-3. Sticky pads called electrodes are attached to the person's chest.

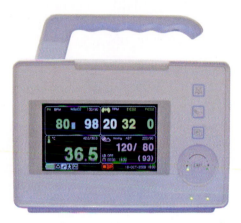

Fig. 26-4. A smaller, portable monitoring unit that can be carried by the person.

Guidelines: Telemetry

G If the alarm sounds, notify the nurse. The alarm may sound with movement, a disconnected electrode, or a low battery.

G Monitor vital signs carefully as ordered.

G Check electrodes regularly and report if they become loose. They can fail to adhere to the skin, and if so, should be replaced.

G Do not get the unit, wires, or electrodes wet during bathing. Report to the nurse if they become wet.

G Check the skin under and around the electrodes for irritation, rashes, broken skin, or cracking. Report these signs to the nurse.

G Remind the resident not to leave the range of the monitoring area during ambulation.

G Notify the nurse if any of the following occurs:

- Change in vital signs
- Rapid pulse (tachycardia)
- Chest pain or discomfort
- Dyspnea or shortness of breath
- Sweating
- Dizziness

6. Explain artificial airways and list care guidelines

An artificial airway is any tube inserted into the respiratory tract for the purpose of maintaining an airway and facilitating ventilation. Artificial airways are used when a person needs assistance with breathing for a prolonged period of time. They keep the airway open. A clear airway is needed for the lungs to perform air exchange.

An artificial airway is needed when the airway is obstructed from illness, injury, secretions, or aspiration, and sometimes it is needed when a person has surgery. Some residents who are unconscious will need an artificial airway.

An artificial airway is inserted during a procedure called **intubation**. It involves a licensed healthcare professional inserting a tube through the mouth, nose, or opening in the neck and into the trachea (windpipe). There are different types of artificial airways.

A common type of artificial airway is a tracheostomy. A tracheostomy is an opening through the neck into the trachea. A tracheostomy tube is inserted through this opening, or stoma, into the trachea. It is also referred to as a *trach tube*. More information on tracheostomies is in the next learning objective. More information on airway management is located in Chapter 15 in the section about bariatrics.

Guidelines: Artificial Airways

G   Observe the resident closely. If tubing falls out, use the call light to notify the nurse immediately. Do not leave the resident.

G   Proper positioning helps reduce the risk of aspiration; orders will depend upon the type of airway, the need for mechanical ventilation, and the level of consciousness. A semi-reclined (semi-Fowler's) or an upright (Fowler's) position may be ordered. Follow orders for positioning of the head and neck; maintain the proper position at all times.

G   Check vital signs as ordered and report any changes.

G   Perform oral care as directed at least every two hours.

G   Watch for biting or tugging on the tube. Report this to the nurse.

G   Use other methods of communication if the resident cannot speak. Communication boards, writing notes, and drawing pictures can be helpful. Watch for hand or eye signals.

G   Be supportive and encouraging. Having an artificial airway can be frightening and uncomfortable. It can cause choking and gagging. Be empathetic; try to imagine how you might feel if you had a tube in your nose, mouth, or throat.

G   Do not move or remove spare artificial airway tubes or other equipment from the bedside.

G   Notify the nurse if any of the following occurs:

- Signs of respiratory distress, including wheezing or other unusual breathing sounds or difficulty breathing

- Cyanosis, pale, gray, or darkening skin or mucous membranes

- Change in vital signs

- Drainage

- Secretions in tubing

- Nervousness or anxiety

7. Discuss care for a resident with a tracheostomy

A tracheostomy is a common type of artificial airway. It may be necessary due to an obstruction, cancer, infection, severe injuries, serious allergic reactions, or coma. It may also be used for a person recovering from facial burns or gunshot wounds and to prevent aspiration in an unconscious person.

Tracheostomy tubes may be held in place by a cuff that attaches to the end of the device in the trachea, or they may be cuffless. A cuffed tracheostomy tube is mostly used with residents who require a mechanical ventilator. The cuff seals the airway to control mechanical ventilation. A cuffless tracheostomy tube is often used for people who are at a low risk for aspiration and who will require the tube for an extended period of time. With a cuffless tube, air flows through and around the tube.

While the tracheostomy is in place, the resident may not be able to speak. Being unable to speak can cause fear and anxiety. Nursing assistants can help by being supportive and carefully observing residents. Keeping call lights within reach and answering call lights promptly is important and may lessen anxiety. Using other methods of communication, such as notepads, communication boards, or hand signals, helps when a resident cannot speak. Speaking valves can be used with tracheostomies to facilitate speech. An SLP may work with residents on the use of speaking valves.

General tracheostomy care includes keeping the skin around the opening, or stoma, clean, assisting with dressing changes, and helping with the cleaning of the inner part of the device. Suctioning is performed by a nurse or respiratory therapist and may be needed frequently.

Gurgling sounds during breathing are one sign that suctioning is needed. NAs do not perform tracheostomy care or suctioning. However, careful observation and reporting is vital to promote health.

Guidelines: Tracheostomies

G Answer call lights promptly.

G Use alternate methods of communication when needed.

G Assist resident into the correct position, as indicated in the care plan. A semi-Fowler's or Fowler's position may be ordered for a conscious resident with a tracheostomy. If the resident is unconscious, a side-lying (lateral) position may be ordered to help drain secretions. Gently move and position residents; always get help if needed.

G Do not tire the resident when performing care.

G Carefully monitor vital signs manually if they are not monitored electronically by a machine.

G Inspect tape or ties often. Do not untie or unfasten the tracheostomy tape or ties.

G Do not get the tracheostomy dressing wet.

G Do not cover the tracheostomy opening.

G Report kinks or disconnected tubing.

G Be careful to prevent aspiration when cleaning the mouth. Use special swabs as needed. Perform mouth care at least every two hours.

G Observe for mouth sores and cracks, breaks, or sores on the skin. Apply lubricant to the lips as needed.

G Provide careful skin care to the site around the tracheostomy. Assist with dressing changes as requested.

G Observe skin carefully for pale, bluish, or darkening skin or mucous membranes.

G Do not move or remove spare tracheostomy tubes or spare bag valve mask (device used to provide ventilation to a person who is not breathing, or not breathing adequately, or during power failures to a person on a mechanical ventilator). A special bag valve mask with a removable mask is needed for use with a tracheostomy.

G Notify the nurse if any of the following occurs:

- Disconnected tubing
- Signs of respiratory distress, including wheezing or other unusual breathing sounds or difficulty breathing
- Cyanosis, pale, gray, or darkening skin or mucous membranes
- Change in vital signs, especially respiratory rate
- Mouth sores or discomfort
- Cracks, breaks, or sores on the skin
- Loose or wet tape or dressings

8. Describe mechanical ventilation and explain care guidelines

A resident in a subacute unit may be on a mechanical ventilator. A ventilator performs the process of breathing for a person who cannot breathe on his own. Many conditions can cause a person to require mechanical ventilation. Injuries that affect the ability to breathe, such as a spinal cord injury, or diseases, such as cancer, are examples.

Once intubated, the ventilator provides oxygen through a tube connected to the person via the mouth, nose, or neck. The ventilator performs the process of moving air in and out of the lungs.

A resident on a ventilator is not able to speak. This is because air no longer reaches the larynx (vocal cords). This can cause intense anxiety. The resident may think that no one will know if he has trouble breathing. Being on a ventilator has been compared to breathing through a straw. While being connected to the ventilator, the resident will need a lot of support. The NA should spend as much time as he can with the resident and should enter the room often so that the resident can see him. This helps to reassure the resident. Clipboards, pads, and communication boards help with communication.

A person requiring mechanical ventilation is usually sedated. **Sedation** is the use of medication to calm a person. Sedation helps reduce anxiety and discomfort that can occur with mechanical ventilation. Whether alert or unconscious, the NA should continue to speak to the resident when providing care and should assume that the resident is able to understand everything going on around him.

Delirium

Delirium, also called *acute confusional state* or *acute brain syndrome*, is a sudden state of severe confusion due to a change in the body. Severe dehydration or malnutrition, fever, pain, poisons, alcohol and drug use, and prescribed medications can cause delirium. Other causes are hypoxia (low blood oxygen), head injuries, and illnesses such as cancer or diabetes. Infections such as pneumonia and urinary tract infections can also cause delirium.

Signs and symptoms of delirium include the following:

- Disorganized thinking
- Inability to concentrate
- Lack of attention span, especially around familiar people
- Decrease in short-term memory
- Problems with speech
- Decrease in the normal ability to move about
- Pulling out tubing, such as a nasogastric tube or a urinary catheter
- Anger or irritability
- Agitation
- Hallucinations
- Drowsiness or sleep disturbances

- Disorientation
- Changes in consciousness

Some effects of delirium are easily treatable with medication, which will reverse or control the delirium. Other causes require emergency care or a hospital stay. Any of these signs and symptoms should be reported to the nurse immediately.

Being on a ventilator puts a person at a higher risk for developing complications, including a type of pneumonia, considered a *ventilator-associated event (VAE)*. An infection can occur if microorganisms reach the lungs from the tube. NAs play an important role in preventing these complications.

Guidelines: Mechanical Ventilator

G Wash your hands thoroughly before providing care.

G Answer the call light promptly.

G Report to the nurse right away if the alarm sounds. Do not turn the alarm off.

G Watch for kinks or disconnected tubing. Tape can loosen, causing the tubing to dislodge. Report kinks, disconnected tubing, or loose tape to the nurse immediately.

G Watch for biting or pulling on the tube. Report this to the nurse.

G Give frequent mouth care as directed. Observe and report mouth sores or discomfort.

G Reposition the resident at least every two hours. Follow instructions carefully when moving and positioning. Keep the resident's head properly elevated, between 30 and 45 degrees, or as ordered. Always get enough help when moving a resident. Have the nurse check the resident after repositioning.

G Give regular skin care to prevent pressure injuries. Observe for cracks, breaks, or sores on the skin, especially at the intubation site. Chlorhexidine (CHG) bathing may be ordered.

G Allow time for rest.

G Follow orders for performing range of motion exercises.

G Be patient during communication. Offer communication aids to assist. Watch for hand or eye signals.

G Provide support during difficult times. Being dependent can cause feelings of despair. Continue to talk to the resident normally and explain things that are happening in the room. Assume the resident can understand everything that is being said.

G Do not move or remove spare artificial airway tubes or bag valve masks from the bedside.

G Residents on ventilators will require one-on-one care during a power failure. A bag valve mask and a portable oxygen tank will need to be used by the caregiver until the power is restored.

G Notify the nurse if any of the following occurs:

- The alarm sounds

- The tube moves or disconnects (the disconnection of a tube is an emergency and possibly life-threatening situation; some facilities allow NAs to reconnect tubing if this situation occurs)

- Signs of respiratory distress, including wheezing or other unusual breathing sounds or difficulty breathing

- Secretions collect in the tubing

- Mouth sores or discomfort

- Cracks, breaks, or sores anywhere on the skin, especially at the site of intubation

- Swollen or red area of an extremity

- Change in vital signs

- Nervousness or anxiety

- Depression

Sepsis

Sepsis is a life-threatening illness caused by an infection, usually bacterial, that requires immediate care. Early, subtle symptoms of sepsis include elevated heart rate, elevated respiratory rate, a slightly elevated temperature or, in some cases, a low body temperature. Being familiar with residents' normal vital signs will help an NA better recognize changes.

Other symptoms are fever, chills, excessive sweating, a general feeling of sickness, abdominal pain, nausea, vomiting, diarrhea, weakness, low blood pressure, decreased urine output or dark urine, headache, skin rash, dyspnea or shortness of breath, a change in mental status, or confusion. If the NA notices any of these symptoms, she should report them immediately.

Some of the risks for sepsis are being over the age of 65; chronic diseases like diabetes, heart disease, liver disease, kidney disease, cancer, or HIV; certain infections; having a transplanted organ; pressure injuries; burns; having a surgical drain; having an indwelling catheter; and recent hospitalization.

Treatment for sepsis depends on the type of infection, but includes antibiotics, other medications, IV fluids, oxygen therapy, and careful monitoring of blood glucose. Surgery to treat some infections and dialysis for people who develop kidney failure may also be needed. A ventilator may be necessary.

9. Describe suctioning and list signs of respiratory distress

Subacute care units include residents who require suctioning by nurses or respiratory therapists. Suctioning is needed when a person has increased secretions that they cannot expel themselves. Suctioning can be performed through the mouth (oropharyngeal), the nasal passages (nasopharyngeal), or the trachea and the bronchi (endotracheal). A person with a tracheostomy may also need suctioning.

Suctioning is normally a sterile procedure. NAs do not perform suctioning; nurses or respiratory therapists will perform suctioning. Suction comes from a wall hook-up or a portable pump (Fig. 26-5). A canister or bottle collects the suctioned material from the airway. Sterile water or sterile saline is normally used to rinse the suction catheter after suctioning has been performed. Nurses will change the tubing at least once daily.

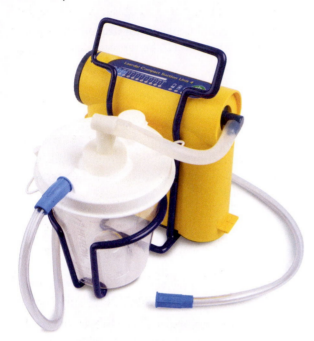

Fig. 26-5. *This is one type of suctioning pump. NAs do not perform suctioning. They help by reporting signs of respiratory distress and monitoring vital signs.* (PHOTO COURTESY OF LAERDAL MEDICAL CORPORATION)

A resident who needs frequent suctioning may show signs of respiratory distress. Signs of respiratory distress include gurgling, an elevated respiratory rate, shortness of breath, difficulty breathing (dyspnea), pallor, or cyanosis.

Guidelines: Assisting with Suctioning

G   Follow Standard Precautions. Wash your hands thoroughly before providing care. Wear gloves, gown, mask, and goggles as directed.

G   Monitor vital signs closely, especially respiratory rate. Report changes.

G   If you note any signs of respiratory distress, report them immediately. An inability to breathe freely causes great anxiety. It is dangerous to remain in respiratory distress for any length of time.

G   Observe skin color carefully for pale, bluish, or darkening skin or mucous membranes.

G   Answer call lights promptly.

G   Place the resident in position as directed by nurse, normally semi-Fowler's or lateral.

G   Place a pad or towel under the chin before the nurse begins suctioning; have a wet washcloth ready.

G   Give mouth and nasal care after suctioning as directed. Apply ordered lubricant to the lips as needed.

G   Be supportive during periods of difficult breathing. Use touch if appropriate.

G   Notify the nurse if any of the following occurs:

  •   Signs of respiratory distress, including wheezing or other unusual breathing sounds or difficulty breathing

  •   Cyanosis, pale, gray, or darkening skin or mucous membranes

  •   Change in vital signs, especially respiratory rate

  •   Change in the color, amount, or quality (thickness/thinness) of secretions coughed up

  •   Nervousness or anxiety

10. Describe chest tubes and explain related care

Chest tubes are hollow drainage tubes that are inserted into the chest during a sterile procedure. They can be inserted at the bedside or during surgery. Chest tubes are placed between the ribs into the pleural cavity or space to drain air, fluid, blood, or pus that has collected inside the cavity. The pleural cavity is the space between the two layers of the pleura, the thin tissue layers covering the lungs. Chest tubes are also inserted to allow full expansion of the lungs. Conditions that require chest tubes include the following:

- Pneumothorax: air or gas in the pleural cavity

- Hemothorax: blood in the pleural cavity

- Empyema: pus in the pleural cavity

- Certain types of surgery

- Chest trauma or injuries

A doctor normally inserts chest tubes. The chest tube is connected to a drainage system. Suction is sometimes attached to the system to encourage drainage. This system must be sealed so that air cannot enter the pleural cavity. The system must be airtight.

When X-rays show that the air, fluid, blood, or pus has been drained, the tube is removed. Medications may be used to prevent or treat infection.

Guidelines: Chest Tubes

G Report signs of respiratory distress or cyanosis to the nurse immediately. Report complaints of pain.

G Check vital signs as directed. Report any changes immediately to the nurse.

G Be aware of the number and location of chest tubes. Tubes may be in the front, back, or side of the body.

G Always keep the drainage system below the level of the resident's chest.

G Make sure the drainage containers remain upright and level at all times. Inform the nurse right away if a container tips over.

G Keep tubing coiled neatly on the bed.

G Report if there are clots in the tubing.

G Observe chest tube drainage for color, amount, and consistency of drainage, and report any changes.

G Observe the dressings for drainage, saturation, or bleeding.

G Certain equipment is kept nearby in case the tube is pulled out. This includes sterile petrolatum gauze, clamps, and containers of sterile fluid. Do not remove these items from the area. If the tubing disconnects, don gloves and call for the nurse immediately. Place the petrolatum gauze over the chest opening and continue to hold the gauze in place until the nurse arrives.

G Follow the repositioning schedule. Be very gentle with turning and repositioning. Move the resident and the tubes at the same time to prevent pulling the tubes out. Always get enough help when moving and positioning.

G If asked to assist with coughing and deep-breathing exercises, be encouraging and patient. These exercises can cause pain.

G Provide rest periods as needed.

G Follow fluid orders carefully. Measure intake and output and weight carefully as ordered.

G Notify the nurse if any of the following occur:

- Disconnected tubing

- Any signs of respiratory distress and cyanosis

- Changes in vital signs

- Change in oxygen level or if pulse oximetry alarm sounds

- Complaints of pain

- Coughing up blood

- Warmth, redness, swelling, sores, or pus

- An increase or decrease in bubbling in the drainage system

- Kinks or clots in the tubing

- Any change in the amount, color, consistency, or odor of chest drainage

- Wet or loose dressings

- Signs of subcutaneous emphysema (crepitus), such as bulging of the skin or skin that produces a crackling sound

Subacute Care

11. Describe alternative feeding methods and related care

When a person is unable to consume food normally due to disease or injury, other methods are used. When a person has difficulty swallowing or is unable to swallow, he may be fed through a tube. A **nasogastric tube** is inserted into the nose, down the back of the throat through the esophagus, and into the stomach. The tube is secured to the nose with dressing tape and to the gown with tape or a clip.

Another type of tube that is placed through the abdominal wall into the stomach is called a **percutaneous endoscopic gastrostomy (PEG) tube**. The surgically created opening in the abdomen and the stomach is called a **gastrostomy** (Fig. 26-6).

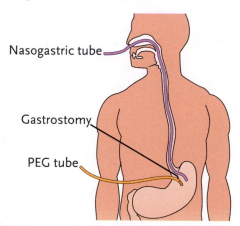

Fig. 26-6. *Nasogastric tubes are inserted through the nose, and PEG tubes are inserted through the abdominal wall into the stomach.*

Tube feedings are used when residents have swallowing difficulties but are able to digest food. Other conditions that may require tube feedings are coma, cancer, stroke, birth defects, or extreme weakness.

NAs do not insert tubes, give the feedings, or clean or suction the tubes. However, they may assist the nurse by assembling equipment, positioning the resident, observing the tube site for signs of infection, and cleaning the tube site. They may also discard or clean and store used equipment and supplies.

Guidelines: Tube Feedings

G   Wash your hands thoroughly before assisting with any aspect of tube feeding.

G   Observe carefully for any signs of aspiration during and after a tube feeding (Chapter 14).

G   Feeding pumps may be used to administer tube feedings. Pumps help regulate the amount of fluid given. Notify the nurse if an alarm sounds.

G   Follow instructions for positioning residents. They will need to sit upright during the feeding and for at least one hour following the feeding to help prevent aspiration. They should never be placed in the supine position while the feeding is occurring.

G   Follow fluid orders and measure weight as instructed. The resident may have an order for nothing by mouth. The resident may need to increase fluid intake due to constipation.

G   Give frequent nose and mouth care to prevent dryness and irritation. Apply lubricant as ordered.

G   Do not pull or tug on the tubing. Make sure that the tubing is not kinked and is securely taped.

G   Observe for the tape or clip falling off the gown.

G   Make conversation or read to residents during tube feedings to help make this time more social.

G   Notify the nurse if any of the following occurs:

   •   Disconnected tubing

   •   Tube comes out of abdomen

   •   Any signs of respiratory distress

   •   Feeding pump alarm sounds

   •   Signs of aspiration

   •   Tube feeding liquid gathering in the mouth

- Cyanosis, pale, gray, or darkening skin or mucous membranes

- Kinked, plugged, cracked, or broken tubing

- Leaking or empty bag or container

- Resident pulling on the tube

- Signs of infection at the tube site, such as warm skin, reddened skin, sores, swelling, or pus

- Bleeding or drainage at the gastrostomy site

- Irritation or sores around the nose or mouth

- Nausea, vomiting, or cramping

- Signs of dehydration (Chapter 14)

If a person's digestive system does not function properly, he is unable to eat, or his nutritional needs cannot be met by tube feedings, **total parenteral nutrition (TPN)** may be ordered. With TPN, a resident receives nutrients intravenously, bypassing the digestive tract. The nutrients are in their most basic forms of carbohydrates, proteins, and fats and are absorbed directly by the cells. Total parenteral nutrition also may be necessary due to surgery, disease, significant weight loss, or coma.

When the need for TPN is expected to continue for a period of time, a central venous line is usually inserted. A **central venous line** is a type of intravenous line (IV) that is placed in one of the larger veins in the body, usually in the upper chest or neck. Another style of central venous line is a peripherally inserted central catheter or *PICC line*. PICC lines allow for the infusion of nutrition, antibiotics and other medications, and chemotherapy. They can remain in place for extended periods of time. There is an increased risk of deep vein thrombosis (DVT) with PICC lines. Central line-associated bloodstream infection (CLABSI) is a bloodstream infection in a central venous line. Ways to prevent this

complication include performing proper hand hygiene and promptly changing dressings using sterile supplies, including sterile gloves.

The NA's responsibilities when caring for a resident receiving total parenteral nutrition (TPN) include the following:

- Observing and reporting fever, headache, swelling, redness, bleeding, or leaking at the insertion site

- Observing and reporting signs of fluctuations in blood sugar, including hyperglycemia and hypoglycemia (Chapter 8 contains information about the signs of hyperglycemia and hypoglycemia)

- Making sure there is no interruption in the delivery of TPN and that it is not turned off

- Making sure the TPN infusion area does not get wet (plastic sheaths should cover the infusion area during bathing or showering)

Tip

Gastric Suctioning

Tubes can be inserted into the stomach for reasons other than feeding. Tubes may be used postoperatively for nausea, vomiting, bloating, and to remove materials from the body via suctioning. In addition, poisons can be removed from the stomach with a special wash that is done via a tube.

12. Discuss care guidelines for dialysis

When the kidneys cannot remove wastes due to acute injury or chronic renal failure (CRF), dialysis is done to clean and filter the blood. Dialysis can be done via a site in the person's arm, neck, abdomen, or leg (Fig. 26-7). Central lines in the neck are generally used for temporary dialysis.

People who are too ill or unstable to have standard dialysis may undergo continuous renal replacement therapy (CRRT) using a machine in a special care unit. CRRT is a significantly slower process and can reduce complications such as hypotension that can occur with dialysis.

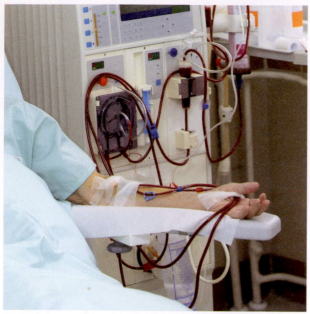

Fig. 26-7. Dialysis being done via a person's arm.

Guidelines: Dialysis

G Follow Standard Precautions. Wash your hands thoroughly before providing care.

G Keep the access arm area clean. Residents should avoid putting pressure on or sleeping on the access arm.

G Help residents dress in proper attire. Loose sleeves may need to be worn.

G Encourage residents to follow their special diets if ordered.

G Follow orders for fluid restrictions. (*RF* is the abbreviation for *restrict fluids*.) Residents on dialysis will have to reduce their fluid intake.

G Measure intake and output (I&O) and weight carefully.

G Check vital signs as ordered. Do not measure blood pressure on the access arm.

G A dialysis session may take several hours. Make sure the resident has reading material, the TV remote, and the call light within reach.

G Notify the nurse if any of the following occurs:

- Any signs of respiratory distress
- Changes in vital signs, especially pulse or blood pressure
- Pain, drainage, redness, swelling, or bleeding from the insertion site
- Abdominal cramps, nausea, or vomiting
- Muscle cramps
- Swelling of extremities (edema)
- Change in intake and output
- Itchy skin

Chapter Review

1. What kinds of conditions require subacute care (LO 2)?

2. What is the purpose of artificial airways (LO 6)?

3. What does tracheostomy care generally involve (LO 7)?

4. Why is it important to enter the room often when a resident is using a mechanical ventilator (LO 8)?

5. What observations should NAs make about chest drainage (LO 10)?

6. What signs and symptoms should the NA report to the nurse when a resident is on dialysis (LO 12)?

Multiple Choice

7. Preoperative fluid restrictions can help prevent (LO 3)
    (A) Blood clots
    (B) Contractures
    (C) Kidney stones
    (D) Vomiting

8. What does a pulse oximeter measure (LO 4)?
    (A) Pulse rate and blood glucose level
    (B) Pulse rate and white blood cell count
    (C) Pulse rate and calcium level
    (D) Pulse rate and blood oxygen level

9. What does a telemetry device monitor (LO 5)?
   (A) The amount of blood stored in the spleen
   (B) The heart's rhythm and rate
   (C) The number of CD4+ lymphocytes in the body
   (D) A person's intake and output of fluids

10. What is one NA responsibility regarding suctioning (LO 9)?
   (A) The NA changes the tubing daily.
   (B) The NA performs the suctioning.
   (C) The NA reports signs of respiratory distress.
   (D) The NA decides when a resident needs suctioning.

11. What is one NA responsibility regarding feeding tubes (LO 11)?
   (A) The NA positions the resident for the feeding.
   (B) The NA performs the feeding.
   (C) The NA inserts the feeding tube.
   (D) The NA cleans the feeding tube.

27
End-of-Life Care

The Ancient Egyptian Art of Embalming the Dead

Many people in ancient Egypt focused on preparing for the afterlife. Their hope was that the afterlife would be a joyful paradise. The art of embalming dead bodies was common, especially for people of "high birth." Embalming consisted of removing and preserving organs, such as the liver and the lungs. They were placed inside jars and then covered. Body cavities were washed out with spices, and then the body was soaked for 70 days with a substance called natron. Natron was made of clay mixed with certain salts. The body was then coated with various gums and wrapped with pieces of fine linen. People who were of "lower birth" were destined to be buried in the sand without any of these preparations.

"As a well-spent day brings happy sleep, so life well used brings happy death."

Leonardo Da Vinci, 1452–1519

"Men fear death as children fear to go in the dark; and as that natural fear in children is increased with tales, so is the other."

Publilius Syrus, circa 42 B.C.

1. Define important words in this chapter

anticipatory grief: a period of mourning when the dying person or his family is expecting the death.

autopsy: an examination of a body by a pathologist to try to determine the cause of death.

bereavement: the period following a loss in which mourning occurs.

cremation: the process of burning a dead body until it turns to ash.

death: the end of life; the cessation of all body functions.

grief: a deeply emotional process that is a response to loss.

grief counseling: therapy to try to help a person cope after someone has died.

grief process: the varying emotional responses to grief.

mourning: the period in which people work to adapt to a loss; influenced by culture, tradition, and society.

palliative care: care that focuses on pain relief, controlling symptoms, preventing side effects and complications, and maintaining quality of life for a person who is very ill and/or is dying.

pathologist: a doctor with advanced training in the examination of organs and tissues.

postmortem care: care of the body after death.

rigor mortis: the Latin term for the condition after death in which the muscles in the body become stiff and rigid.

terminal illness: a disease or condition that will eventually cause death.

2. Describe palliative care

Palliative care is a type of care that is given to people who have serious, chronic diseases, such as cancer, AIDS, and congestive heart failure, as well as to people who are dying. The goals of palliative care are to relieve pain, control symptoms, prevent side effects and complications, and maintain quality of life. Palliative care emphasizes a holistic, person-centered approach. Physical and psychosocial needs, along with personal choices and preferences, are considered when creating the care plan. Keeping the resident engaged in activities when possible is important.

Palliative care works to manage symptoms, not to cure the disease. The care plan will include instructions on how to recognize and treat complications early and how to relieve chronic pain and discomfort. This helps to maintain a person's quality of life. Palliative care involves input from the resident's family and friends. The resident, his family and friends, and various palliative care team members will participate in regularly scheduled care conferences. Doctors, nurses, social workers, dietitians, physical therapists, and nursing assistants are some of the palliative care team members. The team will also provide access to other specialists. Counseling is available to help the resident and his family deal with the stress that accompanies a loved one's serious illness.

3. Discuss hospice care

When an illness is classified as a **terminal illness**, or a disease or condition that will eventually cause **death**, hospice care is often the next step. Hospice care is ordered by a doctor when a person has approximately six months or less to live. This type of care is a compassionate way to care for dying people and their families. Hospice care uses a holistic approach, giving physical and emotional care and comfort. The focus is on pain and symptom management, meeting psychosocial needs, and involving family and friends.

Hospice care can be given in a hospital, at a care facility, or in the home (Fig. 27-1). It is available seven days a week, 24 hours a day. There

is always a nurse on call to answer questions, make an additional visit, or solve a problem. Members of the hospice care team include doctors, nurses, nursing assistants, social workers, counselors, therapists, clergy, dietitians, and volunteers.

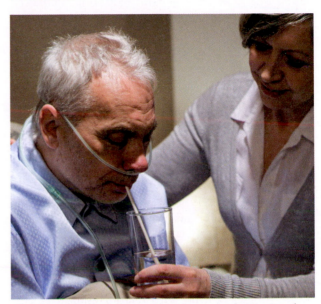

Fig. 27-1. Hospice care can be given anywhere—in a hospital, at a care facility, or in a person's home. The focus of hospice care is on relieving pain and managing symptoms, rather than on curing an illness.

Goals of hospice care include the following:

- Using a holistic, person-centered approach to care

- Focusing on the resident and family as a unit of care

- Offering medically directed, team-managed care

- Offering compassionate care for a person with a terminal illness

- Focusing on comfort care, rather than curative care

- Emphasizing pain and symptom management

- Providing an alternative to traditional hospital care

- Helping the family obtain financial counseling and legal assistance as needed

- Offering assistance in meeting psychosocial needs for the family

Hospice care strives to meet all of the needs of the dying person. The resident and her family and friends are directly involved in care decisions. The resident is encouraged to participate in decision-making as long as possible.

Hospice care focuses on pain relief by monitoring the administration and effectiveness of medications, which are prescribed by a doctor. NAs should report complaints of pain or signs of pain to the nurse immediately. These observations are communicated to the doctor, and adjustments in treatment are made as needed.

Hospice care encourages the involvement of the resident's spiritual or religious leader if the resident has one. Hospice also supports both the family and the dying resident in their continued involvement in social activities. Reading, listening to music, visiting with friends, and learning new skills are encouraged. Residents who are dying need to feel independent for as long as possible. They need to have control over their lives for as long as they are able.

Tip

Hospice Cares

According to the National Hospice and Palliative Care Organization, over 1.4 million people received hospice services in 2016, and there were 4,382 hospices in operation. Hospice volunteers attend a special training program to prepare them for hospice work. The organization's website, nhpco.org, contains more information.

4. Discuss the grief process and related terms

Grief is a deeply emotional response to loss. It is an adaptive, or changing, process and usually involves healing in some way. Grief includes physical, psychological, emotional, social, and spiritual reactions to the loss.

Dr. Elisabeth Kübler-Ross wrote the book *On Death and Dying* in 1969. She developed a theory that dying people experience a common grief process. Her model includes five different emotional stages that a person may experience prior to death. According to Kübler-Ross, the five stages of grief are denial, anger, bargaining, depression, and acceptance. However, not all people go through all of the stages. Some may stay in one stage until death, while others may move back and forth between stages during the process. A brief explanation of the stages follows.

Stage 1. Denial: People in the denial stage may refuse to believe they are dying. They may think a mistake has been made and demand that lab work be repeated. They may avoid discussion about their illnesses and simply act like it is not happening. This is the "No, not me" stage.

Stage 2. Anger: Once people start to face the possibility of death, they may become angry. They may be angry because they think they are too young to die or because they have always taken care of themselves. Anger may be directed at staff, visitors, roommates, family, or friends. Anger is a normal reaction. Even though it may be upsetting, the caregiver must try not to take anger personally. This is the "Why me?" stage.

Stage 3. Bargaining: Once people have begun to believe that they really are dying, they may start trying to bargain with God or a higher power in hope of recovery. They may make promises and try to bargain for the ability to attend an important function, such as a wedding. This is the "Yes me, but . . ." stage.

Stage 4. Depression: As dying people become weaker and their symptoms get worse, they may become deeply sad or depressed. They may cry or become withdrawn (Fig. 27-2). They may be unable to do simple tasks. They need additional physical and emotional support. It is important for caregivers to listen and be understanding.

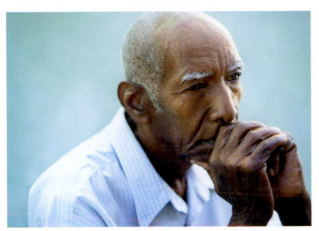

Fig. 27-2. A dying person may become depressed and withdrawn.

Stage 5. Acceptance: Peace or acceptance may or may not come before death. Some people who are dying are eventually able to accept death and prepare for it. They may make arrangements with attorneys, accountants, and loved ones for the care of important people, pets, and belongings. They may prepare for ceremonies before or after death and plan for their last days. At this stage, people who are dying may seem detached.

Experiencing these stages may not be possible for someone who dies suddenly, unexpectedly, or quickly. Caregivers cannot force anyone to move from stage to stage; they can only listen and be ready to offer any help a person needs.

Terms Associated with Death and Dying

Some terms that are associated with death and dying include the following:

anticipatory grief: a period of mourning when the dying person or his family is expecting the death.

bereavement: the period following a loss in which mourning occurs.

grief counseling: therapy to try to help a person cope after someone has died.

grief process: the varying emotional responses to grief; many models have been developed to explain this process.

mourning: the period in which people work to adapt to a loss; heavily influenced by culture, tradition, and society.

5. Explain legal rights for a resident who is dying

NAs can treat residents with dignity when they are approaching death by respecting their rights and preferences. There are some legal rights to remember when caring for people who are dying:

The right to have visitors: Residents who are dying have the right to have visitors of their choosing. They can have visits from family, friends, pets, healthcare providers, clergy, members of the community, and others. Visitors must not be prevented from entering the resident's room unless the resident asks them to leave. Normal visiting hours are generally suspended during this difficult time. Visitors may be at the facility throughout the night. An NA should only report if a visitor is upsetting the resident, if he is purposely disruptive to the unit, or if he becomes a threat to other residents, visitors, or staff members.

The right to privacy: Residents have the right to privacy. They may request that visitors leave their room. They may ask a spouse to leave during an examination or a procedure. These requests must be honored.

The right to be free from pain: Residents who are dying have the right to be free of pain. Pain must be carefully monitored, and medication and pain relief measures must be given to keep the resident as pain-free as possible.

The right to honest and accurate information: Residents who are dying have the right to know the truth about their diagnosis. Information about treatment, possible risks or complications, and side effects must be presented honestly. If residents have questions about their condition or anything else that is beyond an NA's scope of practice, she should notify the nurse.

The right to refuse treatment: Residents have the right to make choices about their care, including refusing treatment for their illness. NAs must not judge these decisions, even if they do not agree with them. The choice belongs to the resident and/or his family. More information on living wills and advance directives may be found in Chapter 2.

Other rights of a dying person are listed below in *The Dying Person's Bill of Rights*. This was created at a workshop, *The Terminally Ill Patient and the Helping Person*, sponsored by Southwestern Michigan In-Service Education Council, and appeared in the *American Journal of Nursing*, Vol. 75, January 1975, p. 99.

I have the right to

- Be treated as a living human being until I die.

- Maintain a sense of hopefulness, however changing its focus may be.

- Be cared for by those who can maintain a sense of hopefulness, however changing this might be.

- Express my feelings and emotions about my approaching death in my own way.

- Participate in decisions concerning my care.

- Expect continuing medical and nursing attentions even though "cure" goals must be changed to "comfort" goals.

- Not die alone.

- Be free from pain.

- Have my questions answered honestly.

- Not be deceived.

- Have help from and for my family in accepting my death.

- Die in peace and dignity.

- Retain my individuality and not be judged for my decisions, which may be contrary to the beliefs of others.

- Discuss and enlarge my religious and/or spiritual experiences, whatever these may mean to others.

- Expect that the sanctity of the human body will be respected after death.

- Be cared for by caring, sensitive, knowledgeable people who will attempt to understand my needs and will be able to gain some satisfaction in helping me face my death.

6. Explain how to care for a resident who is dying

The focus of care for a resident who is dying is to meet all her physical needs, as well as to provide comfort and emotional support. Promoting independence is emphasized in end-of-life care. The resident needs to have as much control over her life as possible. When a resident's ability to perform her activities of daily living decreases, staff will perform these tasks as needed. Family and friends may assist with this care.

Guidelines: Resident Who Is Dying

G **Room environment**: Make sure the room is adequately ventilated. Keep the resident's personal objects, such as photos, religious items, and cards, visible and within reach as requested. Scented items such as fresh flowers may bother the resident. Remove them from the room if requested. Do not wear scented products such as perfume, cologne, or aftershave to work.

G **Skin, nose, and mouth care**: Give frequent skin care. Bathe the resident often if she is perspiring heavily. Change gowns and sheets for comfort. Give incontinence care promptly, and keep the resident clean and dry. Turn and reposition the resident often to prevent pressure injuries. More help may be needed when moving the resident due to fatigue and a decrease in muscle strength. Give mouth care frequently to rinse secretions out of the mouth. Offer ice chips to help keep the mouth moist. Using a light lubricant on the nose and mouth may prevent cracking. A humidifier in the room can help with dryness.

G **Breathing problems**: A resident who is dying may have difficulty breathing. She may have alternating slow, irregular respirations followed by rapid, shallow respirations, called *Cheyne-Stokes respirations*. There may be gurgling or rattling sounds as the resident breathes, which is caused by a buildup of secretions in the throat. Notify the nurse if any of these conditions occur; she may administer medication to help dry the secretions. To ease problems with breathing, elevate the head of the bed and help the resident change position. Give mouth care as necessary. Oxygen therapy and a humidifier may be used.

G **Food and fluid issues**: Remember that the resident has the right to refuse food or fluids. Do not force the resident to eat or drink. When she wants to eat, feed the resident slowly to help prevent choking and aspiration. Small, frequent meals can help. Encourage fluids as requested. Report nausea, vomiting, and diarrhea to the nurse. A clear liquid diet may be ordered. Elevation of the head of the bed can help reduce burping and acid reflux.

If the resident is constipated, the nurse can provide a stool softener or other medication to help. Bowel obstructions can occur in people who are dying. Report any signs and symptoms of a bowel obstruction to the nurse (see Chapter 15).

G **Pain control and comfort**: Residents who are dying may be in pain. Pain relief is critical; observe and report signs of pain to the nurse immediately. Residents may be connected to a patient-controlled analgesia (PCA) device (Chapter 24) that they control themselves. They press a button to give themselves a dose of pain medication. Some residents will not be able to communicate that they are in pain. Watch for body language and other signs that they are in pain (Chapter 13) (Fig. 27-3). Excessive drowsiness can result from pain medication. Report this to the nurse.

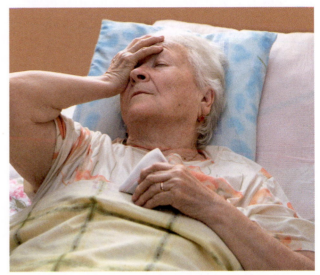

Fig. 27-3. *Observe body language for signs of pain and report them promptly to the nurse.*

If body temperature rises and the resident is perspiring, remove heavier blankets. Fever can cause chills; use extra blankets if the resident needs more warmth.

G **Diminished senses**: Vision may begin to fail as death nears. Keep the room softly lit without glare. Verbal communication may become difficult. Try using communication boards, pictures, or hand or eye signals. The sense of hearing is usually the last sense to leave the body, so continue to speak in a normal tone of voice and tell the resident about care that is being performed. Describe what is happening, but do not expect an answer.

Residents' Rights

The Sense of Hearing

Do not say anything inappropriate around a resident who is dying or her family. The sense of hearing is usually the last sense to leave the body. Continue to be professional, explaining procedures and talking to the resident as you would normally. Assume that the resident can understand you.

7. Discuss factors that influence feelings about death and list ways to meet residents' individual needs

Feelings and attitudes about death differ greatly and are influenced by many factors, including a person's previous experience with death, personality type, religious beliefs, and cultural background.

Some people grieve openly when a loved one is dying, while others show little or no emotion. Some may want to talk and share stories about the person who is ill (Fig. 27-4). Others will not want to discuss their feelings.

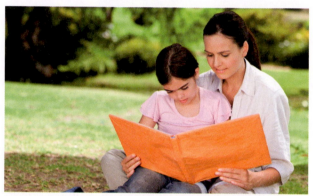

Fig. 27-4. *Looking at photos and sharing stories about a person who is dying is one way family and friends may grieve.*

Cultural and spiritual beliefs may play an important part in activities after death. Some groups share food, play music, and talk about the person who has died. Customs may include burying personal items with the body or specific rules about washing the body after a person has died. Some bury their dead in a coffin, while others prefer cremation. **Cremation** is the process of burning a dead body until it turns to ash. Family or friends may request spiritual or religious leaders, or specific people, to be involved in a ceremony after a person has died.

It is important to understand that no matter how residents and their families deal with dying and death, staff members must respect their wishes, preferences, and behavior. Honoring cultural traditions whenever possible is important. The care team must always respond in a culturally sensitive way to different practices and individual beliefs. This is part of providing person-centered care.

Guidelines: Psychosocial and Spiritual Needs

G   Listen more; talk less. When dealing with a resident who will die soon, listening is often one of the most important things you can do (Fig. 27-5).

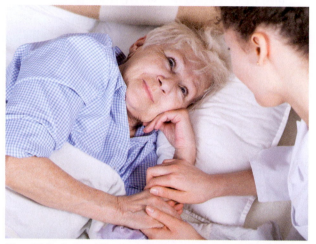

Fig. 27-5. *A good listener can be a great comfort for a resident who is dying.*

G   Provide privacy for visits from family, friends, or clergy. Let the resident and visitors know you will be there if you are needed.

G   Notify the nurse immediately if the resident requests a visit from a clergyperson or any spiritual leader.

G   Do not discuss your religious or spiritual beliefs or lack of beliefs with the resident. Do not try to change or influence the resident's beliefs or cultural traditions.

G   Do not judge anything the resident tells you about her past, beliefs, wishes, or choices.

G   Never share anything private that is said to you by the resident with anyone other than the nurse. Never share anything about the resident, including conversations, appearance, or anything else with anyone other than the nurse. This includes other staff members, volunteers, your own family and friends, or the media.

G Do not isolate or avoid a dying resident; spend as much time as you can with the resident.

G If a resident expresses a fear of dying, inform the nurse. Do not respond with clichés or try to give reassurance using your personal religious or spiritual beliefs. Therapists and other professionals can try to help the resident work through these fears.

8. Identify common signs of approaching death

When a person is dying, all body systems are affected. Common signs of approaching death include the following:

- Cyanotic, pale, or darkening skin or mucous membranes
- Cold skin
- Skin that looks bruised (mottling)
- Heavy perspiration
- Fever
- Low blood pressure
- Increased pulse
- Cheyne-Stokes breathing
- Gurgling and rattling sound when breathing
- Difficulty swallowing
- Decreased appetite and sense of thirst
- Dry mouth
- Nausea, vomiting, and diarrhea
- Decreased sense of touch
- Loss of feeling, beginning in the legs and feet
- Extreme weakness and exhaustion
- Loss of muscle tone

- Fallen jaw, causing the mouth to stay open
- Inability to speak
- Loss of vision
- Dilated pupils and staring eyes
- Urinary and fecal incontinence
- Decreased urinary output
- Hallucinations
- Extreme drowsiness
- Disorientation or confusion
- Loss of hearing

9. List changes that may occur in the human body after death

When death occurs, the body will not have a pulse, respiration, or blood pressure. Other physical signs include the following:

- Eyelids that are partially open, with eyes in a fixed stare
- Fixed and dilated pupils (which means there is no blood flow inside the brain)
- A dropped jaw, which causes the mouth to stay open
- Urinary and fecal incontinence

Though these things are a normal part of death, they can be unsettling. If any of these signs are noted, the NA should tell the nurse immediately so that she can confirm the death.

Tip

Terms to Describe the Body after Death
These Latin terms describe changes in the body after death:

- *Algor mortis* is the cooling of the body after death and the decrease in elasticity of the skin.
- *Livor mortis* is skin discoloration after death in the dependent areas of the body, such as the feet and legs.
- **Rigor mortis** is the stiffness that occurs after death due to a biochemical change that causes muscles to become rigid.

10. Describe ways to help family and friends deal with a resident's death

When a loved one dies, family and friends may experience a range of emotions, including the following:

- Feeling numb or being in shock

- Disbelief or denial of the death

- Intense sadness and crying

- Anxiety or fear

- Anger

- Physical reactions or symptoms, such as pain, especially chest pain, nausea, or difficulty breathing (these should be reported to the nurse immediately)

- Feelings of guilt, especially if there were any unresolved problems or issues with the relationship

- Feelings of relief

Family may direct anger at staff members. They may just be reacting to the loss of a loved one. They may blame staff for a problem that they feel was not addressed. Whatever the reason, NAs should not try to calm a family member or friend who is upset with staff. Those complaints should be referred to the nurse.

Guidelines: Helping the Family Deal with a Resident's Death

G Allowing the family and friends to show their feelings is one of the first steps in the grieving process. Do not ask the family to stop crying or to not be upset about their loss.

G Be available for the family and friends. Talking is an important part of the grieving process. Listen to them if they want to talk (Fig. 27-6). Let them talk, and only respond if needed. Remaining silent can be beneficial.

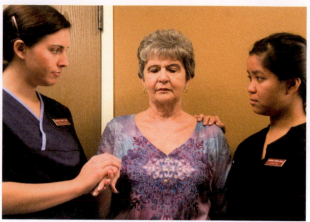

Fig. 27-6. NAs should be available for family and friends if they want to talk and should allow them to express their feelings.

G Do not be afraid to show your feelings for a resident who has died. Family and friends may feel better knowing that their loved one was valued by staff members.

G Do not make inappropriate comments or use clichés, such as, "This will pass," "It is for the best," or "You will get over it." These are painful comments and are not helpful.

G If family or friends make a request to see a spiritual leader or clergyperson, report this to the nurse immediately.

Some facilities have designated staff members available to help families after a resident has died. These people may be social workers, therapists, hospice workers, or spiritual leaders.

11. Describe ways to help staff members cope with a resident's death

Staff members and other residents may be very upset by the death of a beloved resident. Being able to grieve is important. Some facilities offer bereavement therapy, also called grief counseling, to help staff with grieving. Identifying feelings in a formal setting can help staff work through their loss. Many facilities also allow caregivers and residents to participate in memorial or religious services following a death. Some may be held at the facility. If a service is not held at the facility and an NA wants to attend the service, she should check with her supervisor first to make sure it is appropriate.

It is important for those who are grieving not to underestimate their feelings; seeking counseling or bereavement therapy may help during this difficult time. They should grieve at their own pace.

Staff members can cope with the death of a resident by doing the following:

- Not hesitating to express their feelings; sadness and crying are normal responses to grieving

- Getting enough sleep, eating nutritious meals, drinking only in moderation, and not smoking

- Participating in enjoyable activities and exercising regularly; for example, a person may want to spend time outside or take his dog for a walk

- Spending quality time with the people they love (Fig. 27-7)

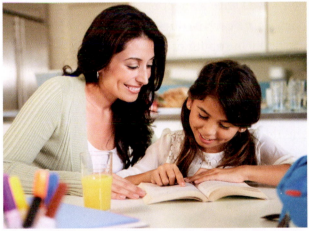

Fig. 27-7. Spending time with a loved one can help a person deal with her grief.

- Sharing important memories about the resident with others

- Joining a special support group for grieving

- Talking to a counselor if the need arises

12. Describe postmortem care

Postmortem care is care of the body after death. It is important for NAs to be sensitive to the needs of the family and friends after death. Family members may wish to stay with the body for some time. They should be allowed to do this. NAs should be aware of religious and cultural practices that the family wants to observe. Facilities will have different policies on postmortem care. The NA should ask the nurse for instructions before beginning this care. A shroud kit containing a large white piece of material for covering the body may be used. It may include special pads, a chin strap, and ID tags. NAs must follow their facility's procedures and only perform assigned tasks.

An **autopsy** is an examination of a body by a pathologist to try to determine the cause of death. A **pathologist** is a doctor with advanced training in the examination of organs and tissues. If the body is to be autopsied, the resident may need to be transferred to another facility. If the resident has designated himself to be an organ donor after death, the body may need to be transported immediately to a hospital. Organ donation is the removal of organs and tissues in order to transplant them into someone who needs them. NAs should follow the nurse's instructions regarding organ donation preparation.

> **Tip**
>
> **Care of the Belongings after Death**
> Every facility has policies for handling residents' personal items, such as jewelry and pictures, after death. NAs should carefully follow their facilities' policies.

Postmortem care

Equipment: two pairs of gloves, drainage pads, shroud kit or sheets, clean gown, washcloths or wipes, wash basin of warm water, mild soap, towel

1. Identify the resident.

2. Wash your hands.

3. Explain procedure to the resident's family and ask them to step outside. Be courteous, respectful, and compassionate at all times.

4. Provide for privacy with a curtain, screen, or door.

5. Adjust the bed to a safe working level, usually waist high. Lock bed wheels.

6. Avoid trauma to the resident's body throughout the procedure. Treat the body with the utmost respect.

7. Put on gloves.

8. Turn off any oxygen, suction, or other equipment if directed by the nurse. Do not remove any tubes or other equipment. A nurse or someone at the funeral home will perform these tasks.

9. Gently close the resident's eyes without putting pressure on them.

10. Position the body in proper alignment, on the back with legs straight. Fold the arms across the abdomen. It is important to position the body before *rigor mortis* occurs, as it will make positioning difficult. The period from two to four hours after death is most common for the development of *rigor mortis*.

11. Close the mouth. Place a rolled towel under the chin.

12. Gently bathe the body using a mild soap (or solution as directed). Be careful to avoid bruising. Replace any dressings only if instructed to do so.

13. Comb or brush hair gently without tugging it.

14. Place drainage pads where needed. Most often this is under the head and/or under the perineal area and buttocks.

15. Put a clean gown on the body.

16. Cover the body to just over the shoulders with sheet. Do not cover the face or head.

17. Tidy the room so family may visit.

18. Remove all used supplies and linen.

19. Follow your facility's policy for handling or removing personal items.

20. Remove and discard gloves properly.

21. Wash your hands.

22. Return bed to a low position if raised. Turn the lights down and allow the family to enter and spend private time with resident.

23. Return after the family leaves and put on clean gloves.

24. Place a shroud on the resident and follow instructions for completing ID tags.

25. Remove and discard gloves properly.

26. Wash your hands.

27. Report and record observations. Document procedure using facility guidelines.

The body will be transported to a morgue or the funeral home. The NA's responsibilities may include transferring the body on a stretcher (with a coworker) to the pick-up area. The body should be covered with a sheet or shroud during transport. Being careful during the transfer helps to avoid any bumping or bruising. The NA should behave professionally and should be courteous and respectful at all times.

After the body has been transported, the NA should return to the room, don gloves, and remove all bed linen and trash. The windows can be opened as needed to air the room. Chapter 10 contains information on unit cleaning.

Tip

Unexpected Sounds or Movements after Death

After a person dies, the body may make sounds or movements. Breathing sounds, movement of the hands or legs, eyes opening, jaws opening, and bouts of incontinence may occur. Although it may be frightening to witness, it is common for these things to happen. Anything of concern, however, should be reported to the nurse.

Two Early Autopsies

Julius Caesar, the well-known Roman leader, was killed on March 15th, known as the *Ides of March*, in 44 B.C. The first recorded autopsy was done on Julius Caesar by a physician named Antistius. Antistius noted 23 stab wounds and is thought to have determined that the chest wound was the fatal blow.

An early autopsy was also performed in 1302 when the nobleman Azzolino died under suspicious circumstances. Bartolomeo da Varignana, a doctor, performed an autopsy to determine the cause of death. He found Azzolino had not died of poisoning, as he had suspected, but from internal bleeding.

Chapter Review

1. What are the goals of palliative care (LO 2)?

2. Briefly describe each of the five stages of grief (denial, anger, bargaining, depression, and acceptance) as defined by Elisabeth Kübler-Ross (LO 4).

3. List five legal rights to remember when caring for a resident who is terminally ill (LO 5).

4. List 20 physical signs that a person is approaching death (LO 8).

5. What should the NA do if he observes physical signs such as a dropped jaw after a resident has died (LO 9)?

6. List four ways that NAs can help families and friends after a loved one has died (LO 10).

7. What is bereavement therapy (LO 11)?

8. Define *postmortem* (LO 12).

Multiple Choice

9. When is hospice care usually ordered by a doctor (LO 3)?
   (A) When a person has a chronic disease
   (B) When a person is not eating normally
   (C) When a person has approximately six months or less to live
   (D) When a person becomes depressed

10. Which sense is usually the last sense to leave the body (LO 6)?
    (A) The sense of hearing
    (B) The sense of smell
    (C) The sense of taste
    (D) The sense of touch

11. Which of the following would be the best way an NA can help meet a dying resident's psychosocial needs (LO 7)?
    (A) Convincing the resident to believe in God
    (B) Bathing the resident
    (C) Making changes in the resident's diet
    (D) Listening to the resident

28
Your New Position

The Good Old Days?

Job descriptions of the distant past included things that seem strange and even laughable today. Nurses had to act as wardens to prevent patients from playing cards, stealing from one another, drinking, or fighting. Nurses spent long hours washing and waxing floors. They even had to carry coal and fill lamps with oil. Sometimes they acted as chimney sweeps, too. Nurses were not allowed to openly smoke, drink, or attend social events. In some places, nursing staff were forbidden to meet or see anyone of the opposite sex.

"When men are employed, they are best contented; for on the days they worked they were good-natured and cheerful, and, with the consciousness of having done a good day's work, they spent the evening jollily."

Benjamin Franklin, 1706–1790

"The superior man is the providence of the inferior. He is eyes for the blind, strength for the weak, and a shield for the defenseless. He stands erect by bending above the fallen. He rises by lifting others."

Robert Green Ingersoll, 1833–1899

1. Define important words in this chapter

conflict resolution: the process of resolving conflicts in a positive way so that everyone is satisfied.

constructive feedback: feedback that involves giving opinions about the work of others in a nonaggressive way.

job description: an outline of what will be expected in a job.

résumé: a summary of a person's education and experience.

stress: a mentally or emotionally disruptive or upsetting condition that occurs due to changes in the environment.

stressor: internal or external factors or stimuli that cause stress.

The first 27 chapters of this book introduce readers to the long-term care setting. They cover the knowledge, skills, and qualities a person needs to work as a nursing assistant. This final chapter is more personal. It has to do with finding and keeping a job. This chapter addresses the reader directly. It includes a step-by-step job-hunting guide and useful advice about building positive relationships with employers and coworkers. It also includes helpful tips for managing stress and staying healthy.

2. Describe how to write a résumé and cover letter

Before beginning a new position as a nursing assistant, you have to look for a job. The first step in any job search is preparing a well-written résumé. A **résumé** is a summary of your education and experience. You will need to include this information when preparing a résumé:

- **Objective:** State your main goals in the field in which you wish to work.

- **Education:** List schools or GED courses completed, beginning with high school and including any college courses. List any certifications you have received, such as CNA, CPR, or first aid certification.

- **Experience**: Identify the work experience you have had to this point, placing your current job first and moving backward. A general rule is to list positions you have held for more than six months.

- **Volunteer Work**: Describe all volunteer work, emphasizing any work related to the healthcare field.

- **Skills**: List all of your special skills, including things like typing, computer skills, and languages that you speak.

- **References**: State that your references are available upon request.

Take time to make your résumé the best it can be. Here are some general rules for writing a résumé:

- Limit your résumé to one page. Use short, precise sentences.

- Do not add borders or color. Use high-quality, white paper.

- Use a basic, 12-point, plain font. Boldface your name (you can also make it larger than a 12-point font), and include your contact information at the top of the page.

- Do not rely on a spell check tool. Use it first, check spelling yourself, and then have a friend or family member check spelling. Read the résumé out loud to make sure you have not made any errors.

- Do not staple anything to your résumé.

A cover letter is a letter that will be included with your résumé. This letter should be brief and serves as your introduction to the interviewer. It should include information about why you are seeking the job and why you are qualified for the position.

After a résumé and cover letter have been created, you will need to identify potential employers. Use the internet and personal contacts to find employers. Ask your instructor for recommendations as well.

3. Identify information that may be required for filling out a job application

Completing a job application can be stressful. Being prepared will help you present yourself well. To save time and avoid mistakes, write down information that you may need for the application. Take this information with you, along with a new copy of your résumé, when you go to complete the application. This information should be included:

- Your address and phone number

- Your email address

- Your social security number

- Salary information from your past and present positions, although some states do not allow employers to ask for this information

- Names, addresses, and telephone numbers of the schools or programs where you were trained and dates you completed training

- Certification numbers and expiration dates from your NA certification card, CPR card, and first aid cards

- Former and present supervisors' and employers' names, titles, addresses, email addresses, and phone numbers

- Exact dates of past and current employment and your reasons for leaving each of your former positions

- Complete names, addresses, email addresses, and phone numbers of personal and professional references

- The days and hours you can work (for example, weekdays, nights, or weekends)

Before going to the facility, think about any potential issues in your job application. For

Your New Position

example, if you have a time when you did not work at all, an interviewer may ask for the reason for the gap in employment. Imagine being the interviewer and consider the questions you might ask yourself.

When you actually fill out the job application, here are a few steps that can make the process run smoothly:

- Fill out the application carefully and neatly. Use a pen to complete it. If you are filling it out at home, check your spelling.

- Never lie on a job application. Tell the truth. Be honest if you have a criminal record. By law, the employer is required to do a complete criminal background check. This law is in place to protect residents at facilities. If you do have a record, write a complete explanation in the appropriate section so that they will have your side of the story.

- Do not leave anything blank on the application. You may write N/A (not applicable) if the question does not apply to you. If you do not understand something on the application, ask about it before filling in the space.

4. Discuss proper grooming guidelines for a job interview

In Chapter 1, professional grooming guidelines were described. Careful grooming is equally important when applying for a job. Creating a positive first impression can increase your odds of success, so you should look and dress appropriately.

Guidelines: Proper Grooming for a Job Interview

G   Bathe beforehand and use deodorant.

G   Do not wear perfume or cologne. Many people dislike or are allergic to scents.

G   Wear simple makeup and jewelry or none at all.

G   Wash your hands and clean and file your nails. Nails should be medium length or shorter. Do not wear artificial nails.

G   Shave or trim facial hair right before the interview.

G   Wear your hair in a simple style.

G   Brush your teeth. Check your teeth right before the interview begins.

G   Do not smoke. You will smell like smoke during the interview.

G   Wear clean, nice clothes. Make sure that skirts, dresses, and pants are wrinkle-free and do not have stains or holes. Dresses and skirts should not be shorter than knee-length. Do not wear jeans or shorts. Do not wear T-shirts or anything with a logo on it. Do not wear low-cut tops that show cleavage.

G   Make sure your shoes are polished. Do not wear sneakers or open-toed sandals.

5. List techniques for interviewing successfully

Use these guidelines to make the best impression at a job interview:

Guidelines: Interviewing Successfully

G   Practice for the interview with a friend. There are websites and books that have commonly asked job interview questions. Practice answering these questions. Write down any questions you have before the interview.

G   Tests may be given during the interview to assess your skills. Find out if there will be a test, and if so, study beforehand to feel better prepared.

G   Get directions to the interview site. If you are taking the bus, make sure you have bus fare the night before. If you are driving, get gas the day before.

G   Do not bring children, other family members, friends, or pets with you.

G   Arrive 10 or 15 minutes early.

G   Turn off your cell phone.

G   Be courteous to other staff members you meet.

G   Introduce yourself to the interviewer. Smile and offer to shake hands. Your handshake should be firm and confident (Fig. 28-1).

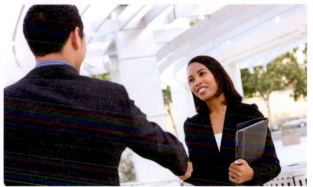

Fig. 28-1. *Smile and shake hands confidently when you arrive at a job interview.*

G   Be positive and look happy to be there.

G   Do not eat or chew gum during the interview.

G   Make eye contact during the interview. Do not look up or down or left or right during the interview. The interviewer may think that you are not telling the truth or are not interested in the conversation. Maintain eye contact to show that you are sincere.

G   Answer questions clearly and completely.

G   Do not use slang or curse words.

G   Do not exaggerate your accomplishments.

G   During the interview, emphasize what you think you will enjoy about your work. Do not speak negatively about a former employer. Ask questions if you are unsure about anything and take notes if needed.

G   Relax. You have worked hard to get this far. You understand the work and what is expected of you. Be confident!

G   After the interview is over, stand up, make eye contact, smile, and shake hands again. Ask when you can expect to hear about the position if you have not already been told. Thank the interviewer for taking the time to meet with you.

Tip

Saying Thank You Makes a Difference

Always mail or email a thank-you note after every job interview. This shows your continued interest in a job and helps to remind the interviewer who you are. If you have not heard from a potential employer within the time frame you discussed, call and politely ask if the job is still available.

6. Describe a standard job description and list steps for following the scope of practice

A **job description** is an outline of what will be expected of you in your job. It can be a long, complex form, and you should read it before you sign it. Ask questions if you do not understand anything in the job description.

The term *scope of practice* was first introduced in Chapter 2. A scope of practice lists the tasks that NAs are permitted to perform as allowed by state or federal law. These tips can help you decide whether or not you should perform a procedure:

•   Do not perform a procedure if it is outside your scope of practice, not listed in your job description, or not listed in the care plan. This is true even if a nurse or doctor asks you to perform the procedure. In that case, politely refuse to perform the procedure and explain why. Refusing to do something that you should not legally do is your right and your responsibility. Doing things that are beyond your scope of practice could injure a resident, you, or another staff member.

•   Do not perform a procedure if you have not been trained to do it.

- Do not perform a procedure if you have forgotten how to do all or part of it. Ask the nurse for a reminder about how to perform the procedure before you do it.

- If you have been trained to perform a procedure that is within your scope of practice, but you believe it may not be appropriate for a certain resident, ask the nurse.

Tip

Organizing Your Days

When you start a new job, you will want to be as organized as possible during your workday. There are several ways to organize your work. You can use a pocket organizer, which can be found online or at uniform stores. Some pocket organizers even have room for a stethoscope.

7. Identify guidelines for maintaining certification and explain the state's registry

In order to meet the Omnibus Budget Reconciliation Act (OBRA) requirements (Chapter 2), several organizations, including the National Council of State Boards of Nursing, created nurse aide training and competency evaluation programs (NATCEP). These programs serve as a guide for each state's development of its NA evaluation (testing) program. OBRA requires that NAs complete at least 75 hours of training before being employed. Many states' requirements exceed the minimum 75 hours.

After completing a state's required number of training hours, NAs may then take the test in that state. A fee may be charged to take this test. Once an NA has passed both the written and manual skills tests, a certificate is issued and mailed to the recipient.

Each state has different requirements for maintaining certification. Know and follow your state's specific requirements. General guidelines on obtaining and keeping NA certification include the following:

- An NA has a certain amount of time from the date he is employed to take the state test. Your employer will supply you with that information when you are hired. Pay attention to the time frame. If you do not take the test during the time given, you will not be able to work until you have passed the test.

- An NA usually must take the state test within 24 months of completing the nursing assisting course. If the test is not taken during that time period, he will have to complete a new training course and state examination.

- An NA must work for pay during the 24-month certification period. If he does not, a new training program and examination must be completed.

- In most states, an NA has three chances to pass the state tests.

- An NA must keep his certification current. File a change-of-address with your state agency if you move to make sure you receive your certification renewal. Some states require that you file a change-of-address form within 30 days.

Your employer will require that you show proof of renewal of your certificate each time it expires. Do not allow your certificate to expire. Respond immediately to your state's request to renew your certification and pay any associated renewal fees.

In the United States, each state keeps a registry for certified NAs (CNAs). This registry keeps track of every NA working in that state. Information kept in this registry includes the following:

- An NA's full name, along with any other names the person may have used

- An NA's home address and other information, such as date of birth and social security number

- The date that an NA was placed in the registry and results from the state testing

- The expiration date of an NA's certificate

- Information about investigations and hearings regarding abuse, neglect, or theft, which becomes a part of an NA's permanent record

NAs can ask for a written statement to be added to the file. This includes information explaining events in the NA's own words. NAs have the right to correct any errors in a state registry file.

It is possible for an NA's certification to be suspended, revoked, or denied. Reasons for this vary. Be familiar with your state's guidelines. An NA can also voluntarily surrender his certification. If an NA surrenders his certification or has his certification revoked, he will not be able to practice in his state and may not be able to work in other states.

8. Describe continuing education for nursing assistants

The OBRA law requires that NAs have 12 hours of continuing education each year in order to keep their certification current. Some states require more hours. These classes help keep your knowledge and skills up to date. Your facility is required to provide and document this continuing, or in-service education. Here are some of the subjects covered in these classes:

- Residents' Rights
- Confidentiality
- Safety
- Fire safety
- Infection prevention
- Bloodborne pathogens
- Tuberculosis
- CPR

Make sure you attend all of the required in-services. Pay attention in class and participate in discussions (Fig. 28-2). Do any required homework or projects. After the in-service is over, keep copies of any certificates and records that show you have successfully completed the class.

> **Tip**
>
> **Hepatitis B Vaccine and TB Tests**
> Employers are required to provide free hepatitis B vaccines to all employees after hire to help protect against the spread of hepatitis. Employers are also required to test newly hired employees for tuberculosis. Follow instructions when notified to take the tests, and return for follow-up as required. Chapters 6 and 20 contain more information on hepatitis and tuberculosis.

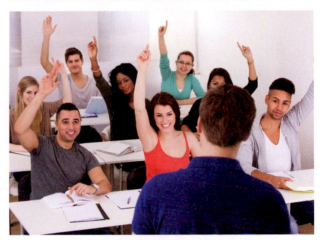

Fig. 28-2. *Students should pay attention and participate during continuing education courses.*

9. Describe employee evaluations and discuss feedback

An annual evaluation, sometimes called a *performance appraisal* or *review*, is used to evaluate the performance of each employee. Some of the things you will be evaluated on are overall knowledge, conflict resolution, and team effort. Flexibility, friendliness, trustworthiness, and customer service skills are other qualities considered in an evaluation. A performance review or appraisal may be done after a three-month probationary period and then annually thereafter. As long as you demonstrate consistent professionalism, excellent customer service, dependability, and ethical behavior, you will usually receive a satisfactory or better evaluation.

Employee evaluations include constructive feedback. **Constructive feedback** involves giving opinions about the work of others, which includes helpful suggestions for change. It may involve both positive and negative feedback, but it is done in a nonaggressive way. Constructive feedback should be given in a private setting. It should be work-related; it should not include personal attacks. It is not the same as hostile criticism. Hostile criticism is angry and negative. Constructive feedback is meant to help you improve in your job.

When receiving constructive feedback, be open to suggestions, as they will help you grow and be more successful in your work. Try to listen without becoming upset or angry. Consider how you can address or fix the problem; offer ideas during the session (Fig. 28-3). If you are not sure how to avoid a mistake you have made, always ask for suggestions. A person who readily accepts constructive feedback can do well in the workplace.

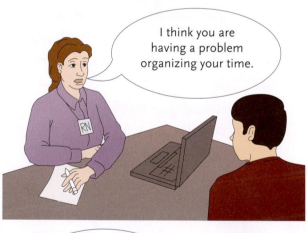

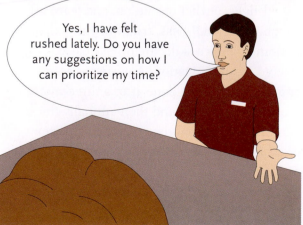

Fig. 28-3. Be open to suggestions when receiving constructive feedback.

It is important for an employee to try each year to improve her performance appraisal score. Performance reviews are frequently the basis for salary increases. In addition, a satisfactory review can increase the chance of advancing within the facility. Ask for and keep a copy of every evaluation you receive.

10. Discuss conflict resolution

When you work with a group of people, conflicts can arise. **Conflict resolution** is the process of resolving conflicts in a positive way so that everyone is satisfied with the result. Most people do not like to disagree; however, sometimes it cannot be avoided. Before reacting, think about possible reasons why someone is behaving in an undesirable way. For example, a coworker may have had a fight with a family member, or an angry resident may be lonely or in pain.

When you disagree with a policy at your facility, know that the management team makes the best and most informed decisions that they can make. If you have a conflict with your boss or supervisor, understand that this person really wants to help you. However, policy cannot be changed for you at the expense of other staff. In short, conflict resolution works best when you are reasonable with your requests.

Sometimes resolving a conflict means you have to compromise. In order to compromise, think about how important the problem is. Making a list of pros and cons may help clarify your options. Identify the benefits of working with others to solve the issue. Think about whether another person, such as an arbitrator or a mediator, could help resolve the conflict. Many organizations have a process for formally resolving conflicts; follow your facility's policy.

Conflicts will occur in the workplace. The key to conflict resolution is to think about the issue before reacting. Think about how to best solve the problem. Know when to stand firm, when to walk away, and when it is time to compromise.

11. Define *stress* and explain ways to manage stress

Many things, both personal and professional, cause stress. **Stress** is a mentally or emotionally disruptive or upsetting condition that occurs due to changes in the environment. Internal factors like worry can also cause stress. Stress causes physical changes in the body. When a person is frightened, anxious, excited, confused, or in danger, stress can occur.

Stress happens because of a stressor. A **stressor** is an internal or external factor or stimulus that causes stress. Anything can be a stressor. Finding out you have a new supervisor can create stress. Being asked to speak in front of fellow employees at a staff meeting can cause stress. A visit from a relative can be stressful.

Stress is linked to many diseases and conditions, including hypertension, depression, ulcers, and migraines. It also increases the risk of developing other chronic diseases. Severe stress that does not go away may be linked to premature death.

If stress is unrelieved, burnout can occur. Burnout is mental or physical exhaustion due to a prolonged period of stress and frustration.

Signs of burnout include arguing frequently, losing patience, being angry, wanting too much control in situations, and obsessing over small, unimportant things. A person who is experiencing burnout may also be rude, irritated, and frustrated. He may have trouble focusing on residents and procedures.

It is important to find ways to manage stress and to take responsibility for your well-being. Learn-

ing how to recognize stress and its causes is helpful. People, situations, places, or things can all cause stress. Try to avoid stressors when possible.

Residents' Rights

Leave Your Stress At Home

When you experience a great deal of stress, it can affect how well you do your job. Not managing stress can cause anger or abusive behavior toward residents, poor relationships with coworkers and residents, and arguments. It is very important to take steps toward managing stress. Seek help when you need it. Deal with your stress at home, not at work. If you feel that you cannot manage your stress, tell your supervisor. He or she may be able to give you some helpful resources.

Guidelines: Managing Stress

G Increase your level of exercise.

G Get enough sleep.

G Eat a healthy diet. Eliminate or reduce caffeine in your diet. Caffeine can cause nervousness and irritability, along with anxiety.

G Do not smoke or take illegal drugs. Drink alcohol only in moderation. Some facilities have mandatory, random drug testing, and you will be required to submit to these tests.

G Do one task at a time, then move on to the next task. Multitasking tends to increase anxiety.

G Develop new hobbies and find time to do something relaxing. Riding a bike, dancing, painting, meditating, listening to music, doing yoga, or taking classes can be relaxing and reduce stress.

G Seek help from others with managing stress (Fig. 28-4). Appropriate people to turn to for help include your supervisor, your doctor, your clergyperson or spiritual leader, your friends, your family, or a local mental health agency. Do not talk to residents or their families about your stress. That is inappropriate.

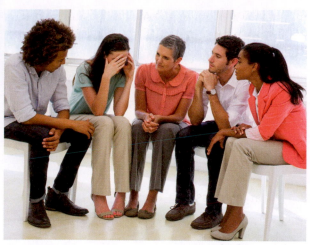

Fig. 28-4. *Support groups can help people deal with different types of stress.*

G Be aware of and understand your emotions. Being a caregiver can be exhausting. Recognize what you have control over and what you are not able to control. Seek counseling if needed. Do not feel embarrassed if you need help. It takes courage to seek help for a problem. Counselors and therapists can suggest a variety of methods to reduce stress.

G Set realistic goals. People can set both short-term and long-term goals for themselves and their families.

G Use a personal reward system. When you accomplish something that makes you happy, do something nice for yourself. See a movie, go out to dinner with friends, visit a loved one, or spend time with a pet.

Tip

Goal-Setting

Setting goals can help manage stress. The key is to make the goals reachable. Do not set only long-term goals. Identify short-term, reachable goals that you can meet in a reasonable time period. The course you are taking right now is an example of a short-term goal, and you are close to meeting this important milestone. If you create long-term goals, do not set a time frame of more than three to five years. Set only long-term goals that you believe you can accomplish.

Relaxation Techniques

Abdominal Breathing:

• Stop, sit down, and breathe.

• Rest your hands on your abdomen and close your eyes.

• Breathe slowly and regularly, pushing your hands out with each breath.

• Do this a few times until you feel yourself begin to relax.

Muscle Relaxation:

• Starting with your head and jaw, relax as many muscles as you can.

• Do this one muscle at a time, moving from the top of your body to the bottom, until you reach your feet and toes.

Tip

Other Ways to Relax

In addition to relaxation ideas discussed in the guidelines, maintaining a sense of humor is important. Laughing causes many physical changes in the body, such as stimulating circulation, increasing the intake of oxygen, improving immune system function, relieving pain, and many other benefits. Try to remember to read, watch, or do something to make yourself laugh when you need to relieve stress. In addition, you can share appropriate humor with residents when the situation is right.

Holding hands with someone special in your life may also decrease stress. Try it and see if it makes you feel calmer and more relaxed.

12. Describe how to be a valued member of the healthcare community

You have now reached the end of your NA course. Very soon you will be a practicing NA. Remember what you have accomplished and know the importance of the work you have chosen to do. You are going to be a valuable member of a care team—a team that literally saves lives every day. It is a noble profession and one that provides a tremendous service to the community. Be very proud of yourself. As you graduate, make sure you thank your family, friends, instructors, and classmates for everything they have done to help you accomplish your goals.

As you move forward in your new profession, never stop learning. Learn new things every day. Stay current in your field. Read materials about health care and other topics. Create your own medical library at home.

Value your profession and treat your new position with all of the respect that it deserves. You worked so hard to get where you are—now it is time to reward yourself (Fig. 28-5)!

> *"Keep close to Nature's heart . . . and break clear away, once in awhile, and climb a mountain or spend a week in the woods."*

John Muir, 1838–1914

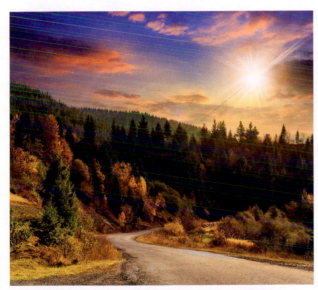

Fig. 28-5. *Reward yourself by taking time to do something meaningful, like exploring nature.*

Chapter Review

1. List six topics that should be included when preparing a résumé (LO 2).

2. How long should a résumé be (LO 2)?

3. Why do you think employers are required to do a criminal background check on NAs (LO 3)?

4. List four ways an NA can make sure she is following her scope of practice before accepting a task (LO 6).

5. List the information about NAs that is kept in the state registry (LO 7).

6. What is constructive feedback (LO 9)?

7. Before reacting to a conflict, what should an NA do (LO 10)?

8. What is stress (LO 11)?

9. List ten ways to manage stress (LO 11).

Multiple Choice

10. Which of the following is part of proper grooming for a job interview (LO 4)?
    (A) Wear a lot of nice jewelry
    (B) Wear a favorite perfume
    (C) Wear comfortable sneakers
    (D) Wear simple makeup

11. After a job interview is over, which of the following would be the best response by the NA (LO 5)?
    (A) The NA should ask, "Will I be hired?"
    (B) The NA should ask, "When can I expect to hear about the position?"
    (C) The NA should ask, "Would you like me to send a thank-you note?"
    (D) The NA should ask, "How soon can I start taking vacation days after I'm hired?"

12. How many hours of continuing education does the federal government require for NAs each year (LO 8)?
    (A) 12
    (B) 25
    (C) 7
    (D) 18

Abbreviations

abd	abdomen
ABR	absolute bedrest
ac, a.c.	before meals
AD	Alzheimer's disease
ad lib	as desired
ADLs	activities of daily living
adm.	admission
AIDS	acquired immuno-deficiency syndrome
AMA	against medical advice, American Medical Association
amb	ambulate, ambulatory
as tol	as tolerated
ax.	axillary (armpit)
BID, b.i.d.	two times a day
BM	bowel movement
BP, B/P	blood pressure
BPM	beats per minute
BR	bedrest
BRP	bathroom privileges
BSC	bedside commode
c̄	with
cath.	catheter
CBR	complete bedrest
CDC	Centers for Disease Control and Prevention
C. diff	*Clostridioides difficile*
CHF	congestive heart failure

ck ✓	check
cl liq	clear liquid
CNA	certified nursing assistant
c/o	complains of
COPD	chronic obstructive pulmonary disease
CPR	cardiopulmonary resuscitation
CRE	carbapenem-resistant *Enterobacteriaceae*
CS	Central Supply
CVA	cerebrovascular ac-cident, stroke
CVP	central venous pressure
CXR	chest X-ray
DAT	diet as tolerated
DM	diabetes mellitus
DNR	do not resuscitate
DOB	date of birth
DON	director of nursing
Dr., DR	doctor
drsg	dressing
Dx/dx	diagnosis
EMS	emergency medical services
exam	examination
FF	force fluids
ft	foot
F/U, f/u	follow-up
FWB	full weight-bearing
geri-chair	geriatric chair
H₂0	water

h, hr, hr.	hour
HBV	hepatitis B virus
HIPAA	Health Insurance Portability and Accountability Act
HIV	human immunodefi-ciency virus
HOB	head of bed
HS/hs	hours of sleep
ht	height
HTN	hypertension
hyper	above normal, too fast, rapid
hypo	low, less than normal
I&O	intake and output
IV, I.V.	intravenous (within a vein)
L, lt	left
lab	laboratory
lb.	pound
lg	large
LOC	level/loss of consciousness
LPN	licensed practical nurse
LTC	long-term care
LVN	licensed vocational nurse
M.D.	medical doctor
MDS	minimum data set
meds	medications
MI	myocardial infarction
min	minute

mm Hg	millimeters of mercury
mL	milliliter
mod	moderate
MRSA	methicillin-resistant *Staphylococcus aureus*
NA	nursing assistant
N/C	no complaints, no call
NG, ng	nasogastric
NKA	no known allergies
NPO	nothing by mouth
NV	nausea and vomiting
NWB	non-weight-bearing
OBRA	Omnibus Budget Reconciliation Act
OOB	out of bed
OSHA	Occupational Safety and Health Administration
oz	ounce
p̄	after
pc, p.c.	after meals
PEG	percutaneous endoscopic gastrostomy
peri care	perineal care
PO	by mouth
PPE	personal protective equipment
p.r.n., prn	when necessary
PWB	partial weight-bearing
q̄	every

q2h	every two hours
q3h	every three hours
q4h	every four hours
qh, qhr	every hour
qhs	every night at bedtime
q.i.d., qid	four times a day
R	respirations, rectal
R, rt.	right
rehab	rehabilitation
res.	resident
resp.	respiration
RN	registered nurse
R/O	rule out
ROM	range of motion
RR	respiratory rate
s̄	without
SDS	safety data sheet
SOB	shortness of breath
SP	Standard Precautions
spec.	specimen
ss	one-half
S&S, S/S	signs and symptoms
stat, STAT	immediately
T., temp	temperature
TB	tuberculosis
TIA	transient ischemic attack
t.i.d., tid	three times a day
TLC	tender loving care
TPR	temperature, pulse, and respiration

U/A, u/a	urinalysis
UTI	urinary tract infection
VRE	vancomycin-resistant *Enterococcus*
VS, vs	vital signs
w/c, W/C	wheelchair
wt.	weight

Symbols

©	copyright
&	and
☣	biohazard
△	change, heat
°	degree
♀	female
♂	male
%	percent
☢	radiation

Appendix

It is important that you continually work on improving yourself and strive to learn something new each day. This section includes a brief review of many basic skills, with which you may already be familiar. Feel free to refer to it any time you need a refresher on writing, studying, note-taking, or math.

Grammar, Punctuation, and Capitalization

It is important to speak well and to use correct grammar. Grammar is the set of rules of a language. Here are some basic grammatical terms and their definitions:

- A noun is a person, place, or thing. Examples: car, home, lipstick, school.

- An adjective is a word that describes a noun. Examples: *blonde* hair, *gray* sweater.

- A pronoun is a word that takes the place of a noun. Examples: I, he, him, she, them, we.

- A verb is a word that expresses an action or the condition of a person. Examples: jumps, drives, lifts.

- An adverb is a word that describes a verb, adjective, or adverb. Examples: He smiled *happily*. She skated *quickly*.

- A conjunction is a connecting word. Examples: and, but, neither, nor, or.

- A sentence is a group of words with a subject and verb that expresses a complete thought. Example: The fireman rescued the cat from the tree.

Punctuation is the use of marks in writing to separate words and ideas. Here are some common punctuation marks and their definitions:

- A period (.) is the punctuation mark placed at the end of sentences and other statements that are considered complete. Examples: Hello. Welcome to the nursing assistant training class.

Periods are also placed after many abbreviations. For example, *Dr.* is an abbreviation for the word *Doctor*.

- A comma (,) separates thoughts or items in a list, such as a list of adjectives. Example: The hospital sat on top of a tall, grassy hill.

- A semicolon (;) connects two sentences with closely related ideas. Example: John is very patient; we appreciate him.

- A colon (:) introduces a list or indicates that an addition is coming. Examples: Kate picked up these items: a comb, a razor, and soap. There was only one thing they needed to make their family complete: a pet.

- An apostrophe (') shows possession (ownership). It also shows where letters are missing in contractions. Examples: Susan took Diana's toy. Elizabeth wasn't trained to do that task (contraction of "was not").

- Quotation marks ("") identify what someone has said or written. Example: The resident said, "I am having pain in my shoulder."

Capitalization is the writing of a word with its first letter as an uppercase letter and the remaining letters in lowercase letters. The following should be capitalized:

- The first word of a sentence, question, or quote. Example: The gate is open.

- Proper names and titles. Example: "Hello, Mr. Dickens. How are you and Margaret today?"

- Names of peoples. Example: Asian

- Names of religious groups and of sacred texts. Examples: Catholic, Buddhist, the Bible, the Koran

- Names of countries, states, cities, or areas. Examples: Italy, Massachusetts, Dallas, the Pacific Northwest

- Names of streets or roads. Example: Thatcher Road

- Names of buildings, organizations, colleges, and schools. Examples: Yale University, the

United Nations, Roosevelt High School, the White House

- Holidays, historical and special events, and holy days. Examples: Labor Day, Passover, the Civil War
- Days of the week and months of the year. Examples: Tuesday, May
- Names of institutions and companies. Examples: the Smithsonian Institution, General Foods

Reading Skills

Reading well is an important part of being a nursing assistant. In the healthcare field, you must be able to read assignments, care plans, menus, activity schedules, and many other documents. Improving your reading skills can help in these situations, and will also help with completing homework and studying for exams.

Choose a place to read where you can concentrate, whether at home or at a public place like the library. When you read your textbook, follow these guidelines:

- Know yourself. Choose the site where you can read best.
- Use eyeglasses or contact lenses if you need them.
- Have enough light to read.
- Sit comfortably so that you do not hurt your back or neck. Use supportive pillows if needed.
- Take notes if you need to.
- Practice saying words you do not know. Do not be embarrassed to ask for help pronouncing a word.
- Refer to a dictionary when you need help.

When reading textbooks, make sure to separate and organize important information. First, look at the objectives for the chapter or unit; this will help you understand its primary goals. Complete each chapter section or learning objective before

moving on to the next one. After all notes are taken and the sections for that chapter are finished, complete the chapter review. If you can successfully answer the questions asked in the review, move on to the next chapter.

Note-Taking

People take notes all the time. You may take notes while in class or while reading this textbook. There are many ways to take notes. Here are some methods that can make this process easier:

1. **Outline Method**: Write down the subject. Then put all sentences about that subject under it in outline form (see the box below). Use a highlighting marker to highlight the subjects and words or points you need to remember.

1. Positioning of Residents
   a. Purpose
   b. Preparation

2. Types of Positions
   a. Supine
   b. Lateral
   c. Dorsal recumbent
   d. Knee-chest
   e. Prone
   f. Sims'
   g. Fowler's/semi-Fowler's
   h. Lithotomy

2. **Index Card Method**: Write down all of your notes neatly on large index cards. Use one card for each topic. To keep cards together, use rubber bands or punch a hole in the corner and use rings (one ring for every chapter).

3. **Rewrite Method**: Rewrite your notes neatly in a spiral notebook to keep them together. Rewriting them may help you remember more material.

You can also take notes on a computer or tablet, which provides some advantages:

- You will be able to read your notes easily.

- You can copy and paste information.
- You can store website links in your file.
- You will be able to cite your work easily if needed.

When making notes on a computer, make sure you carefully label all of your files. For clarity and ease of retrieval, name your files something that corresponds to your class or topic or that you can easily remember. Back up your files to cloud storage or by using an external data storage device.

Studying Effectively

It is not enough to simply sit down and start studying; having the proper tools will help. The following tips may help you study more effectively:

- Keep a large pad of paper to write down questions or notes.
- Use pens and highlighters. After making notes, highlight all important words and main subjects in your notes.
- Record your thoughts and ideas about each chapter. This may help you to remember them. Some people replay their thoughts while resting.
- Take regular breaks, such as every 30 minutes or once per hour. Get a drink of water, take a walk, etc.
- Write new words down in a notepad or on index cards. Look up any terms you do not know, and write down their meanings. Review these words each time you study.

Taking Exams

Sometimes so much effort is put into mental preparation for a test that people forget to prepare their bodies as well. Physical condition affects mental abilities.

Before taking an exam, get plenty of sleep and watch what you eat and drink. On the day of the exam, eat a healthy breakfast. It can be hard to think if you are hungry or if you did not eat a balanced breakfast. Avoid foods that contain simple sugars, such as candy, doughnuts, and soda.

Being in good physical shape allows for more blood to get to the brain. If you get regular physical exercise, your body and mind will use oxygen more effectively than they would if you were out of shape. Even exercising a few days before an exam can make a noticeable difference in your thinking abilities.

Decrease your stress level before an exam. Fill up the car with gas or get correct bus fare the day before. Make lunch the night before. In short, try to avoid stress on the day of an exam. Stress may affect your grade.

When taking the exam, listen carefully to any instructions given. Be sure to read the directions. When taking a multiple-choice test, first eliminate answers you know are wrong. Since your first choice is often correct, do not change your answers unless you are sure of the correction.

Do not spend too much time on any one question. If you do not understand it, move on and go back if time allows. When you are finished with a test, review the entire answer sheet. Make sure you have placed an answer for each question on the answer sheet in the correct space.

Basic Math Skills

Nursing assistants need math skills when doing certain tasks, such as calculating intake and output. A basic math review is listed below:

Addition

$$\begin{array}{r} 3,457 \\ +398 \\ \hline 3,855 \end{array} \qquad \begin{array}{r} 11,999 \\ +7,657 \\ \hline 19,656 \end{array}$$

Subtraction

```
    27,785              179,746
 −   9,358            −  37,437
 ─────────            ─────────
    18,427              142,309
```

Multiplication

```
     3,754                  92
 ×     129            ×      37
 ─────────            ─────────
    33,786                 644
    75,080            +   2,760
 + 375,400                3,404
 ─────────
   484,266
```

Division

```
        49                   33
 26 ⟌ 1,274           16 ⟌  528
    − 1,040                − 480
    ──────                 ─────
       234                   48
     − 234                 − 48
     ─────                 ─────
         0                    0
```

Converting Decimals, Fractions, and Percentages

Decimals, fractions, and percentages are all related. A decimal is a fraction whose denominator is a power of 10. A percentage is a way of expressing a fraction as a whole number, by using 100 as the denominator. To express one-half (½) as a decimal, we would say 0.5. To express one-half (½) as a percentage, we would say 50% or 50/100.

Here are some examples:

Example: ½ = 0.5 = 50%

To get the decimal 0.5 from ½, divide the denominator (2) into the numerator (1).

To change 0.5 into a percent, move the decimal sign two places to the right and add the percent sign.

0.5 = 50%

Example: ¼ = 0.25 = 25%

To change 0.25 into a percent, move the decimal sign two places to the right and add the percent sign.

0.25 = 25%

Example: ¾ = 0.75 = 75%

To change 0.75 into a percent, move the decimal sign two places to the right and add the percent sign.

0.75 = 75%

Other Useful Information

Multiplication Table

1	2	3	4	5	6	7	8	9	10	11	12
2	4	6	8	10	12	14	16	18	20	22	24
3	6	9	12	15	18	21	24	27	30	33	36
4	8	12	16	20	24	28	32	36	40	44	48
5	10	15	20	25	30	35	40	45	50	55	60
6	12	18	24	30	36	42	48	54	60	66	72
7	14	21	28	35	42	49	56	63	70	77	84
8	16	24	32	40	48	56	64	72	80	88	96
9	18	27	36	45	54	63	72	81	90	99	108
10	20	30	40	50	60	70	80	90	100	110	120
11	22	33	44	55	66	77	88	99	110	121	132
12	24	36	48	60	72	84	96	108	120	132	144

Conversions: Volume

1 ounce (oz) = 30 mL

¼ cup = 2 oz = 60 mL

½ cup = 4 oz = 120 mL

1 cup = 8 oz = 240 mL

1 liter (L) = 1000 mL

2 pints = 1 quart (qt) = 960 mL

2 quarts = ½ gallon (gal) = 2 liters (L)

4 quarts = 1 gallon (gal)

Conversions: Weight

1 kilogram (kg) = 2.2 pounds (lb)

1 gram (g) = 1000 milligrams (mg)

1 pound (lb) = 16 ounces (oz)

Conversions: Length

1 inch (in) = 2.54 centimeters (cm)
(or round off to 2.5)

12 inches = 1 foot (ft)

3 feet = 1 yard (yd)

10 millimeters (mm) = 1 centimeter (cm)

100 centimeters (cm) = 1 meter

Glossary

24-hour urine specimen: a urine specimen consisting of all urine voided in a 24-hour period.

abdominal thrusts: a method of attempting to remove an object from the airway of someone who is choking.

abduction: moving a body part away from the midline of the body.

absorption: the transfer of nutrients from the intestines to the cells.

abuse: purposeful mistreatment that causes physical, mental, emotional, or financial pain or injury to a person.

accountable: answerable for one's actions.

acquired immunodeficiency syndrome (AIDS): the final stage of HIV infection, in which infections, tumors, and central nervous system symptoms appear due to a weakened immune system that is unable to fight infection.

active assisted range of motion (AAROM): exercises to put a joint through its full arc of motion that are done by a resident with some assistance from a staff member.

active listening: a way of communicating that involves giving a person one's full attention while he is speaking and encouraging him to give information and clarify ideas.

active range of motion (AROM): exercises to put a joint through its full arc of motion that are done by a resident himself, without help.

activities of daily living (ADLs): daily personal care tasks, such bathing; caring for skin, fingernails, and hair; eating; drinking; caring for the mouth and teeth; dressing; walking; transferring; eliminating; and communicating.

acute care: 24-hour skilled care for short-term illnesses or injuries; generally given in hospitals and ambulatory surgical centers.

additive: a substance added to another substance, changing its effect.

adduction: moving a body part toward the midline of the body.

admission pack: personal care items supplied upon a resident's admission.

adult day services: care for people who need some assistance or supervision during certain hours, but who do not live in the facility where care is given.

advance directives: legal documents that allow people to decide what kind of medical care they wish to have in the event they are unable to make those decisions themselves.

adverse event: an unexpected event that causes serious injury or death; also called *sentinel event*.

ageism: stereotyping of, prejudice toward, and/or discrimination against the elderly.

age-related macular degeneration (AMD): a condition in which the macula degenerates, gradually causing central vision loss.

agitated: the state of being excited, restless, or troubled.

agnostic: a person who believes that he does not know or cannot know if God exists.

airway: the natural passageway for air to enter into the lungs.

allergies: a condition in which the body's immune response is triggered after exposure to a substance called an *allergen*; reactions such as sneezing, difficulty breathing, and skin issues may result.

alveoli: tiny, grape-like sacs in the lungs where the exchange of oxygen and carbon dioxide occurs.

Alzheimer's disease (AD): a progressive, degenerative, and incurable disease that causes proteins to build up in and around nerve cells, which results in memory loss, cognitive impairment, and behavioral changes.

ambulation: the act of moving or walking, with or without an assistive device.

amputation: the surgical removal of an extremity.

anatomy: the study of body structure.

anemia: a condition in which the amount of red blood cells or hemoglobin in the body is less than normal.

angina pectoris: chest pain, pressure, or discomfort.

animal-assisted therapy (AAT): the practice of bringing pets into a facility or home to provide stimulation and companionship.

anticipatory grief: a period of mourning when the dying person or his family is expecting the death.

antiembolic stockings: stockings that are used to prevent swelling and blood clots and to promote circulation; also called *elastic stockings*.

antimicrobial: an agent that destroys, resists, or prevents the development of pathogens.

anxiety: unease or worry, often about a situation or condition.

apathy: a lack of interest.

apical pulse: the pulse on the left side of the chest, just below the nipple.

apnea: the absence of breathing.

artery: vessel that carries blood away from the heart.

arthritis: a general term that refers to inflammation of the joints.

artificial airway: any tube inserted into the respiratory tract for the purpose of maintaining an airway and facilitating ventilation.

aspiration: the inhalation of food, fluid, or foreign material into the lungs.

assault: a threat to harm a person, resulting in the person feeling fearful that he or she will be harmed.

assisted living: residences for people who do not need skilled, 24-hour care, but do require some help with daily care.

assistive devices: special equipment that helps a person who is ill or disabled perform activities of daily living.

asthma: a chronic and episodic inflammatory disease that makes it difficult to breathe and causes coughing and wheezing.

atheist: a person who believes that there is no God.

atria: the upper two chambers of the heart.

atrophy: weakening or wasting away of muscles.

autoclave: an appliance used to sterilize medical instruments or other objects by using steam under pressure.

autoimmune disease: a disease in which the body is unable to recognize its own tissue and begins to attack these tissues.

autopsy: an examination of a body by a pathologist to try to determine the cause of death.

axilla: underarm or armpit area.

bariatrics: branch of medicine that deals with the causes, prevention, and treatment of obesity.

barrier: a block or an obstacle.

baseline: initial value that can be compared to future measurements.

battery: the intentional touching of a person without his or her consent.

bedridden: confined to bed.

benign: noncancerous.

benign prostatic hypertrophy: a disorder that can occur in men as they age, in which the prostate becomes enlarged and causes problems with urination and/or emptying the bladder.

bereavement: the period following a loss in which mourning occurs.

biology: the study of all life forms.

biopsy: a removal of a sample of tissue for examination and diagnosis.

biorhythms: natural rhythms or cycles related to bodily functions.

bipolar disorder: a type of mental illness that causes a person to have mood swings and changes in energy levels and the ability to function.

bloodborne pathogens: microorganisms found in human blood that can cause infection and disease.

Bloodborne Pathogen Standard: federal law requiring that healthcare facilities protect employees from bloodborne health hazards.

body fluids: tears, saliva, sputum (mucus coughed up), urine, feces, semen, vaginal secretions, pus or other wound drainage, and vomit.

body language: all of the conscious or unconscious messages a person's body sends as she communicates; facial expressions, gestures, and posture are examples.

body mechanics: the way the parts of the body work together when a person moves.

body systems: groups of organs that perform specific functions in the human body.

bones: rigid connective tissues that make up the skeleton, lend support to body structures, allow the body to move, and protect the organs.

bony prominences: areas of the body where the bone lies close to the skin.

bowel elimination: the physical process of releasing or emptying the colon or large intestine of solid waste, called *stool* or *feces*.

BPM: the medical abbreviation for beats per minute.

brachial pulse: the pulse inside the elbow, about 1 to 1½ inches above the elbow.

bradycardia: slow heart rate—under 60 beats per minute.

brain: the part of the nervous system housed in the skull that is responsible for motor activity, memory, thought, speech, and intelligence, along with regulation of vital functions, such as heart rate, blood pressure, and breathing.

breakthrough pain: a type of severe pain that happens unexpectedly in people who have cancer.

bridge: a type of dental appliance that replaces missing or pulled teeth.

bronchi: branches of the passages of the respiratory system that lead from the trachea into the lungs.

bronchiectasis: a condition in which the bronchi become permanently dilated (widened) and damaged.

bronchitis: an irritation and inflammation of the lining of the bronchi.

bruise: a purple, black, or blue discoloration on the skin caused by the leakage of blood from broken blood vessels into the surrounding tissues; also called *contusion*.

Buddhism: a religion that follows the teachings of Buddha.

burnout: mental or physical exhaustion due to a prolonged period of stress and frustration.

bursae: tiny sacs of fluid that are located near joints and help reduce friction.

bursitis: a condition in which the bursae become inflamed and painful.

cancer: a general term used to describe a disease in which abnormal cells grow in an uncontrolled way.

capillaries: tiny blood vessels in which the exchange of gases, nutrients, and waste products occurs between blood and cells.

carbapenem-resistant *Enterobacteriaceae* (CRE): bacteria (*Enterobacteriaceae*) that have developed resistance to carbapenems, which is a category of antibiotics.

cardiac arrest: sudden stopping/cessation of the heartbeat.

cardiomyopathy: a weakening of the heart muscle due to enlargement or thickening, which reduces the heart's ability to pump blood effectively.

care conference: a meeting to share and gather information about a resident in order to develop a care plan.

care plan: a plan for each resident created by a registered nurse that outlines the tasks that team members must perform to help the resident reach her goals of care.

care team: the group of people with different kinds of education and experience who provide resident care.

carrier: person who carries a pathogen, usually without signs or symptoms of disease, but who can spread the disease.

cartilage: the protective substance that covers the ends of bones and makes up the discs that are found between vertebrae.

cataract: a condition in which the lens of the eye becomes cloudy, causing vision loss.

catastrophic reaction: reacting to something in an unreasonable, exaggerated way.

catheter: tube inserted through the skin or into a body opening that is used to administer or drain fluid.

catheter-associated urinary tract infection (CAUTI): an infection that occurs in the urethra, bladder, ureter, or kidney when bacteria travels up a catheter.

C. difficile or **C. diff:** an abbreviation for *Clostridioides difficile* (formerly *Clostridium difficile*); a bacterium that is spread by spores in feces that are difficult to kill; it causes symptoms such as diarrhea and nausea and can lead to serious inflammation of the colon (colitis).

cells: the basic structural units of all organisms.

cellulitis: a skin infection caused by bacteria moving into the tissues due to a break in the skin.

Celsius: the centigrade temperature scale in which the boiling point of water is 100 degrees and the freezing point of water is 0 degrees.

Centers for Disease Control and Prevention (CDC): federal government agency responsible for improving the overall health and safety of the people of the United States.

central nervous system: part of the nervous system made up of the brain and spinal cord.

central venous line: a type of intravenous line (IV) that is inserted into a large vein in the body.

cerebrovascular accident (CVA): a condition caused when the blood supply to the brain is cut off suddenly by a clot or a ruptured blood vessel; also called *stroke*.

cervical cancer: a form of female reproductive cancer that begins in the cervix.

chain of command: the order of authority within a facility.

charge nurse: a nurse responsible for a team of healthcare workers.

charting: the act of noting care and observations; documenting.

chemical restraint: medications used to control a person's mood or behavior.

chest percussion: clapping the chest to help lungs drain with the force of gravity.

chest tubes: hollow drainage tubes that are inserted into the chest to drain air, blood, pus, or fluid that has collected inside the pleural space/cavity.

Cheyne-Stokes respiration: alternating periods of slow, irregular respirations and rapid, shallow respirations, possibly along with periods of apnea.

chlamydia: a sexually transmitted infection caused by bacteria.

Christianity: a religion that follows the teachings of Jesus Christ.

chronic: long-term or long-lasting.

chronic obstructive pulmonary disease (COPD): a chronic, progressive, and incurable lung disease that causes difficulty breathing.

chronic renal failure (CRF): a progressive condition in which the kidneys cannot filter certain waste products; also called *chronic kidney failure*.

chyme: semiliquid substance made as a result of the chemical breakdown of food in the stomach.

circadian rhythm: the 24-hour day-night cycle.

cite: in a long-term care facility, to find a problem through a survey.

civil law: private law; law between individuals.

clean: a condition in which an object has not been contaminated with pathogens.

clean-catch specimen: a urine specimen that does not include the first and last urine voided; also called *midstream specimen*.

closed bed: a bed completely made with the bedspread and blankets in place.

closed wound: a type of wound in which the skin's surface is not broken.

code: in health care, an emergent medical situation in which specially trained responders provide the necessary care.

code status: formal documentation of the type and scope of care that should be provided to a particular resident in the event of a cardiac arrest, other catastrophic organ failure, or terminal illness.

critical thinking: the process of reasoning and analyzing in order to solve problems; for the nursing assistant, critical thinking means making careful observations and promptly reporting all potential problems.

code team: group of people chosen for a particular shift to respond to resident emergencies.

cognition: the ability to think clearly and logically.

cognitive behavioral therapy (CBT): a type of psychotherapy that is usually short-term and focuses on skills and solutions that a person can use to modify negative thinking and behavior patterns; often used to treat anxiety disorders.

colon: the large intestine.

colostomy: surgically created opening through the abdominal wall into the large intestine to allow feces to be expelled.

coma: state of unconsciousness in which a person is unable to respond to any change in the environment, including pain.

combative: violent or hostile.

combustion: the process of burning.

communicable disease: an infectious disease transmissible by direct contact or by indirect contact.

concussion: a head injury that occurs from a banging movement of the brain against the skull.

condom catheter: a catheter that has an attachment on the end that fits onto the penis; also called *external* or *Texas* catheter.

conflict resolution: the process of resolving conflicts in a positive way so that everyone is satisfied.

confusion: the inability to think clearly and logically.

congestive heart failure (CHF): a condition in which the heart muscle is damaged and fails to pump effectively.

conscientious: guided by a sense of right and wrong; principled.

conscious: having awareness of surroundings, sensations, and thoughts.

constipation: the inability to eliminate stool, or the infrequent, difficult, and often painful elimination of hard, dry stool.

constructive feedback: feedback that involves giving opinions about the work of others in a nonaggressive way.

contagious disease: a type of communicable disease that spreads quickly from person to person.

contaminated: soiled, unclean; having disease-causing organisms or infectious material on it.

continuity of care: an ongoing coordination of a resident's care over time, during which the care team regularly exchanges information and works toward shared goals.

contracture: the permanent and painful shortening of a muscle, tendon, or ligament that can restrict movement.

coronary artery disease (CAD): a condition in which the coronary arteries become damaged and narrow over time, causing chest pain and other symptoms.

courteous: polite, kind, considerate.

CPR: abbreviation for cardiopulmonary resuscitation; medical procedures used when a person's heart and lungs have stopped working.

cremation: the process of burning a dead body until it turns to ash.

criminal law: public law; related to committing a crime against the community.

critical thinking: the process of reasoning and analyzing in order to solve problems; for the nursing assistant, critical thinking means making careful observations and promptly reporting all potential problems.

Crohn's disease: a disease that causes the lining of the digestive tract to become inflamed (red, sore, and swollen).

cross-infection: the physical movement or transfer of harmful bacteria from one person, object, or place to another, or from one part of the body to another.

cultural competence: an ongoing process of learning about other cultures and applying that knowledge to help provide better health care.

cultural diversity: the variety of people living and working together in the world.

culture: a set of learned beliefs, values, traditions, and behaviors shared by a social or ethnic group.

cyanosis: blue or pale skin and/or mucous membranes due to decreased oxygen in the blood.

dandruff: excessive shedding of dead skin cells from the scalp.

dangle: to sit up with the legs hanging over the side of the bed in order to regain balance.

death: the end of life; the cessation of all body functions.

defamation: any untrue statement (written or oral) that injures a person's reputation and/or damages the person's ability to make a living.

defecation: the process of eliminating feces from the rectum through the anus.

defense mechanisms: unconscious behaviors used to release tension and/or help a person cope with stress.

dehydration: an excessive loss of water from the body; a condition that occurs when fluid loss is greater than fluid intake.

delegation: transferring responsibility to a person for a specific task.

delirium: a sudden state of severe confusion due to a change in the body; also called *acute confusional state* or *acute brain syndrome*.

delusion: a belief in something that is not true, or is out of touch with reality.

dementia: a serious, progressive loss of mental abilities such as thinking, remembering, reasoning, and communicating.

dentures: artificial teeth.

depressant: a substance that causes calmness and drowsiness.

dermatitis: inflammation of the skin.

dermis: the inner layer of the two main layers of tissue that make up the skin.

developmental disability: a chronic condition that restricts physical and/or mental abilities.

diabetes: a condition in which the pancreas does not produce insulin or does not produce enough insulin; causes problems with circulation and can damage vital organs.

diabetic ketoacidosis (DKA): a life-threatening complication of diabetes that can result from undiagnosed diabetes, infection, not enough insulin, hyperglycemia (high blood sugar), eating too much, not getting enough exercise, and stress.

diagnosis: the identification of a disease or other problem by its signs and symptoms and from the results of different tests.

dialysis: a process that cleans the body of wastes that the kidneys cannot remove due to kidney failure.

diarrhea: frequent elimination of liquid or semi-liquid feces.

diastole: phase when the heart muscle relaxes.

diastolic: second measurement of blood pressure; phase when the heart relaxes.

diet cards: cards that list residents' names and information about special diets, allergies, likes and dislikes, and any other dietary instructions.

digestion: the process of converting food so that it can be absorbed into the blood and used by body tissues.

dilate: to widen.

direct contact: way to transmit pathogens through touching the infected person or his or her secretions.

dirty: a condition in which an object has been contaminated with pathogens.

disinfection: process that destroys most pathogens and other types of microorganisms, but not all pathogens.

disorientation: confusion about person, place, or time; may be permanent or temporary.

disposable: only to be used once and then discarded.

disruptive behavior: any behavior that disturbs others.

diuretics: substances that increase urine formation and cause the body to excrete sodium, potassium, and water through the kidneys.

diverticulitis: inflammation of sacs that develop in the wall of the large intestine due to diverticulosis.

diverticulosis: a disorder in which sac-like pouchings develop in weakened areas of the wall of the large intestine (colon).

DNR: an abbreviation for do-not-resuscitate; an order that tells medical professionals not to perform CPR in the event of cardiac or respiratory arrest.

doff: to remove.

domestic violence: physical, sexual, or emotional abuse by spouses, intimate partners, or family members.

don: to put on.

dorsal recumbent: position in which a person is flat on her back with knees flexed and slightly separated and her feet flat on the bed.

dorsiflexion: bending backward.

drainage: flow of fluids from a wound or cavity.

draw sheet: an extra sheet placed on top of the bottom sheet; used for moving residents.

duodenum: the first part of the small intestine, where the common bile duct enters the small intestine.

durable power of attorney for health care: a legal document that appoints someone to make the medical decisions for a person in the event he becomes unable to do so.

dysphagia: difficulty swallowing.

dyspnea: difficulty breathing.

edema: swelling in body tissues caused by excess fluid.

edentulous: lacking teeth; toothless.

electrolytes: chemical substances that are essential to maintaining fluid balance and homeostasis in the body.

electronic health record: the electronic form of a resident's personal and health data that is used to manage and coordinate a resident's health care.

elimination: the process of expelling wastes.

elope: in medicine, when a person with Alzheimer's disease wanders away from a protected area and does not return on his own.

emesis: the act of vomiting, or ejecting stomach contents through the mouth and/or nose.

empathetic: identifying with and understanding another's feelings.

emphysema: a chronic, incurable lung disease in which the alveoli in lungs become filled with trapped air; usually results from smoking and chronic bronchitis.

endometrial cancer: a form of female reproductive cancer that begins in the uterus.

end-stage renal disease (ESRD): condition in which kidneys have failed and dialysis or transplantation is required to sustain life.

enema: a specific amount of water, with or without an additive, introduced into the colon to stimulate the elimination of stool.

epidermis: the outer layer of the two main layers of tissue that make up the skin.

epilepsy: a disorder that causes recurring seizures.

epistaxis: a nosebleed.

erectile dysfunction (ED): the inability to have or maintain a penile erection.

ergonomics: the science of designing equipment, areas, and tasks to make them safer and to suit the worker's abilities.

ethics: the knowledge of right and wrong; standards of conduct.

etiquette: the code of proper behavior and courtesy in a certain setting.

eupnea: normal respirations.

eviction: the involuntary discharge from a facility.

expiration: the process of exhaling air out of the lungs.

exploitation: the act of taking advantage of a person for personal gain.

exposure control plan: plan that outlines specific work practices to prevent exposure to infectious material and identifies step-by-step procedures to follow when exposures do occur.

exposure incident: specific eye, mouth, other mucous membrane, nonintact skin, or parenteral contact with blood or other potentially infectious materials that results from the performance of an employee's duties.

expressive aphasia: difficulty communicating through speech or writing.

extension: straightening a body part.

Fahrenheit: a temperature scale in which the boiling point of water is 212 degrees and the freezing point of water is 32 degrees.

false imprisonment: unlawful restraint that affects a person's freedom of movement; includes both the threat of being physically restrained and actually being physically restrained.

farsightedness: the ability to see distant objects more clearly than objects that are near; also called *hyperopia*.

fasting: a period of time during which food is given up voluntarily.

fecal impaction: a mass of dry, hard stool that remains packed in the rectum and cannot be expelled.

fecal incontinence: an inability to control the muscles of the bowels, which leads to an involuntary passage of stool or gas.

feces: solid body waste excreted through the anus from the large intestine; also called *stool*.

financial abuse: improper or illegal use of a person's money, possessions, property, or other assets.

first aid: care given to an injured person by the first people to respond to an emergency.

first impression: a way of classifying or categorizing someone or something at the first meeting.

flammable: easily ignited and capable of burning quickly.

flatulence: air in the intestine that is passed through the rectum; also called *gas* or *flatus*.

flexion: bending a body part.

fluid balance: maintaining equal input and output.

fluid overload: a condition in which the body cannot eliminate the fluid consumed.

fomite: an object that is contaminated with a pathogen and can spread the pathogen to another person.

foot drop: weakness of muscles in the feet and ankles that interferes with the ability to flex the ankles and walk normally.

Fowler's: semi-sitting body position in which a person's head and shoulders are elevated 45 to 60 degrees.

fracture: a broken bone.

fracture pan: a bedpan that is flatter than a regular bedpan; used for small or thin people or those who cannot lift their buttocks onto a standard bedpan.

full weight-bearing (FWB): a doctor's order stating that a person has the ability to support full body weight on both legs and has no weight-bearing limitations.

functional nursing: method of care that involves assigning specific tasks to each team member.

gangrene: death of tissue caused by infection or lack of blood flow.

gastroesophageal reflux disease (GERD): a chronic condition in which the liquid contents of the stomach back up into the esophagus.

gastrointestinal tract: a continuous tube from the opening of the mouth all the way to the anus, where solid wastes are eliminated from the body.

gastrostomy: a surgically created opening in the abdomen and stomach.

genital herpes: a sexually transmitted, incurable infection caused by herpes simplex viruses type 1 (HSV-1) or type 2 (HSV-2).

genital HPV infection: a sexually transmitted infection caused by human papillomavirus.

gingivitis: an inflammation of the gums.

glands: organs that produce and secrete chemicals called hormones.

glaucoma: a condition in which the pressure in the eye increases, damaging the optic nerve and causing blindness.

glucose: natural sugar.

gonads: the male and female sexual reproductive glands.

gonorrhea: a sexually transmitted infection caused by bacteria.

graduate: container for measuring fluid volume.

grief: a deeply emotional process that is a response to loss.

grief counseling: therapy to try to help a person cope after someone has died.

grief process: the varying emotional responses to grief.

grooming: practices to care for oneself, such as caring for fingernails and hair.

halitosis: bad breath.

hallucinations: seeing, hearing, smelling, tasting, or feeling things that are not there.

hand hygiene: washing hands with either plain or antiseptic soap and water and using alcohol-based hand rubs.

hand rub: an alcohol-containing preparation designed for application to the hands for reducing the number of microorganisms on the hands.

health: state of physical, mental, and social well-being.

healthcare-associated infection (HAI): an infection acquired within a healthcare setting during the delivery of medical care.

hearing aid: a small device placed in the ear that amplifies sound.

heart: four-chambered pump that is responsible for the flow of blood in the body.

heartburn: a condition that results from a weakening of the sphincter muscle which joins the esophagus and the stomach; also known as *acid reflux*.

hemianopsia: loss of vision in one-half of the visual field due to CVA, tumor, or trauma.

hemiparesis: weakness on one side of the body.

hemiplegia: paralysis of one side of the body.

hemoptysis: the coughing up of blood from the respiratory tract.

hemorrhage: bleeding; blood loss.

hemorrhoids: enlarged veins in the rectum that can cause itching, burning, pain, and bleeding.

hepatitis: inflammation of the liver caused by certain viruses and other factors, such as alcohol abuse, some medications, and trauma.

Hinduism: a religion that believes in the unity of everything and that all are a part of God.

HIPAA: an abbreviation for Health Insurance Portability and Accountability Act; a federal law that sets standards for protecting the privacy of patients' health information.

hoarding: collecting and putting things away in a guarded way.

holistic: care that involves the whole person; this includes his or her physical, social, emotional, and spiritual needs.

home health care: care that takes place in a person's home.

homeostasis: the condition in which all of the body's systems are balanced and are working at their best.

homophobia: a fear of homosexuality.

hormones: chemical substances produced by the body that control numerous body functions.

hospice care: care for people who have approximately six months or less to live; care is available until the person dies.

human immunodeficiency virus (HIV): a virus that attacks the body's immune system and gradually disables it; eventually can cause AIDS.

hygiene: practices to keep the body clean.

hyperextension: extending a joint beyond its normal range of motion.

hyperglycemia: high blood glucose (blood sugar).

hypertension: high blood pressure, regularly measuring 140/90 mm Hg or higher.

hyperthyroidism: a condition in which the thyroid gland produces too much thyroid hormone, which causes body processes to speed up and metabolism to increase.

hypoglycemia: low blood glucose (blood sugar); also known as *insulin reaction* or *insulin shock*.

hypotension: low blood pressure, below 90/60 mm Hg.

hypothermia: severe subnormal body temperature; body temperature drops below the level required for normal functioning.

hypothyroidism: a condition in which the body lacks thyroid hormone, which causes body processes to slow down.

hypoxia: a condition in which the body does not receive enough oxygen.

ileostomy: surgically created opening into the end of the small intestine, the ileum, to allow feces to be expelled.

immunity: resistance to infection by a specific pathogen.

impairment: a partial or complete loss of function or ability.

impotence: the inability to have or maintain a penile erection.

incident: an accident, problem, or unexpected event during the course of care.

incident report: a report documenting an incident and the response to the incident; also known as an *occurrence, accident,* or *event* report.

incontinence: the inability to control the bladder or bowels, which leads to an involuntary loss of urine or feces.

incubation period: the period of time between exposure to a pathogen and the time it causes visible signs and symptoms of disease or illness.

indirect contact: way to transmit pathogens from touching something contaminated by the infected person.

indwelling catheter: a catheter that remains inside the bladder for a period of time; urine drains into a bag.

infection: the state resulting from pathogens invading the body and multiplying.

infection prevention: set of methods used to prevent and control the spread of disease.

infectious disease: any disease caused by growth of a pathogen.

ingestion: the process of taking food or fluids into the body.

input: the fluid a person consumes; also called *intake.*

insomnia: the inability to fall asleep or remain asleep.

inspiration: the process of inhaling air into the lungs.

insulin reaction: a life-threatening complication of diabetes that can result from either too much insulin or too little food; also known as *hypoglycemia* or *insulin shock.*

intake: the fluid a person consumes; also called *input.*

integument: natural protective covering.

intergenerational care: caring for children and the elderly in the same setting.

intervention: a way to improve or change an action or development.

intimate partner violence (IPV): physical, sexual, or emotional harm caused by a partner or spouse.

intravenous therapy: the delivery of medication, nutrition, or fluids through a person's vein.

intubation: the insertion of a plastic tube through the mouth or nose and into the trachea or windpipe in order to place an artificial airway.

invasion of privacy: the violation of the right to be left alone and the right to control personal information.

involuntary seclusion: the separation of a person from others against the person's will.

irreversible: unable to be reversed or returned to the original state.

irritable bowel syndrome (IBS): a chronic condition of the large intestine that is worsened by stress.

ischemia: a lack of blood supply to an area.

Islam: a religion that follows the prophet Muhammad and the Five Pillars of Islam.

isolate: to keep something separate, or by itself.

job description: an outline of what will be expected in a job.

Joint Commission: a not-for-profit organization that evaluates and accredits different types of healthcare facilities.

joints: the points where two bones meet; provide movement and flexibility.

Judaism: a religion that follows the teachings of God as given to Moses in laws and commandments.

ketones: chemical substances that the body produces when it does not have enough insulin in the blood.

kilogram: a unit of mass equal to 1000 grams; one kilogram equals 2.2 pounds.

knee-chest: position in which a person is lying on his abdomen with knees pulled up towards the abdomen and with legs separated; arms are pulled up and flexed and the head is turned to one side.

lactose intolerance: the inability to digest lactose, a type of sugar in milk and other dairy products.

lateral: body position in which a person is lying on either side.

laws: rules set by the government to help protect the public.

length of stay: the number of days a person stays in a healthcare facility.

lesion: an area of abnormal tissue or an injury or wound.

liability: a legal term that means a person can be held responsible for harming someone else.

libel: defamation in written form.

licensed practical nurse (LPN) or licensed vocational nurse (LVN): licensed nurse who administers medications, gives treatments, and may supervise daily care of residents.

ligaments: strong bands of fibrous connective tissue that connect bones or cartilage and support the joints and joint movement.

lithotomy: position in which a person is on her back with her hips at the edge of the exam table; legs are flexed and feet are in padded stirrups.

living will: a document that states the medical care a person wants, or does not want, in case he or she becomes unable to make those decisions.

localized infection: an infection that is limited to a specific location in the body and has local symptoms.

logrolling: moving a person as a unit, without disturbing the alignment of the body.

long-term care: 24-hour care provided for people with ongoing conditions who are generally unable to manage their activities of daily living.

lungs: main organs of respiration responsible for the exchange of oxygen and carbon dioxide.

lymph: a clear yellowish fluid that carries disease-fighting cells called lymphocytes.

major depressive disorder: an illness that causes social withdrawal, lack of energy, and loss of interest in activities, as well as other symptoms.

malabsorption: a condition in which the body cannot absorb or digest a particular nutrient properly.

malignant: cancerous.

malnutrition: the lack of proper nutrition that results from insufficient food intake or an improper diet.

malpractice: professional misconduct that results in damage or injury to a person.

mandated reporters: people who are required to report suspected or observed abuse or neglect due to their regular contact with vulnerable populations, such as the elderly in long-term care facilities.

masturbation: to touch or rub sexual organs in order to give oneself or another person sexual pleasure.

mechanical lift: special equipment used to lift and move or lift and weigh a person; also called *hydraulic lift.*

mechanical ventilator: a machine used to inflate and deflate the lungs when a person cannot breathe on his own.

Medicaid: a medical assistance program for people who have low incomes, as well as for people with disabilities.

medical asepsis: refers to practices such as handwashing that reduce, remove, and control the spread of microorganisms.

medical chart: legal record of all medical care a patient, resident, or client receives.

Medicare: a federal health insurance program for people who are 65 or older, are disabled, or are ill and cannot work.

melanin: the pigment that gives skin its color.

melanocyte: cell in the skin that produces and contains the pigment called melanin.

Meniere's disease: a disorder of the inner ear caused by a buildup of fluid, which causes vertigo, hearing loss, tinnitus (ringing in the ear), and pain or pressure.

menopause: the end of menstruation; occurs when a woman has not had a menstrual period for 12 months.

menstruation: the shedding of the lining of the uterus that occurs approximately every 28 days; also known as a *period.*

mental health: the normal functioning of emotional and intellectual abilities.

mental health disorder: a disorder that disrupts a person's ability to function in the family, home, or community and often causes inappropriate behavior.

metabolism: the process of breaking down and transforming all nutrients that enter the body to provide energy and growth.

metastasize: to spread from one part of the body to another.

metric: system of weights and measures based upon the meter and the kilogram.

microbe: a living thing or organism that is so small that it is only visible under a microscope; also called *microorganism.*

microorganism (MO): a living thing or organism that is so small that it is only visible under a microscope; also called *microbe.*

micturition: the process of emptying the bladder of urine; also called *urination* or *voiding.*

Minimum Data Set (MDS): a detailed form with guidelines for assessing residents in long-term care facilities; also details what to do if resident problems are identified.

misappropriation: the deliberate misplacement, exploitation, or improper use of a resident's belongings or money without the resident's consent.

mistreatment: the inappropriate treatment or exploitation of a resident.

mores: the accepted traditional customs of a particular social group.

mourning: the period in which people work to adapt to a loss; influenced by culture, tradition, and society.

MRSA: an abbreviation for methicillin-resistant *Staphylococcus aureus*; bacteria (*Staphylococcus aureus*) that have developed resistance to the antibiotic methicillin.

mucous membranes: the membranes that line body cavities that open to the outside of the body, such as the linings of the mouth, nose, eyes, rectum, or genitals.

multidrug-resistant organisms (MDROs): microorganisms, mostly bacteria, that are resistant to one or more antimicrobial agents that are commonly used for treatment.

multidrug-resistant TB (MDR-TB): a form of tuberculosis that is caused by an organism that is resistant to medication that is used to treat TB.

multiple sclerosis (MS): a progressive disease in which the protective covering for the nerves, spinal cord, and white matter of the brain breaks down over time; causes problems with balance, walking, and many other symptoms.

muscles: groups of tissues that contract and relax, allowing motion, supporting the body, protecting organs, and creating heat.

muscular dystrophy: an inherited, progressive disease that causes a gradual wasting away of muscle, weakness, and deformity.

myocardial infarction (MI): a condition in which blood flow to the heart is blocked and muscle cells die; also called *heart attack*.

myocardial ischemia: a condition in which the heart muscle does not receive enough blood and lacks oxygen; can cause angina pectoris.

nasogastric tube: a feeding tube that is inserted through the nose into the stomach.

NATCEP: an abbreviation for Nurse Aide Training and Competency Evaluation Program; part of the Omnibus Budget Reconciliation Act (OBRA) that sets minimum requirements for training and testing nursing assistants.

nearsightedness: the ability to see objects that are near more clearly than distant objects; also called *myopia*.

necrosis: the death of living cells or tissues caused by disease or injury.

need: something necessary or required.

neglect: failure to provide necessary care or services, resulting in physical, mental, or emotional harm to a person.

negligence: actions, or the failure to act or provide proper care for a person, resulting in unintended injury.

neuron: the basic nerve cell of the nervous system.

nitroglycerin: medication that relaxes the walls of the coronary arteries.

noncommunicable disease: a disease not capable of being spread from one person to another.

nonintact skin: skin that is broken by abrasions, cuts, rashes, acne, pimples, lesions, surgical incisions, or boils.

nonverbal communication: communication without using words, such as through gestures and facial expressions.

non-weight-bearing (NWB): a doctor's order stating that a person is unable to touch the floor or support any weight on one or both legs.

normal flora: microorganisms that normally live in and on the body and do not cause harm in a healthy person, as long as the flora remain in that particular location.

nursing assistant (NA): person who performs assigned nursing tasks and gives personal care.

nursing process: an organized method used by nurses to determine residents' needs, plan the appropriate care to meet those needs, and evaluate how well the plan of care is working; five steps are assessment, diagnosis, planning, implementation, and evaluation.

nutrient: a necessary substance that provides energy, promotes growth and health, and helps regulate metabolism.

nutrition: how the body uses food to maintain health.

objective information: factual information collected using the senses of sight, hearing, smell, and touch; also called *signs*.

OBRA: an abbreviation for Omnibus Budget Reconciliation Act; law passed by the federal government that includes minimum standards for nursing assistant training, staffing requirements, resident assessment instructions, and information on rights for residents.

obsessive-compulsive disorder (OCD): a type of mental health disorder characterized by intrusive repetitive thoughts or behaviors that cause anxiety or stress.

obstructed airway: a condition in which the tube through which air enters the lungs is blocked.

occlusion: a complete obstruction of a blood vessel.

occult: hidden.

Occupational Safety and Health Administration (OSHA): a federal government agency that makes and enforces rules to protect workers from hazards on the job.

occupied bed: a bed made while the person is in the bed.

ombudsman: a legal advocate for residents in long-term care facilities.

open bed: a bed made with linen folded down to the foot of the bed.

open wound: a type of wound in which the skin's surface is not intact.

opportunistic infection: an illness caused by microorganisms that do not affect people with healthy immune systems but cause disease in people with weakened immune systems.

opposition: touching the thumb to any other finger.

organ: a structural unit in the human body that performs a specific function.

orientation: a person's awareness of person, place, and time.

orthopnea: shortness of breath when lying down that is relieved by sitting up.

orthostatic hypotension: a sudden drop in blood pressure that occurs when a person stands or sits up; also called *postural hypotension*.

orthotic devices: devices applied externally to limbs to support, protect, improve function, and prevent complications.

osteoarthritis: a type of arthritis that usually affects weight-bearing joints, especially the hips and knees; also called *degenerative joint disease*.

osteopenia: reduced bone density, but not low enough to be classified as osteoporosis.

osteoporosis: a condition in which the bones become brittle and weak, causing them to break easily.

ostomy: surgical creation of an opening from an area inside the body to the outside.

otitis media: an infection in the middle ear that causes pain, pressure, fever, and reduced ability to hear.

outpatient care: care given to people who have had treatments, procedures, or surgery and do not require an overnight stay in a hospital or other care facility.

output: fluid that is eliminated each day through urine, feces, and vomitus, as well as perspiration; also includes suctioned material and wound drainage.

ovarian cancer: a form of female reproductive cancer that begins in the ovaries.

ovum: female sex cell or egg.

oxygen therapy: the administration of oxygen to increase the supply of oxygen to the lungs.

pacing: walking back and forth in the same area.

palliative care: care that focuses on pain relief, controlling symptoms, preventing side effects and complications, and maintaining quality of life for a person who is very ill and/or is dying.

panic disorder: a disorder that causes a person to have repeated episodes of intense fear, along with physical symptoms such as rapid heartbeat, dizziness, and shortness of breath.

paraplegia: the loss of function of the lower body and legs.

parasomnias: sleep disorders.

Parkinson's disease: a progressive disease that causes a portion of the brain to degenerate; causes rigid muscles, shuffling gait, pill-rolling, mask-like face, and tremors.

partial bath: bath that includes washing the face, underarms, hands, and perineal area.

partial weight-bearing (PWB): a doctor's order stating that a person is able to support some body weight on one or both legs.

PASS: acronym for use of a fire extinguisher; stands for Pull-Aim-Squeeze-Sweep.

passive range of motion (PROM): exercises to put a joint through its full arc of motion that are done by a staff member, without the resident's help.

pathogens: microorganisms that are capable of causing infection and disease.

pathologist: a doctor with advanced training in the examination of organs and tissues.

pathophysiology: the study of the disorders that occur in the body.

pediculosis: an infestation of lice.

percutaneous endoscopic gastrostomy (PEG) tube: a tube placed through the abdominal wall into the stomach to deliver liquid nutrients and medications.

perineal care: care of the genitals and anal area.

peripheral nervous system: part of the nervous system made up of the nerves that extend throughout the body and connect to the spinal cord.

peripheral vascular disease (PVD): a condition in which the legs, feet, arms, or hands do not have enough blood circulation.

peristalsis: muscular contractions that push food through the gastrointestinal tract.

perseveration: the repetition of words, phrases, questions, or actions.

personal protective equipment (PPE): equipment that helps protect employees from serious workplace injuries or illnesses resulting from contact with workplace hazards.

person-centered care: a type of care that places the emphasis on the person needing care and his or her individuality and capabilities.

phantom limb pain: pain in a limb (or extremity) that has been amputated.

phantom sensation: warmth, itching, or tingling from a body part that has been amputated.

phlebitis: inflammation of the veins in the lower extremities.

phobia: an intense, irrational fear of or anxiety about an object, place, or situation.

physiatrists: doctors who specialize in rehabilitation.

physical abuse: any treatment, intentional or not, that causes harm or injury to a person's body.

physical restraint: any method, device, material, or equipment that restricts a person's freedom of movement.

physiology: the study of how body parts function.

plaque: a substance that accumulates on the teeth from food and bacteria.

pneumonia: acute inflammation in the lung tissue caused by a bacterial, viral, or fungal infection or chemical irritants.

policy: a course of action to be followed.

portable commode: a chair with a toilet seat and a removable container underneath that is used for elimination; also called *bedside commode*.

positioning: the act of helping people into positions that promote comfort and health.

postmortem care: care of the body after death.

posttraumatic stress disorder (PTSD): a type of mental health disorder caused by witnessing or experiencing a traumatic event.

posture: the way a person holds and positions his body.

pound: a unit of weight equal to 16 ounces.

prediabetes: a condition in which a person's blood glucose levels are above normal but not high enough for a diagnosis of type 2 diabetes.

prefix: a word part that comes before the root to help form a new term.

pressure injuries: serious wounds resulting from skin breakdown; also known as *pressure sores, decubitus ulcers,* or *bed sores.*

pressure points: areas of the body that bear much of its weight.

primary nursing: a method of nursing care in which the registered nurse provides much of the daily care to residents.

prioritize: to place things in order of importance.

procedure: a method, or way, of doing something.

professionalism: the use of proper standards of behavior at work and in work-related settings.

progressive: something that continually gets worse or deteriorates.

pronation: turning downward.

prone: body position in which a person is lying on his stomach, or the front side of the body.

prostate cancer: a form of male reproductive cancer that begins in the prostate gland.

prosthesis: an artificial device that replaces a body part, such as an eye, hip, arm, leg, tooth, or heart valve; used to help improve function and/or appearance.

protected health information (PHI): information that can be used to identify a person and relates to his or her past, present, or future physical or mental condition, including any health care the patient has had, or payment for that health care.

psoriasis: a chronic skin condition caused by skin cells growing too quickly which results in red, white, or silver patches, itching, and discomfort.

psychological abuse: emotional harm caused by threatening, frightening, isolating, intimidating, humiliating, or insulting a person.

psychosocial needs: needs that involve social interaction, emotions, intellect, and spirituality.

psychotherapy: a method of treating mental illness that involves talking about one's problems with mental health professionals.

puberty: the period during which a person develops secondary sex characteristics.

pulmonary edema: a condition in which there is an accumulation of fluid in the lungs; usually due to heart failure.

pulse oximeter: device that measures a person's blood oxygen level and pulse rate.

puree: to chop, blend, or grind food into a thick paste.

quadriplegia: the loss of function of the legs, trunk, and arms.

RACE: acronym for steps taken during a fire; stands for Rescue-Activate-Contain-Extinguish.

radial pulse: the pulse on the inside of the wrist, where the radial artery runs just beneath the skin.

range of motion (ROM): exercises that put a joint through its full arc of motion.

receptive aphasia: difficulty understanding spoken or written words.

rectal suppository: a medication in a cylindrical shape that is given rectally to cause a bowel movement.

registered nurse (RN): a licensed nurse who assesses residents, creates care plans, monitors progress, provides skilled nursing care, administers treatments and medications, and supervises the care given by nursing assistants and other members of the care team.

rehabilitation: care that is managed by professionals to restore a person to the highest possible level of functioning after an illness or injury.

reinfection: being infected again with the same pathogen.

religion: a set of beliefs concerning the cause and nature of the universe that often includes a moral code and usually involves specific rituals and practices.

reminiscence therapy: type of therapy that encourages people with Alzheimer's disease to remember and talk about the past.

remission: the disappearance of signs and symptoms of cancer or other diseases; can be temporary or permanent.

remotivation therapy: type of group therapy that promotes self-esteem, self-awareness, and socialization for people with Alzheimer's disease.

renal calculi: kidney stones.

resident: a person living in a long-term care facility.

Resident Council: a group of residents who meet regularly to discuss issues related to the long-term care facility.

Residents' Rights: rights identified in the Omnibus Budget Reconciliation Act (OBRA) that relate to how residents must be treated while living in a long-term care facility; they provide an ethical code of conduct for healthcare workers.

resistance: the body's ability to prevent infection and disease.

respiration: the process of inhaling air into the lungs (inspiration) and exhaling air out of the lungs (expiration).

respiratory arrest: stopping/cessation of breathing.

restorative care: care given after rehabilitation to maintain a person's function and increase independence.

restraint: a physical or chemical way to restrict voluntary movement or behavior.

restraint alternatives: measures used in place of a restraint or that reduce the need for a restraint.

restraint-free care: an environment in which restraints are not kept or used for any reason.

restrict fluids (RF): a medical order to limit the amount of fluids a person drinks to the level set by a doctor.

résumé: a summary of a person's education and experience.

rheumatoid arthritis: a type of arthritis in which joints become red, swollen, and very painful; movement is restricted, and deformities of the hands are common.

rigor mortis: the Latin term for the condition after death in which the muscles in the body become stiff and rigid.

root: the main part of a word that gives it meaning.

rotation: turning the joint.

rounds: physical movement of staff from room to room to discuss each resident and his or her care plan.

routine urine specimen: a urine specimen that can be collected any time a person voids.

rummaging: going through items that belong to other people.

Safety Data Sheet (SDS): sheet that provides information on the safe use of and hazards of chemicals, as well as emergency steps to take in the event chemicals are splashed, sprayed, or ingested.

sandwich generation: people responsible for the care of both their children and aging relatives.

sanitation: ways individuals and communities maintain clean, hygienic conditions that help prevent disease, such as the disposal of sewage and solid waste.

scabies: a contagious skin infection caused by mites burrowing into the skin that results in pimple-like irritations, rashes, intense itching, and sores.

scalds: burns caused by hot liquids.

schizophrenia: a form of mental illness that may have acute episodes; affects a person's ability to think, communicate, make decisions, and understand reality.

scope of practice: defines the tasks that healthcare providers are legally permitted to perform as allowed by state or federal law.

sedation: the use of medication to calm a person.

sentinel event: an unexpected event that causes serious injury or death; also called *adverse event*.

sepsis: a serious illness caused by an infection, usually bacterial, that requires immediate care.

sequential compression device (SCD): a plastic, air-filled sleeve that is placed around the leg and inflates and deflates regularly to help improve circulation, reduce fluid buildup, and prevent blood clots.

sexual abuse: nonconsensual sexual contact of any type.

sexual harassment: any unwelcome sexual advance or behavior that creates an intimidating, hostile, or offensive working environment.

sexually transmitted infections (STIs): infections caused by sexual contact with infected people; signs and symptoms are not always apparent.

shearing: rubbing or friction resulting from the skin moving one way and the bone underneath it remaining fixed or moving in the opposite direction.

shingles: a viral infection caused by the same virus that causes chickenpox; results in pain, itching, and rashes.

shock: a condition that occurs when there is decreased blood flow to organs and tissues.

Sims': body position in which a person is lying on his left side with the upper knee flexed and raised toward the chest.

sitz bath: a warm soak of the perineal area to clean perineal wounds and reduce inflammation and pain.

skilled care: medically necessary care given by a skilled nurse or therapist.

skin cancer: the growth of abnormal skin cells.

slander: defamation in oral form.

sleep: natural period of rest for the mind and body during which energy is restored.

sling: a bandage or piece of material that is suspended from the neck for the purpose of holding and supporting a forearm.

social anxiety disorder: a disorder in which a person has excessive anxiety about social situations; also called *social phobia.*

special diet: a diet for people who have certain illnesses or conditions; also called *therapeutic* or *modified diet.*

specific gravity: a test performed to measure the density of urine.

specimen: a sample, such as tissue, blood, urine, stool, or sputum, used for analysis and diagnosis.

sperm: male sex cells.

sphincter: a ring-like muscle that opens and closes an opening in the body.

sphygmomanometer: a device that measures blood pressure.

spinal cord: the part of the nervous system inside the vertebral canal that conducts messages between the brain and the body and controls spinal reflexes.

spirituality: of or relating to the concerns of the spirit, the sacred, or the soul.

sputum: mucus coughed up from the lungs.

stable angina: chest pain that occurs when a person is active or under severe stress.

Standard Precautions: a method of infection prevention in which all blood, body fluids, non-intact skin, and mucous membranes are treated as if they were infected with an infectious disease.

stereotype: a biased generalization about a group that is usually based on opinions and distorted ideas.

sterilization: a measure used to decrease the spread of pathogens and disease by destroying all microorganisms, including those that form spores.

stethoscope: an instrument used to hear sounds in the human body, such as the heartbeat or pulse, breathing sounds, or bowel sounds.

stimulant: a drug that increases or quickens actions of the body.

stoma: an artificial opening in the body.

stool: solid body waste excreted through the anus from the large intestine; also called *feces.*

straight catheter: a catheter that does not remain inside the person; it is removed immediately after urine is drained or collected.

stress: a mentally or emotionally disruptive or upsetting condition that occurs due to changes in the environment.

stressor: internal or external factors or stimuli that cause stress.

subacute care: care for an illness or condition given to people who need less care than for an acute (sudden onset, short-term) illness or injury but more than for a chronic (long-term) illness.

subjective information: information collected from residents, their family members, and friends; information may or may not be true but is what the person reported; also called *symptoms.*

substance abuse: the repeated use of legal or illegal drugs, cigarettes, or alcohol in a way that causes harm to oneself or others.

suffix: a word part added to the end of a root or a prefix to create a new meaning.

suffocation: the stoppage of breathing from a lack of oxygen or excess of carbon dioxide in the body; may result in unconsciousness or death.

sundowning: a condition in which a person gets restless and agitated in the late afternoon, evening, or night.

supination: turning upward.

supine: body position in which a person is lying flat on his back.

surgical asepsis: the state of being completely free of microorganisms; also called *sterile technique.*

surgical bed: a bed made so that a person can easily move onto it from a stretcher.

syncope: temporary loss of consciousness; also called *fainting.*

syphilis: a sexually transmitted infection caused by bacteria.

systemic infection: an infection that is in the bloodstream and is spread throughout the body, causing general symptoms.

systole: phase where the heart is at work, contracting and pushing blood out of the left ventricle.

systolic: first measurement of blood pressure; phase when the heart is at work, contracting and pushing blood out of the left ventricle.

tachycardia: rapid heart rate, over 100 beats per minute.

tachypnea: rapid respirations, over 20 breaths per minute.

tartar: hard deposits on the teeth that are filled with bacteria; may cause gum disease and loose teeth if not removed.

team leader: a nurse in charge of a group of residents for one shift of duty.

team nursing: method of care in which a nurse acts as a leader of a group of people giving care.

telemetry: application of a cardiac monitoring device that transmits information about the heart rhythm and heart rate to a central monitoring station for assessment.

tendons: tough fibrous bands that connect muscle to bone.

terminal illness: a disease or condition that will eventually cause death.

testicular cancer: a form of male reproductive cancer that begins in the testes.

thermometer: a device used for measuring the degree of heat or cold.

thyroid: a butterfly-shaped gland in the neck that is responsible for regulating metabolism and growth.

tinea: a fungal infection that causes red, scaly patches to appear in a ring shape, generally on the upper body or on the hands and feet.

tissues: a group of cells that performs similar tasks.

total hip replacement (THR): a surgical replacement of the head of the femur (long bone of the leg) and the socket it fits into where it joins the hip with artificial materials.

total knee replacement (TKR): a surgical replacement of a damaged or painful knee with artificial materials.

total parenteral nutrition (TPN): the intravenous infusion of nutrients in a basic form that is absorbed directly by the cells, bypassing the digestive tract.

trachea: an air passage that goes from the throat (pharynx) to the bronchi; also called *windpipe.*

tracheostomy: a surgically created opening through the neck into the trachea.

transcultural nursing: the study of various cultures with the goal of providing care specific to each culture.

transfer belt: a belt made of canvas or other heavy material used to help people who are weak, unsteady, or uncoordinated to stand, sit, or walk.

transmission: the way and means by which disease is spread.

trichomoniasis: a sexually transmitted infection caused by protozoa (single-celled animals).

trigger: a situation that leads to agitation.

trustworthy: deserving the trust of others.

tuberculosis (TB): a contagious disease caused by a bacterium called *Mycobacterium tuberculosis* that is transmitted through the air; usually affects the lungs, but other body parts can also be affected, such as the spine, brain, and kidney.

tumor: a group of abnormally growing cells.

ulcerative colitis: a chronic inflammatory disease of the large intestine.

unoccupied bed: a bed made while no person is in the bed.

unstable angina: chest pain that occurs while a person is at rest and not exerting himself.

urinary incontinence: the inability to control the bladder, which leads to an involuntary loss of urine.

urinary tract infection (UTI): an infection of the urethra, bladder, ureter, or kidney.

urostomy: any surgical procedure that diverts the passage of urine by redirecting the ureters.

vaccine: a product that is administered to produce immunity to a specific disease.

vaginitis: an inflammation of the vagina.

validating: giving value to or approving.

validation therapy: a type of therapy that lets people with Alzheimer's disease believe they are living in the past or in imaginary circumstances.

vegans: people who do not eat any animals or animal products, including milk, cheese, other dairy items, or eggs; vegans may also choose not to use or wear any animal products.

vegetarians: people who do not eat meat, fish, or poultry and may or may not eat eggs and dairy products.

vein: vessel that carries blood to the heart.

ventilation: in medicine, the exchange of air between the lungs and the environment.

ventricles: the lower two chambers of the heart.

verbal abuse: the use of language that threatens, embarrasses, or insults a person.

verbal communication: communication involving the use of spoken or written words or sounds.

violence: forceful actions that include attacking, hitting, or threatening someone.

vital signs: measurements—temperature, pulse, respirations, and blood pressure—that monitor the functioning of the vital organs of the body.

voiding: the process of emptying the bladder of urine; also called *urination* or *micturition*.

VRE: an abbreviation for vancomycin-resistant *Enterococcus*; bacteria (*enterococci*) that have developed resistance to the antibiotic vancomycin.

wandering: walking aimlessly around the facility or facility grounds.

wart: contagious hard bump caused by a virus.

wellness: successfully balancing things that happen in everyday life; includes five different types: physical, social, emotional, intellectual, and spiritual.

workplace violence: verbal, physical, or sexual abuse of staff by other staff members, residents, or visitors.

Index